DISSOCIATION

DISSOCIATION
Clinical and Theoretical Perspectives

Edited by
STEVEN JAY LYNN
JUDITH W. RHUE

THE GUILFORD PRESS
New York London

© 1994 The Guilford Press
A Division of Guilford Publications, Inc.
72 Spring Street, New York, NY 10012

Printed in the United States of America

This book is printed on acid-free paper.

Last digit is print number: 9 8 7 6 5 4 3 2 1

Library of Congress Cataloging-in-Publication Data
Dissociation : clinical and theoretical perspectives / edited
   by Steven Jay Lynn, Judith Rhue.
      p.   cm.
   Includes bibliographical references and index.
   ISBN 0-89862-186-0
   1. Dissociative disorders.   2. Dissociation (Psychology)
I. Lynn, Steven J.   II. Rhue, Judith W.
   [DNLM: 1. Dissociative Disorders.   WM 173 6 D611 1994]
RC553.D5D545   1994
616.85'23—dc20
DNLM/DLC
for Library of Congress   94-12041
                                                               CIP

*In memory of
Nicholas P. Spanos,
esteemed colleague
and valued friend*

Contributors

Judith Armstrong, Ph.D., Department of Psychology, University of Southern California, Los Angeles, California

Deirdre L. Barrett, Ph.D., Department of Psychiatry, Harvard Medical School and The Cambridge Hospital, Cambridge, Massachusetts

Robert F. Belli, Ph.D., Survey Research Center/Institute for Social Research, University of Michigan, Ann Arbor, Michigan

Kenneth S. Bowers, Ph.D., Department of Psychology, University of Waterloo, Ontario, Canada

Peter Brown, M.D., F.R.C.P., Department of Psychiatry, Mount Sinai Hospital, Toronto, Canada

Cheryl Burgess, Ph.D., Department of Psychology, Carleton University, Ottawa, Ontario, Canada

Etzel Cardeña, Ph.D., Department of Psychology, USUHS, Bethesda, Maryland

Eve B. Carlson, Ph.D., Department of Psychology, Beloit College, Wisconsin

Fred H. Frankel, M.D., Beth Israel Hospital, Boston, Massachusetts, Department of Psychiatry, Harvard Medical School, Cambridge, Massachusetts

George K. Ganaway, M.D., Department of Psychiatry, Emory University School of Medicine, Atlanta, Georgia, The Ridgeview Center for Dissociative Disorders, Smyrna, Georgia

Joseph P. Green, Ph.D., Department of Psychology, Ohio Univeristy, Lima, Ohio

Ernest Hilgard, Ph.D., Department of Psychology, Stanford University, California

Richard Horevitz, Ph.D., Neuropsych, Libertyville, Illinois, Departments of Psychology and Psychiatry, University of Illinois, Chicago

John F. Kihlstrom, Ph.D., Department of Psychology, Yale University, New Haven, Connecticut

Stanley Krippner, Ph.D., Saybrook Institute, San Francisco, California

Paul M. Lerner, Ed.D., A.B.P.P., Private practice of psychoanalysis, psychotherapy, and psychological testing, Ashville, North Carolina, Department of Psychology, University of Tennessee, Knoxville, Tennessee

Richard J. Loewenstein, M.D., Sheppard and Enoch Pratt Hospital, Baltimore, Maryland, Department of Psychiatry, University of Maryland Medical School, College Park, Maryland

Elizabeth F. Loftus, Ph.D., Department of Psychology, University of Washington, Seattle, Washington

Steven Jay Lynn, Ph.D., Department of Psychology, Ohio University, Athens, Ohio

Jose R. Maldonado, M.D., Department of Psychiatry and Behavioral Sciences, Stanford University School of Medicine, Stanford, California

Paul R. Martin, Ph.D., Wellspring Retreat and Resource Center, Albany, Ohio

Michael R. Nash, Ph.D., Department of Psychology, University of Tennessee, Knoxville

Frank W. Putnam, M.D., National Institute of Mental Health, Bethesda, Maryland

Judith W. Rhue, Ph.D., College of Osteopathic Medicine, Ohio University, Athens, Ohio

David Sandberg, Ph.D., Department of Psychology, Ohio University, Athens, Ohio

Nicholas P. Spanos, Ph.D., (deceased), Department of Psychology, Carleton University, Ottawa, Ontario, Canada

David Spiegel, M.D., Department of Psychiatry and Behavioral Sciences and Psychosocial Treatment Laboratory, Stanford University School of Medicine, Stanford, California

Jane G. Tillman, Ph.D., Department of Psychology, University of Tennessee, Knoxville, Tennessee

Louis Jolyon West, M.D., Department of Psychiatry and Behavioral Sciences, University of California at Los Angeles School of Medicine, Los Angeles, California

Erik Z. Woody, Ph.D., Department of Psychology, University of Waterloo, Ontario, Canada

Nataliya Zelikovsky, Ph.D., Department of Psychology, Ohio Univeristy, Athens, Ohio

Preface

Scientific and popular interest in the topic of dissociation has exploded in the past decade. Clinicians seem to be encountering ever-increasing numbers of clients who present with dissociative experiences, histories of abuse and post-traumatic stress reactions, and even with perplexing symptoms that suggest multiple personality disorder (MPD). What are we to make of this dramatic increase in dissociative disorders, particularly MPD? How do we treat dissociative disorders? How do we work with victims of severe abuse and trauma? How do we evaluate claims of child abuse that seem to have been "repressed" or "dissociated" for many years, only to surface in adulthood during psychotherapy? Are dissociative clients highly hypnotizable and, thus, prone to fall prey to suggestive influences in psychotherapy, perhaps to the point that they begin to enact what they perceive to be the role of a "multiple personality" in a manner consistent with their therapists' diagnoses?

Like virtually every clinician who has worked with severely dissociative clients, we have had to confront these and other questions. Unfortunately, graduate school training failed to fully prepare us for dealing with dissociative clients, who often present with complex character disorders and whose lives are so chaotic as to be almost beyond description and belief. Instead, the knowledge we acquired about dissociative disorders during graduate school derived not from scholarly readings on the topic or from direct contact with persons so diagnosed, but from fictional accounts of MPD, typically in the context of mystery stories or horror movies. In short, we were "educated" by literature and the media.

In more recent years, we have had the opportunity to work with a number of persons with a variety of dissociative disorders. In our efforts to help our clients and to fill in the gaps in our knowledge about treatment, we came to realize that many of the scholarly books and articles that could potentially serve as road maps for treatment were written from the perspective of advocate positions in frankly "either/or" terms. Either multiple personality is "real," for example, and clinicians vastly underestimate its incidence and fail to treat it when it is "staring them in the face," or, alternatively, clinicians are unduly credulous, take their clients' reports at face value, and perhaps even "look for" MPD and suggest its symptoms to a highly suggestible clientele.

Unfortunately, much of what we read was neither founded on research nor grounded in theory. The workshops we attended were equally, if not more so, polarizing and disappointing. Many of the featured "experts" made strong and unsubstantiated claims about the incidence of multiple personality and ritual abuse, models of the mind and "multiplicity," and the therapists' ability to distinguish real from false memories. We left these workshops feeling very frustrated and wondering about the destructive impact of the misinformation that was being imparted to a generation of therapists who were as thirsty for knowledge as we were.

At the same time that our frustration with these forums of "knowledge" mounted, we became fascinated with some of the questions that could potentially be addressed in the process of learning more about dissociative disorders. In our laboratory, we began to examine the relations between and among autobiographical memories, dissociative experiences, hypnotizability, and fantasy proneness; and those between and among rape, posttraumatic experiences, and dissociative experiences, as well as the variables that mediate the creation of false memories. Yet these studies only begged even larger and more important questions such as, "What is the nature of the mind and personality?," "What constraints do dissociative phenomena (e.g., multiple personality) place on the idea of free will?," and "How is memory related to trauma and early life experiences?"

As we became more familiar with both the clinical and research literature, and impressed by the relevance of dissociation to a wide range of issues and questions in the field of psychology, we became increasingly convinced that it would be worthwhile to compile scholarly writings on the topic of dissociation that would be useful to clinicians and researchers. We envisioned a book that would be at once authoritative and provide virtually comprehensive coverage of important aspects of the topic, ranging from the major models of dissociation; to a consideration of diagnostic and treament approaches to dissociative children, adolescents, and adults; to a searching discussion of important research, clinical, and conceptual issues.

We believe that we have succeeded in assembling just such a book. The chapters are written by eminent authorities, who have earned our respect because they have something important to say about dissociation. The scholarly essays advance ideas about dissociation and dissociative disorders from a clinical, theoretical, and research perspective. Many of the chapters are provocative and present entirely novel theories, hypotheses, and syntheses of the research literature.

This collection of writings places the study of dissociation on firm scientific ground by identifying the conceptual domain of dissociation and the research base of clinical work on dissociative disorders. By presenting research evidence alongside examples of clinical work, readers are able to draw their own conclusions about the available evidence and its relevance to clinical practice.

The book is divided into three sections. The first, entitled "Theoretical and Research Perspectives," comprises seven chapters that provide the conceptual and research foundation for the chapters that follow. These chapters outline the domain of dissociation and present major explanatory models ranging from Hilgard's neodissocation theory to a sociocognitive model, which challenges the central tenets of neodissociation theory and traditional thinking about MPD.

The second section, entitled "Diagnosis, Assessment, and Treatment Perspectives," comprises nine chapters that present invaluable information, which will assist clinicians in making diagnostic and treatment decisions with clients suffering from dissociative disorders, post-traumatic stress disorders, and the aftereffects of sexual victimization and cultic involvement. Chapters in this section also foster appreciation for the ways in which social and cultural factors affect the expression of dissociative symptoms, and for the way in which transference and countertransference can have a bearing on the manifestation of dissociation symptoms and the treatment of MPD.

We believe that the third section, "Issues and Controversies," should be required reading for all clinicians who work with clients with dissociative disorders or who intend to expand their practice to do so. The four chapters in this section cover very basic issues and controversies in the field such as whether trauma causes dissociative pathology; whether, and under what circumstances, pseudomemories of child abuse can be created; the relationship between conversion and dissociative disorders, and their respective placement in diagnostic classification schemes; and areas of possible rapproachment between those persons who believe in the "reality" of MPD and those who are skeptical of the disorder.

This book is intended for anyone who wishes to learn about dissociation and the treatment of dissociative disorders. It can also serve as an introduction to the literature on dissociative phenomena and as a more advanced reference guide. The practicing clinician will find that the chapters contain basic information that should be in the foreground of any informed treatment of a person with a dissociative disorder, as well as more sophisticated information about specific diagnostic and treatment techniques and strategies. In short, *Dissociation: Clinical and Theoretical Perspectives* can be used as a primary sourcebook for researchers and students of psychotherapy in a variety of helping professions. We will have achieved some measure of success if our book can stand as a corrective to much of the misinformation that is, unfortunately, all too accessible to the student, clinician, and researcher.

This book has benefitted from the input of many people. Our students' questions, observations, and criticisms clarified and sharpened our thinking about dissociation. We are particularly indebted to the following students for their valuable contributions: Jodi Aronoff, Nicole Bryant, Abigail Matorin, Peter Malinoski, Daniel Martin, David Sandberg, Harry Sivec, Jacqueline Tomac, and Nataliya Zelikovsky. Special thanks go to Jennifer Lynn for her unstinting support, to Martha Kate Rhue for her incredible loyalty and love, and to our young children Jessica Barbara Lynn and Alexandra, Grant, Martha Kate, and Steven Rhue for inspiring our lives. As usual, Sharon Panulla of The Guilford Press was a font of encouragement and wisdom. Thanks to one and all!

Contents

Introduction:
Dissociation and Dissociative Disorders in Perspective

Steven Jay Lynn
Judith W. Rhue

It seems that the topics of dissociation and dissociative disorders provoke fascination and consternation, in roughly equal measure. For many of us, the sense of fascination arises from witnessing and reading about dramatic displays of dissociative symptoms, such as those of multiple personality disorder (MPD). But while whetting our appetite to learn more about dissociation, these puzzling phenomena, as well as the elusive nature of the concept of dissociation itself, also evoke a degree of consternation. No doubt, forces are at work that have stirred a great deal of interest in dissociative phenomena: the national focus on child abuse and victimization, and its purported link with pathological dissociation; the historical association among MPD, dissociation, and hypnosis, an interesting phenomenon in its own right; and increasingly sophisticated attempts to account for dissociation in terms of cognitive models of mental functioning.

It is little wonder, then, that dissociative disorders are the current "rage" in the psychological and psychiatric communities. Indeed, interest in dissociative disorders has increased exponentially in the last decade or so, and harkens back to the prominence dissociative phenomena enjoyed in the field of psychology more than 100 years ago. The circuitous historical path that interest in dissociation has taken is charted in this book. The waxing and waning of interest, and ultimate journey full circle to the present fascination with dissociation, is traced from Janet's (1889) landmark writings on the topic, to the eclipse of dissociation theory by early psychoanalytic theory, to the attack on dissociation and hypnosis by experimentalists later in the century (White & Shevach, 1942; Rosenberg, 1959), to the present-day

1

fascination with dissociation. In no small measure, this renewed interest is attributable to Hilgard's (1973, 1977) neodissociation theory and competing models of dissociation (e.g., Spanos & Burgess, Chapter 7, this volume) and to pressing societal concerns about acknowledging and treating victims of sexual and physical abuse, which have been linked to dissociative pathology.

As will be evident to the reader of this book, some of the most intriguing questions currently addressed by psychological science pivot around some aspect of the study of dissociation: "What is the fundamental nature of personality and the self?" "What is the nature of volition and the will?" "How do people respond in the face of terrible trauma?" "How do we remember and forget?" "Are many memories of sexual abuse fantasies, as Freud suggested long ago?" "Are defense mechanisms like repression, splitting, and dissociation truly distinct, or do they essentially serve the same function, share similar developmental antecedents, and have identical implications for the person?"

In responding to some of these questions, heated controversies within the professional community have emerged, as they have on the larger societal stage, as exemplified by the recent surge of interest in whether delayed recall of memories of sexual abuse are fact or fiction (e.g., Loftus, 1993; Lynn & Nash, 1994). To be sure, readers of this book will not escape being drawn into exciting debates that extend to even the most basic question: "What is dissociation?" In the remainder of this chapter, we overview the contents of the book and consider a number of important issues that the reader will encounter in the pages that follow.

OVERVIEW OF THE BOOK

Theoretical and Research Perspectives

The initial section introduces the reader to important definitional, conceptual, and research issues in the study of dissociation and dissociative disorders. In Chapter 1, Etzel Cardeña, attempts to clear away some of the conceptual confusion about dissociation by describing a domain of dissociation. That is, even if no single hard and fast definition can achieve universal consensus at this time, there can at least be increased precision about the different ways the term can be used, the phenomena included under the rubric of dissociation, and what dissociation is not.

Consistent with the literature, Cardeña describes dissociation in three distinct ways; first, in terms of different mental modules or systems that are not consciously accessible, and/or that may function at least somewhat independently of a person's stream of consciousness. Second, he describes dissociation as representing a fundamental alteration in consciousness, which can involve a disconnection or disengagement between the individual and some aspect of his or her self or the environment, as is apparent in the clinical syndromes of depersonalization and derealization And third, he depicts dissociation as a defense mechanism that accounts for disparate phenomena such as nonorganic amnesia and the warding off of physical and emotional pain, and for the development of severe, chronic conditions such as MPD.

Disagreement exists, however, about just how dissociation operates as a defense, and whether it can be meaningfully distinguished from other defenses. For example, whereas Tillman, Nash, and Lerner argue in Chapter 18 that dissociation is a "complex defensive process, distinct from other defenses such as repression, splitting, and denial," the majority of authors in this book do not make a clear distinction between dissociation and repression (Chapter 18, this volume, p. 401). In contrast to both of these positions, Spanos views dissociation neither as a defense nor as an explanatory mechanism for MPD, while Frankel maintains that dissociation can best be regarded as a metaphor rather than as a mechanism and Lerner (1992) contends that dissociation is more of a descriptive than an explanatory concept.

As is the case with any psychological disorder, dissociative disorders have raised questions about the degree to which their presentation is influenced by historical, biological, intrapsychic, and psychosocial forces. As a result, the first section of the book is devoted to explicating different conceptual models of dissociation and dissociative disorders and presenting a variety of perspectives that are, sometimes, in conflict with one another.

The importance of Ernest Hilgard's neodissociation theory cannot be overestimated. As we have noted (Lynn & Rhue, 1991), his theory has been adopted by a number of researchers and an even greater number of clinicians as a way of explaining hypnotic phenomena. It also has heuristic value in that many experiments have been conducted by proponents and skeptics of neodissociation theory alike.

Hilgard presents his neodissociation theory in Chapter 2. It is based on the idea that there exist multiple cognitive systems or cognitive structures in hierarchical arrangement under some measure of control by an "executive ego." The executive ego, or "central control structure," is responsible for planning and monitoring functions of the personality. Under special circumstances, such as hypnosis, these systems may become independent of or dissociated from each other. During hypnosis, relevant subsystems of control are temporarily dissociated from conscious executive control and are instead directly activated by the hypnotist's suggestions.

One measure of the influence of Hilgard's theory is that it has lead other investigators to extend and refine it, based on empirical evidence. Like Hilgard, Erik Woody and Kenneth Bowers regard hypnosis as a "very useful arena" in which to examine dissociative processes, but they reject the idea that amnestic processes are at the root of hypnotic responses. In Chapter 3, they formulate a neo-neodissociation theory that adapts Norman and Shallice's (1986) theory of willed versus automatic control of behavior. Woody and Bowers construe hypnotic responses as resulting from the diminished function of higher integrative ("supervisory") processes, which normally initiate and maintain deliberate organized attention and control. This weakening of the personality's higher level "supervisory" control system results in a corresponding diminution of the sense of volitional control over novel and particularly complex behaviors related to hypnotic suggestions. While hypnosis weakens the supervisory system, it increases dependence on the lower level contention-scheduling system of the personality, which is responsible for the selection of routine acts that do not require conscious or attentional control. The authors also hypothesize that hypnotic phenomena are associated with the inhibition of prefrontal lobe brain functions.

In Chapter 4, Fred Frankel acknowledges the enormous impact that neodissociation theory has had on the field of psychology, the study of dissociation, and our understanding of hypnosis. Nevertheless, Frankel makes a lucid case for the contention that a complete understanding of hysteria, hypnosis, dissociation, and dissociative disorders, is likely to be difficult if not impossible if they are stripped of their social and interpersonal context, and if the effects of suggestion, imagination, and fantasy are not acknowledged. He argues that the clinical picture of dissociative disorders, in addition to being influenced by the operation of unconscious defense mechanisms and internally generated cues, is also influenced by the psychosocial context, particularly by nuances in interactions with others that convey expectations. The mechanism of dissociation, alone, lacks the explanatory power to account for the wide range of dissociative and hypnotic phenomena observed in the clinical context and the laboratory. Explanations of dissociation that rely on one mechanism are, by implication, limited in scope and in explanatory value.

By focusing his gaze on psychobiological factors, Peter Brown examines dissociative and post-traumatic stress disorders (PTSD) from a very different perspective (see Chapter 5). He correctly notes that the psychobiological study of these disorders and the identification of biological markers and external validating criteria can play an important role in contributing to reliable diagnoses, inasmuch as clinicians are, at present, limited to clinical interviews that lack external validity. In his chapter, he reviews potential models of cerebral function and dysfunction in dissociative states and PTSD. Brown also identifies important ways in which the brain adapts to psychological trauma and summarizes clinical studies of temporal lobe epilepsy and dissociation that implicate specific brain structures in the temporal lobe and limbic system (e.g., hippocampus and amygdala) that are vital to the regulation of attention and the allocation of cognitive resources in response to psychological trauma. In Brown's mind, understanding the biological processes that underlie dissociation will ultimately "resolve the interminable, and largely sterile, dispute between believers and skeptics" (Chapter 5, this volume, p. 113). At the same time, it is necessary to consider psychosocial variables, in that they are germane to a complete understanding of the expression of dissociative and posttraumatic symptoms.

One way that science advances is by a process of analogy (e.g., "the heart is like a pump") and bridge building between different phenomena or fields of study (see Kuhn, 1962; Price & Lynn, 1986). In Chapter 6, Deirdre Barrett makes the provocative claim that dream characters may be thought of as analogous to multiple personality "alters" (i.e., discrete personality entities within the larger organization of the personality) and other dissociated ego states. According to Barrett, this analogy is apparent in the similarity between dreams and dissociative states in terms of amnesia and other alterations of memory, and in terms of specific similarities between dream characters and MPD alters, both of which represent hallucinatory projections of various aspects of the self. In making this claim, Barrett states that "dreaming may also be a more literal precursor, whose physiological mechanisms for amnesia and the projection of dissociated identities get recruited in the development of MPD" (Chapter 6, this volume, p. 123). The author also draws a number of other interesting historical, cognitive, and treatment parallels between dreams and MPD characteristics.

One of the most heated debates in the dissociative-disorder literature, and in the field of psychology more generally, centers around the question of whether MPD is the byproduct of terrible trauma or is, instead, created by helping professionals. Nicholas Spanos has been one of the most active participants in this debate, vigorously challenging the traditional view of MPD. Rather than viewing MPD patients as victims of past injustices and trauma, Spanos and Burgess use experimental data on hypnotic responding and clinical data on MPD to argue that "multiple identities are rule-governed social constructions, which are created, legitimated, maintained, and altered through social interaction" (Chapter 7, this volume, p. 137). Indeed, Spanos and Burgess minimize the historical influences on MPD patients' clinical presentation and emphasize, instead, therapist behaviors with patients that serve to legitimize and maintain symptoms consistent with the enactment of MPD. In short, Spanos and Burgess argue that therapists "create rather than discover multiplicity" (Chapter 7, this volume, p. 139).

Assessment and Treatment Perspectives

In this section of the book, a variety of perspectives on the diagnosis, assessment, and treatment of dissociative disorders are presented. Due to estimates that serious dissociative disorders such as MPD in the inpatient population may range from 2.4% to 11.3%, Eve Carlson and Judith Armstrong argue that it is vitally important that clinicians be well-versed in diagnostic and assessment procedures for dissociative disorders (see Chapter 8). Their chapter takes the reader through the entire diagnostic process, beginning with the special issues that are involved in assessing dissociative-disordered patients, and extending to the use of self-report measures, structured interviews, and standard psychological test instruments for diagnosing dissociative disorders. This chapter is particularly timely insofar as it not only presents data pertinent to understanding the psychometric properties of systematic, standardized measures for assessing dissociative pathology, but also presents information essential to the minimizing of leading questions, suggestive responses, and biased interpretations that can potentially confound test and interview data to the detriment of the patient.

In Chapter 9, Frank Putnam surveys child and adolescent dissociative disorders with regard to their clinical phenomenology, diagnosis, and treatment. Putnam underscores the point that our understanding of these disorders is still at a very early stage, and defines a continuum of dissociation ranging from situation-dependent normative dissociation such as daydreaming, to frequent and prolonged dissociative experiences that can extend to MPD. Putnam outlines the underlying dimensions of dissociation in childhood, including alterations in memory, identity disturbances, passive influence experiences, and trance/absorption phenomena. Putnam addresses important diagnostic and clinical issues including the suitability of applying adult DSM dissociative disorders' criteria to children, the problems with differentiating normative dissociation from more pathological variants, the use of diagnostic scales and interviews, the clinical phenomenology of childhood dissociative disorders, and the issue of applying treatment models to childhood dissociative disorder presentations.

Whereas a causal relation cannot be assumed between childhood abuse and psychopathology, evidence suggests that clinicians need to conduct a careful assessment of psychopathology and dissociation with respect to patients who report a history of physical or psychological abuse. In Chapter 10, Nataliya Zelikovsky and Steven Lynn survey the literature on the aftereffects of abuse and the characteristics that have been associated with physically and psychologically abused children, and describe assessment instruments that can assist clinicians in the evaluation of abused children and adult survivors of abuse.

Many similarities exist between dissociative disorders and PTSD, not the least of which is some overlap in symptoms and the fact that acute dissociative symptoms following a traumatic event predict the later development of PTSD. In their thorough review of treatment methods for PTSD (Chapter 11), Jose Maldonado and David Spiegel discuss the phenomenology and etiology of acute and post-traumatic stress disorders, comorbidity of disorders, and a variety of treatment options that include pharmacotherapy and various forms of psychotherapy (e.g., behavior therapy, cognitive therapy, and group therapy). The authors hold that hypnosis can be particularly useful as an adjuvant to psychotherapy because the components of the hypnotic state (i.e., absorption, dissociation, and suggestibility) resemble the core symptoms of PTSD. Six different techniques (i.e., confrontation, condensation, confession, consolation, concentration, and control) are outlined to bring into the patient's "conscious awareness previously repressed memories" so that he or she can "develop a sense of congruence between past memories and current self images" (see Chapter 11, this volume, p. 234).

There is little doubt that sexual assault can constitute a traumatic experience for the victim. Unfortunately, the incidence and prevalence of sexual assault in the United States is disturbingly high. Yet the high rate at which women suffer repeated victimization is equally disquieting. In Chapter 12, David Sandberg, Steven Lynn, and Joseph Green provide a critical review of research in this area and evaluate three distinct accounts of why women who are sexually assaulted are at increased risk for revictimization. The first explanation suggests that some individuals are motivated to repeat the experience in order to gain a sense of mastery over and/or meaning from the initial experience of victimization. The second explanation suggests that dysfunctional learning about the self, others, and the world in general plays a prominent role in revictimization. And the third hypothesis is that dissociation and denial increase the risk of revictimization. At the conclusion of the chapter, the authors draw out the therapeutic implications for each of the three explanations of revictimization.

With cults proliferating in the United States, and a growing recognition of the fact that many ex-cult members become psychiatric casualties because of their cultic involvement, Paul Martin and Louis Jolyon West's observations of the repercussions of cult participation are timely. In Chapter 13, they examine the ubiquitous and profoundly deleterious effects of cultic involvement on participants, which may remain unrecognized or unacknowledged because of the dissociation fostered by powerful social influence processes at the heart of cult dynamics. By way of case examples, the authors illustrate how dissociation can extend to the development of a "pseudo-identity," which maintains various fictions and illusions about the beneficial aspects of cult participation. This occurs as a direct result of the cult member's dependence on a dominant, charismatic leader, and the cult power structure and group dynamics, which require submersion, if not virtual obliteration, of individual identity to perpetuate the cult and the leader's position of power and authority. In order for the ex-cult member to make a truly adaptive adjustment to society, it is necessary that lingering dissociative symptoms be addressed in psychotherapy, as the survivor reestablishes a healthy and coherent sense of self.

Richard Horevitz and Richard Loewenstein's chapter, "The Rational Treatment of Multiple Personality," is just that: a well-reasoned, logical, and caring approach, which traces the treatment of MPD through three stages of symptom stabilization—the working through of trauma and the resolution of dissociative defenses culminating in integration, and post-integration treatment (see Chapter 14). In elucidating this model, the authors map out basic strategies for affect regulation and the management of self-harm, and for social well-being, social skills, and interpersonal relatedness. These strategies can be imparted to the client in a multimodal treatment that can include cognitive-behavioral, hypnotic, family therapy, and group therapy interventions. Here, as in a number of other chapters, the need for careful assessment and a diagnosis that appreciates the essential diversity of this client population is underscored, along with the necessity of tailoring treatment to each client's special needs.

When a person is sexually assaulted, or experiences the traumatic after-effects of a cultic experience, they often are plagued by trauma-related memories, along with unpleasant, unbidden images. The therapist must deal with a person in crisis, whose images and memories are all too painfully real. The situation is often different, however, when a patient presents with symptoms that are not so readily explicable or traceable to a traumatic event in the past or present. In Chapter 15, George Ganaway sees many parallels between contemporary therapists' search for deeply buried memories of childhood trauma in patients diagnosed as suffering from dissociative disorders, and therapists' uncovering of "traumatic" memories in patients described as suffering from hysteria in Freud and Breuer's era. Ganaway maintains that then, as now, therapists who rely on trauma theory as a straightforward explanation for dissociative symptoms risk shaping the symptoms (e.g., increasing the numbers of "alters" that emerge) that are manifested, in keeping with transference and countertransference processes within the therapeutic dyad. Rather than embrace a simplistic trauma model, Ganaway recommends that therapists appreciate the true complexity of dissociative disorders, which he believes involve an interplay of bio-genetic factors, intrapsychic conflict, defense and compromise formation, object relations disturbances, and sociocultural factors. To work most effectively with a patient population comprised largely of persons with primitive character disorders who are also exceptionally "trance prone," Ganaway believes it is necessary to use modern psychoanalytic principles while fully appreciating and utilizing the interplay of transference and countertransference in the therapeutic relationship.

Stanley Krippner's work has consistently illustrated the wisdom of looking beyond the limited context of our culture to better understand puzzling aspects of the human condition. His cross-cultural examination of the treatment of dissociative disorders, in Chapter 16, is no exception. Here, he compares two examples of dissociation—"possession" by a discarnate entity and multiple personality disorder—which exist within vastly different cultural contexts. His scholarly examination of how the self is constructed in relation to the social milieu ranges from studies of spirit possession and incorporation in Puerto Rico, Haiti, and Brazil, to spiritistic treatment of MPD by Western-oriented psychotherapists. Krippner's study highlights both compelling similarities in the presentation of dissociative disorders across cultures, as well as notable differences, which appear to be intimately related to culture-bound expectations and self-perceptions. Ultimately, what cross-cultural psychology and Krippner's analysis of MPD illustrates is the inherent malleability of the human personality, which can have both adaptive and maladaptive aspects.

Issues and Controversies

This section of the book addresses important diagnostic, clinical, and research issues. In Chapter 17, John Kihlstrom provides a wealth of historical information on hysteria, dissociative disorders, and conversion disorders, while he makes a compelling and spirited case for grouping conversion disorder under the rubric of dissociative disorders in diagnostic classification schemes. Kihlstrom argues that both conversion and dissociative disorders are "fundamentally disorders involving the monitoring and controlling functions of consciousness" (Chapter 17, this volume, p. 378). He maintains that, like dissociative disorders, the symptoms of conversion disorders are essentially mental rather than physical in nature, and are consistent with a disorder in consciousness that affects sensation, perception, and voluntary action. Finally, conversion disorders resemble dissociative disorders in the descriptive sense in that they involve the "exclusion of mental contents and processes from conscious awareness and control" (Chapter 17, this volume, p. 387).

So far, many of the authors have made an implicit, if not an explicit, connection between early life trauma and dissociative pathology. Writing from a psychoanalytic point of view, Jane Tillman, Michael Nash, and Paul Lerner marshal evidence that challenges this widespread assumption (see Chapter 18). Although the trauma–dissociation connection may be intuitively appealing, the authors find little firm support for it in their review of the empirical literature. In addition to citing the problem of the questionable validity of certain child abuse reports, they identify important methodological issues and confounds including problems in defining trauma and dissociation, failure to consider base rates of abuse in all female patients in clinical settings, research design problems, and failure to consider a variety of pathogenic factors in a child's environment that might account for psychopathology. In closing, the authors claim that the relation between dissociation and trauma is far more complex than many workers in the field acknowledge.

In Chapter 19, Robert Belli and Elizabeth Loftus present a source monitoring perspective of recovered memories of childhood abuse. Because dissociative disorders have been associated with repressed or dissociated memories of childhood trauma, it is particularly important for clinicians to be in a position to evaluate the credibility of claims of delayed recall of early traumatic life events. In their chapter, Belli and Loftus carefully review the experimental evidence for the creation of false memories in the laboratory through suggestion and the imagination, and observe that the same factors make it difficult to discriminate real and imagined events in the laboratory and in the clinic. The authors caution that hazards of creating false memories of childhood trauma, very real insofar as childhood memories appear to be particularly vulnerable to pseudomemory creation.

Richard Horevitz's chapter is a fitting conclusion to a collection of chapters that present very different, and sometimes conflicting, perspectives on dissociative disorders and MPD (see Chapter 20). In presenting a cogent analysis of the 100-year-old debate about the "reality" of MPD, Horevitz considers three key areas that represent potential common ground for skeptics and proponents of the "reality" of MPD: (1) a modern flexible process therapy of personal identity and personality; (2) a recognition that differences exist between clinical dissociation and hypnotic dissociation, as well as an acceptance of the importance of suggestibility, fantasy proneness, social influence, and acculturation in the genesis of dissociative symptoms, and (3) an awareness of the fallibility of memory and the vulnerability of the highly hypnotizable person to pseudomemory creation.

Whereas Horevitz explores potential areas of commonality, he also highlights "incommensurabilities" that make it harder to achieve the resolution of conflict or its transformation into reasoned controversy. Some of these incommensurabilities are a product not only of vastly different paradigms held by the skeptics and the proponents in the debate, but of the entwined images, metaphors, and linguistic expressions that frame both sides of the controversy.

In addition to the areas of commonality that Horevitz identifies, our summary of the book indicates that a movement is occurring wherein the researchers and clinicians are taking into consideration multiple determinants (e.g., biopsychosocial, intrapsychic) when assessing and treating MPD and other serious dissociative disorders. Clinicians, in particular, would do well to entertain a number of hypotheses regarding why a patient displays dissociative symptoms, and to question the assumption that a simple cause-and-effect connection exists between trauma and symptom.

Another theme the reader will encounter is that dissociation is not necessarily maladaptive. Krippner, for example, goes so far as to write that in certain contexts, dissociative processes can be thought of as "basic skills or capacities similar to imagination and absorption, as well as a pathological reactions" (Chapter 16, this volume, p. 357). This viewpoint has, with some variations, been adopted by Lynn and his colleagues (Lynn, Rhue, & Green, 1988; Lynn, Neufeld, Green, Sandberg, & Rhue, in press) in other publications.

In conclusion, this book reflects contemporary attempts to define dissociation and a continuum of dissociative disorders and experiences and to discriminate more healthy, adaptive dissociative and imaginal processes (e.g., daydreaming, fantasy) from more pathological variants, which seemingly exist outside the arena of the "will" and voluntary control. The possibility that certain abilities or capacities are at the heart of dissociative disorders, along with the creative treatment approaches represented in this book, raise the hope that increasingly sophisticated treatment technologies will be devised to channel destructive, relatively unregulated imaginative and dissociative tendencies in more self-controlled and adaptation-enhancing directions.

REFERENCES

Hilgard, E. R. (1973). A neodissociation interpretation of pain reduction in hypnosis. *Psychological Review, 80*, 396–411.

Hilgard, E.R. (1977). *Divided consciousness: Multiple controls in human thought and action.* New York: John Wiley.

Janet, P. (1889). *L'automatisme psychologique.* Paris: Felix Alcan.

Kuhn, T. S. (1962). *The structure of scientific revolutions.* Chicago: University of Chicago Press.

Lerner, P. M. (1992). *Some preliminary thoughts on dissociation.* Unpublished manuscript.

Loftus, E. R. (1993). The reality of repressed memories. *American Psychologist, 48,* 518–537.

Lynn, S. J., & Nash, M. R. (1994). Truth in memory: Ramifications for psychotherapy and hypnotherapy. *American Journal of Clinical Hypnosis, 36,* 194–208.

Lynn, S. J., Neufeld, V., Green, J., Sandberg, D., & Rhue, J. (in press). Daydreaming, fantasy, and psychopathology. In R. Kunzendorf, N. Spanos, & B. Wallace (Eds.), *Imagination and hypnosis.* New Jersey: Baywood Press.

Lynn, S. J., & Rhue, J. W. (1991). Theories of hypnosis: An introduction. In S. J. Lynn & J. W. Rhue (Eds.), *Theories of hypnosis* (pp. 1–18). New York: Guilford Press.

Lynn, S. J., Rhue, J., & Green, J. (1988). Multiple personality and fantasy proneness: Is there an association or dissociation? *British Journal of Experimental and Clinical Hypnosis, 5,* 138–142.

Norman, D. A., & Shallice, T. (1986). Attention to action: Willed and automatic control of behavior. In R. J. Davidson, G. E. Schwartz, & D. Shapiro (Eds.), *Consciousness and self-regulation* (Vol. 4, pp. 1–18). New York: Plenum Press.

Price, R. H., & Lynn, S. J. (1986). *Abnormal psychology* (2nd ed.). Homewood, IL: Dorsey Press.

Rosenberg, M.J. (1959). A disconfirmation of the descriptions of hypnosis as a dissociative state. *International Journal of Clinical and Experimental Hypnosis, 7,* 187–204.

White, R. W., & Shevach, B. J. (1942). Hypnosis and the concept of dissociation. *Journal of Abnormal and Social Psychology, 7,* 309–328.

I
THEORETICAL AND RESEARCH PERSPECTIVES

1
The Domain of Dissociation

Etzel Cardeña

Although the term "dissociation" lacks a single, coherent referent or conceptualization that all investigators in the field embrace, it is not premature to identify a domain of dissociation, analogous in certain respects to Hilgard's (1973) concept of a domain of hypnosis. The domain of dissociation can be thought of as a constellation, or a way of thinking about dissociation and its related phenomena, with boundaries that define what lies inside and outside the domain. Thus, even if there is no consistent agreement about precisely what dissociation "is" or about the different theoretical positions that use the concept, we can at least become much more precise about the different uses of and assumptions about the term.

In its broadest sense, "dissociation" (Janet's *désagrégation*) simply means that two or more mental processes or contents are not associated or integrated. It is usually assumed that these dissociated elements should be integrated in conscious awareness, memory, or identity (see, e.g., American Psychiatric Association, 1987; van der Hart & Horst, 1989). However, this assumption is sometimes disregarded, as when overlearned behaviors such as shifting gears while driving and maintaining a conversation are assumed to be instances of dissociation.

Because of the semantic openness of the term, "dissociation" has been used as a descriptive or explanatory concept for such apparently disparate phenomena as hypnosis, perception without awareness, and automatic behaviors (e.g., Hilgard, 1986); to distinguish between various types of memory (e.g., Kihlstrom, 1982); in relation to some forms of psychopathology (e.g., American Psychiatric Association, 1987; Spiegel & Cardeña, 1991), some cognitive responses to trauma (e.g., Cardeña & Spiegel, 1993) and particular neurological syndromes (e.g., Farthing, 1992); and to account for differential performance on word comprehension exercises (e.g., Goodglass & Budin, 1988).

15

Just in the clinical and personality realm, "dissociation" has been viewed as a theoretical construct (i.e., as a defense mechanism) to explain why certain mental contents are not part of an individual's consciousness, as an explanation of the process(es) through which those contents are elided from memory, or as a description of particular contents within the stream of consciousness. While this free use of the term could imply a shared understanding of the connotative and denotative characteristics of the concept, it may also betray conceptual confusion. Partly because of this state of affairs, Frankel (1990) decried the vagueness of the term and proposed that we instead examine the concept of "repression." Unfortunately, his proposed cure is at least as fraught with problems as the terminological malady he sought to treat (cf. Spiegel & Cardeña, 1991).

In this chapter, I examine the various uses of the term "dissociation" in the psychological literature along with their underlying assumptions. Through elaborating the domain of dissociation, and focusing on its specific aspects, theoretical—and often untested—assumptions about the concept of dissociation should come into sharper focus. The reader should also gain a greater understanding of how the various dissociative disorders are related to different formulations of dissociation.

Workers in the field have approached the task of defining dissociation in different ways. Within the field of cognitive psychology, the term "dissociation" has been used to describe differential performance in tasks presumably mediated by distinct mental processes, such as comprehending body parts, colors, numbers, or letters, as well as other categories (Goodglass & Budin, 1988). It has also been used to explain performance in free-recall and word-fragment completion tests (Denny & Hunt, 1992). The term is used here very specifically and does not include the notion that the processes mediating different tasks should be integrated or accessible to the agent. This use of "dissociation" is different from the uses discussed below and will not be elaborated further.

Within the fields of personality and clinical psychology, dissociation has been described in at least three distinct ways. First, dissociation is used to characterize semi-independent mental modules or systems that are not consciously accessible, and/or not integrated within the person's conscious memory, identity, or volition. Second, dissociation is viewed as representing an alteration in consciousness wherein the individual and some aspects of his or her self or environment become disconnected or disengaged from one another. And third, dissociation is described as a defense mechanism that effects such disparate phenomena as nonorganic amnesia, the warding off of current physical or emotional pain, and other alterations of consciousness, including a chronic lack of personality integration, such as with Multiple Personality Disorder (MPD; referred to in the fourth edition of the *Diagnostic and Statistical Manual of Mental Disorders* [DSM-IV; American Psychiatric Association, 1994] as Dissociative Identity Disorder).

Besides describing the various applications of the term "dissociation" and providing representative examples, I will propose that some of these applications are inappropriate. Finally, to illustrate the boundaries of the dissociation domain, I have included an appendix, which gives a number of examples of how dissociation is used, arranged along two orthogonal dimensions of normality/pathology and psychological/neurological causation.

DISSOCIATION AS NONCONSCIOUS OR NONINTEGRATED MENTAL MODULES OR SYSTEMS

Within this category, I propose three subdivisions: (1) dissociation as the absence of conscious awareness of impinging stimuli or ongoing behaviors, (2) as the coexistence of separate mental systems or identities that should be integrated in the person's consciousness, memory, or identity, (3) as ongoing behaviors or perceptions that are inconsistent with a person's introspective verbal report.

It is noteworthy that the view of dissociation as involving parallel, nonconscious systems can overlap with the view of dissociation as involving an alteration of consciousness (see item 2 below). Hilgard (1986) exemplified this when he stated that hypnotic phenomena may involve alterations of consciousness that are the by-product of mental systems working outside of conscious awareness.

1. *Dissociation as the absence of conscious awareness of impinging stimuli or ongoing behaviors*. The notion that humans have fairly limited access to various mental processes pervades all of psychology, from Freud's theories to more recent cognitive (e.g., Baars, 1988) and artificial intelligence (AI) theories (e.g., Minsky, 1985). In its broadest and least distinct application, "dissociation" describes perceptions and behaviors that occur outside of conscious awareness. They range from behaviors in the periphery of a person's awareness (e.g., "unreflective" sequences of motor behavior such as occur when an expert driver shifts gears while simultaneously maintaining an engaging conversation), to behaviors manifested seemingly outside of his or her awareness (e.g., the behaviors that occur while sleepwalking), to the behaviors that result from the reception of subliminal stimuli, which affect the person despite the fact that such stimuli are registered outside of conscious awareness (cf. Hilgard, 1986, pp. 243–244).

As the heading of this subsection suggests, this notion of "dissociation" is indistinguishable from such terms as "preconscious," "subconscious," "subliminal," and "unconscious." In my view, however, the labeling of any form of peripheral awareness, automatic behavior, divided attention, distraction, preconscious process, implicit perception, and so forth, as dissociative, overextends the term, so that it includes any and all of the many processes involving our nonconscious mental executive and monitoring functions (cf. Hilgard, 1986).

The above way of thinking about dissociation disregards whether the individual, although not thinking about or attending to a stimulus or behavior, can bring a stimulus or behavior into conscious awareness, and whether the ability to do so should be expected given ordinary perceptual and information processing capacities. The case in which a driver carries out multiple tasks, only one of which he or she may be reflecting upon at some point, violates this more stringent definition, as the driver can easily turn his or her attention to other driving tasks. This example is not only quantitatively but qualitatively different from the case of a person in a dissociative fugue state, who cannot remember who he or she is despite attempts to do so, and from the case of a person who engages in "automatic writing" wherein purposeful behavior is unclaimed by the person even when he or she attends to the ongoing action. Many years ago Myers (1903/1961) made a similar point when discussing the "disintegration" of personality. He stated that "the *memorability* of an act is, in fact, a better proof of consciousness than its complexity" (p. 37). More recently, Nemiah (1991) proposed that dissociation refers to an "exclusion from consciousness and the *inaccessibility of voluntary recall of mental events*" (p. 250, emphasis added). In a similar vein, Kenneth Bowers (1991) has also made a cogent distinction between purposeful behaviors and those enacted "on purpose," to indicate that dissociation involves purposeful albeit nonvolitional behaviors.

The question of whether to accept reactions to "subliminal stimuli" or "implicit perception" as examples of dissociation is more complicated. These stimuli, by definition, cannot be discriminated at better than chance level and are inaccessible to the perceiver's awareness, although they may have an effect on both his or her waking and dreaming consciousness (cf. Erdelyi, 1985; Kihlstrom, Barnhardt, & Tataryn, 1992). Nonetheless, the term "dissociation" should not be applied to the mere processing of stimuli that are consciously inaccessible because of physical or attentional limitations. Instead, the term might more profitably be applied to a situation wherein current or previous information that should *ordinarily* be accessible to the individual is not. Were we to accept every instance of unawareness, purposeful automatic behavior, or divided attention as an example of dissociation, we would have to conclude that we live our lives in perpetual dissociation, as there are always some stimuli that have a demonstrable effect on us or behaviors that we are not reflectively aware of, but which we nonetheless enact.

In sum, the use of the term dissociation as shorthand for any kind of nonconscious or alternate mental process is of questionable merit.

2. *Dissociation as the coexistence of separate mental systems that should be integrated in the person's consciousness, memory, or identity.* According to this definition, "dissociation" applies to mental processes, such as sensations, thoughts, emotions, volition, memories, and identities, that we would ordinarily expect to be integrated within the individual's stream of consciousness and the historically extended self, but which are not. Dating back to the turn-of the-century and Pierre Janet, whose ideas influenced Breuer and the early Freud, this concept of dissociation has appeared widely in the clinical and personality literature. Currently, this conceptualization of dissociation underlies the notion of dissociative disorders.

In contrast to the definition given in Section 1, dissociation is not conceptualized here as involving the myriad of psychological and physiological processes that are ordinarily inaccessible unless an unusual technique (e.g., biofeedback of a physiological signal) is used. In addition, it does not assume that the mere existence of various psychological systems, some of which we may not be fully aware of (e.g., implicit and explicit memory), is dissociative, unless an unexpected failure of integration occurs. An example of the latter would be an individual who only exhibits implicit memory for an event for which explicit memory would also be expected (e.g., reenacting through play a traumatic memory for which the person claims amnesia).

A related phenomenon, sometimes referred to as "state dissociation" (e.g., Mahowald & Schenck, 1992), involves the notion that material learned or experienced in a particular state of consciousness may be less accessible in other states, or only become accessible when a similar state is reinstated. For instance, one of the main explanations for the amnesia that occurs for mentation during various stages of REM and non-REM sleep centers on the idea that waking and sleeping minds/brains involve different psychobiological states (Farthing, 1992).

Researchers of drug-induced "state dependent learning" have made a similar case. Their research has shown that material learned while under the influence of a particular drug may be more accessible when the person is again under the influence of the drug than when he or she is sober (Overton, 1991). Finally, there is some evidence (Singer & Salovey, 1988) that material learned in a certain mood may be more easily retrievable when that mood is reinstated.

Whether we should view state dependent memory in general as "dissociative" is arguable since it is widespread and no obvious reason exists to assume that the forgotten (or unretrieved) information should ordinarily be integrated into the individual's waking state of consciousness.

Less arguable is the notion that the extraordinary lapses of memory found among patients with dissociative identity disorder (DID; previously referred to as MPD) should be regarded as dissociative and that these lapses are the result of changes in consciousness. Putnam (1988) has reported that individuals with DID undergo alterations in their psychobiological state when shifting to different "alters," which could explain why their memories are compartmentalized. Below are other examples of failures of integration with regard to memory, identity, and volition.

An unexpected failure of explicit or episodic memory, typically brought about by a distressing or traumatic event, underlies dissociative amnesia, dissociative fugue, and DID. Dissociative amnesia involves the inability to recall important personal information that is too extensive to be explained away by ordinary forgetfulness or age, while dissociative fugue also involves a temporary confusion about identity and sudden unexpected travel away from home (Cardeña et al., in press). For example, a 16-year-old male was found amidst shrubbery on a highway, with amnesia for his name, address, and other basic information (Keller & Shaywitz, 1986). In these syndromes, the person is unable to integrate, or consciously recall, basic personal information that should be accessible, although that information may still be affecting the person's behavior (see also Chapter 17, this volume).

DID is characterized by a chronic failure to integrate various experiences and memories into a single identity. From the time of William James to the more recent conceptual work of Natsoulas (1983) and Neisser (1988), *conscious identity* has been viewed as fundamentally related to the ability to recall and connect previous personal experiences. In the case of DID, various forms of memory discontinuity (see Cardeña et al., in press, for a recent review) produce a lack of self-integration, experienced by DID patients as the coexistence of diverse identities that exist more or less independently from the stream of consciousness and bank of memories of the presenting identity or alter.

Because of the experienced presence of coexisting identities among DID patients, Prince chose to use the term coconscious to account for the existence of various identities (1905/1920), although Freud (1915/1984) argued that it was absurd to speak of dual consciousnesses, since the person could only be aware of one identity at any time. Following Freud, one could argue that the term "coconsciousness" should be parsimoniously applied, if at all, when referring to DID patients who have reported that their stream of consciousness may involve the presence of more than one identity or "alter" at times. Nevertheless, even here it would be more precise to speak of the copresence of clusters of ideas/thoughts/identities occurring in a single stream of consciousness at any one point.

A nonpathological example of parallel but distinct forms of "awarenesses" is Hilgard's (1986) "hidden observer" (see Chapter 2, this volume) which refers to a hypnotic phenomenon exhibited by certain highly hypnotizable subjects. While they report diminished or no pain sensitivity following a hypnotic analegesia suggestion and exposure to painful stimuli, they also report an ongoing parallel process, that is, the hidden observer effect, in which an awareness of the dissociated pain is reported. This effect is the result of a suggestion by the hypnotist that they can contact a hidden part of themselves that is aware of things of which the conscious mind is not. Assuming the validity of this explanation (for a contrasting view, see Spanos & Hewitt, 1980, who have argued that the hidden observer is a response created by the demand characteristics of the situation rather than by parallel streams of consciousness), how to regard an awareness that occurs outside of the stream of consciousness remains as problematic now as in Freud's time.

A failure of integration with regard to *volition* can be exemplified by phenomena reported in the anthropological and hypnosis literatures. Present in many cultures, "trance" and "spirit possession" are characterized by the participant's experiencing parts, or the whole, of his or her body carrying out actions seemingly on their own or at the behest of the possessing identity (Cardeña, 1992). Similarly, hypnosis frequently leads to transient forms of dissociation wherein a suggestion by the hypnotist comes to be experienced by hypnotizable individuals as producing behaviors that occur "on their own." For example, when a hypnotist suggests that the participant's arm "will get very light and float," the participant may experience this event as happening "by itself" (P. G. Bowers, 1990). This is an unusual event, not because a motor response is enacted without being purposefully willed by the individual—after all, we engage in unreflective complex motor behaviors all the time—but because the participant experiences his or her arm as rising "on its own," even when he or she attends to the behavior.

3. *Dissociation as ongoing behavior or perception inconsistent with a person's introspective verbal report.* An even more specific use of dissociation defines it as the contradiction between ongoing behaviors or perceptions and the individual's introspective experiential reports about such events. This conceptualization does not refer to the idea that individuals have access to the actual causes of their behavior or perceptions (e.g., Nisbett & Wilson, 1977). Rather, it refers to an inconsistency between individuals' sincere reports about what they are experiencing, and what their physiology or behavior suggests they should be experiencing. Erdelyi (1985) provides a good example of this in his description of a student who would, in a socially embarrassing situation in which she was criticized, break out in a florid rash while concurrently manifesting calmness in her speech and demeanor. Erdelyi writes that the student exhibited a dissociation between her epidermic reaction, suggestive of strong arousal and anger, and other behavioral and verbal indices. Of course, the same description could be used to exemplify the student's putative "repression" of her actual feelings. Indeed, individuals who experience a chronic disconnection between verbal reports and physiological reactivity are known in the literature as manifesting a "repressive" coping style (Weinberger, 1990; see also the section "Dissociation as a Defense Mechanism").

Hypnosis, which can be considered a form of structured and controllable dissociation (Spiegel & Cardeña, 1990), provides numerous examples of a disconnection between reports about experience and related behaviors or perceptions. For example, when given a negative hallucination suggestion (a suggestion *not* to perceive an actual stimulus) very highly hypnotizable individuals may report that they do not see the target object, although they have intact visual capabilities and will behaviorally respond to it (e.g., by walking around a negatively hallucinated chair).

Similar phenomena can be found in the clinical literature. Although not included as a dissociative disorder in the current DSM nosology, conversion syndromes can be viewed as pathological dissociative conditions. In these syndromes, the patient's introspective verbal report of lack of physical sensation or control in a circumscribed part of the body is dissociated from actual anatomical and functional intactness (Nemiah, 1991). A thorough argument for including conversion disorders under the rubric of dissociative disorders is presented by Kihlstrom in Chapter 17.

Some neurological syndromes also exemplify disconnections between a person's phenomenal report and corresponding actions or perceptions. Many neurological conditions have a psychiatric parallel (e.g., organic vs. dissociative amnesia, temporal lobe epilepsy vs. dissociative fugues; hemineglect vs. conversion syndromes). One of the most striking neurological conditions is "blindsight." This is said to be present when patients with striate cortex damage, but an otherwise intact visual system, report "blindness" on the contralateral side of the lesion, even though when given a forced-choice procedure to locate a flash of light or some other stimulus in the "blind" visual field, they may be remarkably, and, to themselves inexplicably, accurate (Weiskrantz, Warrington, Sanders, & Marshall. 1974).

The literature on commissurotomy is also replete with instances of disconnections between introspective verbal reports and behavior. For instance, Gazzaniga (1985) described a commissurotomized individual who, within an experimental setting, did not report having seen a picture of a horse presented tachistoscopically to the left visual field but nonetheless drew such a picture with his left hand.

DISSOCIATION AS AN ALTERATION IN CONSCIOUSNESS WHEREIN DISCONNECTION/DISENGAGEMENT FROM THE SELF OR THE ENVIRONMENT IS EXPERIENCED

While the two previously described concepts of dissociation involve the inability to integrate related mental processes, they do not imply that the person has qualitatively transformed his or her phenomenal experience into a discrete altered state of consciousness (cf. Tart, 1975).

Dissociation, as it is conceptualized here, involves particular alterations in phenomenal experience that are related to a disconnection or disengagement regarding the self and/or the environment (e.g., Noyes & Kletti, 1977; Steinberg, 1991). Although at times the term dissociation is used so loosely, and imprecisely, that it seems to encompass any form of alteration in consciousness, there are, in fact, altered states that do not involve any form of disconnection from the environment. To the contrary, in the case of certain "ecstatic" experiences an enhanced sense of contact with the surroundings and the self is reported (cf. Laski, 1961/1990). To propose that mystical experiences in general are a form of dissociation as Braun (1993) maintains is, in my view, an unwarranted extension of the concept of dissociation.

Even in the midst of an "ordinary" state of consciousness, the extent to which our experiencing self is engaged with various mental processes and its surroundings varies considerably. We may be tired or distracted, we may engage in momentary daydreaming, or we may even choose to adopt a reflective stance, perhaps cultivated through "mindfulness" meditation, so as not to become fully identified and engaged with the phenomenal world. Once again, to assume that any type of disconnection between the experiencing self and various perceptions, emotions, or thoughts is "dissociative" makes the term so overarching that it loses descriptive value. To be useful as a concept, dissociation should not be applied to ordinary instances of less-than-full engagement with one's surroundings, experiences, and actions. Rather, it should pertain to qualitative departures from one's ordinary modes of experiencing, wherein an unusual disconnection or disengagement from the self and/or the surroundings occurs as a central aspect of the experience.

Such disconnection may occur in a number of different ways. A rape victim, for example, may disengage from the ongoing event by seemingly having no sensory experiences or emotions during it, by "observing" it from a perspective at a distance from the physical body (i.e., an out-of-body experience), by becoming fully immersed in an imaginal event, and so forth. Along these lines, a widely used measure of dissociation, the Dissociative Experiences Scale (DES), has been reported to have three stable factors: dissociative amnesia, absorption, and depersonalization/derealization (Carlson & Putnam, 1993).

The literature on hypnosis (Pekala, 1991), and ritually induced states of consciousness (Cardeña, 1989), suggests that altered states involving self-initiated, mostly imaginal events, are qualitatively distinct from those involving a general sense of alteration without imagery. Whether these differences reflect cognitive styles, different forms of induction, or some other process, remains to be determined.

The clinical syndromes of depersonalization and derealization exemplify pronounced dissociative modes of experiencing. Depersonalization refers to a wide range of chronic phenomena, in which the self experiences itself as detached or at an unbridgeable distance from ongoing perceptions, actions, emotions, or thoughts. For example, the depersonalized individual may have the experience that she is physically numb, that bodily sensations happen at a distance from the self, or that the self actually resides outside of the physical body. Further, the person may feel like an automaton, that bodily actions are somehow "happening on their own," or that the self can merely observe instead of experiencing emotions or thoughts (Reed, 1988; Steinberg, 1991). Perhaps the most intriguing and unusual form of depersonalization is the "double" syndrome, in which a person may actually "perceive" and even interact with an external double of him- or herself, a phenomenon that has fascinated writers and psychologists alike including Otto Rank, Edgar Allan Poe, and Fyodor Dostoevsky.

With derealization, the individual may not doubt the reality of the self, but, instead, have the experience that his or her surroundings and fellow inhabitants are not quite real, that he or she inhabits a dreamlike world devoid of substance. In contrast to a delusional individual who may *believe* that the world is unreal, the individual suffering from derealization *experiences* the world or its inhabitants as not quite real.

The clinical literature is replete with anecdotal and systematic accounts of various forms of depersonalization and derealization that result from the use of "dissociative" drugs such as ketamine (Siegel, 1989), natural disasters, serious accidents, or other forms of trauma (e.g., Cardeña & Spiegel, 1993; Noyes & Kletti, 1977), but dissociative phenomenology can also be related to far more benign events. For instance, out-of-body experiences can be accidentally or purposefully elicited by physical relaxation and focusing one's attention internally (Farthing, 1992), particularly among highly hypnotizable (Cardeña, 1988) or fantasy-prone individuals (Wilson & Barber, 1981; Lynn & Rhue, 1988).

Future research should distinguish among the various modes in which individuals can disengage from the environment and clarify the biocognitive processes mediating such alterations in consciousness.

DISSOCIATION AS A DEFENSE MECHANISM

A defense mechanism is a theoretical construct that refers to the intentional disavowing of information that would cause anxiety or pain. (cf. Freud, 1936/1984). The concept of dissociation as a defense mechanism has been used to explain why the phenomena in the above sections came about. Specifically, when confronted with an ongoing danger or threat, a dissociative mechanism is initiated to safeguard the individual's psychological integrity. Within the psychoanalytic framework, such a mechanism is purposeful, although not necessarily conscious, and may be triggered in isolated instances (e.g., when a person is confronted with a disaster) or become a characterological disposition (e.g., the ongoing compartmentalization of memories and identities among the various alters of a person with DID).

While the psychoanalytic notion of defense mechanisms is by definition purposeful and functionalist, Janet, who offered the main competing alternative, did not assume such position. He proposed, in contrast, that dissociation may occur when a person experiences "vehement" emotions, including terror, which narrow attention and disorganize the ordinary integrative functions of consciousness. These experiences and related memories, Janet maintained, are not integrated into the person's identity and long-term memory but become, instead, simple "fixed ideas" (*idées fixes*) or complex alter identities that continue to have a separate mental existence, sometimes affecting the person in insidious ways (van der Hart & Horst, 1989; Putnam, 1989b). This idea is very similar to Jung's concept of mental complexes, which involve semi-independent groups of ideas and feelings.

Although these two theoretical positions may part company with regards to whether dissociative processes are enacted purposefully by a mental structure (the "ego" in the case of psychoanalysis) or not, the most accurate representation of dissociative events probably includes both purposeful and nonpurposeful processes. Dissociative alterations may happen automatically and unwittingly, for instance, when an individual encounters even a benign stimulus that is associated with a traumatic event and automatically engages in internally focused attention, or may purposefully use hypnotic-like techniques to have dissociative experiences, such as unfocusing his or her gaze, focusing attention on an imaginal event, and so on (e.g., Hartman & Burgess, 1993). While attentional processes may be intentionally used to distance the experiencing self from pain, this should not, however, be construed as meaning that dissociative occurrences must necessarily serve a defensive purpose. Dissociative experience can be viewed, instead, as a general mental modality to which some individuals are more predisposed than others, and is elicited by different processes, including the person's deliberate intention. In the same way, humor can be intentionally or automatically used to avoid dealing with anxiety, or it can be experienced for its own pleasurable sake.

While a "defense mechanism" is ordinarily assumed to be an individual's way of warding off anxiety or pain, Ludwig (1983) has proposed an explanation based on evolution. He maintains that dissociative processes bring about an experiential disengagement from overwhelming physical or psychological events because they have had species survival value and served many diverse, adaptation-enhancing functions. He states that the sham death reflex among slow animals may be analogous to dissociation, and that, besides survival, dissociation may have other functions such as the cathartic discharge of feelings and the isolation of catastrophic experiences. In a similar vein, Ironside (1980) concluded that alterations in consciousness and behaviors (e.g., "being in a daze," passivity) that some humans exhibit after a catastrophe is a biological response of conservation/withdrawal to save physical and psychological resources when dealing with inescapable trauma. One of the most important challenges remaining for any researcher or theoretician in the area is to explain how dissociative *processes* and *phenomena*, which may have originally been neutral or even beneficial, become maladaptive. One can speculate that factors such as a benign environment and good psychological resources would lead to a situation in which these processes and phenomena would remain adaptive, but at this point we have much more speculation than actual studies.

Another important issue when talking about dissociation is whether, as a defense mechanism, it actually differs from repression. As Erdelyi (1985) has pointed out, Freud himself used the terms repression and dissociation indistinctly. More recently, only a minority of collaborators in a book on repression and dissociation clearly distinguished between the two terms (Singer & Sincoff, 1990, p. 475). This should not be surprising since when dealing with amnesia, for example, stating that a person has a "dissociated" memory is indistinguishable from stating that he or she has a "repressed" memory, theoretical allegiances aside. Further, Erdelyi (1990) has also shown how metaphors that seem to meaningfully distinguish between dissociation and repression, as when repression is referred to as involving "vertical" splits and dissociation as involving "horizontal" splits, are actually vacuous.

The distinction sometimes made between repression and dissociation, where repression is a defense against anxiety-provoking *internal* stimuli while dissociation is a defense against *external* stimuli, is also problematic. Freud himself used the general term defense mechanism, which he at times equated with repression, to account for the disavowal of material from both "the real external and from the internal world of thoughts and impulses" (Freud, 1936/1984, p. 454). For instance, when a person suffers from dissociative amnesia, the "warded" off material, namely memories, is by definition internal, even though the trigger for the amnesia may have been environmentally caused distress. For any proposed distinction between repression and dissociation to be meaningful, both constructs will have to be operationalized unambiguously. So far, this has not been the case.

At this point, it is beneficial to reiterate that the first two conceptualizations of dissociation discussed in this chapter were mostly descriptive in nature and did not imply any particular theoretical orientation. Going beyond theoretical turf wars, a more fruitful approach to advancing our understanding of dissociation would be to clearly conceptualize what we mean by the term, and to investigate the specific personality and environmental characteristics and the mediating biological and cognitive processes that give rise to and maintain it. For example, there is some evidence from experimental research (Christianson & Loftus, 1987) that, when confronted with distressful events, individuals may narrow their attention and have memory alterations. These attentional changes may, in turn, be involved with alterations in consciousness, including depersonalization and derealization (Cardeña & Spiegel, 1993).

CONCLUSION

The interest in dissociative processes and phenomena has mushroomed in the last decade and is unlikely to abate in the near future. This interest is "overdetermined" and includes the rediscovery of Janet's brilliant proposals, the increasing evidence of some kind of connection between trauma and dissociative phenomena, and current research and theory on the nature and prevalence of the dissociative disorders. As indicated above, dissociation has come to represent different types of phenomena and constructs, from altered experiences of detachment from the self or the surroundings, to a lack of integration between various mental processes, to a presumed defense mechanism, which functions to ward off ongoing anxiety or pain. If we do not tread carefully, the use of the same concept for such diverse entities may come to gloss over the authors' underlying assumptions and may prevent specific research on the actual mental processes involved.

After a period of famine in which distant psychoanalytic concepts or simplistic behavioral conceptions dominated the clinical menu, the concept of dissociation has proved nourishing. However, this feast may become bloating indigestion unless we make explicit how we use the concept of dissociation and what assumptions we buy into.

Ironically, perhaps one of the great appeals of the domain of dissociation is that it allows the investigator and the clinician to connect various areas within psychology (e.g., personality, memory, consciousness, identity) that up until recently have been dissociated.

APPENDIX

Various taxonomies of dissociation have been proposed, including the concept of a dissociation continuum which includes a range from normal dissociative processes, through dissociative episodes and disorders, to the most severe form of

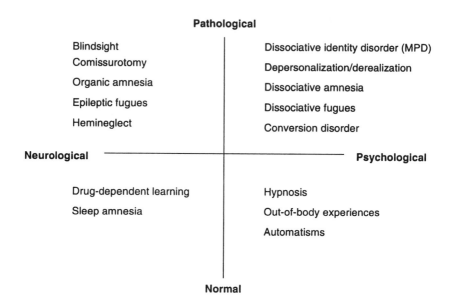

Pathological

Blindsight	Dissociative identity disorder (MPD)
Comissurotomy	Depersonalization/derealization
Organic amnesia	Dissociative amnesia
Epileptic fugues	Dissociative fugues
Hemineglect	Conversion disorder

Neurological ———————————————— **Psychological**

Drug-dependent learning	Hypnosis
Sleep amnesia	Out-of-body experiences
	Automatisms

Normal

FIGURE A.1. Dissociative phenomena.

dissociation, namely dissociative identity disorder (Braun, 1993; also Putnam, 1989a). Others propose that dissociative disorders should be arranged as to the type of mental process not integrated, including sensation, memory, and volition (Kihlstrom, Chapter 17). As a heuristic device, I present in Figure A.1 some of the dissociative phenomena and syndromes discussed in the chapter, arranged as to whether they are considered pathological or normal, and whether their cause is assumed to be primarily neurological or psychological.

In the upper right quadrant of the figure four psychopathological syndromes that the DSM-IV currently categorizes as dissociative are displayed, with the addition of conversion disorders. All of these involve "disruption in the usually integrated functions of consciousness, memory, identity, or perception of the environment" (American Psychiatric Association, 1994, p. 477; Spiegel & Cardeña, 1991), and are not primarily neurological in nature. The upper left quadrant includes various examples wherein a lack of integration between conscious experience (as evaluated through introspective verbal reports) and behaviors is the product of brain injury or malfunction.

In the lower right quadrant are nonpathological phenomena (e.g., hypnotic events) that are primarily produced by psychological and social variables such as deployment of attention, expectations, and such. Finally, the lower left quadrant includes "ordinary" types of amnesia that have been viewed as forms of dissociation involving different psychobiological states.

REFERENCES

American Psychiatric Association. (1987). *Diagnostic and statistical manual of mental disorders* (3rd ed. rev.). Washington, DC: American Psychiatric Association.

American Psychiatric Association. (1994). *Diagnostic and statistical manual of mental disorders* (4th ed.). Washington, DC: Author.

Baars, B. (1988). *A cognitive theory of consciousness.* Cambridge: Cambridge University Press.

Bowers, K. (1991). Dissociation in hypnosis and multiple personality disorder. *International Journal of Clinical and Experimental Hypnosis, 39,* 155–176.

Bowers, P. G. (1990). Examining subjects' experiences during hypnosis. In R. Van Dyck, P. Spinhoven, A. J. Van der Does, Y. R. van Rood, & W. De Moor (Eds.), *Hypnosis: Current theory, research and practice* (pp. 103–111). Amsterdam: VU University Press.

Braun, B. G. (1993). Multiple personality disorder and post-traumatic stress disorder. In J. P. Wilson & B. Raphael (Eds.), *International handbook of traumatic stress syndromes* (pp. 35–47). New York: Plenum Press.

Cardeña, E. (1988, November). *The phenomenology of quiescent and physically active deep hypnosis.* Paper presented at the 38th annual meeting of the Society for Clinical and Experimental Hypnosis, Ashville, NC.

Cardeña, E. (1989). The varieties of possession experience. *Association for the Anthropological Study of Consciousness Quarterly, 5,* 1–17.

Cardeña, E. (1992). Trance and possession as dissociative disorders. *Transcultural psychiatric research review, 29,* 283–297.

Cardeña, E., Lewis-Fernandez, R., Beahr, D., Pakianathan, I., & Spiegel, D. (in press). Dissociative disorders. In *Sourcebook for the DSM-IV* (Vol. 4). Washington, DC: American Psychiatric Press.

Cardeña, E., & Spiegel D. (1993). Dissociative reactions to the Bay Area Earthquake. *American Journal of Psychiatry, 150,* 474–478.

Carlson, E. B., & Putnam, F. W. (1993). An update on the dissociative experiences scale. *Dissociation, 6,* 16–27.

Christianson, S. A., & Loftus, E. F. (1987). Memory for traumatic events. *Applied Cognitive Psychology, 1,* 225–239.

Denny, E. B., & Hunt, R. R. (1992). Affective valence and memory in depression: Dissociation of recall and fragment completion. *Journal of Abnormal Psychology, 101,* 575–580.

Erdelyi, M. H. (1985). *Psychoanalysis: Freud's cognitive psychology.* New York: W. H. Freeman.

Erdelyi, M. H. (1990). Repression, reconstruction, and defense: History and integration of the psychoanalytic and experimental frameworks. In J. L. Singer (Ed.), *Repression and dissociation* (pp. 1–31). Chicago: University of Chicago Press.

Farthing, G. W. (1992). *The psychology of consciousness.* Englewood Cliffs, NJ: Prentice Hall.

Frankel, F. (1990). Hypnotizability and dissociation. *American Journal of Psychiatry, 147*, 823–829.

Freud. S. (1984). The unconscious. In A. Richards (Ed.), *On metapsychology: The theory of psychoanalysis* (pp. 159–222). Middlesex, England: Penguin. (Original work published 1915)

Freud, S. (1984). A disturbance of memory on the Acropolis. In A. Richards (Ed.), *On metapsychology: The theory of psychoanalysis* (pp. 443–456). Middlesex, England: Penguin. (Original work published 1936)

Gazzaniga, M. S. (1985). *The social brain: Discovering the networks of the mind.* New York: Basic Books.

Goodglass, H., & Budin, C. (1988). Category and modality specific dissociations in word comprehension and concurrent phonological dyslexia. *Neuropsychologia, 26*, 67–78.

Hartman, C. R., & Burgess, A. W. (1993). Treatment of victims of rape trauma. In J. P. Wilson & B. Raphael (Eds.), *International handbook of traumatic stress syndromes* (pp. 507–516). New York: Plenum Press.

Hilgard, E. R. (1973). The domain of hypnosis, with some comments on alternative paradigms. *American Psychologist, 28*, 972–982.

Hilgard, E. R. (1986). *Divided consciousness* (expanded ed.). New York: John Wiley.

Ironside, W. (1980). Conservation–withdrawal and action–engagement: On a theory of survival behavior. *Psychosomatic Medicine, 42*, 163–175.

Keller, R., & Shaywitz, B. A. (1986). Amnesia or fugue state: A diagnostic dilemma. *Developmental and Behavioral Pediatrics, 7*, 131–132.

Kihlstrom, J. F. (1982). Hypnosis and the dissociation of memory, with special reference to posthypnotic amnesia. *Research Communications in Psychology, Psychiatry and Behavior, 7*, 181–197.

Kihlstrom, J. F., Barnhardt, T. M., & Tataryn, D. J. (1992). Implicit perception. In R. F. Bornstein & T. S. Pittman (Eds.), *Perception without awareness* (pp. 17–54). New York: Guilford Press.

Laski, M. (1990). *Ecstasy in secular and religious experience.* Los Angeles: Tarcher. (Original work published 1961)

Ludwig, A. M. (1983). The psychobiological functions of dissociation. *American Journal of Clinical Hypnosis, 26*, 93–99.

Lynn, S. J., & Rhue, J. W. (1988). Fantasy proneness: Hypnosis, developmental antecedents, and psychopathology. *American Psychologist, 43*, 35–44.

Mahowald, M. W., & Schenck, C. H. (1992). Dissociated states of wakefulness and sleep. *Neurology, 42*, 44–52.

Minsky, M. (1985). *The society of the mind.* New York: Simon & Schuster.

Myers, F. W. H. (1961). *Human personality and its survival of bodily death.* New York: University Books. (Original work published 1903)

Natsoulas, T. (1983). Concepts of consciousness. *Journal of Mind and Behavior, 4*, 13–59.

Nemiah, J. (1991). Dissociation, conversion, and somatization. In A. Tasman & S. M. Goldfinger (Eds.), *American Psychiatric Press review of psychiatry* (Vol. 10, pp. 248–260). Washington, DC: American Psychiatric Press.

Neisser, U. (1988). Five kinds of self-knowledge. *Philosophical Psychology, 1*, 35–59.

Nisbett R. E., & Wilson, T. D. (1977). Telling more than we can know: Verbal reports on mental processes. *Psychological Review, 84*, 231–259.

Noyes R., & Kletti, R. (1977). Depersonalization in response to life-threatening danger. *Comprehensive Psychiatry, 18*, 375–384.

Overton, D. A. (1991). Historical context of state dependent learning and discriminative drug effects. *Behavioural Pharmacology, 2*, 253–264.

Pekala, R. (1991). Hypnotic types: Evidence from a cluster analysis of phenomenal experience. *Contemporary Hypnosis, 8*, 95–104.

Prince, M. (1920). *The dissociation of a personality*. Norwood, MA: Plimpton Press. (Original work published 1905)

Putnam, F. W. (1988). The switch process in multiple personality disorder and other state-change disorders. *Dissociation, 1*, 24–32.

Putnam, F. W. (1989a). *Diagnosis and treatment of multiple personality disorder*. New York: Guilford Press.

Putnam, F. W. (1989b). Pierre Janet and modern views of dissociation. *Journal of Traumatic Stress, 2*, 413–429.

Reed, G. R. (1988). *The psychology of anomalous experience*. New York: Prometheus.

Siegel, R. K. (1989). *Intoxication*. New York: Dutton.

Singer, J. A., & Salovey, P. (1988). Mood and memory: Evaluating the network theory of affect. *Clinical Psychology Review, 84*, 127–190.

Singer, J. L., & Sincoff, J. B. (1990). Summary: Beyond repression and the defenses. In J. L. Singer (Ed.), *Repression and dissociation* (pp. 471–496). Chicago: University of Chicago Press.

Spanos N. P., & Hewitt, E. C. (1980). The hidden observer in hypnotic analgesia: Discovery or experimental creation? *Journal of Personality and Social Psychology, 39*, 1201–1214.

Spiegel, D., & Cardeña, E. (1990). New uses of hypnosis in the treatment of posttraumatic stress disorder. *Journal of Clinical Psychiatry, 51* (Suppl.), 39–43.

Spiegel, D., & Cardeña, E. (1991). Disintegrated experience: The dissociative disorders revisited. *Journal of Abnormal Psychology, 100*, 366–378.

Steinberg, M. (1991). The spectrum of depersonalization: Assessment and treatment. In A. Tasman & S. M. Goldfinger (Eds.), *American Psychiatric Press review of psychiatry* (Vol. 10, pp. 223–247). Washington, DC: American Psychiatric Press.

Tart, C. T. (1975). *States of consciousness*. New York: E. P. Dutton.

van der Hart, O., & Horst, R. (1989). The dissociation theory of Pierre Janet. *Journal of Traumatic Stress, 2*, 397–412.

Weinberger, D. A. (1990). The construct validity of the repressive coping style. In J. L. Singer (Ed.), *Repression and dissociation* (pp. 337–386). Chicago: University of Chicago Press.

Weiskrantz, L., Warrington, E. K., Sanders, M. D., & Marshall, J. (1974). Visual capacity in the hemianopic field following a restricted occipital ablation. *Brain, 97*, 709–728.

Wilson, S. C. (1981). Vivid fantasy and hallucinatory abilities in the life histories of excellent hypnotic subjects ("somnambules"): Preliminary reports with female subjects. In E. Klinger (Ed.), *Imagery: Vol. 2. Concepts, results, and applications* (pp. 158–172). New York: Plenum Press.

2
Neodissociation Theory

Ernest R. Hilgard

My interest in exploring the significance of dissociation in the understanding of hypnosis goes back to my reading of William James and William McDougall during my graduate student days in the late 1920s, although the interest was little represented in my published work until I began to take a serious interest in hypnosis research in the late 1950s. Even then, my references to dissociation were rather sparse in my first book on hypnosis (Hilgard, 1965). I there presented and discussed the following propositions:

> *The various dissociative experiences activated by hypnotic induction and by suggestions within hypnosis are correlated with specific developmental experiences.* (p. 388)
> *The hypnosis state is characterized by various partial dissociations.* (p. 392)

The first of these two propositions is conjectural, but appears to be plausible in view of the relevant dissociative experiences that can be encouraged in early childhood. Thus, when a mother says, "Come here; I'll rub your head and the bump won't hurt anymore," the suggestion may be effective and the child may indeed no longer feel the pain. This "magic" that the mother performs may provide a readiness for the evoked fantasies in hypnosis.

The mother may also tell some fairy tales prior to bedtime, so that the child learns to enjoy the departures from everyday experiences without being threatened by them. The reality experiences are restored when the mother changes the context and says, "Now it's time to brush your teeth and go to bed."

While writing my first book on hypnosis (Hilgard, 1965) I was aware that there had been attacks upon the dissociation concept in the experimental literature on hypnosis (White & Shevach, 1942; Rosenberg, 1959), but my reply to the criticisms by these authors was that they had been looking for complete dissociation while I was favoring a partial dissociation.

32

Dissociation, in common with many other psychological processes, may be a matter of degree. Thus posthypnotic amnesia, often an aftermath of hypnosis, is commonly incomplete in that subjects or patients (at a signal) recall some, but usually not all, of what happened during hypnosis. This partial recall before the amnesia is cancelled can be viewed as dissociative in that some material recorded in memory is not available to recall. That it has been registered in memory but dissociated is shown by the enhanced recall when the signal to cancel the amnesia is given.

A few years later, I reviewed some of the literature on dissociation in a chapter in which I also discussed its earlier history and later neglect (Hilgard, 1973a). In the same year, I introduced my neodissociation theory (Hilgard, 1973b), this time in relation to the hypnotic reduction of pain. Here, for the first time a careful attempt was made to relate my theory to experimental findings in the Stanford laboratory. Specifically, the development of the neodissociation interpretation was the result of a series of investigations done on the reduction of experimentally induced pain by hypnosis. While these did not involve clinical treatment, some advantage lay in experimentally producing pain over treating clinical pain in that the former could be more carefully calibrated than pain arising through accident or natural causes.

Despite my friendliness to the dissociation concept, I made little direct use of it until the early 1970s, when experimenters in our laboratory initiated some experiments on automatic writing to detect the nature of the dissociations involved. These showed the conflicts that occurred when a person was involved with simultaneous tasks, one of which was done with full awareness, and the other without, (i.e., "automatically") as a consequence of the hypnotic suggestions given to a highly hypnotically responsive subject, who could fulfill the criteria set up for the experiments. Without going into detail here, the two simultaneous tasks were always interfering with each other, depending, in part, on the nature of the tasks (Knox, Crutchfield, & Hilgard, 1975; Stevenson, 1976).

The origin of the concept of a "hidden observer" lay in an observation I made during a demonstration in a class I was offering on hypnotic phenomena, in which the lectures were supplemented with demonstrations on highly hypnotically responsive subjects. I shall repeat the initial observation for those who may not have been acquainted with my earlier writings.

THE UNANTICIPATED APPEARANCE
OF A HIDDEN OBSERVER

At the time, I was offering a course to undergraduate students on hypnosis, which emphasized the variety of phenomena that could be experienced by a responsive hypnotized person. In this instance, the topic was hypnotic deafness. The subject of the demonstration was a blind student of known hypnotic talent, who had volunteered his time. His blindness was not related to the experiment, except that it eliminated any unintended visual cues, although it was important that the subject knew that hypnotic deafness would be temporary because of his acute reliance upon his hearing. After the induction of hypnosis, he was given the suggestion that, at the count of 3, he would become completely deaf to all sounds. He was then told that his hearing would be restored promptly when the instructor's hand was placed upon his right shoulder.

After a slow count to 3, loud sounds made by banging together some wooden blocks close to the subject's head produced no sign of reaction. No reaction was expected because the subject had shown no response to the unexpected shots of a starter's pistol when hypnotically deaf in a previous session. A startle response had been evident when the shots had been fired when his eyes were closed but he was not hypnotized. The students asked him questions and taunted him to see whether they could get a reaction, but no reaction was forthcoming. One student in the class raised the question of whether some part of the subject might know what was going on, for, after all, there was nothing wrong with his ears. It occurred to me to test this by a method of interrogation that I had seen some clinical hypnotists use in seeking information from a hypnotized patient. Following their lead, I addressed the subject in a quiet voice:

"As you know, there are parts of our nervous system that carry on activities that occur without awareness, of which the control of the circulation of the blood, or the digestive processes, are the most familiar. However, there may be intellectual processes of which we also are unaware, such as those that find expression in night dreams. Although you are hypnotically deaf, perhaps there is some part of you that is hearing my voice and processing the information. If there is, I should like the index finger of your right hand to rise as a sign that this is the case."

To both my surprise and that of the class members, the finger rose, and the subject immediately said:

"Please restore my hearing so that you can tell me what you did. I felt my finger rise in a way that was not a spontaneous twitch, so that you must have done something to make it rise." I then placed my hand on his right shoulder, as the prearranged signal for restoring his hearing, and the following conversation took place:

"Can you hear my voice now?"

"Yes, I hear you. Now tell me what you did."

"What do you remember?"

"I remember your telling me that I would be deaf at the count of 3, and could have my hearing restored when you placed your hand on my shoulder. Then everything was quiet for a while. It was a little boring just sitting here, so I busied myself with a statistical problem that I have been working on. I was still doing that when I suddenly felt my finger lift; that is what I wanted you to explain to me."

I assured the subject that he would soon be informed about everything that had transpired. After this demonstration, I dared to introduce what would become an important innovation. As discussed above, my colleagues and I had been conducting some experiments on dissociation, such as the one involving automatic writing. We had found that some of the material not in the hypnotized subject's awareness could be recovered through automatic writing. Hence, through analogy with the automatic writing, it seemed worth testing with this highly hypnotizable subject whether, "automatic talking" might yield similar results. With the subject hypnotized but able to hear and carry on a conversation, I spoke to him as follows:

"When I place my hand on your arm like this [which I demonstrated], I can be in touch with that part of you that listened to me before, while you were hypnotically deaf. But this part of you to whom I am now talking, will not know what you are saying, or even that you are talking, until—when you are out of hypnosis—I shall say, 'Now you can remember everything.' All right, now I am placing my hand on your arm."

The following conversation then ensued: "Do you remember what happened when you were hypnotized and what the hypnotized part of you reported?"

"Yes." (In some instances, hypnotized subjects are thought to be literal in their answers, as in this "Yes," but that is by no means universal. In this instance, the subject had already told me about the experience while he was still hypnotized.) On further questioning, he repeated much of the earlier conversation, including his surprise about his finger's lifting.

I continued, "Does this part to whom I am now talking know more about what went on?"

"Yes."

"Please tell me what went on."

"After you counted to make me deaf, you made some noises as if banging some blocks together behind my head. Members of the class asked me questions to which I did not respond. Then one of them asked if I might really be hearing, and you told me to raise my finger if I was. This part of me responded by raising my finger, so it's all clear now."

I then lifted my hand from his arm to restore his prior condition, according to the directions I had given him.

The next question was addressed to the subject when he was in his usual hypnotic condition following induction.

"Please tell me what happened in the last few minutes."

"You said something about placing your hand on my arm, and some part of me would talk. Did I talk?"

I told him that he would remember everything when hypnosis was terminated and then aroused him by counting backwards, a procedure with which he was familiar. He then recalled all that had happened throughout the demonstration.

This unplanned and, hence, unrehearsed demonstration indicated clearly that a hypnotized subject who is unaware of sensory information (in this case, auditory), may nevertheless be registering and processing it in some manner. Under appropriate circumstances, information that is unknown to the subject while hypnotized can be uncovered and talked about. Instead of using the expression "automatic talking" (the term I had in mind when introducing the demonstration), the degree to which the information was processed led me to introduce the metaphor of a "hidden observer." The metaphor may have been unfortunate because to some it suggested a secondary personality with a life of its own—a kind of homunculus lurking in the head of the conscious person. The "hidden observer" was intended merely as a convenient label for the information source capable of a high level of cognitive functioning, not consciously experienced by the hypnotized person.

THE HIDDEN OBSERVER PHENOMENON

Obviously the results from this one demonstration could not firmly establish that the phenomenon called the hidden observer in fact exists. Hence, a number of investigations were carried out in order that further generalizations could be made. Some findings from one of the investigations of experimentally produced pain performed in the Stanford laboratory are illustrated in Figure 2.1. The pain, known as cold pressor pain, is produced by holding the hand and forearm in circulating ice water.

When hypnotic analgesia had been suggested prior to the insertion of the hand and forearm into the water, subjects chosen for their responsiveness to hypnosis, reported no pain or very little pain at the overt level: On average they reported a level of 2 of pain, where 10 was defined as the level at which they would very much wish to remove their hand from the water. However, they simultaneously reported by automatic key pressing (an equivalent to automatic writing) that on average they were experiencing a pain level of 8, in contrast to the level of 2 they overtly reported. This was slightly below the mean of normal waking pain they reported without analgesic suggestions. Perhaps the lesser reported pain was due, in part, to the general relaxation of hypnosis, as well as to the lack of feedback associated with felt pain such as grimacing, squirming, etc. Why some highly responsive subjects, capable of reducing pain under hypnosis, do not yield the hidden observer reports remains to be explained. For those who do re-

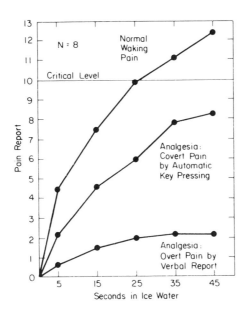

FIGURE 2.1. Pain report of normal waking pain, overt pain, and covert pain with hypnotic analgesia. Results for the 8 most successful subjects of 20 subjects selected for high hypnotizability. From E. R. Hilgard & J. R. Hilgard (1983, p. 172). Copyright 1983 by William Kaufmann. Reprinted by permission.

port differences of the type shown in Figure 2.1, it is appropriate to consider them as evidence of a split in consciousness between the overt (conscious) level and the covert (subconscious) level, and hence as evidence of dissociative processes.

Although this kind of dissociation manifests itself dramatically in experiments on pain, it is by no means limited to pain. Informally, it has been known for a long time that some cognitive system within the hypnotized person processes information beyond that available to him or her that usually painful stimulation does not hurt. William James devoted several pages in his book *Principles of Psychology* to an account of gaps in consciousness. He presented evidence that the mind is active even when it does not seem to be (James, 1890, pp. 201–213). James recorded his own experiment:

> In a perfectly healthy young man who can write with a planchette [a device like a pointer on a Ouija board], I lately found the hand to be entirely anesthetic during the writing act. I could prick it severely without the sub-

ject knowing the fact. The writing on the planchette, however, accused me in strong terms of hurting the hand. (p. 208)

We have been able to demonstrate in our own laboratory that hypnotic blindness and deafness, as well as positive hallucinations can all be penetrated by automatic responses. In other words, the concealed cognitive processing (the "hidden observer") enabled subjects who were experiencing distorted reality because of hypnosis to report the actual physical situation: that is, the numbers not seen, the sentences not heard, and the hallucination of a playful dog, with nothing resembling a dog present.

NEODISSOCIATION THEORY

Three assumptions have been proposed in taking the steps toward elaborating a neodissociation theory that goes beyond the mere fact that dissociations occur. The first assumption is that subordinate cognitive systems exist, each of which has some degree of unity, persistence, and autonomy of function. These systems interact, but occasionally, under special circumstances, may become somewhat isolated from each other. The concept of a totally unified consciousness is an attractive one, but does not hold up under examination. Too many shifts occur in the ordinary course of a day, such as that between waking and dreaming. Furthermore, there are lapses of consciousness in the control of well-learned habits (e.g., driving a car, playing a musical instrument, or reciting the alphabet). Such activities, having been overlearned in the past, can proceed with a minimum of conscious control once the activity is underway.

The second assumption is that some sort of hierarchical control exists that manages the interaction or competition between and among these structures. If no selection process took place, there would be a veritable deluge of thoughts and actions trying to go on at once.

A third assumption is that there must be some sort of overarching monitoring and controlling structure. In the absence of such an assumption, one would have to conclude that the hierarchy is determined by the relative strength of each of the structures (as in the pecking orders of barnyard fowl). I have rejected this proposition because of what we know about human decision making and how humans plan actions to achieve distant goals.

On the basis of the assumptions mentioned above, the theory can be displayed in diagrammatic form (Figure 2.2). This highly generalized diagram is designed to convey the idea of multiple cognitive processing systems or structures (of which only three of the many possible ones are shown). They are arranged in hierarchical order, as suggested by their positions on

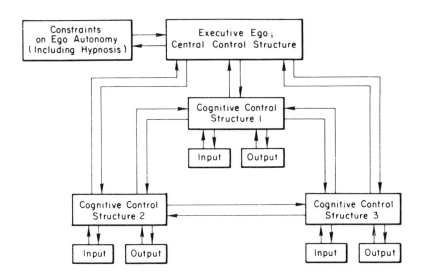

FIGURE 2.2. A hierarchical ordering of subordinate cognitive control structures. Hierarchical positions are subject to change under control of the executive ego. From E. R. Hilgard (1973b, p. 405). Copyright 1973 by the American Psychological Association. Reprinted by permission.

the chart, with the multiple feedback relations between them displayed, but each is also shown to be independent with its own appropriate inputs and outputs. At the top is an "executive ego" or "central control structure," which plans, monitors, and manages functions involving the whole person, so that he or she thinks and acts appropriately.

We may now turn to a fuller characterization of the individual cognitive structures, their hierarchical arrangement, and the role of the central control structure or executive ego.

The Existence of Separate Cognitive Structures

The expression "cognitive structure" was given currency by Tolman (1932) and taken over by Lewin (1935), who acknowledged his debt to Tolman. A related concept, called "schema," was used by Bartlett (1932). Meichenbaum and Gilmore (1984), in their discussion of cognitive structures, found at least nine different terms in the literature used to express the same idea. From a different starting point, Chomsky (1957) implied that innate cognitive structures exist in the brain that permit children to learn language. Hence, when I include cognitive structures in my neodissociation theory, I am not presenting something that familiar theories do not.

The Concept of Hierarchy

The concept of hierarchy has been added to my theory to indicate that one structure can be dominant at a given time, and then succeeded by the activation of another. Consider the bilingual person who has decided to speak in his or her most familiar language, perhaps in reply to a question phrased in that language. At that point, the appropriate vocabulary and grammatical forms of that language become dominant and the other language is inhibited, although still available in latent form.

One of Clark Hull's central concepts was that a habit-family hierarchy exists, which includes a number of habits (each of which may be thought of as a small substructure). More specifically, if the habit highest in the hierarchy cannot function when an organism is seeking to achieve its goals in a given situation, the one next below in the hierarchy is activated (Hull, 1934).

The Presence of an Executive Ego

The idea that the executive ego is a central control structure is important but troublesome. The extreme possibilities are that there is a powerful central control, equivalent to the old idea of a strong will, or that none really exists. If one takes the view that this central control does not exist, one would have to conclude that the control of a final common path is determined by a competition among the parts. In other words, the structure that is strongest at any given moment will win control over those that are weaker. For many years, psychologists evaded the problem of a planning self, so that, in essence, the second of these alternatives was implicitly accepted. If present choices are to be made on the basis of a person's past learned habits instead of willing them, what he or she does must be determined by some sort of compromise depending upon the relative strength of contributions from various learned habits.

The importance of planning was brought to psychologists' attention in a book titled *Plans and the Structure of Behavior* (Miller, Galanter, & Pribram, 1960). Miller et al. proposed the idea that a planner must be inferred given how the activity of planning works. Even such a simple matter as making an appointment for a luncheon is written down or otherwise remembered and acted upon at a later date. The planning person controls his or her behavior so that the plan is fulfilled quite effectively; he or she rejects other invitations and sets aside competing interests in order to give priority to the plan adopted during the prior week. Because appointments of this kind are kept over 90% of the time, the planning function must be taken seriously. It appears to control the hierarchical determinants of specific behavior far in advance. The illustration is trivial, but the implications for the idea of a central control mechanism are not.

Support for an executive function has come from an unlikely source: the computer. Heuristic computer programs commonly have an executive program that monitors the computer's attempt to solve problems (e.g., Newell & Simon, 1972). If a program sets out in one direction and goes on too long without reaching a solution, the executive program calls a halt to it, and a new direction of attack on the problem is entered upon. This close analogy to what a thinker does makes the idea of an executive ego a plausible one (Neisser, 1967).

THE ROLE OF HYPNSOSIS
IN NEODISSOCIATION THEORY

Neodissociation theory is intended to be more general than a theory of hypnosis, but has its origin within hypnosis experimentation. The relevance of hypnosis to this theory becomes apparent when attention is paid to both the prominence of dissociations within hypnosis and to the control hypnosis exerts over cognitive control systems.

That hypnosis impacts upon the hierarchical structure is shown in Figure 2.2 (see the cell labeled "Constraints on Ego Autonomy"). Hypnosis enters the picture because effective suggestions from the hypnotist take much of the subject's normal control away from him or her. More specifically, the hypnotist may influence the executive functions themselves and change the hierarchical arrangements of the substructures. This is what takes place when, in the hypnotic context, motor controls are altered, perception and memory are distorted, and hallucinations are perceived as external reality.

A fuller exposition of the interrelationships that are shown in a general way in Figure 2.2 would provide the essence of the neodissociation theory. Regretfully, I must leave the theory in this incomplete form, so that it is more of a promised than a finished theory. The line of experimental investigation that it has supported may, in the hands of others, provide more nuanced versions of the theory.

APPEARANCE OF THE HIDDEN OBSERVER
IN HYPNOTIC ANALGESIA

As mentioned before, the early experimental evidence on the hidden observer effect was based primarily on experiments dealing with the reduction of pain in hypnosis. More specifically, these experiments used the so-called "cold-pressor" test (e.g., Hilgard, 1973b, 1974; Hilgard, Morgan, & Macdonald, 1975). Later experiments, using the real-simulator design, validated the earlier findings (E. R. Hilgard, J. R. Hilgard, Macdonald, Morgan, & Johnson, 1978). The real-simulator design is a type of control experiment in which the "reals" are highly responsive persons who react as usual to the suggestions of the hypnotist. The "simulators" are persons known to be unresponsive to hypnotic procedures from previous attempts to hypnotize them. When this design is followed, however, they are asked to respond voluntarily as they believe a truly hypnotizable person would respond. In that way the experimenter will find out how much his or her suggestions have placed a demand upon the truly hypnotized to comply in certain ways to his suggestions. This is a control condition for experimental purposes and does not imply that hypnotic responsiveness is merely voluntary compliance. In fact, the simulators may overreact to suggestions under these circumstances (Orne, 1979).

Additional experiments were done with pain involving applying a tourniquet to the upper arm, and then putting it through a series of exercises. Careful earlier experiments by Smith, Egbert, Markowitz, Mosteller, and Beecher (1966) had shown that this was the best method for simulating surgical pain in the laboratory, proven by the fact that it showed a dose sensitivity reaction to morphine. Knox, Morgan, and Hilgard (1974) published an important article on the hidden observer effect. The results they found resembled those found with the cold-pressor experiment, in that the hidden observer responses that followed hypnotic analgesia closely paralleled the responses that resulted when pain occurred in a nonhypnotic condition.

Unlike the experiments on automatic writing, these somewhat more dramatic experiments invited much attention, whether favorable or unfavorable. The most favorable initial attention came from Donald Hebb, who viewed his own theory of cell assemblies as a physiological basis for cognitive structures. In a talk before the Canadian Psychological Association in 1974, he noted a possible correlation between his own proposals and the existence of the hidden observer as I described it (Hebb, 1975). He reiterated his support in an article in *Psychology Today* entitled "Hilgard's Discovery Brings Hypnosis Closer to Everyday Experience" (Hebb, 1982).

At the other extreme were those who totally rejected the theory (Spanos & Hewitt, 1980; Spanos, 1983; Council, 1993). Their main point of contention was that the findings might have resulted from the demand characteristics in the instructions given to the subjects. As we shall see, these objections were adequately answered by other experimenters.

THE HIDDEN OBSERVER'S FREQUENCY AND ITS CORRELATES

Within our laboratory, we had found the phenomenon of the hidden observer only among a small fraction of our very highly responsive hypnotic subjects. In an early study of ice water pain (the cold-pressor response) with 20 highly hypnotizable subjects, all of whom could achieve substantial pain reduction through hypnotically suggested analgesia, clear evidence of covert pain revealed through the hidden observer procedures was significant for the group as a whole. But the mean findings depended very much on the responses of 8 subjects among the 20, who gave the most substantial evidence of having covert pain beyond the pain reported in the usual way following hypnotically suggested analgesia (see Figure 2.1; Hilgard et al., 1975). In another study performed later (although published earlier), the pain known as ischemic pain was produced by applying a tourniquet to the upper arm, and following that with exercise of the occluded hand (Knox et al., 1974). In this study, eight subjects were preselected for exhibiting the hidden observer phenomenon in contexts other than analgesia, so that, as expected, all showed the hidden observer effect in this study. In a later study involving hypnotically suggested hearing loss, only 4 of 16 highly responsive subjects, all of whom showed substantial hearing loss following hypnotic suggestion, gave clear evidence of covert hearing (Crawford, Macdonald, & Hilgard, 1979). The limited number of subjects from whom a hidden observer can be elicited restricts the number of generalizations that can be made regarding this phenomenon. It must be recalled that the highly responsive subjects used in these experiments already constituted a limited sample of the general population of student subjects, so that the 1 in 4 subjects in the deafness experiment who displayed the hidden observer effect represented something less than 5% of a general student sample. Replicating the hidden observer finding in their Montreal laboratory for hypnotically produced analgesia, Laurence and Perry (1981) found hidden observers in only 39% of their highly responsive subjects.

A group in the same laboratory conducted additional experiments that contributed an important finding about who among highly responsive subjects report and do not report hidden observers (Nogrady, McConkey, Laurence, & Perry, 1983). Aware of attacks by others who regarded the hidden observer as a possible laboratory creation (Spanos & Hewitt, 1980), Nogrady et al. (1983) were meticulous in controlling for "demand characteristics" that might produce the phenomena through pressure of compliance. By making use of the "real-simulator" design of Orne (1979), who discovered that if compliance cues are prominent those simulating hypnosis will respond to them, they were able to show that these cues were not operative. To avoid any experimenter bias in interpreting what the subject experienced, one of the experimenters (McConkey, who had done none of the hypnotizing) conducted a postsession interview. He was unaware of which of the subjects were highly hypnotizable and which were merely acting "as if" highly hypnotizable, since they were selected for not being hypnotically responsive. He made use of the Experiential Analysis Technique of Sheehan, McConkey, and Cross (1978), which he had helped develop. The technique consisted (and consists) of showing a subject, some time after a session, a videotape of all that took place—what was done and what was said by both the hypnotist and the subject. At predetermined points, the videotape was stopped, and the subjects were encouraged to comment on the observed material that they found meaningful. They could also request that the tape be stopped at other points when they wished to comment. McConkey occasionally asked specific questions. For example, with regard to the hidden observer experience, he asked, "Is this an experience you had following the instructions, or is it one you were having throughout the session?" Another member of the investigative team, unfamiliar with the subjects' hypnotizability or with the ratings made by the interviewer, rated aspects of the subjects' experience bearing on dissociation and the hidden observer phenomena. This carefully designed experiment confirmed our results (Hilgard et al., 1978) and those of Laurence and Perry (1981) by finding a hidden observer response in 5 of 12 highly hypnotizable subjects, in none of 10 high–medium subjects, and in none of 10 low hypnotizables simulating hypnosis.

The study by Laurence and Perry (1981), and confirmed by Nogrady et al. (1983), in addition to showing the validity of the findings, threw some light on the problem of why some "highs" showed hidden observers and others did not. In the course of hypnotic testing, these investigators included age regression, in which the subjects were to experience themselves as children again of 5 years of age. Age regression may take one of two different forms. In one form, the subject becomes completely absorbed in being a child again, in a manner convincing to him or her and to an observer present. Sometimes this is reported in statements, such as the following: "I felt sorry for that child [the person as a child] because I was lost and frightened lest my mother would not find me, but I knew all along that she would return soon." The experience can be considered as one of duality—the subject is at once a child and an adult. In the Montreal experiments, regression was recorded before an opportunity existed to test for a hidden observer. It turned out, however, that the presence or absence of the duality experience was almost perfectly correlated with the subsequent experience of the hidden observer effect.

What would be the expected relationship? Would duality be predictive of a hidden observer or the absence of one? Let us take the position that people tend to conform to expectations. When someone suggests that a subject become a child of 5 again, clearly no demand has been made that an adult observer appear. Hence, duality would not be the expected result. Further, if the hidden observer is a result of responses by the most compliant subjects, one would expect the hidden observer phenomenon to occur with those who do not undergo the duality experience—that is, with those who comply strictly with the wording of the suggested age regression. If, on the other hand, the hidden observer effect is an aspect of genuinely dissociated experiences, then the duality in age regression that occurs can be taken as a mark of spontaneous dissociation and as a sign that a hidden observer may be more readily manifested. This was, in fact, what was found: Those who had the duality experience also manifested the hidden observer.

Care is needed when advancing interpretations, however plausible, when sufficient experimentation is lacking. The possibility that some sort of amnesic process is involved in these less severe dissociations, as it often is in reported cases of multiple personality, has led to a search for such amnesic correlates. In a subsequent paper, Perry (1983) reported new data showing that amnesia was more profound in highly hypnotizable subjects with hidden observers than in those not demonstrating hidden observers. Why, one might ask, should there be a greater incidence of amnesia among "highs" with hidden observers? A possible conjecture is that they more readily store marginal experiences behind a cloak of amnesia, which are ready to be recovered when amnesia is reversed. Put differently, those with less access to amnesia (i.e., those without a hidden observer) fail to record and store in memory events not in focus. Because events are complex, supplementary experiments are needed to clarify the kinds of individual differences involved in amnesia and the hidden observer.

FURTHER SUPPORT FOR AND ELABORATION OF NEODISSOCIATION THEORY

The unfinished theory represented in Figure 2.2 was further elaborated by Kihlstrom (1984) in an article entitled "Conscious, Subconscious, Unconscious: A Cognitive Approach." Here, he tied the dissociation theory closely to modern cognitive psychology by including the interpretations of models of memory and the distinctions between procedural and declarative knowledge. In his elaboration of neodissociation theory, he strongly supported it, and indicated regret that many cognitive theorists had failed to take the implications of dissociation into account (see Bowers & Meichenbaum, 1984, for other articles on cognitive conceptions of unconscious processes).

THE INTERACTION BETWEEN EXECUTIVE AND MONITORING FUNCTIONS

It is artificial to sharply separate executive from monitoring functions since all initiated action is monitored. When the relationships between executive and monitor functions are harmonious, their interplay seems entirely natural and sensible, as in any "trial-and-error" setting.

Hence, if one course of action does not work, another may be tried. Whether the second course works better is determined by the monitoring function; the executive function then acts on this information. If a harmonious relationship always existed, little more than academic interest would be served by separating the two functions. Often, however, the two functions are not well balanced, which is demonstrated particularly well in hypnosis. In some cases outside of hypnosis, an alert monitoring function will be helpless in modifying executive action through feedback. In obsessive compulsive behavior, for example, when executive control is weak, the monitoring function may be well aware of the negative behavior and critical of it, yet unable to alter it by way of the information available. On other occasions, the monitor in its role as critical may be more persuasive and thereby modify executive functioning. If, for example, a person is tempted to engage in antisocial behavior, the monitor may throw its weight against yielding and be successful. Internal conflicts of this sort are familiar enough. Hence, it is appropriate to describe some of them as conflicts between the monitoring and executive functions.

These familiar illustrations are intended to show that executive control and monitoring are part of a general system that can be recognized in our ordinary lives. There are always interrelations between more immediate and more long-range goals, and consequently the need for feedback occurs continuously. When specific activities are initiated by the central control mechanisms, the activated subsystem achieves some degree of independence from them, at least the conscious representations of these systems appear to retreat as the person becomes absorbed in what he or she is doing. This calls for further discussion.

SUBSYSTEMS OF ACTIVITY: LATENT AND ACTUATED

A person's life is made up of an almost infinite number of activities, from trivial responses to stimuli (e.g., brushing a fly off one's face), to those consuming more time but still with definable beginnings and endings (e.g., writing a letter, playing a game of golf, listening to a symphony), to activities that endure over many years and interact in a complex fashion with each other (e.g., raising a family, doing housework, saving for retirement).

Psychologists have found it difficult to decide on the best level of analysis to make psychology a coherent science, and the search for a satisfactory unit of behavior or experience to be most widely applicable still goes on. There is widespread agreement that the sensation and the reflex are too reductive as units to be focused upon. The hope that a unit of information, referred to as a "bit," might serve proved disappointing as well, since the "bit" also proved to be too reductive. Specifically, "chunks" of information had to be added to it in order to describe how information is actually handled (Miller, 1956). The TOTE unit (Test–Operate–Text–Exit) was later proposed as a more meaningful unit than the reflex, since it allowed for information concepts, as implied by the repeated "testing" within the unit of behavior (Miller et al., 1960). Examining habits and cognitive structures is another example of an attempt to "package" experience and behavior to permit the consideration of one topic at a time in the midst of complexity.

For the purposes of the present discussion, the identifiable activities that a person can be engaged in are referred to as *subsystems* to distinguish them from the larger control and monitoring functions that regulate them. These subsystems are the visible or reportable behaviors that occur when a person is engaged in any definable activity—reading a book, operating a machine, scratching his or her head, solving a problem.

Because these subsystems are so numerous, yet with only a few visibly going on at any time, it is possible to distinguish between those that are active and those that are inactive. Those that are not operative, but available, are referred to as *latent*, whereas those that are active in the present are described as *actuated*. A latent subsystem can become actuated in many ways, such as as a consequence of the impact of the physical or social environment, by bodily changes that influence organic motivational systems, or by self-initiation, which occurs through the cognitive activities of reflection and planning.

Hypnotic suggestion is one of the ways of actuating a specific set of subsystems. It is particularly useful because it permits the manipulation of the hierarchies according to which subsystems are controlled. The subsystems actuated in hypnosis—the behaviors and experiences represented by the usual hypnotic "items" or "tests" of ideomotor action, hallucinations, age regression, amnesia, and the rest—are sufficiently limited to be studied repeatedly and in detail, thereby providing data that can serve as a basis for theoretical interpretation. Hypnotic fantasies may be extensive, but such fantasies are typically under the control of and limited to the hypnotic period. Hence, they serve to illuminate the roles of simultaneous cognitive activities.

THE ACTUATED SUBSYSTEM IN RELATION TO CENTRAL CONTROLS

Accepting the idea of central controls, in the form of executive and monitoring functions, does not mean that one has to view all behavior and experience as under their dominion. We need not return to a new form of the older self-psychology that always found a self in every act of introspection. What happens is that once an activity is under way it becomes relatively self-sustaining. Woodworth (1918) recognized this in his principle that any activity once aroused may generate its own "drive." Similarly, Allport (1937) indicated that motives may lose connection with their origins and become "functionally autonomous" in sustaining behavior.

It is readily observed that a person absorbed in a skilled task may have little consciousness of him- or herself. The task and its completion are indirectly self-monitored once the activity has been initiated. The subsystem's own monitoring and control system operates through habit as mediated by feedback; these activity-related controls permit the high degree of autonomy with which the skilled act is performed. Of course the individual absorbed in his or her work may now and then step back to admire it, at which time the monitoring function is active both as observer and as critic. Observation, as such, ties the monitor to perceptual operations; criticizing the work according to standards of value ties the monitor to aesthetic appreciation, rationality, and conceptions of right and wrong. Hence, the monitor, as part of the central control system, is a member of the family of controls that includes the conscience and the superego. The conceptual problem of distinguishing a general monitoring function from a specific one arises because, as noted, the activated subsystem has its own internal executive monitoring function. The typist, for example, must attend to the copy and observe the proprioceptive feedback from the keys as well as occasional visual feedback from the typed material. These controls belong to the typing subsystem itself and are a result of the interplay between the typist and the typewriter. The superordinate control systems in which the behavior of typing from copy is imbedded include such larger contexts as the typist's self-image and his or her interactions with the superior who assigned the work and will judge the end product. If the control and monitoring functions are difficult to understand in the familiar experiences of daily life, it is not surprising that something as unfamiliar as hypnosis might produce insurmountable difficulties. Curiously, the controls within hypnosis, as studied in the laboratory, are exhibited in such dramatic form as to make the task easier rather than more difficult.

CONCLUDING REMARKS

The roles of central control processes, here characterized as executive and monitoring functions, recently have been increasingly recognized by both experimental and social psychologists. After the many years it suffered because of the narrow perspective of behaviorism, the idea of consciousness has finally been accepted, although somewhat haltingly. It is still somewhat more acceptable to talk about information processing and decision making, using mathematical formulations of the transitions taking place, than to examine the internal characteristics of the central agencies that are inferred. However, changes in conceptualization are emerging in many areas, including attention, memory, psycholinguistics, problem solving, and creativity and are the result of influences derived from the wider culture and from the science of psychology itself.

An account of hypnotic phenomena must necessarily involve itself with these issues because of the dramatic alterations in physical and mental functions that take place in the hypnotic interaction and the equally dramatic restoration of normality when hypnosis is terminated. The concept of dissociation necessarily comes into play considering how control processes operate in normal behavior and how they differ within hypnosis. The hidden observer phenomena give evidence that more usual intellectual activity may be occurring with altered cognition at the overt level.

The fractionation of the monitoring function can be observed in the three stages of the hidden observer phenomena as they occur: (1) the preserved normal intellectual functioning which is initially concealed beneath an amnesia-like barrier but may later be recovered; (2) a distorted, relatively uncritical function—a typical function of hypnotic suggestion that usually accepts distorted reality as though it were physical reality; and (3) the control processes, as affected by hypnosis, whereby the covert material is recovered and used as evidence for a hidden observer. The executive and monitoring functions, whether in the usual normal condition, or as modified within hypnotic practices, imply that the intellectual processes involved are conscious or can be made conscious.

REFERENCES

Allport, G. W. (1937). *Personality: A psychological interpretation.* New York: Holt.

Bartlett, F. C. (1932). *Remembering.* Cambridge: Cambridge University Press.

Bowers, K. S., & Meichenbaum, D. (Eds.). (1984). *The unconscious reconsidered.* New York: John Wiley.

Chomsky, N. (1957). *Syntatic structures.* The Hague: Mouton.

Council, J. R. (1993). Context effects in personality research. *Current Directions in Psychological Science, 2,* 31–34.

Crawford, H. J., Macdonald, H., & Hilgard, E. R. (1979). Hypnotic deafness: A psychophysical study of responses to tone intensity as modified by hypnosis. *American Journal of Psychology, 92,* 193–214.

Hebb, D. O (1975). Science and the world of imagination. *Canadian Psychological Review, 16,* 4–11.

Hebb, D. O. (1982, May). Hilgard's discovery brings hypnosis closer to everyday experience. *Psychology Today,* pp. 52–54.

Hilgard, E. R. (1965). *Hypnotic susceptibility.* New York: Harcourt, Brace & World.

Hilgard, E. R. (1973a). Dissociation revisited. In M. Henle, J. Jaynes, & J. Sullivan (Eds.), *Historical conceptions of psychology* (pp. 205–219). New York: Springer.

Hilgard, E. R. (1973b). A neodissociation interpretation of pain reduction in hypnosis. *Psychological Review, 80*, 396–411.

Hilgard, E. R. (1974). Toward a neo-dissociation theory: Multiple cognitive controls in human functioning. *Perspectives in Biology and Medicine, 17*, 301–316.

Hilgard, E. R. (1991). A neodissociation interpretation of hypnosis. In S. J. Lynn & J. W. Rhue (Eds.), *Theories of hypnosis: Current models and perspectives* (pp. 83–104). New York: Guilford Press.

Hilgard, E. R. (1992). Dissociation and theories of hypnosis. In E. Fromm & M. R. Nash (Eds.), *Contemporary hypnosis research* (pp. 69–101). New York: Guilford Press.

Hilgard, E. R., & Hilgard, J. R. (1983). *Hypnosis in the relief of pain* (2nd ed.). Los Altos, CA: William Kaufmann.

Hilgard, E. R., Hilgard, J. R., Macdonald, H., Morgan, A. H., & Johnson, L. S. (1978). Covert pain in hypnotic analgesia: Its reality as tested by the real-simulator design. *Journal of Abnormal Psychology, 87*, 239–246.

Hilgard, E. R., Morgan, A. H., & Macdonald, H. (1975). Pain and dissociation in the cold pressor test: A study of hypnotic analgesia with "hidden reports" through automatic key-pressing and automatic talking. *Journal of Abnormal Psychology, 84*, 280–289.

Hull, C. L. (1934). The concept of habit-family hierarchy and maze learning. *Psychological Review, 41*, 33–54, 134–152.

James, W. (1890). *Principles of psychology* (2 vols.). New York: Henry Holt.

Kihlstrom, J. F. (1984). Conscious, subconscious, unconscious: A cognitive perspective. In K. S. Bowers & D. Meichenbaum (Eds.), *The unconscious reconsidered* (pp. 149–211). New York: John Wiley.

Knox, V. J., Crutchfield, L., & Hilgard, E. R. (1975). The nature of task interference in hypnotic dissociation. An investigation of hypnotic behavior. *International Journal of Clinical and Experimental Hypnosis, 23*, 305–323.

Knox, V. J., Morgan, A. H., & Hilgard, E. R. (1974). Pain and suffering in ischemia: The paradox of hypnotically suggested anesthesia as contradicted by reports from the "hidden observer." *Archives of General Psychiatry, 39*, 1201–1214.

Laurence, J.-R., & Perry, C. (1981). The "hidden observer" phenomenon in hypnosis: Some additional findings. *Journal of Abnormal Psychology, 90*, 334–344.

Lewin, K. (1935). *A dynamic theory of personality.* New York: McGraw-Hill.

Meichenbaum, D., & Gilmore, J. B. (1984). The nature of unconscious processes: A cognitive-behavioral perspective. In K. S. Bowers & D. Meichenbaum (Eds.), *The unconscious reconsidered* (pp. 273–298). New York: John Wiley.

Miller, G. A. (1956). The magical number seven plus or minus two: Some limits on our capacity for processing information. *Psychological Review, 63*, 81–97.

Miller, G. A., Galanter, E., & Pribram, K. H. (1960). *Plans and the structure of behavior.* New York: Henry Holt.

Neisser, U. (1967). *Cognitive psychology.* New York: Appleton-Century-Crofts.

Newell, A., & Simon, H. A. (1972). *Human problem solving.* Englewood Cliffs, NJ: Prentice-Hall.

Nogrady, H., McConkey, K. M., Laurence, J.-R., & Perry, C. (1983). Dissociation, duality, and demand characteristics in hypnosis. *Journal of Abnormal Psychology, 92*, 223–35.

Orne, M. T. (1979). On the simulating subject as a quasi-control group in hypnosis research: What, why, and how. In E. Fromm & R. E. Shor (Eds.), *Hypnosis: Developments in research and new perspectives* (2nd ed., pp. 519–566). New York: Aldine.

Perry, C. (1983). *Dissociative phenomena and hypnosis.* Address presented at the Annual Convention of the American Psychology Association, Anaheim, CA.

Rosenberg, M. J. (1959). A disconfirmation of the descriptions of hypnosis as a dissociative state. *International Journal of Clinical and Experimental Hypnosis, 7*, 187–204.

Sheehan, P. W., McConkey, J. M., & Cross, D. (1978). Experimental analysis of hypnosis: Some new observations on hypnotic phenomena. *Journal of Abnormal Psychology, 87*, 570–573.

Smith, G. M., Egbert, L. D., Markowitz, P. A., Mosteller, F., & Beecher, H. K. (1966). An experimental pain method sensitive to morphine in man: The submaximum effort tourniquet technique. *Journal of Pharmacological and Experimental Therapeutics, 154*, 324–332.

Spanos, N. P. (1983). The hidden observer as an experimental creation. *Journal of Personality and Social Psychology, 44*, 170–176.

Spanos, N. P., & Hewitt, E. C. (1980). The hidden observer in hypnotic analgesia: Discovery or experimental creation? *Journal of Personality and Social Psychology, 39*, 1201–1214.

Stevenson, J. (1976). The effect of posthypnotic dissociation on the performance of interfering tasks. *Journal of Abnormal Psychology, 85*, 398–407.

Tolman, E. C. (1932). *Purposive behavior in animals and men.* New York: Appleton-Century-Crofts.

White, R. W., & Shevach, B. J. (1942). Hypnosis and the concept of dissociation. *Journal of Abnormal and Social Psychology, 7*, 309–328.

Woodworth, R. S. (1918). *Dynamic psychology.* New York: Columbia University Press.

3

A Frontal Assault
on Dissociated Control

Erik Z. Woody
Kenneth S. Bowers

In English literature, the most famous instance of dissociation is surely *The Strange Case of Dr. Jekyll and Mr. Hyde* (Stevenson, 1886/1967). The circumstances that surrounded the writing of this work are quite interesting. No stranger to dissociation himself, Stevenson described the process that led to some of his best writing as one in which the characters took on an independent life of their own and seemed to move about and speak for themselves, completely unaided. In addition, he was sometimes haunted by serial dreams in which he nightly played out a dreadful second life that seemed every bit as real as his daytime one. Indeed, the story of Jekyll and Hyde originated as a nightmare. At the point in the story at which Jekyll is first transformed into Hyde, Stevenson began screaming so loudly that his wife woke him up, whereupon he scolded her, saying that he had been dreaming "a fine bogey tale" (Pope-Hennessey, 1974).

He wrote down the story feverishly in the next 3 days, and then exultantly read it aloud to his wife. She, it turns out, was very unimpressed, and "finally blurted out that Louis had missed the point of his own story, and that it was an allegory that he should have written, and not a straight piece of sensationalism" (Pope-Hennessey, 1974, p. 180). After a furious argument, Stevenson threw the 40,000-word manuscript into the fire. Then he started over from the beginning, completely refashioning the story, particularly with regard to its central theme.

What had been a straightforward horror tale, in which a drug induces a pathology that produces a new and evil, second self, turned in the new version into something quite different. Stevenson's revised theme emerges clearly in the following statement from the chastened Jekyll: "Man is not truly one, but truly two. . . . I hazard the guess that man will be ultimately known for a mere polity of multifarious, incongruous and independent denizens" (Stevenson, 1886/1967, p. 68). In other words, the action of the drug in the story is simply to bring to light divisions that were *already* within: The action tendencies elicited in Hyde, horrific as they are to Jekyll, always lay dormant within Jekyll. The drug, rather than creating a second personality, weakens the integrative mechanisms by which the gaping cracks in a personality are papered over and normally hidden from view.

Accordingly, in the present chapter we contrast two psychological views of dissociation:

1. One view of dissociation starts with the assumption that mental processes normally represent some kind of unity. However, this unity may be uncharacteristically disrupted by an unusual and special mechanism (dissociation), in which mental processes become divided. (This might be dubbed the "bogey tale" view.)
2. The second view of dissociation begins with the assumption that some multiplicity of mental process is typical and normal, in the sense of coexisting levels of control that are usually well-coordinated by higher conscious functioning. Circumstances in which dissociation becomes evident, therefore, are ones in which this higher functioning is weakened, laying bare some of the underlying "multifarious" architecture of the mind. (This is, properly, the Stevensonian view.)

Our specific task will be to apply these conceptions of dissociation to an understanding of hypnosis. Hypnosis, for our present purposes, serves as a very useful arena in which dissociative processes are commonly assumed to be evident.

AMNESTIC BARRIERS AND PARALLEL PROCESSORS

The "bogey tale" view of dissociation has a long history in psychology. Interestingly, it originated in the same era as Stevenson's work, with Janet (1901, 1907/1965). For Janet, dissociation—the splitting off of various mental contents from consciousness—was something that occurred under stress, particularly to individuals who were congenitally predisposed to dissociate. The implication was that there was some particular kind of mental deficit or biological weak-mindedness in people disposed to dissociation.

Janet's biologizing has fallen out of favor. However, a strictly psychological view of dissociation is difficult to differentiate from the concept of repression. Indeed, Erdelyi (1985, 1990) has argued that there is no difference—in both cases, ideas or information have an unconscious status. However, historically, at least, repression has always implied that information was *motivated* into an unconscious status, whereas this was not necessarily the case for dissociation. Moreover, E. R. Hilgard's neodissociation theory (1977), which was partially inspired by Janet's work, elaborated on the distinction between dissociation and repression by arguing that the repressed unconscious was dominated by primary-process thinking that made it unrealistic and illogical in nature. In contrast, he considered dissociation to pertain to a system of ideas that were disconnected from consciousness by an "amnestic barrier," but which maintained realistic, logical relations amongst themselves.

This amnestic-barrier conception of dissociation also has the implication that a "split" in consciousness can exist, such that two parallel streams of consciousness can coexist. The classic demonstration of this supposed splitting of consciousness in the sphere of hypnosis is E. R. Hilgard's (1973, 1977) "hidden observer" phenomena, in which a part of a person (the hidden observer) knows about the presence of pain that the other, conscious part of him or her knows nothing about. On a larger scale, this consciousness-splitting function of dissociation has long been invoked as the basis for multiple personality disorder (MPD). Specifically, dissociation is allegedly a likely defense mechanism against child abuse: the child who cannot escape physically from the abuse escapes psychologically, by imagining him- or herself elsewhere, perhaps as another person, while his or her body remains behind to receive the abuse unfeelingly. This conceptualization of dissociation as a defense mechanism clearly seems to presuppose that an amnestic barrier is central to its functioning (although here again the differentiation of dissociation from repression seems to become rather problematic).

The implication typically is that when one of the parallel streams is conscious the other is not. However, this is not always the case. For example, a secondary "personality" is often nonamnestic for a primary personality (though the reverse is not true), and, likewise, the hidden observer remains in touch with the hypnotized person (though, again, not the reverse).

The amnestic-barrier conception of dissociation has played an often tacit, but nevertheless pervasive role in the neodissociation conception of hypnotic responding. For example, it has commonly been assumed that the experiences of involuntariness and effortlessness that virtually define hypnotic responding are *entirely* illusory; that is, the subject enacting a hypnotic suggestion is thought to exert considerable effort and self-mediated control, which is, however, hidden from consciousness (e.g., Bowers & Brenneman, 1981).

A vigorous expression of this view appears in a very recent review essay on hypnosis by Kihlstrom (1992). He quotes approvingly a memorable statement by Shor (1979):

Although the hypnotic subject may look as if he is no longer in control of his own volitional activities—for example, he may behave as if he is unable to bend his hypnotically stiffened elbow—that is only because at some deeper level than is operative within the bounds of consciousness, he is actively, deliberately, voluntarily keeping his elbow stiff while simultaneously orchestrating for himself the illusion that he is really trying his best to bend it. (p. 124)

Kihlstrom (1992) himself then goes on to explain in the language of neo-dissociation theory that

when the cognitive control system that executes the response to a hypnotic suggestion is dissociated from conscious awareness, S will experience that response as automatic and nonvolitional . . . however, that experience is illusory—obviously, there is *some* executive control involved in hypnotic responding, even if the hypnotized S does not experience it as such. (p. 308)

Clearly the point expressed above is that hypnotic behavior is controlled and executed like any nonhypnotic behavior; however, the subject's *experience* of why the act occurred is incomplete and incorrect. Kihlstrom does not explicitly mention any kind of amnesia-like barrier behind which the cognitive control system hides. However, unless we presume such a mechanism, this explanation of the nature of hypnosis is virtually indistinguishable from the misattributional explanation of the social-psychological theorists (Spanos, 1986; Lynn, Rhue, & Weekes, 1990) that he is trying to argue against.

In any case, defining the essence of hypnosis in terms of such amnesia-like barriers and consequent distortions of experience is problematic. To see why, it is useful to distinguish between strong and weak senses of the notion of amnestic barrier.

In the strong sense of amnestic barrier, hypnotic performances may be viewed as requiring *spontaneous amnesia*, in which some information that should normally be available to consciousness is lost. For example, the fact that a subject cannot remember his or her *deliberate* failure to bend his or her arm may be seen as a mild instance of spontaneous amnesia for the events occurring during a hypnotic session. However, despite the strong association of hypnosis with spontaneous amnesia historically and in the popular imagination, such spontaneous amnesia is quite rare (E. R. Hilgard & Cooper, 1965); hence, we have the unappealing prospect of attempting to explain routine hypnotic behaviors in terms of a very rare one. More telling is the fact that such unsuggested amnesias would need to be arbitrarily selective. To illustrate, Bowers (1992) has pointed out that "the pain and cognitive effort involved to reduce it is hidden behind an amnestic barrier, but not the original suggestions for analgesia, nor the goal-directed fantasies that typically accompany the reductions in pain" (pp. 261–262). Finally, it may be pointed out that individual differences in hypnotically *suggested* amnesia seem to be only rather peripherally associated with the core of individual differences in hypnotic ability; for example, there are many subjects who show strong hypnotic performances of most other kinds, but little or no amnesia (e.g., Monteiro, Macdonald, & Hilgard, 1980). This pattern of association is, of course, not what we would expect if amnestic processes were at the root of other kinds of hypnotic tasks.

In the weak sense of amnestic barrier, it may be argued that we are only talking about temporary occlusions of some information that might have been available to consciousness—in other words, a process more like disattention than spontaneous amnesia. However, unless one assumes some kind of unity of mental process and accompanying transparency of consciousness, this more modest notion does not appear to tell us anything very interesting, and little about hypnosis per se. Consider that current conceptions of the mind (e.g., Baars, 1988) involve very numerous, distributed, specialized modules that work in parallel, are typically unconscious, and jointly have enormous information-processing capacity. In contrast, consciousness involves a single, serial flow of information of quite limited capacity. This might be likened to a televised event, in which a great variety of events are occurring simultaneously, but in which only one thing at a time may appear on the television screen, and the sequence of events is orchestrated so as to form a coherent narrative. Hence, even outside of hypnosis, there are virtually always many layers of "amnestic barrier" occurring in the performance of any reasonably complex behavior, in the sense parallel ongoing processes and materials are present that are necessarily deleted from the conscious accounting. Furthermore, the conscious experience of the causes of one's behavior is therefore necessarily incomplete and frequently incorrect, again, with or without hypnosis (cf. Nisbett & Wilson, 1977). In short, consciousness is such a narrow window on mental processes that we cannot rely on any notion of dissociated experience to explain its uncountable lacunae.

This tension between an unconscious mind of multiple, reasonably independent modules and a conscious mind that somehow integrates these diverse modules and makes them appear as one is of great importance. It harkens back to what we labeled as "the Stevensonian view"—that is, of the mind as a "mere polity of multifarious, incongruous and independent denizens" (Stevenson, 1886/1967, p. 68), whose apparent unity is, at least in part, an illusion of normal consciousness. Stevenson focused on the very high level of personal identity, but of course the notion of the mind as consisting of parallel modules applies even more readily and broadly to lower levels of functioning.

According to this view, the mind is already, in a sense, deeply divided (among many parallel modules), and higher conscious functioning somehow acts to bridge these gaps. As Baars (1991) has argued, the chief function of consciousness may be to "help integrate otherwise dissociated functions" (p. 440). Thus, if higher conscious functioning is weakened, the already-dissociated nature of mind, so to speak, should become more frankly evident.

It will come as no surprise that a hypnotic induction, with its typically relentless monotony and many allusions to sleep, may be thought of as releasing lower-level functions from the integration that is normally imposed on them by consciousness. In fact, a widely recognized effect of hypnosis is a reduced "general reality orientation" (Shor, 1959). Therefore, rather than viewing hypnotic responses as being due to the onset of a special amnestic barrier that *hides* control processes from consciousness, we may alternatively think of them as resulting from a partial loss of the higher integrative functioning normally associated with consciousness.

The notion that hypnosis weakens higher integrative functioning has an extremely important implication: hypnosis alters not just the experience of behavior, but how it is *controlled*. Let us refer one more time to the Stevenson story, as the metaphor is quite apt. The effect of the drug, which we may think of for present purposes as an analogue of hypnosis, is not simply to provide Jekyll with some novel experiences, but to release patterns of behavior that would have been entirely suppressed when in his normal state.

Perhaps partly due to the specter of its Jekyll–Hyde-like implications, there has long been considerable ambivalence in the hypnosis literature concerning the possibility that hypnosis can alter the control of behavior. With his highly influential neodissociation model of hypnosis, E. R. Hilgard (1977) made use of a current view in cognitive psychology that there is a hierarchy of levels of control involved in the generation of behavior. He proposed that hypnosis allows the bypassing of the highest level of control, an executive level associated with the willful planning, monitoring, and coordination of behavior. Thus, he argued, hypnotic suggestions may directly activate lower subsystems of control, such as those which enact specific behavior sequences. The hypnotic subject's experience of nonvolition and effortlessness, then, would accurately correspond to a genuine alteration in the usual hierarchy of control that governs behavior.

Nonetheless, in this and subsequent accounts of hypnotic phenomena, Hilgard has shown a consistent tendency to revert back to the older, amnestic-barrier account, in which no genuine alteration of control is implied. This tendency unfortunately obscures the fact that in crucial ways the amnestic-barrier and the altered-control accounts of hypnosis are quite inconsistent with each other, despite being lumped together under the protean term "dissociation." In addition, the cautiousness about admitting any genuine alterations of control in hypnosis has been widely influential, as is reflected in the very clear views of Shor and of Kihlstrom quoted earlier, as well as in the views, until fairly recently, of one of us (e.g., Bowers & Brenneman, 1981).

More recently, Bowers (1990, 1992) has advanced a modified version of Hilgard's neodissociation model of hypnosis, in which he rejects the amnestic-barrier concept of dissociation and emphasizes the altered-control concept. This modification, in effect, amputates the seemingly less viable part of Hilgard's theory—namely, the part that maintained the historically important link between hypnosis and amnesia-based dissociation—while retaining the more modern hierarchical-control model of the mind. Indeed, Bowers (1990) makes explicit that what remains is a theory of *dissociated control*, rather than one of *dissociated experience*. With regard to the latter, he points out that "dissociation is not intrinsically a matter of keeping things out of consciousness—whether by amnesia, or any other means" (Bowers, 1992, p. 267). Instead, with regard to dissociated control, Bowers (1992) has maintained Hilgard's original neodissociation language, as seen in the following definition of the theory: "Dissociation is primarily concerned with the fact that subsystems of control can be directly and automatically activated, instead of being governed by high level executive control" (p. 267). In other words, in hypnotic behavior what is "dissociated" is lower from higher, executive levels of control.

Despite what we, naturally enough, perceive to be its many strengths, this account of the altered-control theory can appear to have a number of potential shortcomings, including the following:

1. When applied to specific hypnotic behaviors, the language of *subsystems of control* can seem to strain credibility. For example, when Miller and Bowers (1993) argue that hypnotic analgesia is due to the direct activation of subsystems of control, one might wonder what sort of preexisting subsystem of control could be in place for the reduction of pain, and what sense it makes to refer to its being *directly* (vs. indirectly) activated. In a way, invoking dissociated control might just seem to postpone the problem of explaining hypnotic responding, rather than really solving it.

2. What specifically could it mean to "dissociate" lower levels of control from executive control? At present, this kind of dissociation seems to be defined chiefly in a dangerously circular manner. For example, Hilgard (1977) claims of a hypnotic response that the "less it is felt to be under the subject's control the more it has been dissociated from the normal executive functions" (p. 228). Nonetheless, in the passages quoted earlier from Shor and from Kihlstrom, it was held to be self-evident that there is some degree of higher executive control in any hypnotic behavior, irrespective of the subject's report.

3. What happens to amnesia in light of this theory? Certain classical

and widely recognized hypnotic phenomena involve suggested (rather than spontaneous) amnesia. Hence, surely these remain important to explain. How can a theory of dissociated control account for these hypnotically mediated amnestic phenomena?

We will attempt to address these questions in the rest of this chapter by relating the dissociated-control theory to some current cognitive and neuropsychological models of mental functioning. Our aims are both to substantiate the plausibility of such a theory, and in the process of fleshing it out, to suggest some novel directions for further work.

WILLED VERSUS AUTOMATIC CONTROL OF BEHAVIOR

In ordinary conditions when people do as they are told, we do not call their cooperativeness "hypnosis." The essence of hypnotic respond-ing, as seen in the so-called "classic suggestion effect" (Weitzenhoffer, 1953), is that the subject's carrying out of the suggestion is experienced as invol-untary. Hence, alterations in the experience of volition are perhaps the single most crucial thing to explain in understanding hypnosis.

The different ways in which an action may be experienced, from willed to automatic, has been a major concern, likewise, for some cognitive psy-chologists. A recent theory by Norman and Shallice (1986), for example, attempts to explain how these different ways of experiencing an action come about, and does so by relating them to differences in underlying control processes.

Let us briefly review Norman and Shallice's model. On the basis of a wide variety of findings in cognitive and neuropsychology (see Shallice, 1988), they argue that there are two complementary control systems for the initiation and control of action. The lower-level control system, which they term "contention scheduling," is decentralized and takes care of the routine selection of routine acts that do not require conscious or attentional control. Contention scheduling works through the competitive and coop-erative activation of schemas. The activation level of a particular schema is affected partly by various environmental triggers and partly by other schemas, of both a supporting and conflicting nature, that are being acti-vated at the same time. Once the activation level of a particular schema exceeds a threshold, the schema is selected and the corresponding action ensues. The essence of this process is conveyed well in the following quote: "For well-learned, habitual tasks an autonomous, self-sufficient strand of processing structures and procedures can usually carry out the required ac-tivities without the need for conscious or attentional control" (Norman & Shallice, 1986, p. 4).

However, in cases where the required action is novel or complex, or a strong habitual response must be overcome, the contention-scheduling system may fail to make appropriate schemas available. A second, higher-level control system, which Norman and Shallice term the "supervisory attentional system," assists with such nonroutine actions in a qualitatively different, and centralized way. The supervisory system not only can monitor processes taking place in the contention-scheduling system, but also has access to its own relatively unique information, including the individual's goals and intentions. Nonetheless, this higher-level control system is held to operate only indirectly, by modulating the lower-level control system, rather than by directly controlling behavior. Through the addition of extra activation and inhibition to particular schemas, the supervisory system biases the selection of schemas by the contention-scheduling system.

Because higher executive control is normally experienced as dominant (rather than supplementary), the indirect role that Norman and Shallice assign to the supervisory system can at first seem rather counterintuitive. However, the role of the supervisory system might be likened to that of a chief executive officer, who guides and redirects the activities in a company with memos and so forth. The CEO's function is not to directly execute any action (e.g., roll up his or her sleeves and shovel), but is mainly to manage the initiation and termination of actions, especially when some novel adjustment of usual operating procedures is required. In addition, despite the CEO's dominant role, workers will sometimes fail to carry out some directives successfully, and will sometimes act on their own in ways that may be inconsistent with the CEO's intentions.

Regarding the phenomenology of the individual from the perspective of this two-tier model of control, how an action is experienced depends on the nature of the involvement of the supervisory system. When the supervisory system is actively modulating the selection of schemas, we have the phenomenal experience of will, or deliberate conscious control. In contrast, when the supervisory system is neither modulating nor monitoring the contention-scheduling system, the action is experienced as automatic. Between these two extremes, a range of other states of awareness of an action is possible. For example, if the supervisory system is monitoring the contention-scheduling process but not actively modulating it, then the experience is one wherein the action immediately followed the idea of it in the mind—what William James (1890/1981) called an "ideo-motor act," to distinguish it from a genuinely willed act.

It is reasonably straightforward to apply this cognitive model to an understanding of the altered experience of volition in hypnosis. For reasonably highly hypnotizable subjects, hypnosis may be thought of as weakening the operation of the supervisory system; that is, hypnosis may partly disable the higher-level control system, associated with the phenomenal experience of will, by which the contention-scheduling system may normally be modulated. This weakening of the supervisory system, then, explains what we mean by "dissociating" lower levels of control from higher-level, executive control.

According to this conception, hypnosis results in a genuine change in the control of behavior—namely, the hypnotized individual is especially dependent on the contention-scheduling level of control, and this control can not be modulated readily in a willful manner. One should keep in mind that routine control of action can occur without the intervention of the supervisory system (the one weakened by hypnosis), for instance, with action that is triggered directly by environmental stimuli and coactive schemas. Control at the level of the contention-scheduling system, then, would be what is meant—in the language of the neodissociation theory of hypnosis—by "subsystems of control," which may be "directly activated."

It is important to point out that this increased dependence on the lower-level of control does not rule out a vast repertoire of possible behavior. Norman and Shallice (1986) argue that although well-learned action sequences and cognitive skills can be modulated by deliberate conscious control, they do not *require* this higher-level control system. In short, it is mainly an individual's capacity for novel or particularly complex behaviors that could be diminished under hypnosis, as well as, more generally, behavior that requires the exertion of his or her will.

Finally, while there may be unsolved mysteries about the nature of some of the subsystems of control referred to in neodissociation theory, the general notion that such systems lie outside of higher executive control is nevertheless quite unproblematic. Recall that the supervisory system is held to have only a relatively indirect influence on action—that is, through biasing the selection of schemas by the lower-level system. Thus, although the supervisory system may strongly affect the selection of actions, it does not have any direct role in carrying them out. Because the supervisory system (i.e., the one weakened by hypnosis) does not directly control any action, a system of control for virtually any action must lie elsewhere.

Thus, the dissociated-control theory of hypnosis can be seen to be highly consistent with the Norman and Shallice model of willed versus automatic control of behavior. In addition, the Norman and Shallice model can shed some interesting light on our understanding of various hypnotic phenomena, of which we here give a few examples.

First, if the effect of hypnosis is to weaken the supervisory system, we would expect hypnotized subjects to show two seemingly contradictory patterns of behavior: a behavioral rigidity characterized by a lack of spontaneous, self-generated action; and a tendency for thought and behavior to be triggered inappropriately by irrelevant stimuli and associations. Despite the preservation of the ability to carry out routine actions when specifically requested, a general impoverishment of spontaneous, self-generated behavior would be expected because spontaneous voluntary behavior requires an active supervisory system, whereas the responding to reasonably routine requests does not. That a paucity of spontaneous voluntary behavior characterizes hypnotized subjects will be evident to anyone who has ever conducted a group hypnosis scale—the spontaneously behaving subjects are almost certainly the ones who are not hypnotized. Another intriguing illustration of the impoverishment of spontaneous behavior in hypnosis comes from studies by Orne (1979), in which he compared the behavior of hypnotized subjects to that of simulators in response to a novel circumstance, such as an apparent power outage. Hypnotized subjects seemed to respond much more slowly to such altered circumstances, even though the conditions make the continuation of the experiment nonsensical.

A weakened supervisory system may also lead to disinhibition of control, and hence the eliciting of inappropriate or irrelevant associations and behavior (Shallice, 1988). When circumstances threaten to trigger an inappropriate or irrelevant schema, a major function of the supervisory system is ordinarily to inhibit this activation. Loss of supervisory control due to hypnosis, then, would be expected to disable such inhibition, so that peculiar associations and behavior might be activated if triggers are present. The hypnotic circumstance, however, at least in laboratory conditions, seems typically to present few such possible triggers. Hence, such disinhibition is infrequently reported, and the operative triggers are found to be quite idiosyncratic to particular subjects. J. R. Hilgard (1974) noted that people who had previously had bad experiences with drugs sometimes found themselves reexperiencing these events when being hypnotized. More generally, the phenomenon of sequelae—relatively rare, but sometimes striking effects of hypnosis that were not suggested by the hypnotist (Coe & Ryken, 1979; Crawford, Hilgard, & Macdonald, 1982; Reyher, 1967)—seems consistent with the theory that the disinhibition of tangential associations is due to a loss of supervisory control.

Second, the Norman and Shallice model seems to be quite helpful in disentangling what is going on in hypnotic performances of the easy to moderate range of difficulty. Particularly for the easiest kinds of suggestions traditionally associated with hypnosis, it is difficult to resist the impression that it does not take any special dissociative capacity to pass them. Instead, passing relatively easy hypnosis items would seem only to require some social-psychological influencibility or compliance-like attribute. Nonetheless, previous attempts to show a consistent relationship between such nonhypnotic variables and hypnotizability have not been successful (Bowers, 1976).

Accordingly, in a recent study, Woody, Oakman, and Drugovic (1992) took a new approach to devising a nonhypnotic measure of susceptibility. Borrowing a paradigm used in alcohol research to study expectancy effects, they asked subjects to consume two drinks that purportedly contained a moderate dose of alcohol, but were actually alcohol-free. Later, subjects rated the extent to which they had experienced each of 13 suggested effects, that is, alterations in sensation, perception, and thinking that might plausibly have ensued from the consumption of alcohol. These suggested effects paralleled those typically attributed to hypnosis—for example, checking for a "feeling of sluggishness or immobilization" in one's limbs, and producing a daydream to check for "more vivid or more fluid images than normal." Ratings on the 13 suggested effects showed high internal consistency and were summed to form an overall nonhypnotic suggestibility score.

This nonhypnotic suggestion measure showed a strongly differential pattern of correlation with the individual items of the Harvard Group Scale of Hypnotic Susceptibility, Form A (Shor & Orne, 1962). Namely, the easier the A-Scale item, the more strongly it correlated with the alcohol expectancy measure. Indeed, for the easiest A-Scale items, the correlations with the alcohol expectancy measure approached the items' corrected item-total correlations, indicating that these items tap little more than such expectancy effects. By contrast, the most difficult A-Scale items had virtually nothing to do with such expectancy effects.

More specifically, the great majority of items on the Harvard A-Scale consist of suggestions for motor behaviors, which are of two quite distinct types—direct motor items, which tend to be the easiest ones, and motor inhibition or challenge items, which tend to be somewhat harder to pass. The relationship of the alcohol-expectancy measure to each of the direct motor items was quite strong, whereas the measure's relationship to the challenge items was weaker and trailed toward zero as the challenge items became harder. Hence, the processes that underlie the ability to pass each type of item appear to be quite different.

The Norman and Shallice model provides an intriguing approach to understanding how direct motor and challenge items differ. To begin, consider that a direct motor suggestion can be carried out automatically and requires so little attentional effort that the role of the will is ambiguous or indeterminate. As Norman and Shallice (1986) specifically point out, "introspection fails in determining whether the will is involved in the voluntary lifting of the arm" (p. 15). Thus, the relevant characteristic of direct motor items in hypnosis appears to be this ambiguity, or indeterminacy, of the role of the will and attention. The hypnotic context, then, offers the subject a plausible hypothesis concerning the nature of this ambiguous experience—namely, the hypothesis that it is happening because of hypnosis (rather than one's own will). It is this attribution that makes the experience potentially impressive and conveys at least some sense of involuntariness. What is happening in the alcohol-expectancy measure, arguably, is very similar, except that the context offers the subject a somewhat different kind of plausible attribution—namely, that the ambiguous experience is happening due to alcohol. The connecting individual difference, then, would have to do with the propensity to interpret an ambiguous experience in terms of a plausible hypothesis offered by the context. Although some subjects high in hypnotic ability may well pass direct motor suggestions via a different mechanism from this, many subjects without much genuine hypnotic talent can probably pass such items in this nondissociative way.

It is worth reflecting for a moment on how different this explanation of passing a direct motor item is from the classic amnestic-barrier or "dissociated experience" explanation. According to the classic account, the suggested behavior is actually enacted by the subject voluntarily, but the activities of his or her higher-level control system are blocked from consciousness, and the act is therefore experienced as nonvolitional. However, according to the Norman and Shallice model, it is not necessary for the hypnotic subject to dissociate the fact of higher-level control from consciousness for such simple actions, due to the simple reason that no such higher-level control is necessary for the occurrence of the act.

Turning now to the motor inhibition or challenge suggestions, these typically consist of a simple motor suggestion followed by the instruction to *try* to oppose or overcome it. This circumstance is quite different from the direct motor suggestion, in that to carry out the instruction to try, the subject must attempt to exert will; in the language of the Norman and Shallice model, he or she must involve the supervisory system in activating the appropriate schema. Consider how different the instruction "Raise your arm" is from the instruction "*Try* to raise your arm"—in the latter case, attentional effort is unmistakable, and the role of volition unambiguous. Recall that according to the Norman and Shallice model, this phenomenal experience of will is the indicator that the supervisory system is making a bid to modulate schema selection.

It would appear that in response to a motor inhibition suggestion, some hypnotic subjects would still respond in the fashion described previously for direct motor items by remaining "role consistent" and not exerting effort to bend their arm, or whatever (e.g., the subject might think, "If I really try to bend my arm, it might spoil the effect"). If some subjects do not actually attempt to exert will, the ambiguity of the experience is maintained, so that they might look to the context for a reasonable explanation, as described earlier for direct motor suggestions. However, as soon as a subject genuinely *tries* to carry out the challenge suggestion, thereby invoking supervisory control, the process involved must be quite different. If we conceive of the "genuine" effect of hypnosis as the weakening of the supervisory system, it follows that when a hypnotized subject really tries to exert will, he or she might have the experience that such effortful attention is notably less effective—that is, less tied to action—than it normally is outside of hypnosis. In other words, compared to the lower, contention-scheduling level of control, which is evoked by suggestion, effects of the supervisory system, or executive level of control, are uncharacteristically weak. Of course, this is a very different explanation of the experience of nonvolition than the one we argued for with regard to direct motor items, and it is closely allied with what Bowers (1990, 1992) has termed the capacity for "dissociated control."

Finally, although the Norman and Shallice model and the remarks here have focused on the control of action, we may use the example of hypnotic analgesia to illustrate similar insights about the control of perception. Indeed, paralleling (and in fact antedating) the distinction between automatic and willed control of action is the distinction between "automatic" and "controlled" processing of perceptual inputs (Shiffrin & Schneider, 1977).

It is interesting in this regard to compare hypnotic analgesia with cognitive-behavioral approaches to the control of pain (Turk, Meichenbaum, & Genest, 1983). First, cognitive-behavioral interventions involve the maintenance of deliberate attentional control over the experience of a pain-evoking stimulus, using such strategies as actively diverting attention away from the stimulus, imaginatively transforming it, engaging in a counter-pain fantasy, and inhibiting negative thoughts. In terms of the model proposed by Norman and Shallice, these strategies require strong ongoing activation of the supervisory system, and the experiential equivalent for this state of high demand for attentional activation, as they point out, is *concentration* (rather than simply will). The hallmark of such a state is that a lapse in its effortful maintenance brings failure of the perceptual control. (Such control of perception is no different in kind from control of action—for example, in a sport or game, where a momentary lapse of concentration can bring about a highly inappropriate action.)

One view of hypnotic analgesia is that it, too, is basically a deliberate, effortful, strategic controlling of attention (e.g., Spanos, 1986; Wagstaff, 1991). Nonetheless, according to the conception of hypnosis proposed here, hypnotic analgesia and cognitive-behavioral pain control might better be characterized as opposites. If we view hypnosis as weakening the supervisory system, then its ultimate effect should be to *diminish* the capacity for initiating and maintaining a well-organized set of deliberate attentional strategies (i.e., strong activation of the supervisory system), not to increase it. In this sense, hypnosis and cognitive-behavioral strategies would seem to be antithetical; that is, hypnotized subjects should not be very good at self-generating attentional control strategies nor at effortfully maintaining them.

Indeed, several findings in a set of recent studies by Bowers and his colleagues indicate that hypnotic analgesia is quite unlike cognitive-behavioral pain control. In particular, subjects who show hypnotic analgesia do not typically report spontaneously using any deliberate cognitive strategies; and highly hypnotizable subjects tend to show substantially greater benefit from hypnotic analgesia than from a nonhypnotic cognitive-behavioral approach (Miller & Bowers, 1986; see Miller & Bowers, 1993, for a result to the contrary). Furthermore, unlike cognitive-behavioral pain reduction, hypnotic analgesia is not accompanied by signs of cognitive effort, as measured by impairment on a competing task (Miller & Bowers, 1993). Finally, Hargadon and Bowers (1992) have shown that hypnotic analgesia can be obtained in the absence of any deliberate cognitive strategies, such as engaging in counter-pain imagery. A completely unelaborated hypnotic suggestion for the reduction of pain seems sufficient to produce analgesia in highly hypnotizable subjects, and many of these subjects report no strategic embellishment or amplification of the suggestion at all.

Thus, deliberate attentional control does not appear to be the mechanism underlying hypnotic analgesia; but, then, what is? Miller and Bowers (1993) argued that such results are consistent with a dissociated-control model of hypnosis, in which "suggestive communications more or less directly activate subsystems of control and thereby minimize the influence of executive initiative and effort" (p. 37). For our present purposes, an attractive aspect of this proposal is that it is quite congruent with the notion that hypnosis weakens supervisory system functions, as advanced here. However, a somewhat unattractive aspect is that it appears to presume the existence of a subsystem of control over pain, one that somehow tends to remain unactivated under normal, nonhypnotic conditions. A potential criticism of Miller and Bowers's proposal, then, is that while it makes clear that hypnotic analgesia differs from effortful, nonhypnotic pain-control strategies, it does not quite succeed in advancing a specific alternative mechanism.

Once again, we turn to the Norman and Shallice model to sketch some intriguing, if as yet incomplete, possibilities. The important aspect of a pain stimulus is its peremptory quality. Even though unbidden, it hogs attentional resources in a fashion that is difficult to overturn (McCaul & Malott, 1984). In addition, this attention-grabbing characteristic of pain is closely linked to its distressing and unpleasant quality, whereas other aspects of a pain stimulus such as its sensory location appear to be mediated by other mechanisms (Pribram, 1991). Norman and Shallice discuss such automatically attention-demanding characteristics of some stimuli in terms of the computer-science notion of an *interrupt*. Specifically, in addition to whatever impact a triggering stimulus may have on schema activation, there are occasions when it also produces an interrupt in the supervisory system—loosely meaning, a "moment of emergency" that breaks in upon any ongoing deliberative activity.

In accordance with the idea that the effect of hypnosis is to weaken supervisory system functions, hypnotic analgesia could possibly result from the fact that hypnosis reduces the sensitivity of the supervisory system to interrupts. In other words, due to hypnosis, some kinds of triggers may have a diminished capacity to break in at the supervisory level. (Note that this idea is quite consistent with the notion of reduced spontaneous behavior in hypnosis, as discussed earlier.) Given that much of the disturbing aspect of pain results from interrupts, hypnosis would attenuate such discomfort. Indeed, hypnosis might make the pain unnoticeable because it no longer draws attention to itself. However, if attention were directed to the pain stimulus by an external agent, such as the hypnotist, it makes sense to assume that the supervisory system could still monitor the pain stimulus, as in the case of the hidden observer.

There is another interesting, if rather more tentative, implication of this interrupt concept of pain. The supervisory system operates in such a way as to allow some kinds of triggers to have more broadly distributed consequences than they might have without its presence; that is, via the supervisory system, a stimulus may come to have an impact on schema selection that it otherwise would not have had. For example, a pain stimulus, via supervisory functions, may come to have an inhibiting effect on a particular schema—say, a numerical cognitive operation—that would have been relatively easy to execute in the absence of supervisory input. The important point, then, is that by weakening supervisory functions, hypnosis may reduce such distributed consequences of a pain stimulus, making it easier for the subject to engage in concurrent, relatively routine behavior.

What this line of reasoning leaves unclear is the role of *suggestions* for pain reduction in hypnotic analgesia. Recent work by Hargadon and Bowers (1992) shows that such analgesic suggestions may be surprisingly simple and straightforward, and may not require any amplification by suggested imagery, as is commonly assumed. Yet the specific instruction for the subject to reduce the pain still seems to be important for obtaining hypnotic analgesia. In contrast, the present reasoning would appear to imply that hypnosis alone (unaccompanied by suggestions for pain reduction) might be sufficient for analgesia. One tentative proposal would be that to some degree all subjects have at their disposal a mechanism for the temporary suppression of pain (as seen, e.g., in emergency situations), but that this mechanism is ordinarily overturned fairly rapidly by the interrupt phenomenon described above. Hypnotic analgesia, then, might result from evoking this mechanism through suggesting a reduction of pain, and making the mechanism much more lastingly effective by inhibiting its being over-turned by the supervisory system. This proposal at least has the merit of seeming broadly consistent with the basic theme of dissociated control—that is, of lower levels of control becoming decoupled from higher-level functions. It is, however, obviously speculative and somewhat incomplete.

A DISSOCIATED-CONTROL VIEW
OF HYPNOTIC AMNESIA

One of the classic and most striking effects of hypnosis is sug-gested amnesia. Clearly, this phenomenon represents an alteration in *re-trieval*, rather than in the encoding processes of memory (Kihlstrom, 1985). That is, after the suggestion for amnesia, the hypnotized subject fails to bring to mind some material, but this material returns to mind when the suggestion is canceled. Indeed, one likely reason for the persistence of the amnestic-barrier conception of hypnosis, discussed earlier, is that it is very appealing to view such reversible lapses in memory in terms of a tempo-rary barrier that blocks material that would normally emerge easily into consciousness. It is at first much less clear how a dissociated-control model of hypnosis could account for such a phenomenon.

Nonetheless, Shallice (1988) has developed a model that will provide the bridge we need, which describes how the supervisory system affects memory processes. He argues that the well-known distinction between semantic and episodic memory (Tulving, 1972) reflects not just a differ-ence in the kinds of information needed or in the subsystems where the information is stored, but a crucial difference in the retrieval procedures that are employed. Specifically, episodic memory tasks require the utiliza-tion of *"specialized retrieval procedures directable by only the supervisory system,"* whereas semantic memory tasks simply involve "accessing the relevant information through the operation of the schemata that control routine processing" (Shallice, 1988, p. 372). Hence, for memory, as with action, the supervisory system is hypothesized to function as a higher-control sys-tem, one which, again as with action, enables the negotiation of nonroutine problems—that is, ones that cannot be handled by standard memory re-trieval routines.

Shallice suggests that although most information would not be stored in the supervisory system, some features of memories may be specially stored there—namely, those aspects "necessary for effective integration of the memory into the overall structure of a person's life history" (1988, p. 372). However, the more important point about the supervisory system is *how* it approaches retrieval tasks. Drawing on a theory by Norman and Bobrow (1979), Shallice proposes that when confronted by a nonroutine problem, the supervisory system first formulates descriptions of what the relevant memory records might be like if they existed. Next these descriptions are matched with records, and then those candidate records that have been retrieved are checked to verify that they are indeed relevant.

The process of remembering, as directed by the supervisory system, would consist, then, of cycles of description, matching, and verification. This process might be likened to using CD-ROM resources to locate any psychological literature possibly relevant to a particular question—material about which one has as yet, or retains, only a rough idea. One might need to try a variety of descriptions of what is desired, and at various stages, the verification process may reveal that most or even all of the candidate records (which are sometimes maddeningly numerous!) are actually totally irrelevant. Naturally, there are many other times when desired records can be accessed much more directly and simply than this—using our analogy, these would be comparable to the use of standard semantic memory retrieval routines.

This theory of supervisory system memory functions can be quite readily, if as yet somewhat tentatively, applied to an understanding of memory alterations in hypnosis. If hypnosis weakens the supervisory system, as we have argued, then it should tend to interfere with control over some memory functions while leaving other functions unaffected. Specifically, we would expect hypnosis to affect both the description and verification phases in the cycles, as they are directed by the Supervisory System, leading to at least the following two sorts of effects.

First, there should be relatively poor access to memories that require the formulation of preliminary descriptions—for example, ones for which there is no overlearned access routine. One way this change would likely be evident is that cases of hypnotically reduced free-recall memory should be accompanied by relatively well-preserved cued-recall and recognition memory. Memory tasks that provide external cues should be relatively unaffected because to some extent they supply the needed description; thus the formulation of descriptions by the supervisory system would be less important or even unnecessary with such tasks. Indeed, the evidence on hypnotic amnesia is strikingly consistent with these implications: hypnotic amnesia selectively impairs free recall, rather than recognition and implicit-memory tasks such as word associations (Evans, 1979; Kihlstrom, 1980; Kihlstrom & Shor, 1978; McConkey & Sheehan, 1981; McConkey, Sheehan, & Cross, 1980; Spanos, Radtke, & Dubreuil, 1982).

Second, hypnotized subjects should show poor verification—that is, diminished ability to discriminate appropriate or correct records from inappropriate or incorrect ones. Specifically, they should mistake irrelevant and inappropriate associations for the required memories, and be incorrectly confident that these incorrect associations "match" with the required material. Indeed, such distorting effects of hypnosis on memory have been shown in a number of studies (Dywan & Bowers, 1983; Laurence & Perry, 1983; Orne, Whitehouse, Dinges, & Orne, 1988). One striking example of impoverished verification is the "discovery" made during hypnotic age-regression of elaborate previous lives, which obviously consist of a mish-mash of irrelevant memories and fantasies.

To summarize, the essential point is that a dissociated-control theory of hypnotic amnesia is possible, even if, admittedly, much work remains to be done. Such a theory emphasizes hypnotic alteration in the control over memory processes, such as the description and verification phases of super-visory system processing—rather than the erection of amnestic barriers.

THE HYPNOTIZED SUBJECT
AS A FRONTAL LOBE PATIENT

That a dissociated-control theory of hypnosis would implicate change in frontal lobe functioning is almost obvious, since the essence of dissociated control is the bypassing of high-level executive control, and the frontal cortex is strongly believed to be the site of such executive control (e.g., Pribram, 1973). More specifically, the prefrontal cortex is thought to be the site of the highest level of control in the hierarchy of motor con-trol, and is thought to provide a system for the overall organization, regu-lation, and verification of activity (Kolb & Whishaw, 1985).

Indeed, Norman and Shallice (1986) developed the conceptual frame-work of the supervisory system in large part to account for uniquely fron-tal functions. Furthermore, there is a very close parallel between how we have used this framework to explain hypnotic behavior and how Norman and Shallice use it to explain the behavior of patients with frontal lobe dis-orders. In particular, we have argued that hypnosis, in highly susceptible subjects, weakens the supervisory system and increases dependence on the contention-scheduling level of control. Similarly, Shallice (1988) points out that damage to the supervisory system, resulting in "reliance on conten-tion scheduling alone," gives rise to "the symptoms classically associated with frontal lobe disorders" (p. 335).

Let us examine this parallel in greater detail. Bowers (1992) has re-cently illustrated the principle of dissociated control through examining the nonhypnotic example of a person being distracted and inadvertently dialing a familiar telephone number rather than the intended one. As in the case of hypnotic behavior, a controlled action sequence seems to have escaped from higher executive control. Interestingly, Shallice (1988) uses the same capture-error action lapses in distracted normal subjects as an illustration of what happens when action is unaided by the supervisory system, and hence as the normal analogue of pathological behavior that ensues from damage to the supervisory system:

> Depending on the pattern of trigger-schema relations, a system of contention scheduling without supervisory control may show one of two apparently contradictory types of behaviour. Behavioural rigidity (a tendency to perseverate) should occur in some situations; in others, a distractibility and a tendency to be side-tracked by irrelevant associations. (p. 339)

There are a number of specific ways in which the hypnotic phenomena we described earlier suggest the inhibition of frontal functions. First, the general impoverishment of spontaneous, self-generated behavior we noted in hypnotized subjects is also one of the classic hallmarks of patients with frontal lobe lesions (Kolb & Whishaw, 1985; Hécaen & Albert, 1975). Such patients, like hypnotized subjects, are capable of carrying out most any action when urged to do so, yet spontaneously initiate little activity. Similarly, the weakening of volitional control we noted in hypnotized subjects is also a classic hallmark of frontal lobe dysfunction. Indeed, one of the first systematic reviews of patients with frontal lobe lesions noted their peculiar "other-directedness" (Feuchtwanger, 1923, as cited in Teuber, 1964). Further, there is general agreement that such patients typically show an inability to select and execute self-mediated plans (Kolb & Whishaw, 1985).

The fact that the most distressing aspect of pain (as opposed to its sensory location aspect) is associated with the frontal lobes is of further relevance to hypnotic analgesia (Pribram, 1991). Indeed, in cases of intractable pain, removal of the frontal cortex ameliorates the distress (Bouckoms, 1989).

Finally, hypnotic amnesia may be likened to what Shallice (1988) has termed "frontal amnesia." Patients diagnosed with this are unable to distinguish true memories from irrelevant associations elicited by stimuli, are highly confident about their incorrect memories, and are prone to confabulation, especially when prompted by leading questions—all characteristics of hypnotically influenced memory, as well. Shallice (1988) contrasts frontal amnesia with classical amnesia as follows:

> *Frontal amnesia*, then, appears to be an impairment of that part of the Supervisory System concerned with formulating the description of any memories that might be required and of verifying that any candidate memories that have been retrieved are relevant. *Classical amnesia*, by contrast, would arise from an interruption of the flow of memory information from the processing systems to the Supervisory System. (p. 378)

This contrast provides an intriguing and fairly direct parallel to the distinction between a dissociated-control model of hypnotic amnesia, as presented here, and the classic amnestic-barrier model. According to the dissociated-control model, hypnosis alters high-level controls over memory functions, so that material is more difficult to retrieve under conditions that require the control system to generate preliminary descriptions, and verification of retrieved material is faulty. This model is in contrast to the view that hypnosis blocks access to memories in a barrierlike, comparatively all-or-nothing fashion.

In addition, Kolb and Whishaw (1985) argue that the best established effect on memory of frontal lobe damage is impaired memory for recency, or the temporal ordering of events. Correspondingly, there is quite a body of evidence to indicate that hypnotized subjects show a disorganization in the temporal or sequential organization of events in memory (e.g., Evans & Kihlstrom, 1973; Geiselman et al., 1983; Kihlstrom & Evans, 1979; Kihlstrom & Wilson, 1984; Spanos & Bodorik, 1977; Spanos, Radtke-Bodorik, & Stam, 1980; Tkachyk, Spanos, & Bertrand, 1985; Wilson & Kihlstrom, 1986).

In summary, it is quite attractive to link a dissociated-control theory of hypnosis to the inhibition of functions subserved by the prefrontal cortex. There remains, however, the question of how best to proceed in making something useful out of the hypothesis of such a brain–behavior relationship. One approach to take is to do neuropsychophysiological studies that examine regional specificities of brain function during hypnosis. This is the approach predominantly employed by Crawford and by Gruzelier (for a review, see Crawford & Gruzelier, 1992). Based on a rather complex hypothesis of changes in hemispheric laterality with hypnosis, these researchers and their colleagues, as well as others, have produced a maze of complex and sometimes conflicting findings, using a variety of procedures such as sophisticated EEG analyses and brain imaging techniques. Toward the end of the review, however, Crawford and Gruzelier (1992) seem to have pulled away somewhat from the complex shift-in-laterality position and moved toward a simpler position quite in line with what has been argued here. They write: "With hindsight, what may be more central to hypnosis is the inhibition of anterior frontal lobe functions" (p. 265).

Another approach to take is a more cognitive-functional one, which would emphasize the construction and evaluation of explanatory cognitive models, and deemphasize (due to its prematurity) the issues of regional specificity in the brain. There are many testable hypotheses about hypnosis that might emerge from comparing it to frontal lobe disorders, of which the following are some examples:

1. The notion that frontal functions are inhibited in hypnosis suggests that hypnotized subjects should show some of the problem-solving behaviors of frontal lobe patients: for example, the "stuck-in-set" perseveration

on such tasks as the Wisconsin Card-Sorting Task (Milner, 1963), the relatively poor performance on tasks that require a planning or self-organizing component (e.g., Milner, Petrides, & Smith, 1985), and the relatively high rate of bizarre answers on tasks that require thinking of a nonroutine approach and checking the plausibility of a potential response (e.g., Shallice & Evans, 1978; Smith & Milner, 1984). Such findings would be consistent with the general hypothesis that under hypnosis, subjects show a reduced capacity to overcome routine responses and cope with novel problem-solving demands (the principal contribution of the supervisory system).

2. The notion that the effects of hypnosis on memory processes are akin to frontal amnesia suggests that hypnotized subjects should have more difficulty with certain kinds of memory tasks—for example, with accurately retrieving events that are long past and therefore not part of any standard semantic-memory retrieval routine (e.g., Sanders & Warrington, 1971; Shallice, 1988). Such findings would be consistent with the general hypothesis that under hypnosis, subjects show less capacity to engage in the description and verification procedures subserved by the supervisory system.

CONCLUSION: WHAT SORT OF CONTROL IS DISSOCIATED CONTROL?

To return finally to an issue raised much earlier in this chapter, let us begin by citing Kihlstrom's (1992) assertion, "The experience of automaticity, like so much else about hypnosis, is illusory" (p. 308). In light of the present dissociated-control account of hypnosis, this statement is quite interesting because it appears to be wrong in one way, and right in another. It is wrong in the sense that alterations of control in hypnosis are quite like automatized actions, in that they both involve the minimizing of supervisory system functions. Rather than simply colluding in the construction of an illusion of nonvolition, the hypnotized subject, within the context of the present account, undergoes a real change in the control of behavior—simply put, a shift down in the hierarchy of control. One important implication of a genuine change in control, as opposed to a collusive illusion, is that a subject could act quite unlike his or her "usual self" under hypnosis, in conflict with consciously represented standards. Such discrepant acts would perhaps be particularly likely when the behavior in question is well-learned or "deeply ingrained," but the person (outside hypnosis) is typically exerting a high degree of deliberate attentional control to inhibit it (e.g., a bad habit).

However, Kihlstrom's statement is right in the sense that there is no reason to think a hypnotic induction could make a behavior automatized that was not ever automatized before; for example, hypnosis cannot substitute for learning or practice. Indeed, the present view of what happens in hypnosis to highly susceptible subjects may be regarded as far less flattering than some other views of hypnosis (e.g., Crawford, 1991), it suggests that, for the most part, hypnosis simply allows already routinized behaviors to be run off without the volitional level of control.

How, then, does the notion of dissociated control allow hypnosis to add anything new say of potential clinical utility to a subject's behavioral repertoire? Consider that despite its wonderful flexibility, deliberate attentional control, with its serial processing steps, hypnosis is slow, limited in capacity, and unwieldy. Hence, in circumstances as varied as performing music and managing social interactions, effortful control at the level of the supervisory system can become counterproductive and lead to maladaptive "overcontrol." As Norman and Shallice (1986) remark, "deliberate control of skilled performance leads to deterioration of performance" (p. 11). Thus, hypnosis may be viewed as a therapeutic opportunity to relinquish some kinds of control in order to further others—of a more parallel and less centralized sort. In addition, by exerting some outboard planning and control functions, the hypnotist may sometimes promote the eliciting of novel solutions and responses, ones for which the subject has not yet quite "put together the pieces" (e.g., Talmon, 1990).

Given the current interest in the likely relation between hypnotizability and multiple personality disorder (e.g., Bliss, 1984; Bowers, 1992), it is intriguing to speculate about whether a process of dissociated control could produce something as new and novel as a second personality. Consider that by inhibiting supervisory system functions, hypnosis should lead to some temporary loss of personality integration, in the sense of how well behavior is integrated with overarching goals, and events with an overall life structure. However, the result would seem to be a state of attenuation, in which the sense of personal identity is weakened, rather than that a "new" personality is created. Given the link we have drawn between supervisory functions and the frontal lobes, it is also worth recalling the classic case of Phineas Gage, which truly involves a real-life Jekyll-to-Hyde transformation. After an accident that damaged Gage's left frontal lobe, the dramatic change in his behavior was described in words that might have come straight out of Stevenson's story:

> The equilibrium or balance, so to speak, between his intellectual faculties and animal propensities seems to have been destroyed. He is fitful, irreverent, indulging at times in the grossest profanity, manifesting but little deference to his fellows, impatient of restraint or advice when it conflicts with his desires, at times pertinaciously obstinate, yet capricious and vacillating. (Harlow, 1868, cited in Blumer & Benson, 1975, p. 153)

Here, too, Gage's condition seems better described as a severe loss of personality integration than as involving the emergence of a well-organized new personality. In short, one might well be skeptical of the idea that the mechanism of dissociative control, with its weakening of high-level executive functions, would account for the development of a true second personality, as opposed to loosened personality integration.

However, that may not quite be the end of the story. Shallice (1988) has noted that the concept of the supervisory system parallels Johnson-Laird's (1983) notion of consciousness as the operating system of the mind. Pursuing this computer metaphor, it is an intriguing fact that nothing can prevent the possibility of two operating systems coexisting on the same hardware—for example, Windows and OS/2, either of which could be "brought up" during a particular session. (It is amusing in the present context to note that Windows and OS/2 began as the same operating system, and then split apart rather late in their development.) Returning to people, normally one good supervisory or operating system is all that is needed; but perhaps in rare cases, two alternative, coexisting executive control systems, each with its own memory-management processes and access to unique records, may develop. They should be distinguishable in terms of different implicit self-knowledge, and so on. Admittedly, such demonstrations have been extremely rare. Nonetheless, within the context of this speculative model, the essence of MPD would not involve the erection of amnestic barriers, nor poor personality integration expressed metaphorically as "multiple personalities," but the development of alternative executive-control systems, each of which operates independently.

REFERENCES

Baars, B. J. (1988). *A cognitive theory of consciousness*. Cambridge: Cambridge University Press.

Baars, B. J. (1991). Consciousness and modularity. *Behavioral and Brain Sciences, 14*, 440.

Bliss, E. L. (1986). *Multiple personality, allied disorders and hypnosis*. New York: Oxford University Press.

Blumer, D., & Benson, D. F. (1975). Personality changes with frontal and temporal lobe lesions. In D. F. Benson & D. Blumer (Eds.), *Psychiatric aspects of neurologic disease* (pp. 151–170). New York: Grune & Stratton.

Bouckoms, A. J. (1989). Psychosurgery for pain. In P. D. Wall & R. Melzack (Eds.), *Textbook of pain* (2nd ed., pp. 868–881). Edinburgh: Churchill Livingstone.

Bowers, K. S. (1976). *Hypnosis for the seriously curious*. Monterey, CA: Brooks/Cole.

Bowers, K. S. (1990). Unconscious influences and hypnosis. In J. L. Singer (Ed.), *Repression and dissociation: Implications for personality theory, psychopathology, and health* (pp. 143–178). Chicago: University of Chicago Press.

Bowers, K. S. (1992). Imagination and dissociation in hypnotic responding. *International Journal of Clinical and Experimental Hypnosis, 40,* 253–275.

Bowers, K. S., & Brenneman, H. A. (1981). Hypnotic dissociation, dichotic listening, and active versus passive modes of attention. *Journal of Abnormal Psychology, 90,* 55–67.

Coe, W. C., & Ryken, K. (1979). Hypnosis and risks to human subjects. *American Psychologist, 34,* 673–681.

Crawford, H. J. (1991, October). *The hypnotizable brain: Attentional and disattentional processes.* Presidential address delivered at the annual meeting of the Society for Clinical and Experimental Hypnosis, New Orleans.

Crawford, H. J., & Gruzelier, J. H. (1992). A midstream view of the neuropsychophysiology of hypnosis: Recent research and future directions. In E. Fromm & M. R. Nash (Eds.), *Contemporary hypnosis research* (pp. 227–266). New York: Guilford Press.

Crawford, H. J., Hilgard, J. R., & Macdonald, H. (1982). Transient experiences following hypnotic testing and special termination procedures. *International Journal of Clinical and Experimental Hypnosis, 30,* 117–126.

Dywan, J., & Bowers, K. S. (1983). The use of hypnosis to enhance recall. *Science, 222,* 184–185.

Erdelyi, M. H. (1985). *Psychoanalysis: Freud's cognitive psychology.* New York: W. H. Freeman.

Erdelyi, M. H. (1990). Repression, reconstruction, and defense: History and integration of the psychoanalytic and experimental frameworks. In J. L. Singer (Ed.), *Repression and dissociation: Implications for personality theory, psychopathology, and health* (pp. 1–31). Chicago: University of Chicago Press.

Evans, F. J. (1979). Contextual forgetting: Posthypnotic source amnesia. *Journal of Abnormal Psychology, 88,* 556–563.

Evans, F. J., & Kihlstrom, J. F. (1973). Posthypnotic amnesia as disrupted recall. *Journal of Abnormal Psychology, 82,* 317–323.

Geiselman, R. E., Fishman, D. L., Jaenicke, C., Larner, B. R., MacKinnon, D. P., Shoenberg, S., & Swartz, S. (1983). Mechanisms of hypnotic and nonhypnotic forgetting. *Journal of Experimental Psychology: Learning, Memory, and Cognition, 9,* 626–635.

Hargadon, R., & Bowers, K. S. (1992, October). *High hypnotizables and hypnotic analgesia: An examination of underlying mechanisms.* Paper presented at the annual meeting of the Society for Clinical and Experimental Hypnosis, Arlington, VA.

Hécaen, H., & Albert, M. L. (1975). Disorders of mental functioning related to frontal lobe pathology. In D. F. Benson & D. Blumer (Eds.), *Psychiatric aspects of neourologic disease.* New York: Grune & Stratton.

Hilgard, E. R. (1973). A neodissociation interpretation of pain reduction in hypnosis. *Psychological Review, 80,* 396–411.

Higard, E. R. (1977). *Divided consciousness: Multiple controls in human thought and action.* New York: Wiley-Interscience.

Hilgard, E. R., & Cooper, L. M. (1965). Spontaneous and suggested post-hypnotic amnesia. *International Journal of Clinical and Experimental Hypnosis, 13,* 261–273.

Hilgard, J. R. (1974). Sequelae to hypnosis. *International Journal of Clinical and Experimental Hypnosis, 22,* 138–156.

James, W. (1981). *The principles of psychology*. Cambridge, MA: Harvard University Press. (Original work published 1890)

Janet, P. (1901). *The mental state of hystericals*. New York: Putnam.

Janet, P. (1965). *The major symptoms of hysteria*. New York: Hafner. (Original work published 1907)

Johnson-Laird, P. N. (1983). *Mental models*. Cambridge, MA: Harvard University Press.

Kihlstrom, J. F. (1980). Posthypnotic amnesia for recently learned material: Interactions with "episodic" and "semantic" memory. *Cognitive Psychology, 12*, 227–251.

Kihlstrom, J. F. (1985). Hypnosis. *Annual Review of Psychology, 36*, 385–418.

Kihlstrom, J. F. (1992). Hypnosis: A sesquicentennial essay. *International Journal of Clinical and Experimental Hypnosis, 40*, 301–314.

Kihlstrom, J. F., & Evans, F. J. (1979). Memory retrieval processes during posthypnotic amnesia. In J. F. Kihlstrom & F. J. Evans (Eds.), *Functional disorders of memory* (pp. 179–218). Hillsdale, NJ: Lawrence Erlbaum.

Kihlstrom, J. F., & Shor, R. E. (1978). Recall and recognition during posthypnotic amnesia. *International Journal of Clinical and Experimental Hypnosis, 26*, 330–349.

Kihlstrom, J. F., & Wilson, L. (1984). Temporal organization of recall during posthypnotic amnesia. *Journal of Abnormal Psychology, 93*, 200–208.

Kolb, B., & Whishaw, I. Q. (1985). *Fundamentals of human neuropsychology* (2nd ed.). New York: W. H. Freeman.

Laurence, J.-R., & Perry, C. (1983). Hypnotically created memory among highly hypnotizable subjects. *Science, 222*, 523–524.

Lynn, S. J., Rhue, J. W., & Weekes, J. R. (1990). Hypnotic involuntariness: A social cognitive analysis. *Psychological Review, 97*, 169–184.

McCaul, K. D., & Malott, J. M. (1984). Distraction and coping with pain. *Psychological Bulletin, 95*, 516–533.

McConkey, K. M., & Sheehan, P. W. (1981). The impact of videotape playback of hypnotic events on hypnotic amnesia. *Journal of Abnormal Psychology, 90*, 46–54.

McConkey, K. M., Sheehan, P. W., & Cross, D. G. (1980). Posthypnotic amnesia: Seeing is not remembering. *British Journal of Social and Clinical Psychology, 19*, 99–107.

Miller, M. E., & Bowers, K. S. (1986). Hypnotic analgesia and stress inoculation in the reduction of pain. *Journal of Abnormal Psychology, 95*, 6–14.

Miller, M. E., & Bowers, K. S. (1993). Hypnotic analgesia: Dissociated experience or dissociated control? *Journal of Abnormal Psychology, 102*, 29–38.

Milner, B. (1963). Effects of different brain lesions on card-sorting. *Archives of Neurology, 9*, 90–100.

Milner, B., Petrides, M., & Smith, M. L. (1985). Frontal lobes and the temporal organization of memory. *Human Neurobiology, 4*, 137–142.

Monteiro, K. P., Macdonald, H., & Hilgard, E. R. (1980). Imagery, absorption, and hypnosis: A factorial study. *Journal of Mental Imagery, 4*, 63–81.

Nisbett, R., & Wilson, T. D. (1977). Telling more than we can know: Verbal reports on mental processes. *Psychological Review, 84*, 231–254.

Norman, D. A., & Bobrow, D. G. (1979). Descriptions: An intermediate stage in memory retrieval. *Cognitive Psychology, 11*, 107–123.

Norman, D. A., & Shallice, T. (1986). Attention to action: Willed and automatic control of behavior. In R. J. Davidson, G. E. Schwartz, & D. Shapiro (Eds.), *Consciousness and self-regulation* (Vol. 4, pp. 1–18). New York: Plenum Press.

Orne, M. T. (1979). On the simulating subject as a quasi-control group in hypnosis research: What, why, and how. In E. Fromm & R. E. Shor (Eds.), *Hypnosis: Developments in research and new perspectives* (pp. 519–565). Chicago: Aldine.

Orne, M. T., Whitehouse, W. G., Dinges, D. F., & Orne, E. C. (1988). Reconstructing memory through hypnosis: Forensic and clinical implications. In H. M. Pettinati (Ed.), *Hypnosis and memory* (pp. 21–63). New York: Guilford Press.

Pope-Hennessey, J. (1974). *Robert Louis Stevenson.* London: Jonathan Cape.

Pribram, K. H. (1973). The primate frontal cortex—executive of the brain. In K. H. Pribram & A. R. Luria (Eds.), *Psychophysiology of the frontal lobes* (pp. 293–314). New York: Academic Press.

Pribram, K. H. (1991). *Brain and perception: Holonomy and structure in figural processing.* Hillsdale, NJ: Lawrence Erlbaum.

Reyher, J. (1967). Hypnosis in research on psychopathology. In J. E. Gordon (Ed.), *Handbook of clinical and experimental hypnosis* (pp. 110–147). New York: Macmillan.

Sanders, H. I., & Warrington, E. K. (1971). Memory for remote events in amnestic patients. *Brain, 94,* 661–668.

Shallice, T. (1988). *From neuropsychology to mental structure.* Cambridge: Cambridge University Press.

Shallice, T., & Evans, M. E. (1978). The involvement of the frontal lobes in cognitive estimation. *Cortex, 14,* 294–303.

Shiffrin, R. M., & Schneider, W. (1977). Controlled and automatic human information processing: II. Perceptual learning, automatic attending, and a general theory. *Psychological Review, 84,* 127–190.

Shor, R. E. (1959). Hypnosis and the concept of the generalized reality-orientation. *American Journal of Psychotherapy, 13,* 582–602.

Shor, R. E. (1979). The fundamental problem in hypnosis research as viewed from historic perspectives. In E. Fromm & R. E. Shor (Eds.), *Hypnosis: Developments in research and new perspectives* (2nd ed., pp. 15–41). Chicago: Aldine.

Shor, R. E., & Orne, M. T. (1962). *Harvard Group Scale of Hypnotic Susceptibility, Form A.* Palo Alto, CA: Consulting Psychologists Press.

Smith, M. L., & Milner, B. (1984). Differential effects of frontal lobe lesions on cognitive estimation and spatial memory. *Neuropsychologia, 22,* 697–705.

Spanos, N. P. (1986). Hypnotic behavior: A social psychological interpretation of amnesia, analgesia, and "trance logic." *Behavioral and Brain Sciences, 9,* 449–467.

Spanos, N. P., & Bodorik, H. L. (1977). Suggested amnesia and disorganized recall in hypnotic and task-motivated subjects. *Journal of Abnormal Psychology, 86,* 295–305.

Spanos, N. P., Radtke, H. L., & Dubreuil, D. L. (1982). Episodic and semantic memory in posthypnotic amnesia: A reevaluation. *Journal of Personality and Social Psychology, 43,* 565–573.

Spanos, N. P., Radtke-Bodorik, H. L., & Stam, H. J. (1980). Disorganized recall during suggested amnesia: Fact not artifact. *Journal of Abnormal Psychology, 89,* 1–19.

Stevenson, R. L. (1967). *The strange case of Dr. Jekyll and Mr. Hyde.* New York: Franklin Watts. (Original work published 1886)

Talmon, M. (1990). *Single-session therapy: Maximizing the effect of the first (and often only) therapeutic encounter.* San Francisco: Jossey-Bass.

Tkachyk, M. E., Spanos, N. P., & Bertrand, L. D. (1985). Variables affecting subjective organization during posthypnotic amnesia. *Journal of Research in Personality, 19,* 95–108.

Teuber, H.-L. (1964). The riddle of frontal lobe function in man. In J. M. Warren & K. Akert (Eds.), *The frontal granular cortex and behavior.* New York: McGraw-Hill.

Tulving, E. (1972). Episodic and semantic memory. In E. Tulving & W. Donaldson (Eds.), *Organization of memory* (pp. 381–403). New York: Academic Press.

Turk, D., Meichenbaum, D. H., & Genest, M. (1983). *Pain and behavioral medicine: A cognitive-behavioral perspective.* New York: Guilford Press.

Wagstaff, B. F. (1991). Compliance, belief, and semantics in hypnosis: A nonstate, sociocognitive perspective. In S. J. Lynn & J. W. Rhue (Eds.), *Theories of hypnosis: Current models and perspectives* (pp. 362–396). New York: Guilford Press.

Weitzenhoffer, A. M. (1953). *Hypnotism: An objective study in suggestibility.* New York: John Wiley.

Wilson, L., & Kihlstrom, J. F. (1986). Subjective and categorical organization of recall during posthypnotic amnesia. *Journal of Abnormal Psychology, 95,* 264–273.

Woody, E. Z., Oakman, J. M., & Drugovic, M. (1992, October). *Fleshing out a two-component view of individual differences underlying hypnotic responsiveness.* Paper presented at the annual meeting of the Society for Clinical and Experimental Hypnosis, Arlington, VA.

4

Dissociation in Hysteria and Hypnosis: A Concept Aggrandized

Fred H. Frankel

The views discussed below take into account the origin of psychotherapy at the turn of the century, and its development in this one. Furthermore, the directions facilitated by the third and the revised third editions of the *Diagnostic and Statistical Manual of Mental Disorders* (DSM-III and DSM-III-R; American Psychiatric Association, 1980, 1987), and Hilgard's neodissociation theory (Hilgard, 1973, 1977) will be reviewed. These sources, in my view, have helped propel dissociation and the "dissociative disorders" into the clinical forefront. Wilson (1993) in a review of the history of DSM-III noted that as the essential focus of psychiatric knowledge shifted from the clinically based biopsychosocial model to a research-based medical model, a return to descriptive psychiatry was inaugurated, beginning in DSM-III. While this has had some positive consequences for the profession, it at the same time represents a significant narrowing of psychiatry's clinical gaze. More specifically, it has seriously limited our clinical understanding of many individuals, and for our purposes here, of many of the patients described as having a dissociative disorder. I also believe that in important ways the neodissociation theory has been enlarged upon and aggrandized by clinical theorists, which I will expand on later.

The terms hysteria and hysterical behavior have in the past embraced much of what is now described as dissociative. Protean and complicated, hysteria has been difficult to understand at most times, and especially so when stripped of its psychosocial context, which has occurred in recent years. We have an even deeper appreciation of this restricted view when we consider what has been mandated by the DSM. The introduction to DSM-III-R contains the disclaimer: "It should also be noted that the DSM-III-R classification of mental disorders does not attempt to classify disturbed dyadic, family or other interpersonal relationships" (American Psychiatric Association, 1987, p. xxv). It is my contention that a reasonable understanding of hysteria and hysterical behavior minus its context of interpersonal interaction is likely to be difficult if not impossible, and this refers not only to the interaction between patients and their families, but also to that between patients and their caretakers.

The supplanting of the DSM-II category Hysterical Neuroses, Dissociative Type with Dissociative Disorders in DSM-III, was part of a conscious plan to reassemble the psychiatric constituents of hysteria under other labels (Hyler & Spitzer, 1978). Removing dissociation per se from its neurotic psychosocial matrix, and presenting it as if a widespread understanding of its clinical nature exists, and as if it were observable and measurable without confounding variables, will in all likelihood prove historically to be an impressive piece of legerdemain. Rather than viewing the dissociation concept as a useful point of departure for investigative studies as suggested by Hilgard's theory (1977), the clinical field has embraced a reified version of it, which attempts to define and account for several clinical behaviors. The concomitant interest in post-traumatic stress disorder in recent years, and the emphasis on victimization and survival have brought considerable energy to this clinical exercise. Clinicians now devote much effort and time to searching for memories of childhood physical and sexual abuse. The assumption is that those early events encouraged the initial use of dissociation as a defense, and paved the way for repeated dissociative behaviors. At the same time, questions that examine meaning are rarely raised because of the emphasis on descriptive criteria, and factors that might contribute to the dissociative systems such as the circumstances of the interview and the expectations of the examiner, plus the role of suggestion and contagion in the unfolding of the history, are rarely addressed. This situation leads me rather directly to a revisitation of hysteria, and then to a review of dissociation and hypnosis.

HYSTERIA

It is interesting, and probably no coincidence, that the only disorders in the DSM-III and DSM-III-R that still have theoretical mechanisms as their basis are the *conversion* and *dissociative disorders*. While some disorders that formerly fell under the rubric "hysterical" have been dispersed among the somatoform disorders, the eating disorders and others, the two categories mentioned above bear the major legacy of hysteria, now banned from the lexicon. The uncertainties surrounding what constitutes hysteria still bedevil these purposefully contrived successors.

The term "hysteria" has a long and colorful history, with roots in ancient Greek and Egyptian medicine. Several monographs and papers in recent years (Chodoff, 1974; Merskey, 1979; Micale, 1990; Slavney, 1990), and edited papers (Roy, 1982), have focused on the clinical presentations, history, and theoretical understanding of the phenomenon. Influenced no doubt by their preferred perspectives, writers have either approved of the diminishing dependence on this term to describe a clinical presentation (Slavney, 1990), spoken of its indestructibility (Lewis, 1982), or encouraged the continued recognition of the psychological motives behind the clinical picture (Merskey, 1979).

Many symptoms included in Briquet's syndrome and polysymptomatic bodily complaints have, by and large, demanded more attention from the nonpsychiatric physician than from those in our field. On the other hand, the hysterical symptoms demanding our neurological and psychiatric attention during this past century include seizures, motor and sensory disabilities, and disturbed mental states. With these latter cases, the hysterical presentations have generally been characterized by drama, or exaggerated, volatile, or unconstrained emotionality on the part of the patients, and incredulity at times balanced by fascination on the part of their caretakers. Further, the question of whether these patients were pretending to be ill not infrequently permeated the clinical assessment. In short, hysteria and hysterical behavior have presented a challenge to the great majority of clinicians.

Because the clinical picture of hysteria is still not understood in pathophysiological terms (since no "broken part" can be discerned), its right to be listed as a disease entity has been seriously questioned (Slavney, 1990). Further, it is often frustrating to professionals who are trained to look for causal mechanisms to try to understand and treat the presenting clinical chaos that accompanies hysteria. As a result, many routine treatment procedures have failed to affect the course of the behavior or the symptoms in a predictable manner, and the not infrequent conclusion has been that the affected individuals had no real desire to get well. Censure, reproach, and devaluation are not unusual in the clinician's ultimate response.

In explaining their understanding of hysteria and hysterical behavior from both a medical and psychiatric perspective, authors have ranged from being highly critical of the concept of a disease entity per se, to being extremely sensitive to the suffering and unspoken needs of the patients. Symonds (1979) saw but little to distinguish hysteria from malingering, and Kendell (1982) recommended that once laboratory procedures indicated a patient had no organic defect, the best method of treatment was to ignore the symptoms that enabled him or her to use the sick role to gain his or her ends. A more compassionate view takes into account the fact that if the patient is being deceptive, he or she is largely deceiving him- or herself (Ey, 1982) in an attempt to ward off the harshness of his or her own reality. Chodoff, in his lucid and creative papers on the treatment of hysteria and the hysterical personality (1974, 1978), has drawn attention to our need to develop a flexible approach rather than an absolute one. He referred to the need to measure carefully how much to respond, to match the demands for direct gratification that emerge in the interaction with these patients, whose symptoms and behavior are most often a way of communicating their needs to society and the therapist. History confirms the breadth of early neuropsychiatric attempts to understand hysteria, from Charcot's emphasis on the organic basis of the disease (Ellenberger, 1970) to Janet's idea that those who suffer from it have a constitutional deficiency (Janet, 1925/1976), to initial Freudian theorizing in which hysterical symptoms are viewed as the result of sexual fantasies and memories.

While the heterogeneity of the conceptualizations and poorly understood clinical behaviors previously included under the category of "hysteria" or "hysterical," at the least, partially contributed to their exclusion from the DSM-III, there is reason to regret the excision of the category. The terms captured to a large extent the psychosocial implications of the disease and the importance of the unspoken dialogue between patient and caretaker. It is apparent that several of the current DSM-III and DSM-III-R disorders, which are constituents of hysteria that have been reassembled under new labels such as somatoform, eating, and dissociative disorders, contain behaviors that still illustrate this unspoken dialogue. In my opinion, much of what in this century had become part of an essentially psychiatric perspective, namely the meaning behind the symptom, has been abandoned. Currently, the emphasis is on the purely observable and measurable phenomena, which has resulted in the discrediting of the older and more inclusive term "hysteria." Psychodynamic understanding embraced the principle that things are not always what they appear to be nor how they are initially perceived by the patient, an idea implicit in the concept of hysteria. Admittedly not always characterized by precision, "hysteria" was a richer and more three-dimensional term than the current descriptive terms that have displaced it.

Reynolds (1869), in discussing complaints he heard following railway accidents, referred to the importance of the *patient's ideas* in the creation of the clinical picture. Some years later Janet (1901) reemphasized the importance of the "fixed" or strongly held idea to the hysteric. The history of incidents of mass hysteria attest not only to the influence of ideas but to the receptivity of people, and the role of contagion or imitation, all of which are directly attributable to *suggestion, suggestibility,* and the *imagination.* These factors are all surprisingly forceful in that they readily imprison the patient's attention and direct it to his or her own creations. The ideas, suggested or imagined, are not quite the equivalent of delusions, perhaps because they are not usually as permanent, fixed, or incorrigible. It has been assumed that *dissociation*, *denial*, and/or *repression* are among the mental mechanisms facilitating this process, which depends upon the suspension of critical judgment and the diminished influence of counterarguments.

For a deeper understanding of hysteria, it is important to bear in mind that the clinical picture is influenced by cues generated both internally, and by the psychosocial context, that is, by nuances in the *interaction* with others, particularly those conveying expectations. Careful clinicians have long recognized the adverse consequences of leading questions, shared assumptions, or lists of the possible side effects of procedures and new medications. *Thus, in addition to the influence of ideas, suggestibility, and the imagination on the inner experience of the patient, the clinical picture is affected by the nature and determinants of his or her interactions and unspoken dialogue with relevant others. Further, what is pertinent to hysteria should be viewed as of equal importance to our grasp of the dissociative disorders.*

Whereas most observers and writers recognized a demand or manipulative intent in the clinical presentation of hysteria, Merskey (1979) was more compassionate than some in that he suggested that the simplest and best paradigm to explain this disorder which is characterized by an infinite variety of human motives and circumstances is that of the "small child within the adult frame . . . protesting weakness and debility to secure love and affection" (p. 243). He also contended that "hysteric" behaviors are keenly sensitive to the reactions of those who witness them.

DISSOCIATION

The clinical roots of dissociation lie embedded in the history of hypnosis. The lucid sleep or artificial somnambulism described by de Puységur direct our attention to an aspect of the hypnotic experience that is different from the motor, sensory, and convulsive events that developed around the *baquet* under the influence of Mesmer (Kravis, 1988). De Puységur's subject, a young man who served on de Puységur's estate, spoke critically of a member of his family when under the influence of the magnetism, but once awakened failed to remember that he had done so (Ellenberger, 1970). This was taken as evidence that the conscious mind could be disconnected from parts of itself in ways different from simple forgetting, an observation Janet elaborated considerably upon a century later, in his comments on *désagrégation* or dissociation (Janet, 1925/1976). A considerable literature at the turn of the last century (Azam, 1892; James, 1890; Prince, 1914/1921; Sidis & Goodhart, 1905) focused on constructs that "explained" dissociation and its clinical manifestations, which were believed to be dependent on levels and compartments of consciousness. Hysteria, multiple personality disorder

(MPD), and hysterical fugue were at the center of attention. Under Janet's aegis, hysteria and hypnosis were considered to be almost identical, and dissociation the mechanism accountable for both of them. It was postulated that lost or disconnected function and sensation, as well as lost memories, occurred spontaneously in hysteria or were elicited in hypnosis—possible in both circumstances because of a deficiency or weakness in the nervous system to which some individuals were prone. With hysteria, the patients' vulnerability was activated by an external event, usually of a traumatic nature, which paved the way for the dissociative behavior.

Against this backdrop of persuasive postulating about levels and compartments of consciousness, Freud developed his psychoanalytic explanation that hysteria represented an active defense against conflict, which he labeled repression (Freud, 1895/1953). This conceptualization came to eclipse Janet's passive defense theory. The subsequent history on hysteria is both unclear at times and subject to revisionism (Masson, 1985). What is clear, however, is that until the early 1970s the English-speaking Western world focused almost exclusively on the Freudian explanation, with its emphasis on defense mechanisms, with little mention of Janet's dissociation theory. Ellenberger (1970) is probably largely responsible for reintroducing and explaining Janet to those unfamiliar with the French theorist, and for encouraging the academic world to revisit and reexamine the essential differences between the theories of the two men.

While the more recent sequence of events might well be better understood by the historians of the future, it appears to me that the rise of academic interest in hypnosis over the past 30 years has contributed in a major way to an appreciation of its importance (Hilgard, 1965; Orne, 1959). Emphasis on the hypnotic state, as well as on Hilgard neodissociation theory (Hilgard, 1977), also has contributed to the intellectual license that resulted in the emergence of the dissociative disorders in DSM-III. Descriptive psychiatry seized on the elaborated concept of dissociation as if it were a clearly observable sign, or a well-understood symptom.

No account of these developments is complete without acknowledging the importance of Hilgard's views on dissociation. In his book entitled *Divided Consciousness* (1977), he expanded on the idea that multiple controls influence human thought and action. His opening sentences lucidly anticipate his subsequent remarks: "The unity of consciousness is illusory. Man does more than one thing at a time—all the time—and the conscious representation of these actions is never complete" (p. 1). On reexamining turn-of-the-century dissociation theory, which was rooted in psychopathology, Hilgard attempted to develop an updated version, to be taken seriously within general as well as abnormal psychology. The neodissociation concept as he described it thus covered a spectrum of behaviors and experiences from the normal at one end (such as learned skills like typing or bicycle riding), to the abnormal, where painful thoughts, which were concealed from awareness, were viewed as "dissociated" from the person. Although out of conscious awareness, they could still continue to exert an influence on the individual's thoughts and actions. Divided consciousness was seen to be reflected in the way registered experiences or memories were disconnected from consciousness. Hilgard further postulated that the separation or dissociation of the executive or monitoring functions from actions could account for the sense of involuntariness in a hypnotic arm levitation, as well as the uncontrollable, destructive clinical behavior MPD patients deny responsibility or claim amnesia for, or both. The multiple and various manifestations of dissociation supported the view that different levels of hypnotic tasks or achievements, as well as differing clinical behaviors, call for varying degrees of dissociation or dissociative capacity, depending on their level of difficulty or complexity.

Hilgard's careful observations and analyses provided a wealth of opportunity for further investigative studies. However, time functions differently for the intellectual world than it does for the political or pragmatic one. It is generally acknowledged that careful laboratory studies accumulate slowly, and that a clinical field challenged by critics and pressured by the needs of patients outpaces these studies. Hilgard's postulates appear to have been adapted to support the theoretical infrastructure of the dissociative disorders (Spiegel & Cardeña, 1991), which was arbitrarily adopted by the consensus or majority of a committee. In thus extrapolating from and exaggerating a creative concept, clinicians have oversimplified the clinical picture and drawn linear relationships where the realities are considerably more complex. In keeping with Janet's writings of a century ago, trauma, particularly early childhood abuse, has emerged as the major trigger of dissociative disorders, and blame has displaced shame as the predominant modern psychodynamic force.

In 1990, in a review of the history of the use of the term "dissociation," I pointed out that in the clinical arena clarity was conspicuous by its absence (Frankel, 1990). Although the core of dissociative phenomena is fairly readily recognizable with dramatic clinical behavior, as soon as one moves to consider other shades of clinical experience matters become less clear. For example, when considering psychogenic fugues or amnesia, the existence of a disconnection or dissociation seems clear-cut. But when we wander further afield to consider other types of clinical behavior such as phobias or post-traumatic symptoms, influences such as suggestibility, denial, flattened affect, or emotional detachment are deserving of attention. Indeed, the symptoms might well be accounted for by these mental mechanisms, as well as by alterations in attention and perception, motivation, imagination, and memory. In short, it is not at all clear that a dissociative mechanism always plays the central role.

Events in the clinical field over the past decade or more, however, appear to have been propelled by their own momentum. Supported by several publications (Ross, 1989; Herman, 1992), clinicians have claimed for dissociation a large series of observable clinical behaviors and reported experiences that could equally well, if not more persuasively, be explained by other mechanisms. The term has been invoked by clinicians to account for the following at least: (1) the "flashback," that is, a sudden reexperiencing or remembering of a past event, usually in the presence of some observing ego; (2) childlike speech and behavior, for instance, that of a four year old, wherein current adult identity is pushed to the periphery of awareness if not beyond; (3) uncontrollable and destructive behavior for which a person subsequently denies responsibility because she or he has no memory of it— even though in most instances a patient will subsequently admit when questioned sympathetically that he or she might have some guilt related to the behavior; (4) binge eating, and other impulsive or compulsive behaviors; (5) becoming preoccupied with a thought or memory, and staring off into space while in this state; (6) experiencing some limitation in the ability to concentrate or behave purposefully, or feeling a sense of emotional numbness at the time of and during the subsequent days or weeks following a trauma or crisis; (7) experiencing incongruity in how an event is reacted to and the event itself; and (8) degrees of analgesia, muscle weakness, and forgetfulness.

The clinical domain claimed for dissociation has thus broadened, with the term being freely used by both patients and therapists to describe experiences of which many are more usefully attributed to factors such as regression, fantasy-proneness, suggestibility, altered memory, or selective inattention. Furthermore, the term is used to imply that dissociation happens to the individual often precipitously, and that the experience is rarely under his or her control. It has almost assumed the characteristics of demonic possession, or as if consciousness suddenly fell off a precipice. In such instances, little attention is clinically paid to the degrees of the disconnectedness, to alternative explanations, or to the motivations and meanings behind the behavior, other than that it results from the replay of a reaction to childhood trauma.

Although this wide clinical dependence on the term dissociation conveys a sense of understanding or even certainty, we soon gain insight into the unsettled characterization of the mechanism when we turn to the theoretical debate. Janet's original postulate was based on the concept that a deficiency in the personality structure is the prerequisite for dissociation. He thought that a part of the mind separates in the presence or aftermath of emotional trauma, which carries the memory of the trauma with it. The Freudian view that an active defense, repression, is created to remove the conflict or pain from conscious awareness, appears on the surface to be somewhat different. Perhaps the two terms are not that far apart. If we now attribute an active defensive purpose to dissociation, we must logically reevaluate all the commonly invoked defense mechanisms such as isolation, projection, and reaction formation to determine whether and how they might differ from one another and from dissociation. Indeed, Erdelyi (1990) proposed that Freud's defense mechanisms are nothing other than frequent types of reconstructed memories observed in the clinic—the result of both intellective and emotional factors that transform memories not merely into the more reasonable but also into the more palatable. Kihlstrom and Hoyt (1990) pointed out that several theorists of the past have refused to choose between the two terms, dissociation and repression, seeing value and utility as well as vagueness in both concepts. In the past, both seemed necessary to account for memory disturbances in the clinic.

Hilgard (1977), utilizing the topographical model of depth psychology, has described repression as the result of the separation of consciousness by means of a horizontal barrier, and dissociation by means of a vertical barrier. The contents below the horizontal barrier, he contended, can be known only indirectly by their effects on observable behavior. The vertical separation in dissociation interferes with communication between the two sets of consciousness, and the individual operations function in parallel.

In their review of dissociation, Spiegel and Cardeña (1991) emphasized that the apparent automaticity of normal behavior is not the only factor involved in the dissociative disorders; the intentionality of dissociative processes and the concurrent inability to integrate those separated aspects of experience are also important factors. In their review, they referred to dissociation "as involving at least momentarily unbridgeable compartmentalization of experiences" (1991, p. 367). Regarding the issue of underlying intentionality, the curious reader must ponder the degree of voluntariness, that shapes that compartmentalization. This then leads to a major question about the conscious or unconscious nature of the compartmentalization that is seen to account for repression and/or dissociation. Despite the more traditional psychoanalytic view that repression must be unconscious, Erdelyi (1990) made a strong argument for allowing it to be either. It can be unconscious, but is not necessarily totally so. A series of questions arises from this explanation. What is the judgment on dissociation if it is, in fact, different from repression. Can it also take place either at a conscious or unconscious level, and to what extent is selective inattention consciously or unconsciously driven? How should we categorize whistling in the dark? Cognitive events may remain in consciousness fleetingly, to be overtaken by forgetfulness almost immediately. If this has been observed with regard to repression, can it also be associated with dissociation? To what extent does this illuminate the question of responsibility when a nonpsychotic patient's behavior runs out of control, and influence how it should be managed clinically?

The debate deepens as we consider the differences between suppression and repression, such as which is the less unconscious of the two, and what is their relationship. Although we have tended to believe that suppression is conscious and repression generally unconscious, Singer and Sincoff (1990) drew attention to the uncertainties involved in this conclusion, and indicated the considerable need for further study. Furthermore, is dissociation always a defensive strategy, or can it be neutral at times and defensive at others, and is repression a defensive variant of dissociation? If dissociation involves an alteration in the integrative functions of consciousness as well as in identity, does gambling or other addictive behaviors, such as binge eating, that are associated with being out of control belong with the dissociative disorders? Singer and Sincoff raise the interesting question of whether shifts in thought to other fantasy roles provide practice for dissociative behavior. For that matter, at what point does daydreaming become a dissociative disorder, and under what circumstances should it be viewed as primarily regressive rather than involuntarily dissociative? It is apparent that any simple explanation about the true nature of a disconnection between executive control and function, or about any linked processes, in the clinical disorders is likely to be insufficient and when presented as primary, even misleading.

This is well illustrated when one considers involuntariness and responsibility, factors that are important in the clinical management of patients with dissociative-like behaviors, as hinted above. If both dissociation and repression can be either out of conscious awareness or in it, at what point is involuntariness and a lack of responsibility for one's own behavior no longer acceptable? This is especially relevant to the disclaimed, and often negative, activities of the "alters" that present with MPD. Are the clinical behaviors involving dissociation or the compartmentalization of experiences thoroughly involuntary if the underlying mechanism is partially accessible to consciousness? To what extent can they be accounted for by selective inattention? How does the therapist most effectively navigate these shoals? I believe that he or she does so largely by acknowledging the shifting levels of involuntariness, and viewing dissociation as a *metaphor* rather than as a *mechanism*.

With this amount of uncertainty and ambiguity, dissociation appears to deserve only a modest role in explaining clinical behavior, not the important one it has been assigned more recently of being a forceful causal factor. This is reaffirmed by a consideration of hypnosis and its uncertainties, thus far one of the more useful models to help us conceptualize dissociation, and a phenomenon whose acceptability has somehow run parallel to that of dissociation.

HYPNOSIS

Contrary to what many clinicians prefer to believe, the term hypnosis carries a wealth of meanings and implications, some very different from others. Largely because of that, the phenomenon continues to attract accomplished investigators, who are seeking an opportunity to study a range of psychological topics of importance to general psychology. Whatever the most widely accepted definition of the term, which I shall not attempt here, clinical practitioners feel licensed to speak about it and apply hypnotic techniques as if it is a clear-cut entity. They most often utilize an induction procedure within the context of a trusting relationship, and then proceed with the therapy as if the hypnotic trance has occurred as part of a relatively simple and linear process. It should be noted, however, that external psychosocial factors, in addition to intrapsychic ones, are an essential part of the hypnotic event. Furthermore, no one has been able to define with any precision the point at which the "trance" begins. We also know that with many susceptible subjects, formal induction is irrelevant, and that hypnoticlike behaviors can occur without it if certain contextual factors such as a good rapport with the therapist are in place. The broad range of behaviors included in the hypnotic spectrum, such as sensorimotor changes, hallucinations, posthypnotic suggestions and amnesia, to mention some, affirm the multidimensional nature of the phenomenon. Clinical goals include not only relaxation and relief from pain, but also autonomic effects such as relaxed breathing, as well as improved ways of thinking about habits like overeating and smoking. Hilgard (1965) met this challenge by stating that the several distinguishable manifestations are all part of the "domain of hypnosis," and Coe (1992) has recently expanded on the complexities involved in trying to define what hypnosis is.

In moving toward an explanation of the mechanisms underlying the phenomenon, emphasis has been placed on the role of suggestibility as well as on dissociation. Some writers (Weitzenhoffer, 1989; Woody, Bowers, & Oakman, 1992) have tended to consider the more unusual achievements in hypnosis as dependent on dissociation, and the common and perhaps less difficult ones on suggestion. If we focus for a moment on positive hallucinations, it becomes clear that even that analysis is inadequate. Negative hallucinations and analgesia can be theoretically accounted for by a process such as separation, disconnectedness, or dissociation; neither positively hallucinating a tingling feeling in the fingers (which is relatively easy), nor a voice or a person (which is relatively difficult) can be accounted for in that way. In other words, does it make sense that what is disconnected or dissociated can *create* a positive hallucination? Zamansky (personal communication, 1993), who has also pointed out this distinction, draws attention to the lacunae in the constructs assembled thus far to explain the full spectrum of hypnotic behaviors.

Experimental work in recent years has increasingly acknowledged the importance of several mechanisms and forces in influencing hypnotic performance. Suggestibility and dissociation are but two. Imagination, absorption, fantasy and fantasy-proneness, as well as psychosocial factors such as expectations and anticipation are among them (Lynn & Rhue, 1991). Involuntariness is assumed to be a major criterion of hypnotic behavior (Weitzenhoffer, 1989), but this is not consistently true since even reasonably good subjects will oftentimes voluntarily initiate behaviors, which then seem to take on a life of their own (e.g., consider the arm levitation phenomenon).

As stated above, hypnosis provides a useful theoretical model for our understanding of dissociation and suggestibility. This is supported by the finding that patients with clinical symptoms often ascribed primarily to either dissociation or suggestibility, such as MPD, bulimia, and phobic behavior, tend to show high levels of hypnotizability (Frankel, 1990). But it bears repeating that these clinical conditions were placed under the rubric of hysteria a century ago, and persuasively presented by Janet (1925/1976) as the spontaneous equivalents of hypnotic behavior. The articulation of the concepts of dissociation, hysteria, and hypnosis continues to elude us, probably largely because the concepts themselves are imprecise.

SUMMARY

The theoretical perspectives on dissociation discussed above demand that we be more modest in our clinical dependence on the term, and that we avoid the frequent error of oversimplification. For any reasonable understanding of the phenomenon of dissociated identities such as occurs with MPD or psychogenic fugue, one must take into account suggestibility, the imagination, and the meaning of the social communications. Indeed, these factors should command equal if not more attention than that of the separation or dissociation between linked processes. To do otherwise would be comparable to searching for a car key under the nearest street lamp rather than the place where it was dropped, simply because of the light.

Hysteria has given way to dissociation, a concept which derived much of its clinical importance from what we had learned from hypnosis. The dimensions of imagination, suggestibility, and psychosocial influences, to name but a few, appear to be woven into the fabric of both hypnotic behavior and dissociative disorders, and carry us full circle back to the uncertainties surrounding hysteria, which led to its dismissal from DSM-III in the first place. It is apparent that DSM-III and DSM-III-R have not succeeded in eliminating hysteria from our midst even though the term has been banished from the manual; nor has the emphasis on the simplistic notion of trauma-triggered dissociation improved our understanding or treatment of many of the patients previously considered to be suffering from hysteria.

Thus, in taking advantage of the neodissociation construct, our field has been audacious in its reach. Regrettably, DSM-III and DSM-III-R, by diligently replacing hysteria with the dissociative disorders, have failed to take into account the complexities of the clinical picture. Of importance is how this problem will be redressed in the future.

REFERENCES

American Psychiatric Association. (1980). *Diagnostic and statistical manual of mental disorders* (3rd ed.). Washington, DC: Author.

American Psychiatric Association. (1987). *Diagnostic and statistical manual of mental disorders* (3rd ed., rev.). Washington, DC: Author.

Azam, E. (1892). Double consciousness. In D. Tuke (Ed.), *A dictionary of psychological medicine* (pp. 401–406). Philadelphia: Blakiston.

Chodoff, P. (1974). The diagnosis of hysteria: An overview. *American Journal of Psychiatry, 131,* 1073–1078.

Chodoff, P. (1978). Psychotherapy of the hysterical personality disorder. *Journal of the American Academy of Psychoanalysis, 6,* 497–510.

Coe, W. C. (1992). Hypnosis: Wherefore art thou? *International Journal of Clinical and Experimental Hypnosis, 40,* 219–237.

Ellenberger, H. (1970). *The discovery of the unconscious.* New York: Basic Books.

Erdelyi, M. H. (1990). Repression, reconstruction, and defense: History and integration of the psychoanalytic and experimental frameworks. In J. L. Singer (Ed.), *Repression and dissociation: Implications for personality theory, psychopathology and health* (pp. 1–31). Chicago: University of Chicago Press.

Ey, H. (1982). History and analysis of the concept. In A. Roy (Ed.), *Hysteria* (pp. 3–19). New York: John Wiley.

Frankel, F. H. (1990). Hypnotizability and dissociation. *American Journal of Psychiatry, 147,* 823–829.

Freud, S. (1953). Studies on hysteria. In J. Strachey (Ed. and Trans.), *The standard edition of the complete psychological works of Sigmund Freud* (Vol. 2, p. 23). London: Hogarth Press. (Original work published 1895)

Herman, J. L. (1992). *Trauma and recovery USA.* New York: Basic Books.

Hilgard, E. R. (1965). *Hypnotic susceptibility.* New York: Harcourt, Brace & World.

Hilgard, E. R. (1973). Dissociation revisited. In M. Henle, J. Jaynes, & J. J. Sullivan (Eds.), *Historical conceptions of psychology* (pp. 205–219). New York: Springer.

Hilgard, E. R. (1977). *Divided consciousness: Multiple controls in human thought and action.* New York: John Wiley.

Hyler, S. E., & Spitzer, R. L. (1978). Hysteria split asunder. *American Journal of Psychiatry, 135,* 1500–1504.

James, W. (1890). *Principles of psychology.* New York: Henry Holt.

Janet, P. (1901). *The mental state of hystericals* (C. R. Carson, Trans.). New York: Putnam.

Janet, P. (1976). *Psychological healing.* New York: Arno Press. (Original work published 1925)

Kendell, R. E. (1982). A new look at hysteria. In A. Roy (Ed.), *Hysteria* (pp. 27–36). New York: John Wiley.

Kihlstrom, J. F., & Hoyt, I. P. (1990). Repression, dissociation, and hypnosis. In J. L. Singer (Ed.), *Repression and dissociation: Implications for personality theory, psychopathology and health* (pp. 181–208). Chicago: University of Chicago Press.

Kravis, N. M. (1988). James Braid's psychophysiology: A turning point in the history of dynamic psychiatry. *American Journal of Psychiatry, 145*, 1191–1206.

Lewis, A. (1982). The survival of hysteria. In A. Roy (Ed.), *Hysteria* (pp. 21–26). New York: John Wiley.

Lynn, S. J., & Rhue, J. W. (1991). An integrative model of hypnosis. In S. J. Lynn & J. W. Rhue (Eds.), *Theories of hypnosis: Current models and perspectives* (pp. 397–438). New York: Guilford Press.

Masson, J. M. (1985). *The complete letters of Sigmund Freud to Wilhelm Fliess 1887–1904.* Cambridge: The Belknap Press of Harvard University Press.

Merskey, H. (1979). *The analysis of hysteria.* London: Baillière Tindall.

Micale, M. S. (1990). Hysteria and its historiography: The future perspective. *History of Psychiatry, 1*, 33–124.

Orne, M. T. (1959). The nature of hypnosis: Artifact and essence. *Journal of Abnormal and Social Psychology, 58*, 277–299.

Prince, M. (1921). *The unconscious: The fundamentals of human personality normal and abnormal* (2nd ed.) New York: Macmillan. (Original work published 1914)

Reynolds, J. R. (1869). Remarks on paralysis and other disorders of motion and sensation dependent on idea. *British Medical Journal, 2*, 483–485.

Ross, C. (1989). *Multiple personality disorder: Diagnosis, clinical features, and treatment.* New York: John Wiley.

Roy, A. (Ed.). (1982). *Hysteria.* New York: John Wiley.

Sidis, B., & Goodhart, S. P. (1905). *Multiple personality: An experimental investigation into the nature of human individuality.* New York: Appleton.

Singer, J. L., & Sincoff, J. B. (1990). Summary chapter: Beyond repression and the defenses. In J. L. Singer (Ed.), *Repression and dissociation: Implications for personality theory psychopathology and health* (pp. 471–496). Chicago: University of Chicago Press.

Slavney, P. R. (1990). *Perspectives on hysteria.* Baltimore: Johns Hopkins University Press.

Spiegel, D., & Cardeña, E. (1991). Disintegrated experience: The dissociative disorders revisited. *Journal of Abnormal Psychology, 100*, 366–378.

Symonds, C. (1970). Hysteria (Appendix C). In H. Merskey (Ed.), *The analysis of hysteria* (pp. 258–265). London: Baillière Tindall.

Weitzenhoffer, A. M. (1989). *The practice of hypnotism* (Vols. 1 & 2). New York: John Wiley.

Wilson, M. (1993). DSM-III and the transformation of American psychiatry: A history. *American Journal of Psychiatry, 150*, 399–410.

Woody, E. Z., Bowers K. S., & Oakman, J. M. (1992). A conceptual analysis of hypnotic responsiveness: Experience, individual differences, and context. In E. Fromm & M. R. Nash (Eds.), *Contemporary hypnosis research* (pp. 3–33). New York: Guilford Press.

5

Toward a Psychobiological Model of Dissociation and Post-Traumatic Stress Disorder

Peter Brown

The controversy surrounding the wider clinical acceptance of the dissociative disorders stems, in part, from the absence of external validating criteria that can reliably establish the presence of the disorder outside of the clinical interview (cf. Bowers, 1991). The identification of biological markers, which may predict vulnerability for the development of a disorder ("trait" markers) or accompany the onset of the disorder ("state" markers), is important in defining nosological boundaries and may ultimately be useful in identifying underlying brain mechanisms. It seems timely, therefore, to review the potential models of cerebral function and dysfunction in dissociative states in an attempt to establish which research strategies might prove to be the most profitable. The relatively few direct studies of brain function in dissociative disorders only serves to underline the complexity of the problem (Spiegel, 1991; Putnam, 1991). However, we can examine evidence from two related areas: (1) the psychophysiological studies of post-traumatic stress disorder (PTSD), which can serve as the beginning of an understanding of the way in which the brain adapts to psychological trauma; and (2) clinical studies of the similarities and differences between temporal lobe epilepsy and dissociation. Ultimately, an approach that integrates psychological and biological models offers the best opportunity to understand the nature of dissociation.

POST-TRAUMATIC STRESS DISORDER
AND DISSOCIATION

A steady accumulation of data over the past decade has suggested a strong association between childhood physical and sexual abuse and the subsequent development of dissociation (Sanders, McRoberts, & Tollefson, 1989; Sanders & Giolas, 1991; Terr, 1991). As a result of the growing popularity of this etiological model, interest has focused on how psychological trauma may produce subsequent prolonged effects on brain function. This focus leads us to consider the applicability of the model of PTSD to the understanding of dissociation.

Post-Traumatic Stress Disorder

DSM-III-R organizes the symptoms of PTSD around three dimensions of stress response: (1) the reexperiencing of intrusive images and feelings surrounding the trauma, (2) a general numbing of responsiveness through emotional blunting, avoidance, or amnesia, and (3) an altered state of physiological arousal (Brett, Spitzer, & Williams, 1988). The symptoms' patterns alternate in two phases. In the denial phase, patients experience restricted cognition and fantasy, memory disturbances, emotional numbing, withdrawal from social interactions, and a general inhibition in many areas of behavior (Krystal, 1984; Horowitz, 1986). In contrast, during the intrusive phase, the person may be flooded by vivid nightmares, waking fantasies, overwhelming fear, and preoccupation with reenacting or reliving aspects of the experience. There is an impressive body of neurobiologic research related to each of the dimensions of PTSD (Krystal et al., 1989; ver Ellen & van Kammen, 1990; Jones & Barlow, 1990; Pitman, 1993).

There is also strong suggestive evidence of an association between PTSD and dissociation (Brett, 1985). In patients with PTSD dissociative symptoms, including decreased concentration and level of functioning, unexplained chronic pain, episodes of amnesia or confusion, emotional numbing, and "flashbacks" (brief, vivid hallucinations of the traumatic situation) are common (Benedikt & Kolb, 1986; Horowitz, 1986; Spiegel, Frischholz, Spiegel, et al., 1989). For example, in a sample of 180 women with PTSD, there was a high frequency of visual (57%), auditory (31%), and tactile (29%) flashbacks (Resnick, Kilpatrick, & Lipovsky, 1990). Such hallucinations occur more frequently with patients who score highly on scales of vividness of mental imagery and on impact of the event (Bernstein & Putnam, 1986). PTSD patients report significantly higher levels of dissociative symptoms than do matched controls both at the time of the original trauma and subsequently (Bremner, Southwick, Brett, et al., 1992; Bremner, Steinberg, Southwick, et al., 1993b). Finally, patients seeking treatment for combat-related PTSD report significantly higher rates of childhood physical abuse than do veterans without PTSD, suggesting that psychological trauma may increase an individual's vulnerability to subsequent traumatic events (Bremner, Southwick, Johnson, et al., 1993a).

Neurochemical Changes in Post-Traumatic Stress Disorder

Catecholamines

The catecholamines norepinephrine, epinephrine, and dopamine are chemical messengers that are released in response to stress as part of the "fright, fight, or flight" response both within the brain itself and, via the peripheral nervous system, throughout the rest of the body (Snyder, 1985). Brain function can be studied indirectly by measuring (1) the blood or urinary levels of these substances and their metabolites, (2) changes in receptor number and activity on circulating white blood cells or platelets (Nutt, & Lawson, 1992), or (3) the resultant alterations in autonomic nervous system (ANS) activity as reflected by physiological measures of arousal such as increases in heart rate, blood pressure, respiratory rate, muscle tension, skin conductance, and changes in electroencephalographic (EEG) rhythm (Kolb, 1987; van der Kolk, Greenberg, & Boyd, 1985). Newer brain imaging techniques will eventually provide a more direct way of studying activity within the living brain. Most studies of PTSD patients have examined the following three different aspects of arousal:

1. *Baseline studies*: Most studies have reported elevations of baseline measures of heart rate, systolic blood pressure, and forehead electromyograph (EMG; Dobbs, 1960; Blanchard, Kolb, & Pallmeyer, 1982; Blanchard, Kolb, & Gerardi, et al., 1986; Pitman, Orr, Forgue, et al., 1987). These changes are associated with slightly higher resting levels of plasma and urinary catecholamines (Hamner & Diamond, 1990a; McFall, Murburg, Veith, et al., 1990) and their metabolites (Giller, Koster, Wahby, et al., 1989; Kosten, Mason, Giller, et al., 1987; Krystal, Kosten, Southwick, et al., 1989; Southwick, Yehudi, Perry, et al., 1990; Yehuda, Southwick, Giller, et al., 1992). Changes in plasma catecholamines and their metabolites in response to exercise are also different when compared to controls (Hamner et al., 1990b). Yehuda and coworkers reported that higher urinary excretion levels of dopamine and norepinephrine were correlated with severity of PTSD symptoms in general and the intrusive symptoms in particular (1992).

2. *Pharmacological studies*: PTSD patients show greater increases in heart rate, blood pressure, and anxiety than do controls following the administration of epinephrine (Pitman et al., 1987). In the brain, norepinephrine release is regulated by negative feedback from alpha-2 receptors (Hyman,

1988). In controls, administration of the alpha-2 receptor antagonist yohimbine results in mild stimulation, whereas PTSD patients experience anxiety, panic attacks and dissociative experiences including flashbacks and increased norepinephrine turnover (Krystal, Southwick, & Charney, 1990; Southwick, Krystal, Morgan, et al., 1993). PTSD patients have a 40% decrease in the platelet alpha-2 receptors on platelets when compared with controls, and a fourfold greater "down regulation" or decrease in sensitivity to norepinephrine compared with controls (Perry, Southwick, & Giller, 1989; Perry, 1990). (In contrast, patients with major depression show increased binding activity or "up regulation.") Also in keeping with alterations in catecholamine function, the platelet monoamine oxidase (MAO; the principle peripheral enzyme involved in catecholamine metabolism) is found in lower levels in PTSD patients (Davidson, Lipper, Kilts, et al., 1985; Lerer, Ebstein, Shestatsky, et al., 1987). In addition to the increased norepinephrine levels and reduced receptor activity, impaired transduction of the signal across the cell membrane by the adenylate cyclase system, associated with beta-adrenergic receptors in platelets and lymphocytes, is found in PTSD (Lerer, Bleich, Solomon, et al., 1990). Giller and coworkers (Giller, Perry, Southwick, et al., 1990) suggest that such changes may reflect a noradrenergic system both more sensitive to, and less able to "damp down," input. The net result appears to be a heightened response to stimuli and difficulty in maintaining consistent levels of arousal.

3. *Responses to specific stimuli*: The physiological changes that accompany PTSD most prominently reveal themselves in response to cues that recall the stressful events. Vietnam veterans who are exposed to violent films or audiotapes of combat sounds, or who have accounts of their own combat experiences read back to them, show higher levels of arousal than do controls (McFall, et al., 1990; Pitman, et al., 1987; van der Kolk et al., 1985; van der Kolk, Pitman, Orr, et al., 1989). These changes include increases in blood pressure, heart rate, and emotional lability, and peripheral blood levels of epinephrine (Murburg, McFall, Veith, et al., 1990) and norepinephrine (Blanchard, Kolb, Prins, et al., 1991). Desensitization for specific imagery will result in the normalization of the responses but the new learning does not easily extend to related imagery, suggesting a deficit in the ability to generalize (Shalev, Orr, & Pitman, 1992b).

"PTSD develops out of a complex interaction between biological and psychological predispositions, the occurrence of stressful events alarms, the development of anxiety, and the adequacy of coping strategies and social support" (Jones & Barlow, 1990, p. 324). Krystal et al. (1989) notes similarities between the symptoms (including altered baseline levels of arousal, learned alarm responses to specific stimuli, disturbances in memory regulation, and reduction of arousal avoidance behavior) of PTSD and the "learned helplessness" syndrome that follows exposure to inescapable shock (IS) in animals. The noradrenergic system plays an important role in tuning the level of arousal to facilitate learning and to integrate internal and external cues, and appears to be activated in response to threat (Sara, 1985). Most noradrenergic neurons originate in the locus coeruleus, a center in the brain stem involved in activating both brain and body (or both central and peripheral) changes in arousal. Massive increases in the activity of these pathways in IS results in increased baseline levels of arousal, increased startle responses, and behavioral "freezing." Persistent changes in arousal and behavior are the result of alterations in the "second messenger" system, including cyclic adenosine $3',5'$ monophosphate (cAMP), which result in changes in the structure and number of synaptic connections. In mammals, such structural changes in the hippocampus and amygdala are associated with memory consolidation, conditioned fear responses, increased sensitization to subsequent stressors, and a resistance of fear to extinction with new learning (Charney, Deutch, Krystal, et al., 1993).

Kolb (1987) suggests that these neurochemical changes result in instabilities in maintaining arousal and a bias in perception and information processing, which prevents habituation (the ability to adapt to new stimuli) in both PTSD and IS. PTSD patients experience a pattern of chronic changes in their levels of arousal, which narrows attention, produces pervasive distortions in the processing of related information, and reinforces patterns of avoidance. This combination paradoxically ensures that related stimuli will continue to trigger the alarm response through a combination of reduced sensitivity to unrelated cues and heightened responses to specific stimuli (Kramer, Kinney, & Schoen, 1989). The flashbacks and panic symptoms that follow lactate infusion in subjects with PTSD suggest that the level of arousal serves as a cue for state related intrusive imagery and anxiety symptoms (Rainey, Aleem, Ortiz, et al., 1987). Changes in the level of arousal are paralleled by disturbances in orienting responses, difficulties in maintaining the level of sleep, with longer REM periods, a greater REM density, and a greater variance in REM latency (the time between falling asleep and the onset of the first REM episode), supporting the notion of a central disturbance in attentional processes and level of arousal (R. J. Ross et al., 1989; Ross, Ball, Dinges et al., 1990).

The PTSD patients show significantly greater eye-blink reflex EMG response (a component of the startle reaction) amplitudes at intermediate levels of acoustic stimulation (Butler, Braff, Rausch, et al., 1990). When the stimuli were increased the differences were nonsignificant. In addition to supporting the notion of hypervigilance and a lowered threshold in PTSD, the authors suggest that such changes in startle reflex may be related to the dissociative symptoms and altered sense of self and of reality experienced by some PTSD patients. PTSD patients also show greater eye-blink, gal-vanic skin response (GSR), and heart-rate responses than patients with anxi-ety disorders, suggesting that the changes are not simply related to the coincident level of arousal (Shalev, Orr, Peri, et al., 1992a).

Corticosteroids

The systems that ordinarily dampen the prolonged effects of increased cate-cholamine levels are impaired with PTSD. The 24-hour urinary cortisol excretion levels (which increase during acute stress) are chronically reduced with PTSD (Mason, Giller, Kosten, et al., 1986; Southwick et al., 1990; Yehuda, Southwick, Nussbaum, et al., 1990). In animals, severe or pro-longed uncontrollable trauma gradually depletes corticosteroid and cat-echolamine responses and hypersensitizes the animal to subsequent expo-sure through kindling (changes in response threshold) (MacIntyre & Edson, 1982). In humans, low urinary cortisol may be related to denial, emotional blunting, or other attempts to minimize the intensity of intrusive imagery or affect (Mason, Kosten, Southwick, et al., 1990). The combination of high norepinephrine and low cortisol levels distinguishes individuals with PTSD from those with other psychiatric diagnoses (Giller et al., 1989; Mason et al., 1990).

Patients with PTSD will also show a greater than normal suppression of cortisol to dexamethasone, in contrast to about 40% of patients with major depression, who show a failure of normal suppression (Yehuda, South-wick, Krystal, et al., 1993). These findings support the notion of a distinc-tive disregulation of cortisol release in PTSD patients (Yehuda et al., 1993). This is supported by evidence that PTSD patients show alterations in the system that regulates cortisal levels despite having normal cortisol responses (Smith, Davidson, Ritchie, et al., 1989) and decreased beta-endorphin levels (Hoffman 1989). PTSD patients have an increased greater number of cor-tisol receptors on circulating lymphocytes (Mason et al., 1986; Southwick et al., 1990; Yehuda, Lowy, Southwick, et al., 1991). The number of lym-phocytes glucocorticoid receptors is strongly correlated with the number of glucocorticoid receptors in the CNS, particularly in the hippocampus. Yehuda and coworkers also found that the increase was strongly associated with the degree of anxiety. While the average PTSD patient has a lower than average baseline of cortisol, increased cortisol activity is found when some patients are experiencing a marked increase in intrusive symptoms (Mason et al., 1990). Thus PTSD patients may show both reduced baseline levels of cortisol and exaggerated responses to ACTH or emotional stimuli, suggesting a chronic alteration in cortisol regulation (Mason et al., 1990). Given the link between lowered cortisol levels and the use of denial and emotional blunting, and increased levels with anxiety and intrusive symptoms in PTSD, it would seem important to determine whether a connection exists between the use of dissociation as a defense mechanism and persistently lowered cortisol levels in dissociative-disordered patients as well.

We are accustomed to thinking about the value of the acute stress response in mobilizing the individual. However, the benefits of prolonged responses to severe or chronic stressors are less certain. These responses may be related to protective maneuvers that modify attention (e.g., dissociation), cognition (e.g., denial or repression), behavior (e.g., withdrawal), affect (emotional numbing), and sensation (analgesia). Emotional numbing may be particularly related to an absence of response to positive events, and is associated with difficulties in concentration, complaints of fatigue, and a lack of emotional involvement in the patient's surroundings (Litz, 1992). Biologically, emotional numbing may be related to catecholamine depletion as a result of hyperreactivity to conditioned stimuli, behavioral constriction (with the consequent loss of curiosity and involvement resulting in a further dampening of responses), immunosuppression, and analgesia related to the release of endogenous opioids during conditioned fear responses (Pitman et al., 1990; van der Kolk et al., 1985; van der Kolk, 1987). The model of stress-related analgesia may be relevant in understanding these phenomena.

Stress-Induced Analgesia and Endogenous Opiates

Pain sensitivity is an important variable in determining animals' response to stress (Lewis, Cannon & Liebeskind, 1980; Lewis, 1986). Stress-induced analgesia in experimental animals appears to be mediated by endogenous opioids (Akil, 1985) and can be blocked by the administration of the opioid antagonist naloxone (Calcagnetti, Helmstetter, & Fanselow, 1987). In humans, stress-induced analgesia is heightened by the belief that the stress is uncontrollable (Bandura, Cioffi, Taylor, et al., 1988; Foa, Zinbarg, & Rothbaum, 1992). Observing that a similar lack of control over disturbing imagery distinguishes PTSD patients from controls, Pitman and his coworkers (Pitman et al., 1990) compared the pain responses of eight Vietnam veterans with PTSD with those of eight controls, following either neutral or combat videotapes. After seeing the combat videotape, the PTSD patients showed a 30% decrease in pain intensity ratings in response to a standardized heat source. This decrease disappeared when naloxone was administered. In another study, almost 1/3 of a sample of PTSD patients reported significant decreases in pain responses following naxloxone administration (van der Kolk et al., 1989). PTSD patients also display greater elevations of serum levels of beta-endorphin when exercising than do controls (Hamner, Hitri, & Appelbaum, 1989). In light of recent findings that analgesic response may be a component of the acute dissociative response (Cardeña & Spiegel 1993), it would be of great interest to examine the analgesic response of MPD patients following reexposure to pertinent stimuli. Reduction of the analgesic response might also provide a quantitative measure of the effectiveness of the therapeutic "working through" of traumatic material.

Opiate release may be related to a decreased response to pain, which at the same time reinforces disturbances in arousal. Similarities between chronic PTSD and narcotic withdrawal suggest opioid depletion affects in PTSD patients (van der Kolk et al., 1985). An attempt to raise endogenous opioid levels may account for the need of many PTSD patients to overstimulate themselves. Periods of heightened arousal, increased sensitivity to specific stimuli, and the phasic reexperiencing of trauma-related imagery alternating with emotional numbing and the development of dissociative symptoms might be associated with a persistent imbalance between the systems that regulate both the catecholamines and the endogenous opiates (Burges, Watson, Hoffman, & Wilson, 1988; Spiegel, Hunt, Dondershine, 1988). A biological dynamic instability appears to underlie the psychological changes, in which heightened activity in the noradrenergic systems of the hippocampus and amygdala (Margulies, 1985) is accompanied by surges in endogenous opiate release during reexposure to traumatic situations (Friedman 1988; van der Kolk et al., 1985; van der Kolk, 1989). This brief storm is followed by periods of emotional numbing in which amine and opioid depletion are accompanied by parasympathetic dominance (van der Kolk et al., 1985).

There is evidence for linking specific hormonal patterns with both enduring coping styles and transient emotional states with overall symptomatology. Mason and his coworkers (Mason et al., 1990) report a combination of both abnormally high and abnormally low hormonal levels when a number of neuroendocrine variables are measured simultaneously, with both significantly lower levels of cortisol and higher levels of norepinephrine, epinephrine, testosterone, and thyroxine in PTSD patients when compared with other patients. Acute elevations of epinephrine and norepinephrine in response to stressful experiences are typically associated with elevations of cortisol and the lowering of testosterone levels. Lowered testosterone levels are often seen in actively stressful situations, particularly with individuals who have high preexisting levels of anxiety, hostility, or depression (Mason et al., 1990). Elevated testosterone levels may be associated with repressed anger, a sense of mastery, impulsivity, suspicion, and general aggression, but the relationships are not simple ones (Mason et al., 1986, 1990).

A divergence of epinephrine and norepinephrine levels may occur in response to particular aspects of stress. High norepinephrine levels have been associated with sustained alertness, feelings of competence and coping in response to acute stress, and the expression of angry feelings, violent fantasies, or overtly aggressive behavior (so-called "anger out") (Mason et al., 1990). Increased norepinephrine levels are also associated with feelings of competence and coping. There may be an inverse relationship between overall severity of symptomatology and norepinephrine levels in PTSD. High levels of epinephrine are associated with uncertainty and ambiguity (Frankenhauser & Lundsberg, 1985) and self-critical or passive behavior (so-called "anger in"), and are found to be more common in suicidal patients (Ostroff, Giller, Bonese, et al., 1982). The older studies on anger and its "direction" had many methodological problems but recent work, particularly in the areas of anger and hypertension, suggests that the results of the former studies could be extended. It would be of interest to compare baseline hormonal patterns with changes to them that occur during episodes of dissociation. In particular, differences in the feeling tones of various "alters" (e.g., paranoid, aggressive, fearful, or submissive) could reasonably be expected to show significant differences in the norepinephrine/epinephrine ratio and cortisol and testosterone levels as part of their overall "personalities" or coping styles.

There is a great deal of individual variability for any single physiological response, while the presence of an overall pattern of disturbed response appears to be constant. Consequently, evaluating multiple measures of different variables with multivariant analysis is critical. Combining a variety of responses appears to dramatically increase the accuracy of discriminating patients from controls. For example, the hormonal profile can be used to improve the differential diagnosis of PTSD. With several samples of patients, a single hormone correctly identified 60% of the PTSD patients, the norepinephrine/cortisol ratio identified 78%, and when three or more of the hormones were used in stepwise discriminant analysis, 95% of the PTSD patients were correctly identified (Mason et al. 1986, 1990).

A further example involves one of the few studies that includes male and female civilian PTSD patients. Shalev and coworkers (Shaler, Orr, & Pitman, 1993) read scripts of the traumatic event to 26 subjects who had been previously exposed to a major trauma (half of the subjects had consequent PTSD while the other half did not). Multivariate analysis revealed that the composite physiological response (including heart rate, EMG, and skin conductants) was significantly greater for the PTSD group. Overall, the female PTSD subjects responded to imagery for the personal traumatic events far more strongly than the male subjects did (about 1/3 higher). These findings were very similar to those found with combat veterans. Interestingly, and perhaps significantly from a therapeutic point of view, the PTSD group also showed significantly greater reductions of skin conductance during positive imagery.

The Response to Trauma and Dissociation

Current attempts to understand PTSD have emphasized an information processing model, wherein the features of the post-traumatic syndrome consist of an attempt to integrate and assimilate the experience with preexisting models of self and the world (Horowitz, 1986). Bioinformational theory postulates that the experience of a trauma results in the formation of a coherent memory network, which changes the threshold of arousal and serves to maintain an increased vigilance for cues related to the trauma (Creamer, Burgess, & Pattison, 1992; Foa et al., 1992). PTSD symptoms such as arousal, feelings of vulnerability and loss of control, intrusive images and thoughts, flashbacks and nightmares, result from the product of activation of the memory structure by stimuli that resemble the original trauma. Periods of intrusive imagery with very high levels of arousal may lead to the consolidation of the experience and prompt the avoidance of reminders of the trauma while emotional and cognitive blinking can be seen as a temporary way of limiting the distress. Psychobiologic healing may involve a blend of both aspects. Trauma can be processed during a manageable reexperiencing so that levels of arousal are reduced while new information is presented so that the memory structure can be altered.

Reviewing the evidence that suggests that these phases of high arousal may be associated with the enhancement of learning and memory, Rossi compared the phenomenon of state-dependent learning to both traumatic dissociation and therapeutic hypnosis (Rossi & Cheek 1988). Intrusive memories, feelings, and flashbacks can be conceptualized as state-bound patterns of information, that are released whenever arousal reaches a certain critical level. This would account not only for the vividness of intrusive imagery and affect at certain times but also for the way in which such material can emerge in subsequent periods of arousal. This model also parsimoniously accounts for the frequency of both affective disturbance and somatic symptoms (either as the direct consequence of ANS disturbance or as a physical reexperiencing of the intrusion of traumatic memories), and for the decreased threshold for subsequent dissociation (Spiegel et al., 1989).

Integration occurs in stages in which reexperiencing alternates with self-protective blunting mechanisms. Psychobiological studies are helping in the reformulation of the significance of these two stages and their relation to dissociation. In a series of six cases, hypnotically induced traumatic imagery of events was associated with increased left-sided electrodermal responses (reflecting increased right hemisphere activity), while emotional blunting was related to decreased left-sided electrodermal responses, suggesting differential hemispheric activation in PTSD in each of the two stages, which may account for the phasic alternation (Brende, 1982). The ultimate goal of these repeating cycles is both to reduce the distress that results from the trauma and to achieve a new equilibrium. Emotional blunting, amnesia, avoidance, and dissociation are seen as attempts to modulate the consequences of both the trauma and the subsequent reexperiencing of it. Similarly, the intrusion of imagery and affect related to the trauma represent either a further assault or a gradual reintegration, depending on both the intensity and the meaning of the experience for the individual. Dissociation, typically with attendant amnesia, and alteration of perceptions, cognitive style, and behavior, may thus be conceptualized as both a protective mechanism and an intermediate or transitional step between these two extremes and a coming to terms with the traumatic event (Horowitz, 1986). In this sense, dissociation may be analogous to Rothenberg's (1988) study of creative processing in which two images with strong and competing emotional valences are briefly linked by the brain, resulting in a transient, unstable intermediate step toward creative resolution.

The treatment process, whether for combat veteran or incest victim, extends beyond the clinical setting to involve the attitude of society toward the patient (Wilson, 1989). Many cultures effectively support the treatment process by prescribing not only cognitive restructuring and emotional support, but highly patterned rituals for altering the veteran or victim's level of arousal (Wilson, 1989). Rossi (1982) has proposed that hypnosis and dissociation are similar in structure to the spontaneous ultradian rhythms in cognition, affect, and behavior that occur on a regular rhythm of between 90 and 120 minutes. These rhythms appear to be important not only in regulating physiological function but in promoting constructive daydreaming, problem solving, and emotionally positive personal experiences (Brown 1991a, 1991b). These processes allow not only for the deconditioning of the traumatic responses but for a resynchronization at both the physiological and social levels.

These "tuning and attuning" influences on attention and learning appear to be mediated by biogenic amine and opiate pathways, which connect to temporal lobe and limbic structures. In particular, the hippocampus and amygdala are highly responsive to contextual cues and appear to be altered by ongoing learning (Brown, 1991a, 1991b). From this perspective, the widespread use of ritual to recognize and modulate possession states may also be a cultural attempt at using spontaneous dissociative phenomena in the service of the individual and the society (Frecska & Kulscar, 1989). It also prompts us to consider in further detail the neurological pathways that may be involved in dissociation.

CEREBRAL FUNCTION AND DISSOCIATION

The standard EEG records the spontaneous fluctuations in voltage of the entire brain as they are recorded from the surface leads. The inherent difficulties of establishing a normal range due to the large interindividual variation, variations in inter-rater agreement, the presence of artifact (such as eye movements), the difficulty in localizing abnormal foci, the relative inaccessibility of deep structures, and the sheer mass of electrical activity being recorded, all make interpretation of EEG results notoriously difficult (Kohrman, Sugioka, Huttenlocher, et al., 1989; McNamara, 1991; Ray, 1990; Spencer, 1988; Williams, Luders, Brickner, et al., 1985). Despite all of the limitations, the standard EEG is highly stable in a particular individual over time and offers the possibility of an ongoing record of brain activity that is as yet without parallel (Ray, 1991). Computer-enhanced EEG analysis provides us with one answer to the problem of separating critical features from background activity (Ray, 1990). A wide variety of techniques have been used to improve the utility of the EEG, including specialized leads, the surgical implantation of electrodes for depth recordings, topographical EEG mapping, magnetoencephalography, brain electrical activity mapping (BEAM), dipole localization, and ambulatory cassette EEG (McNamara, 1991). In addition, as adjuncts to the EEG, there are a number of new technologies, including regional cerebral blood flow studies, computerized axial tomography (CAT scan), positron emission tomography, nuclear magnetic resonance, electron spin resonance, and impedance imaging, which may eventually be of a great value in studying brain function (Ray, 1990).

Perhaps the most widely used enhancement of EEG technology is the study of event-related potentials, in which a barrage of stimuli (typically auditory or visual) are used to evoke potentials (electrical changes) in the EEG (Coles, Gratton, & Fabiari, 1990). These specific patterns show us time-related changes in the brain in preparation for, or in response to particular events, allowing us to study the ways in which attention is focused, sensory channels process information, and responses change with new information. In other words, the patterns reveal how cognitive resources are allocated. Further, evoked potentials have the advantage of being highly specific to particular stimuli.

With these caveats in mind, it is possible to understand the difficulties in interpreting the results of studies of brain activity in dissociation. EEG studies in this area have revolved around two key questions: (1) does a relationship exist between dissociative symptoms and temporal lobe epilepsy (TLE), and (2) can distinctive features be discerned in the EEG when a MPD subject is either at rest or in the process of "switching" from one personality to another?

Complex Partial Seizures (Temporal Lobe Epilepsy)

Complex partial seizures, particularly those involving temporal limbic structures, are a poorly understood and difficult to diagnose collection of brain dysfunctions (McNamara, 1987). The temporal lobe is composed of several functionally distinct regions that integrate the functions of a number of cortical and subcortical structures (Mesulam, 1985). The temporal lobes are highly vulnerable to a variety of physical traumas, including hypoxia, mild head injury, viral infection, and cerebral vascular accident (McNamara, 1987). Moreover, the temporal lobes normally exert a strong inhibitory effect on one another and damage of one is likely to produce dysfunctions in both (McNamara, 1991).

Dissociation and complex partial seizures may share certain neurophysiological or neuroanatomical features without sharing a common etiology. Patients with TLE frequently report transient episodes of disorientation, amnesia, and dramatic behavioral and emotional changes (Tucker, Price, Johnson, et al., 1986). Schenk and Bear (1981) reported that 12 of 23 female TLE patients demonstrated dissociative symptoms, which had developed after the onset of the seizure disorder. Similarly, Mesulam (1981) described 12 cases involving multiple personality or delusions of possession that were shown to have clinical and EEG manifestations of TLE.

A history of seizures does appear to occur more frequently with MPD than might otherwise be expected. In a careful descriptive study of EEG recordings of six MPD patients with epilepsy, Devinsky and his colleagues (Devinsky, Putnam, Grafman, et al., 1989) reported a very high instance of additional nonspecific abnormalities independent of seizure activity. Coons also found that a greater than expected number of patients with dissociative disorders have been reported to have EEG abnormalities, and TLE or other seizure disorders (1988). However, there appears to be little diagnostic overlap between carefully diagnosed populations. Ross and coworkers (C. A. Ross, Heber, Anderson, et al., 1989) demonstrated that MPD patients could be clearly distinguished from patients with complex partial seizures or a neurological control group when carefully standardized diagnostic instruments are used. While TLE and dissociation are two distinct diagnostic phenomena, there still may be important clues to learn with regard to clinical features, anatomical localization, and risk factors for the development of a dissociative disorder. In medicine, it is not unusual for two different illnesses that affect the same organ systems to have many of the same signs and symptoms.

Signs of temporal lobe dysfunction may exist in the absence of a complex partial seizure diagnosis. In a study of 414 university students, Persinger and Makarec (1992) found a strong association between complex partial epileptic signs and reports of "paranormal" experiences as well as distinctive cognitive styles, certain personality attributes, and levels of anxiety. Ross and Persinger (1987) have reported a positive correlation between frequency of temporal lobe symptoms and hypnotic susceptibility. Reports of memory of previously unrecognized trauma in hypnosis may be more common in individuals with neuropsychological dysfunction in the frontal, parietal, and right temporal hemispheres (Persinger, 1992).

Persinger (1983) has postulated that a proportion of the population may exhibit a "sensory–limbic, hyper-connection syndrome," in which physical or psychological stressors exacerbate electrical instabilities within the hippocampal and amygdala structures that regulate attention and concentration. A continuum of sensitivity would account for the clinical pictures ranging from the large number of individuals who only show transient symptoms briefly following a stressor to a small percentage with a greater temporal lobe lability who show more severe symptoms over a prolonged course. Indeed there may be an association between temporal dysfunction and the development of PTSD, further implicating the temporal lobes in some individuals' response to trauma (Persinger, 1992). While there is little evidence to suggest a one-to-one link between dissociation and TLE, future EEG studies should include a focus on temporal lobe activity. A reliable physiological marker of distinctive states of mind would be enormously useful both in understanding the mechanisms involved and also in further studying the variety of cognitive-behavioral and emotional phenomena that are observed clinically. Studies of brain function in dissociation has not yet established the existence of such a marker.

The Neurophysiology of Multiple Personality Disorder and Dissociation

While there have been at least 15 reports of EEG results in MPD, most of these have been case studies that lack adequate controls (Coons, 1988). To date there is neither consistent evidence for a distinctive EEG abnormality in MPD patients (trait) nor for a shift in EEG activity (state) when a patient experiences a "shift" between personalities. The substantial differences in alpha activity occurring with the switch from one personality to another initially reported are nonspecific and may be related to level of alertness (Cocores, Bender, & McBride, 1984), task demands, subject expectancies, muscle tension, or artifact produced by movement during the study (Coons, Milstein, & Marley, 1982).

Similar reservations can be made concerning the relatively few reports of cerebral blood flow, GSR, evoked potentials, EMG, and brain mapping (Bahnson & Smith, 1975; Brende, 1982; Hughes, Kuhlman, Fichtner, et al., 1990; Larmore, Ludwig, & Cain, 1977; Ludwig, Brandsma, Wilbur, et al., 1972). Change in personality state was associated with increased blood flow to the right temporal lobe in one MPD patient when compared with three controls (Mathew, Jack, & West, 1985).

The rapidly growing focus on evoked potentials appears to be a promising approach to the study of dissociative phenomena. Evoked potentials may be more sensitive to relatively subtle shifts in attention and may tell us more about differences in information processing strategies than the power spectrum EEGs have done (Coles et al., 1990; Spiegel, 1991). There are five published reports of evoked potential studies in MPD on a cumulative total of only five subjects. Larmore and colleagues (Lamore et al., 1977) and Ludwig and coworkers (Ludwig et al., 1972) reported differences in latency and amplitude of the early components of visual evoked responses across various states, Coons and colleagues (Coons et al., 1982) reported no differences in two patients when compared with a control, and Putnam (1984) reported equivocal results. In his study of cerebral evoked potential responses to visual stimuli in 10 patients compared to simulating controls, Putnam reported differences with respect to both the amplitude and the latency of the responses, suggesting a more durable and innate difference than those found in the case reports (1984).

Therapeutic integration in MPD has also been associated with change in the pattern of evoked potentials. Braun (1983) presented strikingly different topographical maps of visual evoked potentials for a patient with MPD prior to and following treatment. However, methodological limitations prevent any conclusions as to whether the reported changes are related to the effects of treatment or result from difficulties in standardizing the technique, intra-individual variation, or other causes (Braun, 1983). Thus, while there is some evidence of neurophysiological alterations with MPD, the intriguing studies to date are too small and too limited methodologically to provide any conclusions.

There are reports of autonomical dysfunction in MPD patients, as well as an altered threshold for arousal. Bahnson and Smith (1975) reported dramatic changes in respiratory and heart rates, accompanying the switch process in an MPD patient. While case reports have suggested evidence of state specific asymmetries in autonomic activity (Brende, 1984), the only controlled study failed to confirm the finding. Putnam and coworkers (Putnam, Zahn, & Post, 1990) compared the psychophysiological responses of nine MPD patients with five simulating subjects. Eight of the nine patients and three of the five controls were able to produce physiologically distinct responses.

There have been reports of differences with a variety of measures of visual function in MPD patients. Further, MPD patients do appear to be more variable in these responses than do matched controls. In a pair of carefully designed studies of visual changes in a total of 30 MPD patients and matched simulating controls, Miller and coworkers (Miller, 1989; Miller,

Blackburn, et al., 1991) reported a variety of changes in visual acuity, refraction, visual fields, and eye-muscle balance that the simulating patients did not demonstrate. These are some of the best designed studies to date but our limited knowledge of how the brain controls visual function makes interpretation of these findings difficult.

DISCUSSION

While the studies that have been done allow for only the barest of outlines, that outline does suggest a way of exploring the underlying biological processes in dissociation. There are two specific lines of inquiry that appear to be particularly promising: the evidence for the localization of brain function with regard to the regulation of attention and the integration of affect, memory, and behavior in the temporal–limbic structures; and the possible value of the psychophysiological markers found in PTSD to a study of the dissociative disorders.

Methodologically sound studies are required to examine the neurology of dissociation. Measures of cerebral blood flow, electroencephalographic studies, and the use of modern brain imaging techniques may all eventually be useful. Of particular importance is the need to establish whether or not patients with dissociative disorders show a significant difference in brain function when compared with normal controls during hypnotically induced or spontaneous dissociative states (so-called "state" markers, which can reliably identify dissociation). Similarly, studies are needed to determine whether patients with a propensity for dissociation can be neurologically distinguished from controls in those time periods between dissociative episodes (so-called "trait" markers, which can indicate an underlying vulnerability) (Lerer et al., 1990). The relationship between such markers and validated measures of dissociation, hypnotizability, absorption, or intensity of mental imagery may ultimately be useful in the identification of an underlying common vulnerability across the variety of dissociative diagnoses.

While the new technologies of brain imaging are still in their infancy, they are already capable of identifying changes in cerebral blood flow related to relatively subtle changes in cognitive (Volkow & Tancredi, 1991) or emotional (Pardo, Pardo, & Raichle, 1993) states. However, the core of psychobiological research in dissociation for the near future will continue to be based on established techniques such as evoked potentials, the power spectrum EEG (with specialized leads), and blood samples of neuroendocrine variables. Perhaps the most important priority is not more elaborate technology but a continued refinement of research questions and methodological issues for the effective use of existing techniques.

The second issue is the possible link between the psychophysiological

alterations found in PTSD and the development of dissociation. If dissociative phenomena are related to the alternating stages of intrusion and
avoidance, then it is not unreasonable to expect that dissociative patients
will show many of the biological changes which differentiate PTSD patients
from controls. In particular, the altered regulation of catecholamine, endogenous opioids, and cortisol release have been implicated. The alterations
appear to be reflected not only in changes in baseline neurochemical levels,
but even more so in the response of these systems to specific pharmacological or psychological challenges. Evidence for altered physiological function
in PTSD has played an important part in establishing the validity of the
diagnostic criteria in the minds of most clinicians. Similar studies may help
in defining the boundaries of dissociative disorders and testing the validity of the diagnosis. Further work is also needed to chart the change from
the acute reaction to trauma to its possible long-term consequences. In order
to separate out these differences, studies not only of adult populations but
of children who have been exposed to trauma are of particular importance.
Given the nature of the instabilities that have been reported, more specific
psychophysiological and psychopharmacological challenges (to further
measure the response of the various systems to subsequent stresses) will be
of particular interest.

   The study of the response to trauma allows us to begin to create a bridge
between biological and psychological models. We are beginning to understand that significant trauma represents a special case of learning, in which
chemicals are produced and, eventually, in which structural changes take
place in the brain. Learning not only alters behavior, it can also result in
structural changes in the synaptic connections of neuronal circuits (Kissin,
1986). A growing body of evidence implicates temporolimbic structures,
particularly the amygdala–hippocampus in the regulation of attention,
memory, emotion, and autonomic activity. This system integrates information from all of these sources and plays an important role in the allocation of cognitive resources in problem solving (Brown, 1991a; Gray 1990).
It appears that stressors, by activating the high neuroendocrine and neurotransmitter levels, can "reset" the system so that subsequent behavior is
changed (Sapolsky, 1990). Thus, long-lasting changes in responsivity are
the result of self-perpetuating circuits that can strengthen themselves with
a subsequent reexposure (Charney et al., 1993; Post, 1992). The "psycho-
endocrine window" provides us with a way of studying these changes.

   Mason and colleagues (1990) have summarized the overall consensus
in the field as follows:

> A number of guiding principles have emerged from basic psychoendocrine
> research in the past 30 years which indicate how hormone levels may be
> helpful in the study of psychological and social aspects of stress. Some ex-

amples of these principles are: (a) many hormonal systems are keenly sensitive to both acute and chronic social and psychological influences; (b) the social environment can exert a "tonicity" effect upon basal hormonal levels in a continuing background fashion; (c) hormonal levels can undergo phasic adaptations in relation to prolonged, severe stress exposure; (d) hormonal levels are related not only to emotional or state changes, but also to trait and cognitive variables, including the style, organization and effectiveness of defensive and coping mechanisms; (e) there is a bidirectional relationship between the brain and hormones the later being capable of reflecting as well as modulating psychological mechanisms; and (f) different hormones are linked in a specific way with different and distinctive sets of psychological dimensions. (p. 1823)

In measuring psychophysiological variables, we have to be cautious in interpreting the results. In addition to often having only sketchy information as to what constitutes the "normal" range and the way in which these variables may change over time in the general population, there is also an important question with regard to interpretation. An abnormal result may be related to a specific disorder either directly (as an etiological factor) or indirectly as a marker of severity, chronicity, or an associated disorder (e.g., when PTSD is associated with alcohol or drug abuse), or may be related to treatment (e.g., receptor changes that are related to prolonged sedative or antidepressant use). Comorbidity is also an important and underrecognized issue. Because of the potential overlap with other psychiatric disorders, it is essential that dissociative-patient populations be carefully characterized with standardized diagnostic interviews to identify the existence of other psychiatric diagnoses (including anxiety and depressive disorders, alcoholism, personality disorders, and substance abuse) if biological variables are to be studied. In all of these cases, it is necessary to have longitudinal studies with designs that include appropriate control groups in order that the results be interpreted properly.

Diagnostic issues in both PTSD and dissociation are related to questions of vulnerability and prevalence. For example, in a survey of 1,400 women, the frequency of PTSD was far lower than one might expect given the number who reported exposure to a significant trauma (Cottler, Compton, Mager, et al., 1992). Attempts to explain why all those who are exposed to trauma are not at equal risk have focused on the interaction between the type or severity of the stress or on a vulnerability, possibly related to previous stressors, in the individuals who developed the disorder (Jones & Barlow, 1990). In animals, the response to exposure to stress has been found to be influenced by previous exposure to stress, as well as whether the stress is escapable or inescapable (Foa et al., 1992). This would suggest that both a history of previous exposure to stress and the degree to which the stress is perceived as being controllable are critical for the development of the disorder. In humans, children and adolescents who have been abused physically or sexually demonstrated higher baseline heart rates and blood pressures and down-regulated alpha-2 receptors, which were similar to findings from studies on adult PTSD patients (Perry, 1990). Furthermore, women with a history of childhood sexual abuse have significantly blunted cortisol and prolactin responses to intravenous clomipramine challenge (Corrigan, Garbutt, Gillette, et al., 1990), suggesting that the biological fingerprint of trauma may indeed persist for decades.

Transient dissociative symptoms such as alterations in cognition, memory, somatic sensation, distortions of time, and feelings of depersonalization and derealization may be more frequent than has been appreciated in populations exposed to a significant stress such as a natural disaster. Following the San Francisco earthquake of October 1989, a population of university students reported significantly more dissociative symptoms 1 month after the event than 4 months after (Cardeña & Spiegel, 1993). Cardeña and Spiegel suggest that further epidemiological studies of baseline rates of dissociation within the general population and of the identification of particular populations (e.g., the highly hypnotizable, children, individuals with a previous history of exposure to trauma or abuse) will be useful in understanding the scope of dissociation. The suggestion is an important one. Most of the studies to date have focused on MPD because of the assumption that this represents the prototype of dissociative disorders. In fact, by focusing on one end of the continuum, we may run the risk of getting a distorted view of dissociative processes. Dissociative responses to natural disasters, major stressors, and the general calamities of life may give us a clearer vision of the uncomplicated natural history of dissociation.

Unfortunately, disasters are only all too frequent in the life of humankind, and so we are presented with the possibility of studying the populations affected by these calamities both to learn more about dissociation and, hopefully, to enable us to ameliorate distress. The natural history of a traumatized patient is a series of repeated stresses as the pain of the original trauma is reevoked by subsequent events. Intrusive imagery, associated cues, anniversaries, and the general vicissitudes of life can all have a measurable impact. Even treatment programs, such as admission to an inpatient unit or regular psychotherapy (or even the testing conditions in a study), are likely to produce measurable changes in the system insofar as memory of the original event is activated.

All of the models reviewed suggest that the specific deficits associated with trauma are most likely to be in evidence when patients are reexperiencing memories and/or hyperaroused states associated with the trauma. Reexposing patients to the trauma (albeit in a progressively more manageable way) is a critical component of any therapeutic approach. Desensitization and exposure appears to reduce both emotional distress and physiological responses to traumatic imagery (Foa et al., 1992; Shalev, Orr, & Pitman, 1992). Consequently, studies of patients during therapy with longitudinal repeat of measures, would appear to be both a humane and effective way of examining not only dissociative symptoms but the natural history of their resolution. Neurobiological approaches may contribute significantly to improving our diagnostic and therapeutic capacities as the therapeutic milieu provides the opportunity to observe the great natural experiment in the self-healing capacities of the human mind.

The study of the psychobiology of dissociation is in its infancy, but it can avoid some of the "developmental delays" that other growing fields have encountered. A careful consideration of the methodological issues is paramount. At this stage, a single carefully designed study is infinitely more important than any number of intriguing but flawed reports. Similarly, there is an urgent need for investigators in the field to coordinate their efforts and agree upon general lines of approach so that results from different studies can be legitimately compared. There is no area of brain research that has progressed without this kind of consensus. To this end, there needs to be agreement about technical standardization (e.g., EEG leads) and testing procedures, sample selection, length of follow-up, study methodology (e.g., repeat measures and counterbalanced designs), and decisions as to appropriate controls. Population differences, gender effects, practice effects, and a host of other potentially confounding variables must be addressed. For example, many psychoendocrine studies in PTSD have involved male Vietnam veterans admitted to an inpatient unit while the majority of patients with dissociative disorders are female outpatients.

Despite their inherent difficulties, psychophysiological studies promise a number of advantages. Such studies may well be able to ultimately establish a neurophysiological basis for the clinical observation of dissociative disorders, and resolve the interminable, and largely sterile, dispute between believers and skeptics. By providing external validating criteria, psychophysiological measures can define the extent and nature of this continuum of disorders and help to refine diagnosis and treatment issues. Conversely, the study of dissociation is a two-way street. Further elucidation of the neural substrate of dissociation may also increase our understanding of memory, of the selection of perceptual and cognitive strategies and, for clinicians, that most important question of the nature of the individual's response to psychological trauma.

REFERENCES

Akil, H., Young, E., Walker, J. M., et al. (1985). The many possible roles of opioids and related peptides in stress-induced analgesia. *Annals of the New York Academy of Sciences, 467,* 140–153.

Bahnson, C. B., & Smith, K. (1975). Autonomic changes in a multiple personality patient. *Psychosomatic Medicine 37*, 85–86.

Bandura, A., Cioffi, D., Taylor, C. B., et al. (1988). Perceived self-efficacy in coping with cognitive stressors and opioid activation. *Journal of Personality and Social Psychology, 55*, 479–488.

Benedikt, R. A., & Kolb, L. C. (1986). Preliminary findings on chronic pain and post-traumatic stress disorder. *American Journal of Psychiatry, 143*, 908–910.

Bernstein, E. M., & Putnam, F. W. (1986). Development, reliability, and validity of a dissociation scale. *Journal of Nervous and Mental Disease, 174*, 727–735.

Blanchard, E., Kolb, L., Gerardi, R. J., et al. (1986). Cardiac response to relevant stimuli as an adjunctive tool for diagnosing post-traumatic stress disorder in Vietnam veterans. *Behavior Therapy, 17*, 592–606.

Blanchard, E., Kolb, L., Pallmeyer, T., et al. (1982). The development of a psychophysiological assessment procedure for post-traumatic stress disorder in Vietnam veterans. *Psychiatric Quarterly, 54*, 220–229.

Blanchard, E. B., Kolb, L. C., Prins, A., et al. (1991). Changes in plasma norepinephrine to combat-related stimuli among Vietnam Veterans with posttraumatic stress disorder. *Journal of Nervous and Mental Disease, 179*(6), 371–373.

Bowers, K. S. (1991). Dissociation in hypnosis and multiple personality disorder. *International Journal of Clinical and Experimental Hypnosis, 31*(3), 155–176.

Braun, B. G. (1983). Neurophysiologic changes in multiple personality due to integration: A preliminary report. *American Journal of Clinical Hypnosis, 26*, 84–92.

Bremner, J. D., Southwick, S., Brett, E., et al. (1992, March). Dissociation and posttraumatic stress disorder in Vietnam combat veterans. *American Journal of Psychiatry, 149*(3), 328–332.

Bremner, J. D., Southwick, S. M., Johnson, D. R., et al. (1993a, February). Childhood physical abuse and combat-related posttraumatic stress disorder in Vietnam veterans. *American Journal of Psychiatry, 150*(2), 235–239.

Bremner, J. D., Steinberg, M., Southwick, S. M., et al. (1993b, July). Use of the structured clinical interview for DSM-IV dissociative disorders for systematic assessment of dissociative symptoms in posttraumatic stress disorder. *American Journal of Psychiatry, 150*(7), 1011–1014.

Brende, J. O. (1982). Electrodermal responses in post-traumatic syndromes: A pilot study of cerebral hemisphere functioning in Vietnam veterans. *Journal of Nervous and Mental Disease, 170*, 352–361.

Brende, J. O. (1984). An educational-therapeutic group for drug and alcohol abusing combat veterans. *Journal of Contemporary Psychotherapy, 14*, 122–136.

Brett, E. A., & Ostroff, R. (1985, April). Imagery and post-traumatic stress disorder: An overview. *American Journal of Psychiatry, 142*(2), 417–424.

Brett, E. A., Spitzer, R. L., & Williams, J. B. W. (1988). DSM-III-R criteria for post-traumatic stress disorder. *American Journal of Psychiatry, 145*, 1232–1236.

Brown, P. (1991a). *The hypnotic brain: Hypnotherapy and social communication.* New Haven, CT: Yale University Press.

Brown, P. (1991b). Ultradian rhythms of cerebral function and hypnosis. *British Journal of Experimental and Clinical Hypnosis, 8*(1), 17–24.

Brown, D. P., & Fromm, E. (1986). *Hypnotherapy and hypnoanalysis.* Hillsdale, NJ: Lawrence Erlbaum.

Burges, P., Watson, I. P., Hoffman, L., & Wilson, G. V. (1988). The neuropsychiatry of post-traumatic stress disorder. *British Journal of Psychiatry, 152*, 164–173.

Butler, R. W., Braff, D. L., Rausch, J. L., et al. (1990). Physiological evidence of exaggerated startle response in a subgroup of Vietnam veterans with combat-related PTSD. *American Journal of Psychiatry, 147*, 1308–1312.

Calcagnetti, D. J., Helmstetter, F. J., & Fanselow, M. S. (1987). Quaternary naltrexone reveals the central mediation of conditional opioid analgesia. *Pharmacology, Biochemistry and Behavior, 27*, 1529–1531.

Cardeña, E., & Spiegel, D. (1993, March). Dissociative reactions to the San Francisco Bay area earthquake of 1989. *American Journal of Psychiatry, 150*(3), 474–478.

Charney, D. S., Deutch, A. Y., Krystal, J. H., et al. (1993, April). Psychobiologic mechanisms of posttraumatic stress disorder. *Archives of General Psychiatry, 50*, 294–305.

Cocores, J. A., Bender, A. L., & McBride, E. (1984). Multiple personality, seizure disorder, and the electroencephalogram. *Journal of Nervous and Mental Disease, 172*(7), 436–438.

Coles, M. G. H., Gratton, G., & Fabiani, M. (1990). Event-related brain potentials. In J. T. Cacioppo & L. G. Tassinary (Eds.), *Principles of psychophysiology: Physical, social and inferential elements* (pp. 413–455). New York: Cambridge University Press.

Coons, P. M. (1988, March). Psychophysiological aspects of multiple personality disorder: A review. *Dissociation, 1*(1), 47–53.

Coons, P. M., Milstein, V., & Marley, C. (1982). EEG studies of two multiple personalities and a control. *Archives of General Psychiatry, 39*, 823–825.

Corrigan, M. H., Garbutt, J. C., & Gillette, G. M., et al. (1990, May). *Serotonin and victims of childhood sexual abuse.* Paper presented at the annual meeting of the American Psychiatric Association, New York.

Cottler, L. B., Compton, W. M., Mager, D., et al. (1992). Posttraumatic stress disorder among substance users from the general population. *American Journal of Psychiatry, 149*, 664–670.

Creamer, M., Burgess, P., & Pattison, P. (1990). Cognitive processing in post-trauma reactions: Some preliminary findings. *Psychological Medicine, 20*, 597–604.

Creamer, M., Burgess, P., & Pattison, P. (1992). Reaction to trauma: A cognitive processing model. *Journal of Abnormal Psychology, 101*(3), 452–459.

Davidson, J., Lipper, S., Kilts, C. D., et al. (1985). Platelet MAO activity in posttraumatic stress disorder. *American Journal of Psychiatry, 142*(11), 1341–1343.

Devinsky, O., Putnam, F. W., Grafman, J., et al. (1989). Dissociative states and epilepsy. *Neurology, 39*, 835–840.

Dobbs, D., & Wilson, W. P. (1960). Observations on persistence of war neurosis. *Diseases of the Nervous System, 21*, 686–691.

Dobkin de Rios, M., & Winkelman, M. (1989). Shamanism and altered states of consciousness: An introduction. *Journal of Psychoactive Drugs, 21*, 1–7.

Dunn, G. E., Paolo, A. M., Ryan, J. J., et al. (1993, July). Dissociative symptoms in a substance abuse population. *American Journal of Psychiatry, 150*(7), 1043–1047.

Field, T. (1985). Attachment as psychobiological attunement: Being on the same wavelength. In M. Reite & T. Field (Eds.), *The psychobiology of attachment and separation* (pp. 415–454). New York: Academic Press.

Foa, E. B., Zinbarg, R., & Rothbaum, B. O. (1992). Uncontrollability and unpredictability in post-traumatic stress disorder: An animal model. *Psychology Bulletin, 112*(2), 218–238.

Frankenhaeuser, M., & Lundsberg, U. (1985). Sympathetic-adrenal and pituitary-adrenal response to challenge. In P. Pichot, P. Berner, R. Wolf & K. Thau (Eds.), *Psychiatry* (Vol. 2, pp. 699–704). London: Plenum Press.

Frecska, E., & Kulcsar, Z. (1989). Social bonding in the modulation of the physiology of ritual trance. *Ethos, 17*, 70–87.

Friedman, M. J. (1988). Toward rational pharmacotherapy for post-traumatic stress disorder: An interim report. *American Journal of Psychiatry, 145*, 281–285.

Giller, E. L., Kosten, T. R., Wahby, V., et al. (1989, May). *Psychoendocrinology of PTSD.* Paper presented at the annual meeting of the American Psychiatric Association, San Francisco.

Giller, E. L., Perry, B. D., Southwick, S., et al. (1990). Psychoendocrinology of post-traumatic stress disorder. In M. E. Wolf & A. D. Mosnaim (Eds.), *Posttraumatic stress disorder: Etiology, phenomenology, and treatment* (pp. 158–169). Washington, DC: American Psychiatric Press.

Gray, T. S. (1990). Limbic pathways and neurotransmitters as mediators of autonomic and neuroendocrine responses to stress: The amygdala. In M. Brown, G. Koob, & C. Rivier (Eds.), *Stress neurobiology and neuroendocrinology* (pp. 73–89). New York: Dekker.

Halbreich, U., Olympia, J., Carson, S., et al. (1989). Hypothalamo–pituitary–adrenal activity in endogenously depressed post-traumatic stress disorder patients. *Psychoneuroendocrinology, 14*, 365–370.

Hamner, M. B., & Diamond, B. I. (1990a, May). *Elevated plasma dopamine levels in PTSD.* Paper presented at the annual meeting of the American Psychiatric Association, New York.

Hamner, M. B., Diamond, B. I., & Hitri, A. (1990b, May). *Plasma catecholamine response to exercise in PTSD.* Paper presented at the annual meeting of the American Psychiatric Association, New York.

Hamner, M. B., Hitri, A., & Appelbaum, B. (1989, May). *Plasma beta-endorphins in PTSD.* Paper presented at the annual meeting of the American Psychiatric Association, San Francisco.

Herbert, W. (1983). The three brains of Eve: EEG data. *Science, 121*, 356.

Hofer, M. A. (1984). Relationships as regulators: A psychobiologic perspective on bereavement. *Psychosomatic Medicine, 46*, 183–197.

Hoffman, L., Burges-Watson, P., Wilson, G., & Montgomery, J. (1989). Low plasma bendorphin in posttraumatic stress disorder. *Australian and New Zealand Journal of Psychiatry, 23*, 269–277.

Horowitz, M. J. (1986). *Stress response syndromes* (2nd ed.). Northvale, NJ: Jason Aronson.

Hughes, J., Kuhlman, D., Fichtner, C., et al. (1990). *Clinical Electroencephalography, 21*(4), 200–209.

Hyman, S. E. (1988). Recent developments in neurobiology: Part II. Neurotransmitter receptors and psychopharmacology. *Psychosomatics, 29*, 254–263.

Jones, J. C., & Barlow, D. H. (1990). The etiology of post-traumatic stress disorder. *Clinical Psychology Review, 10*, 299–328.

Kissin, B. (1986). *Psychobiology of human behaviour: Vol.1. Conscious and unconscious programs in the brain.* New York: Plenum Medical Book Company.

Kohrman, M. H., Sugioka, C., Huttenlocher, P. R., et al. (1989). Inter-versus intra-subject variance in topographic mapping of the electroencephalogram. *Clinical Electroencephalography, 20,* 248–253.

Kolb, L. C. (1987). A neuropsychological hypothesis explaining post-traumatic stress disorders. *American Journal of Psychiatry, 144,* 989–995.

Kosten, T. R., Mason, J. W., Giller, E. L., et al. (1987). Sustained urinary norepinephrine and epinephrine elevation in posttraumatic stress disorder. *Psychoneuroendocrinology, 12,* 13–20.

Kramer, M., Kinney, L., & Schoen, L. S. (1989, May). *Vigilance during sleep in PTSD.* Paper presented at the annual meeting of the American Psychiatric Association, San Francisco.

Krystal, H. (1984). Psychoanalytic views on human emotional damages. In B. A. van der Kolk (Ed.), *Post-traumatic stress disorder: Psychological and biological sequelae* (pp. 2–28). Washington, DC: American Psychiatric Press.

Krystal, J. H., Kosten, T. R., Southwick, S., et al. (1989). Neurobiological aspects of PTSD: Review of clinical and preclinical studies. *Behavior Therapy, 20,* 177–198.

Krystal, J. H., Southwick, S. M., & Charney, D. S. (1990, May). *Yohimbine effects in PTSD patients.* Paper presented at the annual meeting of the American Psychiatric Association, New York.

Kudler, H., Davidson, J., Meador, K., et al. (1987). The DST and posttraumatic stress disorder. *American Journal of Psychiatry, 144,* 1068–1071.

Larmore, K., Ludwig, A. M., Cain, R. L. (1977). Multiple personality: An objective case study. *British Journal of Psychiatry, 131,* 35–40.

Lerer, B., Bleich, A., Solomon, Z., et al. (1990). Platelet adenylate cyclase activity as a possible biologic marker for posttraumatic stress disorder. In M. E. Wolf & A. D. Mosnaim (Eds.), *Post-traumatic stress disorder: Etiology, phenomenology, and treatment* (pp. 148–157). Washington, DC: American Psychiatric Press.

Lerer, B., Ebstein, R. P., Shestatsky, M., et al. (1987). Cyclic AMP signal transduction in post-traumatic stress disorder. *American Journal of Psychiatry, 144,* 1324–1326.

Lewis, J. W. (1986). Multiple neurochemical and hormonal mechanisms of stress-induced analgesia. *Annals of the New York Academy of Sciences, 467,* 194–204.

Lewis, J. W., Cannon, J. T., & Liebeskind, J. C. (1980). Opioid and nonopioid mechanisms of stress analgesia. *Science, 208,* 623–625.

Linn, L. (1985). Clinical manifestations of psychiatric disorders. In H. I. Kaplan & B. J. Sadock (Eds.), *Comprehensive textbook of psychiatry* (4th ed., Vol. 4, pp. 550–590). Baltimore: Williams and Wilkins, 1985.

Lipper, J., Davidson, J. R., Grady, T. A., et al. (1986). Preliminary study of carbamezepine in posttraumatic stress disorder. *Psychosomatics, 27,* 849–854.

Litz, B. T. (1992). Emotional numbing in combat-related post-traumatic stress disorder: A critical review and reformulation. *Clinical Psychology Review, 12,* 417–432.

Ludwig, A. M., Brandsma, J. M., Wilbur, C. R., et al. (1972). The objective study of a multiple personality: Or are four heads better than one? *Archives of General Psychiatry, 26,* 298–310.

MacIntyre, D., & Edson, N. (1982). Effect of norepinephrine depletion on dorsal hippocampus kindling in rats. *Exploratory Neurology, 77*, 700–704.

Maier, S. F. (1986). Stressor controllability and stress-induced analgesia. In D. D. Kelly (Ed.), *Stress-induced analgesia: Annals of the New York Academy of Sciences* (Vol. 467, pp. 55–72). New York: New York Academy of Sciences.

Margulies, D. M. (1985). Selective attention and the brain: A hypothesis concerning the hippocampalventral striatal axis, the mediation of selective attention, and the pathogenesis of attentional disorders. *Medical Hypotheses, 18*, 221–264.

Mason, J. W., Giller, E. L., Kosten, T. R., et al. (1986). Urinary free-cortisol levels in post-traumatic stress disorder patients. *Journal of Nervous and Mental Disease, 174*, 145–149.

Mason, J. W., Kosten, T. R., Southwick, S. M., et al. (1990). The use of psycho-endocrine strategies in post-traumatic stress disorder. *Journal of Applied Social Psychology, 20*(21), 1822–1846.

Mathew, R. J., Jack, R. A., & West, W. S. (1985, April). Regional cerebral blood flow in a patient with multiple personality. *American Journal of Psychiatry, 142*(4), 504–505.

Mathew, R. J., Weinman, M. L., & Barr, D. L. (1984). Personality and regional cerebral blood flow. *British Journal of Psychiatry, 144*, 529–532.

McFall, M. E., Murburg, M. M., Veith, R. C., et al. (1990, May). *Psychophysiologic investigations of PTSD*. Paper presented at the annual meeting of the American Psychiatric Association, New York.

McNamara, M. E. (1987). Neurology. In A. Stoudemire & B. S. Fogel (Eds.), *Principles of medical psychiatry* (pp. 521–552). Orlando, FL: Grune and Stratton.

McNamara, M. E. (1991). Advances in EEG-based diagnostic technologies. In A. Stoudemire & B. S. Fogel (Eds.), *Medical psychiatric practice* (pp. 163–189). Washington, DC: American Psychiatric Press.

Mesulam, M.-M. (1981). Dissociative states with abnormal temporal lobe EEG: Multiple personality and the illusion of possession. *Archives of Neurology, 38*, 176–181.

Mesulam, M.-M. (Ed.). (1985). *Principles of behavioral neurology*. Philadelphia: F. A. Davis Company.

Miller, S. D. (1989). Optical differences in cases of multiple personality disorder. *Journal of Nervous and Mental Disease, 177*, 480–486.

Miller, S. D., Blackburn, T., et al. (1991). Optical differences in cases of multiple personality disorder: A second look. *Journal of Nervous and Mental Disease, 179*, 132–135.

Murburg, M. M., McFall, M. E., Veith, R. C., et al. (1990, May). *Plasma catecholamine response to stressors in PTSD*. Paper presented at the annual meeting of the American Psychiatric Association, New York.

Nutt, D., & Lawson, C. (1992). A neurochemical overview of models and mechanisms. *British Journal of Psychiatry, 160*, 165–178.

Ostroff, R. B., Giller, E., Bonese, K., et al. (1982). Neuroendocrine risk factors of suicidal behavior. *American Journal of Psychiatry, 139*, 1323–1325.

Ostroff, R. B., Giller, E., Harkness, L., et al. (1985). The norepinephrine/epinephrine ratio in suicide attempters. *American Journal of Psychiatry, 142*, 224–227.

Panksepp, J., Siviy, S. M., & Normansell, L. A. (1985). Brain opioids and social emotions. In M. Reite & T. Field (Eds.), *The psychobiology of attachment and separation* (pp. 3–49). New York: Academic Press.

Pardo, J. V., Pardo, P. J., & Raichle, M. E. (1993, May). Neural correlates of self-induced dysphoria. *American Journal of Psychiatry, 150*(5), 713–719.

Perry, B. D. (1990, May). *Adrenergic receptors in child and adolescent PTSD.* Paper presented at the annual meeting of the American Psychiatric Association, New York.

Perry, B. D., Southwick, S., & Giller, E. J. (1989). Adrenergic receptor regulation in PTSD. In E. L. Giller (Ed.), *Biological assessment and treatment in PTSD* (pp. 87–114). Washington, DC: American Psychiatric Press.

Persinger, M. A. (1983). Religious and mystical experiences as artifacts of temporal lobe function: A general hypothesis. *Perceptual and Motor Skills, 57*, 1255–1262.

Persinger, M. A. (1992). Neuropsychological profiles of adults who report "sudden remembering" of early childhood memories: Implications for claims of sex abuse and alien visitation/abduction experiences. *Perceptual and Motor Skills, 75*, 259–266.

Persinger, M. A., & Makarec, K. (1986). Temporal lobe epileptic signs and correlative behaviors displayed by normal populations. *Journal of General Psychology, 114*(2), 179–195.

Persinger, M. A., & Makarec, K. (1992). The feeling of a presence and verbal meaningfulness in context of temporal lobe function: Factor analytic verification of the muses? *Brain and Cognition, 20*, 217–226.

Pitman, R. K., Orr, S. P., Forgue, D. F., et al. (1987). Psychophysiologic assessment of post-traumatic stress disorder imagery in Vietnam combat veterans. *Archives of General Psychiatry, 44*, 970–975.

Pitman, R. K., van der Kolk, B. A., Orr, S. P., et al. (1990). Naloxone-reversible analgesic response to combat-related stimuli in post-traumatic stress disorder: A pilot study. *Archives of General Psychiatry, 47*, 541–544.

Pitman, R. K., Orr, S. P., van der Kolk, B. A., et al. (1990). Analgesia: A new dependent variable for the biological study of posttraumatic stress disorder. In M. E. Wolf & A. D. Mosnaim (Eds.), *Posttraumatic stress disorder: Etiology, phenomenology, and treatment* (pp. 140–147). Washington, DC: American Psychiatric Press.

Pitman, R. (1993). Biological findings in posttraumatic stress disorder: Implications for DSM-IV classification in posttraumatic stress disorder. In J. Davidson & E. Foa (Eds.), *Posttraumatic stress disorder: DSM-IV and beyond* (pp. 173–190). Washington, DC: American Psychiatric Press.

Post, R. M. (1992, August). Transduction of psychosocial stress into the neurobiology of recurrent affective disorder. *American Journal of Psychiatry, 149*(8), 999–1010.

Putnam, F. W. (1984, March). The psychophysiologic investigation of multiple personality disorder: A review. *Psychiatric Clinics of North America, 7*(1), 31–39.

Putnam, F. W. (1991). Dissociative phenomena. In A. Tasman & S. M. Goldfinger (Eds.), *American Psychiatric Press review of psychiatry* (pp. 145–160). Washington, DC: American Psychiatric Press.

Putnam, F. W., Zahn, T. P., & Post, R. M. (1990). Differential autonomic nervous system activity in multiple personality disorder. *Psychiatry Research, 31*, 251–260.

Rainey, J. M., Aleem, A., Ortiz, A., et al. (1987). A laboratory procedure for the induction of flashbacks. *American Journal of Psychiatry, 144*, 1317–1319.

Ray, W. J. (1990). The electrocortical system. In J. T. Cacioppo & L. G. Tassinary (Eds.), *Principles of psychophysiology: Physical, social, and inferential elements* (pp. 385–412). New York: Cambridge University Press.

Resnick, H. S., Kilpatrick, D. G., Lipovsky, J. A., et al. (1990, May). *Sensory modalities of flashbacks: post-trauma.* Paper presented at the annual meeting of the American Psychiatric Association, New York.

Rogers, L. (1976, May). *Human EEG response to certain rhythmic pattern stimuli, with possible relations to EEG lateral asymmetry measures and EEG correlates of chanting.* Unpublished doctoral dissertation, University of California, Los Angeles.

Ross, R. J., Ball, W. A., Sullivan, K. A., et al. (1989). Sleep disturbance as the hallmark of post-traumatic stress disorder. *American Journal of Psychiatry, 146,* 697–707.

Ross, R. J., Ball, W. A., Dinges, D. F., et al. (1990, May). *REM sleep disturbance as the hallmark of PTSD.* Paper presented at the annual meeting of the American Psychiatric Association, New York.

Ross, C. A., Heber, S., Anderson, G., et al. (1989). Differentiating multiple personality disorder and complex partial seizures. *General Hospital Psychiatry, 11,* 54–58.

Ross, J., & Persinger, M. A. (1987). Positive correlations between temporal lobe signs and hypnosis induction profiles: A replication. *Perceptual and Motor Skills, 64,* 828–830.

Rossi, E. L. (1982). Hypnosis and ultradian cycles: A new state(s) theory of hypnosis? *American Journal of Clinical Hypnosis, 25,* 21–32.

Rossi, E. L., & Cheek, D. B. (1988). *Mind–body therapy: Methods of ideodynamic healing in hypnosis.* New York: W.W. Norton.

Rothenberg, A. (1988). *The creative process of psychotherapy.* New York: W.W.Norton.

Sanders, B., & Giolas, M. H. (1991, January). Dissociation and childhood trauma in psychologically disturbed adolescents. *American Journal of Psychiatry, 148*(1), 50–54.

Sanders, B., McRoberts, G., & Tollefson, C. (1989, March). Childhood stress and dissociation in a college population. *Dissociation, 2*(1), 17–23.

Sapolsky, R. M. (1990). Effects of stress and glucocorticoids on hippocampal neuronal survival. In M. Brown, G. Koob, & C. Rivier (Eds.), *Stress neurobiology and neuroendocrinology* (pp. 293–322). New York: Dekker.

Sara, S. J. (1985). The locus coeruleus and cognitive function: Attempts to relate noradrenergic enhancement of signal/noise in the brain to behavior. *Physiology Psychology, 13,* 151–162.

Schenk, L., & Bear, D. (1981). Multiple personality and related dissociative phenomena in patients with temporal lobe epilepsy. *American Journal of Psychiatry, 138,* 1311–1316.

Schottenfeld, R. S., & Cullen, M. R. (1985). Occupation-induced post-traumatic stress disorders. *American Journal of Psychiatry, 142,* 198–202.

Shalev, A. Y., Orr, S. P., Peri, T., et al. (1992, November). Physiologic responses to loud tones in Israeli patients with posttraumatic stress disorder. *Archives of General Psychiatry, 49,* 870–875.

Shalev, A. Y., Orr, S. P., & Pitman, R. K. (1992, September). Psychophysiologic response during script-driven imagery as an outcome measure in posttraumatic stress disorder. *Journal of Clinical Psychiatry, 53*(9), 324–326.

Shalev, A. Y., Orr, S. P., & Pitman, R. K. (1993, April). Psychophysiologic assessment of traumatic imagery in Israeli civilian patients with posttraumatic stress disorder. *American Journal of Psychiatry, 150*(4), 620–624.

Silverman, J. J., Hart, R. P., Garrettson, L. K., et al. (1985). Post-traumatic stress disorder from pentaborane intoxication. *Journal of the American Medical Association, 254,* 2603–2608.

Smith, M. A., Davidson, J., Ritchie, J., et al. (1989). Corticotropin-releasing hormone tests in patients with PTSD. *Biological Psychiatry,* 349–355.

Snyder, S. H. (1985). Basic science of psychopharmacology. In H. I. Kaplan & B. J. Sadock (Eds.), *Comprehensive textbook of psychiatry* (4th ed., Vol. 4, pp. 42–55). Baltimore: Williams and Wilkins.

Solomon, Z., Garb, R., Bleich, A., et al. (1987). Reactivation of combat-related posttraumatic stress disorder. *American Journal of Psychiatry, 144,* 51–55.

Southwick, S. M., Krystal, J. H., Morgan, C. A., et al. (1993, April). Abnormal noradrenergic function in posttraumatic stress disorder. *Archives of General Psychiatry, 50,* 266–274.

Southwick, S. M., Yehudi, R., Perry, B. D., et al. (1990, May). *Sympathoadrenal dysfunction in PTSD.* Paper presented at the annual meeting of the American Psychiatric Association, New York.

Spanos, N. P., Weekes, J. R., Menary, E., et al. (1986). Hypnotic interview and age regression procedures in the elicitation of multiple personality symptoms: A simulation study. *Psychiatry, 49,* 298–311.

Spencer, S. S., Williamson, P. D., Bridgers, S. L., et al. (1988). Reliability and accuracy of localization by scalp ictal EEG. *Neurology, 35,* 1567–1575.

Spiegel, D. (1986). Dissociating damage. *American Journal of Clinical Hypnosis, 29,* 123–131.

Spiegel, D. (1991, Fall). Neurophysiological correlates of hypnosis and dissociation. *Journal of Neuropsychiatry, 3*(4), 440–444.

Spiegel, D., Frischholz, E. J., Spiegel, H., et al. (1989, May). *Dissociation, hypnotizability and trauma.* Paper presented at the annual meeting of the American Psychiatric Association, San Francisco.

Spiegel, D., Hunt, T., & Dondershine, H. E. (1988). Dissociation and hypnotizability in post-traumatic stress disorder. *American Journal of Psychiatry, 145,* 301–305.

Spiers, P. A., Schomer, D. L., Blume, H. W., et al. (1985). Temporolimbic epilepsy and behavior. In M.-M. Mesulam (Ed.), *Principles of behavioral neurology* (pp. 289–326). Philadelphia: F. A. Davis Company.

Steklis, H. D., & Kling, A. (1985). Neurobiology of affiliative behaviour in nonhuman primates. In M. Reite & T. Field (Eds.), *The psychobiology of attachment and separation* (pp. 93–134). New York: Academic Press.

Stewart, J. T., & Bartucci, R. J. (1986). Post-traumatic stress disorder and partial complex seizures. *American Journal of Psychiatry, 143,* 113–114.

Stutman, R. K., & Bliss, E. L. (1985). Post-traumatic stress disorder, hypnotizability, and imagery. *American Journal of Psychiatry, 142,* 741–743.

Terr, L. C. (1991, January). Childhood traumas: An outline and overview. *American Journal of Psychiatry, 148*(1), 10–20.

Tucker, G. J., Price, T. R. P., Johnson, V. B., et al. (1986). Phenomenology of temporal lobe dysfunction: A link to atypical psychosis—A series of cases. *Journal of Nervous and Mental Disease, 174,* 348–356.

van der Kolk, B. (1987). *Psychological trauma.* Washington, DC: American Psychiatric Press.

van der Kolk, B. A., Greenberg, M. S., Boyd, H., et al. (1985). Inescapable shock, neurotransmitters and addiction to trauma: Towards a psychology of post traumatic stress. *Biological Psychiatry, 20,* 314–325.

van der Kolk, B. A., Pitman, R. K., Orr, S. P., et al. (1989, May). *Endogenous opioids and post-traumatic stress.* Paper presented at the annual meeting of the American Psychiatric Association, San Francisco.

ver Ellen, P., & van Kammen, D. (1990). The biological findings in post-traumatic stress disorder: A review. *Journal of Applied Social Psychology,* 1789–1821.

Volkow, N. D., & Tancredi, L. R. (1991, April). Biological correlates of mental activity studied with PET. *American Journal of Psychiatry, 148*(4), 439–444.

Wallace, R., & Benson, H. (1972). The physiology of meditation. *Scientific American, 226*(2), 84–90.

Williams, G. W., Luders, H. O., Brickner, A., et al. (1985). Interobserver variability in EEG interpretation. *Neurology, 35,* 1714–1719.

Wilson, J. P. (1989). *Trauma, transformation, and healing: An integrative approach to theory, research, and post-traumatic therapy* (Brunner/Mazel Psychosocial Stress Series No.14). New York: Brunner/Mazel.

Winkelman, M. (1986). Trance states: A theoretical model and cross-cultural analysis. *Ethos, 14,* 174–203.

Yehuda, R., Lowy, M. T., Southwick, S. M., et al. (1991). Lymphocyte glucocorticoid receptor number in posttraumatic stress disorder. *American Journal of Psychiatry, 148,* 499–504.

Yehuda, R., Southwick, S., Giller, E. L., et al. (1992). Urinary catecholamine excretion and severity of PTSD symptoms in Vietnam combat veterans. *Journal of Nervous and Mental Disease, 180*(5), 321–325.

Yehuda, R., Southwick, S. M., Krystal, J. H., et al. (1993, January). Enhanced suppression of cortisol following dexamethasone administration in posttraumatic stress disorder. *American Journal of Psychiatry, 150*(1), 83–86.

Yehuda, R., Southwick, S. M., Nussbaum, G., et al. (1990). Low urinary cortisol excretion in patients with post-traumatic stress disorder. *Journal of Nervous and Mental Disease, 178,* 366–369.

6

Dreaming as a Normal Model for Multiple Personality Disorder

Deirdre L. Barrett

> *One trembles to think of that mysterious thing in the soul,*
> *which seems to acknowledge no human jurisdiction, but in*
> *spite of the individual's own innocent self, will still dream*
> *horrid dreams and mutter unmentionable thoughts.*
> —HERMAN MELVILLE (1852/1971, p. 67)

We manufacture others out of parts of ourselves each night when we dream. Dream characters, at the very least, may be seen as analogous to multiple personality disorder (MPD) alters and other dissociated ego states. This chapter will suggest that dreaming may also be a more literal precursor, whose physiological mechanisms for amnesia and the projection of dissociated identities get recruited in the development of MPD. There are constellations of cognitive and personality processes that operate outside conscious awareness and normally are observable primarily in dreams. Extreme early trauma may mutate or overdevelop these dissociated parts and call upon them to "wake up" and function in the external world. I will describe how this dream model parallels the observed phenomena of MPD more directly than do explanations relying on waking fantasy processes.

HISTORICAL PERSPECTIVES ON DREAMS AND DISSOCIATION

There is a long history of equating dreams with symptoms of mental illness. Freud concurs with Schopenhauer, who called dreams "a brief madness and madness a long dream" (quoted in Freud, 1900/1965, p. 122). Although the analogy was picked up and applied more specifically as a model for schizophrenia during the middle of this century (Fischer & Dement, 1963), this has now been rejected as not fitting closely enough the cognitive deficits or biochemistry of schizophrenia.

However, Freud and his contemporaries did not use the term "madness" to mean schizophrenia specifically but to cover all major mental illnesses; the patients they saw largely consisted of those with conversion hysteria and/or dissociative symptoms. What was discarded in terms of schizophrenia deserves to be reconsidered in terms of dissociative phenomena. After all, Kluft (1987) found patients with MPD even likelier than schizophrenics to show Schneiderian first-rank symptoms, including auditory hallucinations. Consider in that context a passage Freud (1900/1965) quotes from Radestock to make a point about "madness" and dreams:

> In dreams the personality may be split—when for instance, the dreamer's own knowledge is divided between two persons and when, in the dream, the extraneous ego corrects the actual one. This is precisely on par with the splitting of personality that is familiar to us in [auditory hallucinations]; the dreamer too hears his own thoughts pronounced by extraneous voices. (p. 123)

Breuer and Freud (1895/1955) and Janet (1929) referred to patients' waking symptoms, which we would now describe as dissociative episodes, with the term "dreams." Prince (1910) published a theory that explicitly described nocturnal dreams as a dissociated state of consciousness having much in common with both hypnosis and MPD. Two recent papers by Gable (1989, 1990) address relationships between dreams and dissociation, although he emphasizes duality, right brain activation, and concepts of dissociation arising from Sperry and Gazzaniga's "split-brain," postcommissurotomy patients.

Ernest Hilgard produced a dreaming/dissociation equation when he unexpectedly evoked the first occurrence of his hidden observer phenomena in a hypnotized subject:

> There may be intellectual processes also of which we are unaware, *such as those that find expression in night dreams.* Although you are hypnotically deaf, perhaps there is some part of you that is hearing my voice and processing the information. If there is, I should like the index finger of your right hand to rise as a sign that this is the case. (E. Hilgard, 1992, p. 75, emphasis added; see also Chapter 2, this volume)

Analogies recur throughout these comparisons of dreams and dissociative states, which can be distilled into two major categories: (1) those in which general similarities are found between dreaming and states such as amnesia and those involving other alterations of memory, and (2) those in which more specific similarities between dream characters and MPD alters are found, such as the hallucinatory projection of aspects of the self. Table

6.1 summarizes these shared characteristics. We will start with amnesia because it has the most obvious similarities, but will not dwell on it long for the same reason.

AMNESIA

Current biological dream theorists claim a better understanding of amnesia than of most other dream characteristics. They conceptualize the failure to recall dreams as the result of a lack of transfer from short- to long-term memory, that transfer being one in which waking aminergic neuronal activity seems to play a crucial role (Hobson, 1988). If awakened in a lab toward the end of each REM period, most people remember some part of most dreams. If allowed to sleep through the night, only a small percentage of dreams are recalled. Upon awakening, aminergic modulation resumes rapidly and the last part of a REM period may be processed into

TABLE 6.1. Similarities between Dream and MPD Characteristics

	Normal dreams	MPD and related states
Historical	Called "dissociative" in nature by Prince and Gable	Called "dreams" by Janet, Breuer, and Freud
Amnesia	Often present Sometimes breachable Some motivated Much state-dependent	Often present Sometimes breachable Motivated initially State-dependent later
Hypermnesia	Occasionally	Occasionally
Continuity with normal waking	Discontinuous	Discontinuous; may be remembered as a dream
	Dream characters	MPD alters
Cognitive abilities	Occasionally exceed normal waking ones	Often exceed normal waking ones
Personality	Traits rejected for normal waking self	Traits rejected for normal waking self
Most common	Persona Shadow Puer Anima/us	Host "Bad" alter Child alter Cross-gender alter
Movement	Only very rarely when REM paralysis breached	Yes when out, inhibited when other alters out
Therapy	Communication facilitates integration	Communication facilitates integration

long-term memory, fitting the observation that usually only the part of REM present just before awakening is retained.

However, this short-term/long-term model of memory has generally come into question as new research on implicit memory and state-dependent learning demonstrates that memories are not lost as completely as the older paradigm claimed (Schacter, 1984). In terms of dreaming, the short-term/long-term model also does not fit the observation that—at anytime during the day—something can trigger a sudden "déjà vu" or "tip-of-the-tongue" experience, and then a whole dream floods back from the night before or even from several nights previously. Obviously, the forgetting of dreams is neither instant nor complete and is subject to cueing. Dreaming is beginning to appear to be much more analogous to the amnesia of dissociative disorders in which an experience is gone from consciousness until something activates the ego state associated with that experience and it returns suddenly sometimes with flashback intensity, and—in the case of MPD—with a switch to an alter who holds the memory. Although repression has fallen into disrepute as the major saboteur of dream recall (Cohen & Wolfe, 1973), some recent evidence suggests that a significant amount of dream forgetting does have a repressive aspect similar to that found with the dissociative disorders (Erdelyi & Goldberg, 1979).

HYPERMNESIA

Not all alterations of memory in dreams or dissociation are in the direction of less recall than that of normal waking consciousness. Another observation noted by Freud's time was that both processes could at times enhance memory. Radestock, for instance, wrote, ". . . in dreamers, memories arise from the remote past; both sleeping and sick men recollect things which waking and healthy men seem to have forgotten" (quoted in Freud 1900/1965, p. 122).

Freud gave several examples of what he termed "hypermnestic dreams" —many of which involve another character as the repository of forgotten memories (1900/1965). He quotes Maury, who described how a dream character gave him accurate geographical information about a place he had been trying to recall. He also describes how the poet Scalinger had a man calling himself Brugnolus show up in a dream to complain of being overlooked in Scalinger's epic about Verona; the poet later confirmed Brugnolus had existed. Freud also recounts how a certain Marquis de St. Denys had two dreams, the first of which contained a character he believed might exist in waking life. In the second one, the character reappeared and St. Denys asked her where they had met. She named a time and place years before, about which St. Denys then recalled more detail upon awakening.

Schatzman (1992) describes a hypermnestic dream in which an entire chorus sang a passage from Monteverdi's *Vespers* to the dreamer, which she recalled in enough detail to write down. She later confirmed it as correct. Compare that to Schreiber's (1974) account of Sybil listening to a tape recording of her alter playing the piano and being amazed that music she was taught in childhood had been retained outside of awareness all those years.

Dreams and dissociative disorders also may take traumatic episodes that are already clearly recalled awake and replay them more vividly in the altered state. Only in severe post-traumatic stress disorder (PTSD) does one have full-blown flashbacks during the day. However, the majority of people who experience a trauma have recurring dreams in which they relive it rather literally (van der Kolk, Blitz, Burr, Sherry, & Hartmann, 1984).

One group of theorists (Ross, Ball, Sullivan, & Caroff, 1989) goes so far as to suggest that all trauma sequela are due to long-term impairments to the barriers between waking and REM sleep. They reviewed the sleep laboratory studies of combat veterans in which some degree of disruption or fragmentation of REM was found with them all. They concluded that these veterans' PTSD symptoms are normal phenomena for REM, but abnormal when they manifested as non-REM nightmares—such as waking flashbacks and a level of autonomic arousal that is dysfunctional for waking but would be normal in REM. These non-Rem nightmares do not occur in nontrauma populations.

The thesis of the present chapter is that this adult trauma sequelae of REM fragmentation resembles that which results from repeated early childhood trauma. However, early fragmentation of REM has more implications for disordered development since dreaming, waking cognition, and their boundaries are still evolving during childhood (Foulkes, 1872).

In a survey of 48 dissociative-disordered patients (Barrett, 1994), 74% were observed to have some of the same repressed memories accessible in their dissociated ego states as were accessible in their dreams. These included memories of childhood traumas and content of recent fugue episodes. One dream phenomenon specific to the MPD patients studied is of special relevance to memory and is described in the next section.

ALTER'S EXPERIENCE RECALLED AS A DREAM

*If you could pass through Paradise in a dream, and have a
flower presented to you as a pledge that your soul had really
been there, and if you found that flower in your hand when
you awoke. . . . What then?*

—COLERIDGE (1895, p. 326)

It is hardly Paradise that multiple personalities are visiting in their dreams, but a subset of the dissociative-disordered patients in the survey expressed an additional way in which memory in dreams and dissociative states resemble each other. Four of the 23 MPD patients in the sample, or 17%, reported what later turned out to be actual waking experiences of their alters as "dreams," which they at first believed had occurred only in their sleeping psyche. The most common way they found out that the "dream" event had really happened was through some external evidence equivalent to Coleridge's flower.

One woman, who had recurring "nightmares" of catching evil cats by the throat and stuffing them in garbage cans, awoke from one of these dreams to find the velour jogging suit in which she slept covered in cat hair. She did not own a cat and was so disturbed by what the hairs suggested that she both searched trash cans in her neighborhood and brought in the top of the jogging suit so that her therapist would also see the hair on it.

Sizemore and Pittillo (1977, pp. 64–65) describe a certain "Eve" as having a Coleridge-type experience as a child. This "Eve" lay down for a nap and "dreamed" of watching a redheaded girl steal and smash her cousin's coveted new watch "only to awaken to find the ruined treasure in her own hand."

PROJECTION OF PARTS OF THE SELF ONTO OTHER IDENTITIES

In addition to the similarities between how memory functions in dreams and dissociative states, MPD alters and dream characters share the further distinction of being the two most dramatic examples of a splitting off of parts of the self, which are fashioned into somewhat autonomous-looking entities. The thesis of the present chapter is that this process occurs naturally in REM sleep and can also mutate and move out into the waking state in response to extreme early traumas.

The claim here is not that dream characters are the only antecedents of MPD alters, but that they are the strongest. Certainly imaginary companions and other waking fantasy content are somewhat analogous to alters, but dreams universally feature formed, autonomous characters of hallucinatory vividness. Fantasized characters rarely surprise—much less frighten—their authors while dream characters routinely do so. Only very extreme imagers or hypnotic virtuosos experience their daydreams this way. Furthermore, research has found that these virtuosos have such a high rate of childhood abuse that a number of them should be viewed as pathologically dissociative, rather than as merely having a precursor ability (J. Hilgard, 1970; Frischholz, 1985; Barrett, 1991, in press-a).

Schatzman's (1983a, 1983b, 1986) accounts of problem-solving dreams include some dramatic examples of dream characters that are in possession of cognitive abilities or knowledge that both the dream ego and the waking self lack. His procedure involved having subjects study a "brain-teaser" type problem at bedtime for 10 minutes and then notice whether their dreams contained solutions. After working on the problem of what English words both begin and end with the letters "*he*," one subject dreamed of a doctor, or "word specialist," who prompted him to describe his angina in plain English (as *he*artac*he*), and then to name his *he*adac*he*, all the while laughing "hee-hee-hee" at him. Schatzman (1983a) observed:

> It was as though during the dream, some component of the dreamer's mind, knowing the answer, played hide-and-seek with him. Possibly before the dream began, part of the dreamer's mind of which he was unaware had already solved the problem, and the dream used a dramatic means of presenting the solution to ensure that the dreamer's attention was called to it. (p. 693)

With other examples Schatzman gave, characters stated solutions more directly. A man trying to solve a problem about what was distinctive about a certain sentence (where the first word contained one letter, the second two, etc.) dreamed that he was typing and his supervisor told him to stop using words and to type instead "123456789" (1983b, p. 417). A woman working on a problem whose solution was that one sentence forms another when the first letter of each word is removed ("Show this bold . . ."→"How his old . . .") had a dream character tell her "Too many letters!" (1986, p. 37). And a subject who had read two of Schatzman's puzzles dreamed of Michael Caine taking the puzzles in hand and miming the correct answers to each in turn, as in the game of charades (1986, p. 38).

The dream character Caine is behaving much like the subset of alters who hold cognitive faculties because intellectual pursuits were associated with traumatic punishment. It is common for people with MPD to report experiences in school of hearing voices in their head say answers to exam questions that are eluding the host.

Although the dream examples above are somewhat unusual in the specific cognitive details of their characters' separateness, several major dream theories have as their central premise the idea that dream characters are projected parts of the dreamer's self that have been denied expression in the waking personality. Jung (1916–1945/1974) conceptualized dream characters as "archetypes," archetypes being enduring constellations of traits within the psyche.

Jung's four main archetypes "persona," "shadow," "puer," and "anima/us" correspond almost exactly to the four most common personality types to be found in MPD (Putnam, 1989). Similar to the "persona" archetype, the host personality is usually nice, socially compliant, and of a conforming nature. Most people with MPD also have an alter who is "bad," in the sense that he or she manifests forbidden sexuality and aggression. Many have one that is even "evil" and identified with an abuser, as with the "shadow" archetype. The majority also have at least one child alter, like the "puer" archetype. The other common alter is a cross-gender one who manifests gender-stereotyped traits of the opposite sex that have been denied to him or her—the "anima/us" archetype. Jung believed that these archetypes exist in the psyche at all times, but are most obviously manifested in the dream state.

Gestalt therapy (Perls, 1969) takes a very similar view of dream characters. Again, the idea is that these characters represent split-off parts of the self that exist with some autonomy all the time and manifest most clearly in dreams. The main purpose of Gestalt dream work is to open a dialogue between these parts so that they can eventually integrate. Note the language used by a Gestalt therapist in describing dream work with a person *who does not have a dissociative disorder*: "This method seems to be useful in the treatment of 'rejected subpersonalities,' of 'parts' that do not 'want' to contact each other" (Pisarevitch, 1992, p. 1).

These theorists frequently emphasize that recurring dream characters are especially strong manifestations of repressed archetypes or dissociated selves trying to communicate. In the trauma literature, recurring characters have also been noticed to be associated with a higher rate of childhood abuse (Zadra, in press). Trauma seems to give dream characters more autonomy. With milder cases of abuse, characters gain in strength and persistence in dreams, with extreme cases they move into the waking world.

Theories on dreams suggest that dream characters are not entirely a product of the dream state. Schatzman's examples indicate that temporary constellations of memories, emotions, or information processing systems formed around transient problems may work to solve them in a waking state but present the results in a dream. More importantly, Jung and Perls suggest that dream characters—especially recurring ones—consist of fairly permanent ego states, which exist at other times but are released into consciousness predominantly in REM sleep. Such characters are occasionally hypmnestic because they hold dissociated memories, but are more often amnestic, or have weaker associational links to experiences that could be easily cued in the normal waking state.

One issue relevant to the dream character/MPD alter analogy is that dream characters obviously often draw on real people as their sources. When one dreams about one's grandmother, characteristics of the real grandmother are likely to significantly determine what the dream grandmother is like. At the same time, some aspects of the self that empathasize with and understand (or even misunderstand) the grandmother must be called into play to manufacture the dream character. Jung described archetypes as often being represented by a real person with the archetypal traits. However, this is not so dissimilar from MPD alters; a number of them are often based on a real external person such as a childhood friend or relative. Occasionally, they are based on a fictional character.

It may seem that I am at risk of overstating the primacy of dream origins to make my point here. Clearly, these dissociative processes for both cognition and personality compensation do go on quietly outside of REM. However, the discrete, autonomous, personification of these processes is normally a REM phenomena, and it seems to take early trauma to disrupt this boundary. Below, I will review what various therapists have noted about their MPD patients' dream characteristics (Barrett, in press-b) to further explore what a high degree of trauma does to the dream process and how well MPD alters fit the dream character model.

ALTERS AS DREAM CHARACTERS

Thirteen of twenty-three patients (57%) in a survey (Barrett, 1994) reported that their alters appeared as dream characters. One dreamed of a blond little girl, who begged her repetitively, "Don't let them hurt me; take me home with you." The patient was not yet in touch with this child alter but the therapist recognized that the description fit an alter that had come out in moments when the host was amnestic. The alter had used exactly those words with the therapist. Two patients who had made suicidal gestures that they attributed to accidents or intoxication had dreams that later played a great role in explaining the gestures. One had dreamed of a woman determined to commit suicide; the other of one vowing to kill the dreamer. These turned out to be alters that were responsible for self-mutilation and a drug overdose.

Six patients (26%) had personalities who reported the same dream from different perspectives, and experienced each other as characters in it. Sometimes, one personality only watched and was not observed as a character by the others. When they met in a dream early in treatment, the host and sometimes the alter did not recognize each other until the dream experiences were discussed. Further into the therapy process, they were likely to recognize each other in the dream as soon as each appeared. This may actually happen much more often than assumed because, in many cases, the therapist asks only the host about the dreams and not the alters. In the following case example, the therapist had inquired extensively:

> The host personality, Sarah, remembered only that her dream from the previous night involved hearing a girl screaming for help. Alter Annie, age four, remembered a nightmare of being tied down naked and unable to cry

out as a man began to cut her vagina. Ann, age nine, dreamed of watching this scene and screaming desperately for help (apparently the voice in the host's dream). Teen-age Jo dreamed of coming upon this scene and clubbing the little girl's attacker over the head; in her dream he fell to the ground dead and she left. In the dreams of Ann and Annie, the teen-ager with the club appeared, struck the man to the ground but he arose and renewed his attack again. Four year old Sally dreamed of playing with her dolls happily and nothing else. Both Annie and Ann reported a little girl playing obliviously in the corner of the room in their dreams. Although there was no definite abuser-identified alter manifesting at this time, the presence at times of a hallucinated voice similar to Sarah's uncle suggested there might be yet another alter experiencing the dream from the attacker's vantage. (Barrett, 1994, p. 171)

Other writers also mention that alters appear as dream characters. Schreiber (1974, p. 335) described Sybil, at an early stage of therapy, dreaming of a house where she could go to "escape doom" in which she met 15 children, who she later recognized to be her 15 alters. Paley (1993) described how a persecutory alter appeared in a patient's dreams as a recurring character. Salley (1988, p. 153) described alters that were able to appear to hosts strategically to influence their behavior or communicate information. Gruenwald (1971, p. 44) reported asking an alter to introduce herself to a host in a dream, which the alter proceeded to do successfully.

BOUNDARIES BETWEEN WAKING AND REM SLEEP

Usually dream characters disappear upon waking, but there are two disorders in which at least some of the physiological aspects of REM spill over into waking. With narcolepsy, patients may continue to hallucinate some aspects of the dream—including dream characters—upon first awakening. In other words, the material is superimposed on their real environment. With chronic behavior disorders of REM sleep, the usual paralysis that accompanies dreaming is absent; these patients move around their bedroom acting out their dreams in the real world, often with dangerous consequences (Schneck et al., 1986). Many more people experience some partial motor disinhibition, occasionally during sleep walking and talking episodes. Some, although not most of this behavior occurs during dreaming.

It is usually assumed that the actions occurring with the disinhibition of REM movements are those of the dream ego; however, there are two instances I know of that demonstrate this is not always the case. The first dream involves a clinical psychologist, who in waking life was evaluating an inpatient who displayed a distinctive motor pattern. She traced the outline of one hand and then the other repetitively. The psychologist had a dream in which she was watching the patient do this and trying to learn what it meant by playing on an old Victrola the patient's hospital "record." At this point, the therapist's partner woke her up and told her that she had been tracing the fingers of each hand alternately as she slept. She had not made any movements suggestive of the dream ego's use of the phonograph.

The second anecdote comes from an undergraduate psychology major. She dreamt of a boating trip with friends, which was pleasant until a shark appeared, leapt out of the water, and grabbed the dreamer's forearm in its jaws, biting hard. She felt pain and struggled with the shark; it held its grip until she awoke in a panic. She found she had bitten her own arm hard enough to leave deep red marks, which subsequently lingered as bruises.

I have seen one dissociative-disordered patient who regularly manifested a dream character engaged in overt action. The patient's major complaint was that he had nightmares about alien beings appearing. While dreaming, he also spoke out loud in the character of these entities, rather than as himself, although he was otherwise immobilized.

Full-blown MPD can be seen as an extension of the phenomena described above. Normal dissociative cognitive and personality processes that operate largely outside consciousness manifest as dream characters. They can be crystallyzed by trauma into permanent constellations that become recurring characters. Extreme and early enough trauma disrupts REM so greatly and demands such extraordinary defenses that these dream characters, who hold important skills and memories, begin to manifest when the victim is awake. As stated earlier, at the very least, these dream characters who "wake up" represent the closest existing normal analogy to MPD, but the REM state also may prove to be the concrete physiological precursor of MPD.

REFERENCES

Barrett, D. L. (1991) Deep trance subjects: A schema of two distinct subgroups. In R. Kunzendorf (Ed.), *Mental imagery*, (pp. 101–112). New York: Plenum Press.

Barrett, D. L. (1994). Dreams in dissociative disorders. *Dreaming*, 6, 165–175.

Barrett, D. L. (in press-a). Fantisizers and dissociaters: Two types of high hypnotizables, their developmental antecedents, and relationship to other dimensions of hypnotizibility. In R. Kunzendorf, N. Spanos, & B. Wallace (Eds.), *Hypnosis and imagination*. Amityville, NY: Baywood.

Barrett, D. L. (in press-b). Dreams in multiple personality disorder. In D. L. Barrett (Ed.), *Trauma and dreams*. Cambridge, MA: Harvard University Press.

Breuer, J., & Freud, S. (1955). Studies on hysteria. In J. Strachey (Ed. and Trans.), *The standard edition of the complete psychological works of Sigmund Freud* (Vol. 2, pp. 3–305). London: Hogarth Press. (Original work published 1895)

Coleridge, S. T. (1895). Anima poetae. In J. D. Campbell (Ed.), *The collected poetical and dramatic works* (p. 326). London: W. Heinemann.

Cohen , D. B., & Wolfe, G. (1973). Dream recall and repression: Evidence for an alternative hypothesis. *Journal of Consulting and Clinical Psychology, 41*, 349–355.

Erdelyi, M H., & Goldberg, B. (1979). Let's not sweep repression under the rug: Toward a cognitive psychology of repression. In J. F. Kihlstrom & F. J. Evans (Eds.), *Functional disorders of memory* (pp. 355–402). Hillsdale, NJ: Lawrence Erlbaum.

Fisher, C., & Dement, W. (1963) Studies on the psychopathology of sleep and dreams. *American Journal of Psychiatry, 119*, 1160–1168.

Foulkes, D. (1982). *Children's dreams: Longitudinal studies*. New York: John Wiley.

Freud, S. (1965). *The interpretation of dreams*. New York: Avon. (Original work published 1900)

Frischholz, E. J. (1985). The relationship among dissociation, hypnosis, and child abuse in the development of multiple personality. In R. P. Kluft (Ed.), *Childhood antecedents of multiple personality* (pp. 99–120). Washington, DC: American Psychiatric Press.

Gable, S. (1989). Dreams as a possible reflection of a dissociated self-monitoring system. *Journal of Nervous and Mental Disease, 177*(9), 560–568.

Gable, S. (1990). Dreams and dissociation theory: Speculations on beneficial aspects of their linkage. *Dissociation, 3*(1), 38–47.

Gruenewald, D. (1971). Hypnotic techniques without hypnosis in the treatment of multiple personality. *Journal of Nervous and Mental Disease, 153*, pp. 41–46.

Hilgard, E. (1992). Dissociation and theories of hypnosis. In E. Fromm & M. Nash (Eds.), *Contemporary hypnosis research* (pp. 69–101). New York: Guilford Press.

Hilgard, J. (1970). *Personality and hypnosis: A study of imaginitive involvement*. Chicago: University of Chicago Press.

Hobson, J. A. (1988). *The dreaming brain*. New York: Basic Books.

Janet, P. (1929). *The major symptoms of hysteria* (2nd ed.). New York: Macmillan.

Jung, C. G. (1974). *Dreams* (R. Hull, Trans.). Princeton, NJ: Princeton University Press. (Original work published 1916–1945).

Kluft, R. P. (1987). First-rank symptoms as a diagnostic clue to multiple personality disorder. *American Journal of Psychiatry, 144*, 293–298.

Melville, H. (1971). *Pierre*. Chicago: Northeastern University Press. (Original work published 1852)

Paley, K. S. (1993). Dream wars: A case study of a woman with multiple personalities. *Dissociation, 6*(1), 67–74.

Perls, F. (1969). *Gestalt therapy verbatim*. Moab, UT: Real People Press.

Pisarevitch, M. H. (1992, July). *On the use of Erikson's hypnosis in the treatment of dreams*. 12th International Congress of Hypnosis Book of Abstracts, Jerusalem, Israel.

Prince, M. (1910). The mechanism and interpretation of dreams. *Journal of Abnormal Psychology, 5*, 139–195.

Putnam, F. W. (1989). *Diagnosis and treatment of multiple personality disorder*. New York: Guilford Press.

Ross, R. J., Ball, W. A., Sullivan, K. A., & Caroff, S. N. (1989). Sleep disturbances as the hallmark of posttraumatic stress disorder. *American Journal of Psychiatry, 146*, 697–707.

Salley, R. D. (1988). Subpersonalities with dreaming functions in a patient with multiple personalities. *Journal of Nervous and Mental Disease, 176*(2), pp. 112–115.

Schacter, D. (1984). Toward the multidisciplinary study of memory: Ontogeny, phylogeny, and pathology of memory systems. In L. Squire & N. Butters (Eds.), *Neuropsychology of memory* (1st ed., pp. 13–24). New York: Guilford Press.

Schatzman, M. (1983a, June 9). Solve your problems in your sleep. *New Scientist*, 692–693.

Schatzman, M. (1983b, Aug. 11). Sleeping on problems can really solve them. *New Scientist*, pp. 416–417.

Schatzman, M. (1986, Dec. 25). The meaning of dreams. *New Scientist*, pp. 36–39.

Schatzman, M. (1992, June). *Hypermnestic dreams*. Paper presented at the 9th international conference of the Association for the Study of Dreams, Santa Cruz, CA.

Schneck, C. H., Bundlie, S. R., Ettinger, M. G., & Mahowald, M. W. (1986). Chronic behavior disorders of human REM sleep: A new category of parasomnia. *Sleep, 9*, 293–308.

Schreiber, F. R. (1974). *Sybil*. New York: Warner Paperbacks.

Sizemore, C. C., & Pittillo, E. S (1977). *I'm Eve*. Garden City, NY: Doubleday.

Zadra, A. (in press). Recurrent dreams: Their relation to life events and well-being. In D. L. Barrett (Ed.), *Trauma and dreams*. Cambridge, MA: Harvard University Press.

van der Kolk, B. A., Blitz, R., Burr, W., Sherry, S., & Hartmann, E. (1984). Clinical characteristics of traumatic and lifelong nightmare sufferers. *American Journal of Psychiatry, 141*, 187–190.

7

Hypnosis and Multiple Personality Disorder: A Sociocognitive Perspective

Nicholas P. Spanos
Cheryl Burgess

People who are diagnosed as suffering from multiple personality disorder (MPD) behave as if they possess two or more distinct personalities. They exhibit a relatively integrated interpersonal style (i.e., a distinct personality) when referring to themselves with one name and different interpersonal styles when referring to themselves with other names. Frequently, MPD patients behave as if their alter personalities have their own unique memories and experiences, and as if some of their alters are unaware of and have no memory of other alters.

MPD patients are usually women. They exhibit a wide range of chronic psychiatric problems that predate their MPD diagnosis (e.g., Ross, Norton, & Wozney, 1989), and they usually claim to have been severely physically and/or sexually abused in childhood (Ross, Miller, Bjornson, Reagor, & Fraser, 1991; Young, Sachs, Braun, & Watkins, 1991). It is now commonly argued that MPD is caused by severe childhood abuse (e.g., Bliss, 1986; Braun, 1990; Putnam, 1989; Ross, 1989). According to this hypothesis, severe trauma during childhood produces a mental splitting or "dissociation," as a defensive reaction to the trauma. These dissociated "parts" of the person develop into alter personalities that, in adulthood, periodically manifest themselves in order to help the individual cope with stressful situations, and express resentments or other feelings that are disavowed by the primary personality. Thus, from this perspective, the development of alter personalities is something that happens to the person as a result of early traumas and other experiences over which he or she has no control and often no memory, rather than something that he or she does in response to current contingencies, goals, and understandings. Historically, MPD has been closely tied to hypnotic phenomena, and many modern investigators argue that similar psychological processes underlie MPD and hypnosis (e.g., Bliss, 1986; Braun, 1990). For instance, early trauma supposedly produces an "hypnotic state" in predisposed individuals that facilitates the development of alter personalities (Bliss, 1980, 1986). Purportedly, these alters remain separated from normal consciousness by a process akin to hypnotic amnesia (Bliss, 1986; Ross, 1989). Moreover, individual differences in hypnotizability supposedly reflect differences in the capacity for dissociation. The high hypnotizability scores frequently attained by MPD patients are used to support this idea (Bliss, 1986).

In this chapter, we argue that MPD theorists are correct in concluding that some of the psychological processes underlying MPD and hypnotic responding are similar. However, we further argue that MPD theorists fundamentally misunderstand the nature of both MPD enactments and hypnotic responding. More specifically, we use experimental data concerning hypnotic responding and clinical data concerning MPD to argue that multiple identities are rule-governed social constructions, which are created, legitimated, maintained, and altered through social interaction.

According to this sociocognitive formulation, patients learn to construe themselves as possessing multiple selves, learn to present themselves in terms of this perception, and learn to reorganize and elaborate upon their personal biography so as to make it congruent with their understanding of what it means to be a multiple (Spanos, 1994).

This perspective suggests that psychotherapists play a prominent part in the generation and maintenance of MPD. Indeed, therapists routinely encourage patients to construe themselves as having alter personalities, provide them with information about how to convincingly enact the role of "multiple personality patient," and provide official legitimation for the different alters that their patients enact (Spanos, 1993).

THE NATURE OF HYPNOTIC RESPONDING

Hypnosis has been viewed historically as an altered state of consciousness in which responsiveness to suggestions greatly increases and in which, with highly hypnotizable subjects, the recall of hidden memories is facilitated. This view of hypnosis has almost always uncritically been accepted in the MPD literature (e.g., Bliss, 1986; Ross, 1989). In the last 40 years, however, a great deal of empirical evidence has challenged this view (for reviews see Spanos, 1986; Spanos & Chaves, 1989; Wagstaff, 1981). Contrary to the assumption frequently found in the MPD literature, over a century of research has failed to uncover unambiguous behavioral, physiological, or subjective report criteria that would conclusively affirm that a uniquely "hypnotic state" exists (Barber, 1979; Sarbin & Coe, 1972). In addition, a large number of studies indicate that even the seeming dramatic behaviors associated with hypnosis (e.g., displays of analgesia and amnesia) can be accomplished by motivated control subjects who have not been administered hypnotic induction procedures, and who do not give the appearance of being in a "trance state" (Barber, 1979; Wagstaff, 1981). Contrary to a general assumption in the MPD literature, hypnotic procedures do not facilitate the accurate recall of memories and, under some circumstances, may enhance the confidence people place in their incorrect recall (Smith, 1983; Wagstaff, 1989).

Descriptions of hypnotic responding in the MPD literature frequently imply that hypnosis is a "state" that happens to people or that people go into (Bliss, 1986). Instead, much data supports the hypothesis that hypnotic behaviors are goal-directed enactments, and that highly hypnotizable subjects are cognizing individuals who are attuned to even subtle interpersonal cues, and who are invested in meeting the social demands of hypnotic situations in order to present themselves as "good" subjects (Sarbin & Coe, 1972; Spanos & Coe, 1992). Hypnotic suggestions are communications that call for the construction of "as if" situations. Thus, suggestions for arm levitation, hallucination and amnesia are, in effect, tacit requests to use imaginative and other cognitive abilities to behave as if one's arm is rising by itself, as if one sees a nonexistent object, or as if one is unable to remember. Behaving as if an imaginary scenario is true involves creating the requisite subjective experiences as well as generating the requisite behaviors (Sarbin & Coe, 1972; Spanos, Rivers, & Ross, 1977). For instance, suggestions for amnesia require not only that subjects fail to report target material, but also that they define themselves as having forgotten that material. Subjects who are unable to generate the subjective experiences called for by suggestions frequently admit their failures rather than fake their responses. On the other hand, hypnotic responding is exceedingly easy to fake (Orne, 1979), and some subjects do purposely misdescribe their experiences to meet test demands, a tendency most likely to be seen with highly hypnotizable subjects (Spanos, Flynn, & Gabora, 1989; Burgess, Spanos, Ritt, Hordy, & Brooks, 1993; Wagstaff, 1981).

THE CREATION OF MULTIPLE IDENTITIES

Occurrence rates for MPD have differed dramatically from one historical epoch to another, and from one country to another. For instance, cases that today would be classified as MPD were infrequently diagnosed in the first three-quarters of the 19th century, increased dramatically in frequency between about 1876 and 1920, dwindled to a trickle between 1920 and 1970, and since 1970 have increased astronomically. However, the huge increase in cases since 1970 has been largely restricted to North America. Few cases have been reported in Japan, India, France, England, Switzerland, or Russia (for reviews of MPD occurrence rates see Aldridge-Morris, 1989; Spanos, 1994). The large majority of patients who are eventually diagnosed with MPD do not display symptoms of multiplicity before they enter treatment, and are unaware that they possess alter personalities until the therapist helps them "uncover" their multiplicity (Kluft, 1985). The therapeutic procedure most commonly used to uncover evidence of multiplicity involves hypnotic interviewing, in which the existence of alter personalities is directly suggested to patients (Allison, 1978; Bliss, 1980; Wilbur, 1984). From a sociocognitive perspective, these findings, taken together, suggest that therapists very frequently create rather than discover multiplicity.

The Experimental Creation of Alter Identities

Hilgard (1979, 1991; see also Chapter 2, this volume) conducted a well-known series of studies that led to the hypnotic elicitation of "hidden selves" from normal college students who were high in hypnotizability. In these experiments, subjects were given suggestions for analgesia or deafness and were then instructed that they possessed a hidden self that remained aware of sensory experiences their "hypnotically analgesic" or "hypnotically deaf" part remained unaware of. During later testing, these subjects behaved as if they possessed both a hypnotic self and a hidden self. When reporting as their hypnotic self, subjects indicated that their sensations were greatly diminished. However, when reporting as their hidden self, these subjects reported high levels of sensory experience.

Hilgard (1979, 1991) argued that hidden reports do not result from suggestions or from experimental demands. Instead, he hypothesized that hypnotic subjects who respond to suggestions for reduced sensations continue to experience the sensations outside of consciousness even though they are unaware of these "dissociated" sensations. Supposedly, these hidden sensations remain concealed behind an amnesic barrier unless and until the experimenter obtains hidden reports. According to this view, the explicit hidden observer instructions used in these experiments did not provide subjects with the idea that they had a hidden self or with the idea that hidden reports and overt reports should differ from each other. Instead, Hilgard (1979) argued that these instructions simply provided a structured setting, which allowed a preexisting hidden cognitive subsystem to come to light.

A sociocognitive perspective suggests instead that reports of hidden sensations and of a hidden self reflect interpretations that subjects place on the instructions used in hidden observer experiments (Coe & Sarbin, 1977; Spanos, 1982, 1991; Wagstaff, 1981). A number of experiments now provide strong support for this sociocognitive position (Spanos, Flynn, & Gwynn, 1988; Spanos & Hewitt, 1980; Spanos, Gwynn, & Stam, 1983). Basically, these experiments demonstrated that the characteristics subjects attributed to their hidden selves, and the reports associated with these self-enactments varied as a function of the expectations conveyed to subjects by the experimental instruction. These findings also indicated that the frequency with which subjects displayed hidden selves reflected the explicitness of the instructions subjects were administered. When these were vague and ambiguous, rates of hidden self responding were low, whereas when instructions were explicit, rates of hidden self responding were high (Spanos, 1986). In short, the findings of hidden observer experiments indicate that hidden self responding is goal-directed action that is shaped by the demands conveyed in the instructions. The instructions provide subjects with the idea that they possess a hidden self with particular characteristics, and subjects generate the interpretations, experiences, and behaviors that confirm the expectations conveyed by their instructions.

Several studies have examined those factors that influence the formation of multiple selves when the phenomenon of past-life hypnotic regression is employed. Although some believers in reincarnation hold that people can be hypnotically regressed back past their birth to previous lives (e.g., Wambaugh, 1979), the available evidence provides no support whatsoever for this notion. Instead, the available data suggest that past-life experiences and enactments are fantasy constructions (Baker, 1992; Spanos, Menary, Gabora, DuBreuil, & Dewhirst, 1991). Past-life constructions are important because they are similar in many respects to the multiple identities of MPD patients. Like MPD patients, subjects who exhibit past-life identities behave as if they are inhabited by more than one self. Like the alter personalities of MPD patients, those exhibited by past-life responders often display moods and personality characteristics that are different from the person's primary self, have a different name than the primary self, and report memories that the primary self was unaware of. Just as MPD patients come to believe that their alter identities are real personalities rather than self-generated fantasies, many of the subjects who enact past lives continue to believe in the reality of their past lives after termination of the hypnotic procedures.

On the basis of work by Kampman (1976), Spanos, Menary, and colleagues (1991) conducted a series of experiments on hypnotic past-life identity enactments. After being given suggestions to regress back to a time before their birth, many subjects exhibited elaborate past-life identities. These identities had their own names and often described their lives in detail. Significantly, subjects who exhibited past-life identities scored higher on measures of hypnotizability and fantasy-proneness, but no higher on measures of psychopathology than those who did not report a past life.

The social nature of past-life identities was underscored by the finding that the characteristics that subjects attributed to these identities was influenced by expectations transmitted by the experimenter. In one study (Spanos, Menary, et al., 1991, Experiment 1) subjects in one group were informed before hypnotic regression took place that their past lives were likely to differ from their current ones in several important respects (e.g., they might be of a different sex). Control subjects were administered the same hypnotic regression procedures but given no prehypnotic information about the characteristics of their past lives. Subjects provided with prehypnotic information about the characteristics of their past identities were much more likely than controls to incorporate these characteristics into their past-life descriptions.

In a different study, Spanos, Menary, et al. (1991, Experiment 3) manipulated prehypnotic information that concerned the reality of past-life identities. Subjects in one condition were informed that past-life identities were interesting fantasies but were certainly not evidence of past lives. Those in another condition were provided with background information suggesting that reincarnation was a scientifically credible notion, and that past-life identities were real people who had lived previously. Subjects in the two conditions were equally likely to enact past-life identities. For instance, while enacting their past-life identities subjects in these two groups were equally likely to call themselves by a different name, provide a different life history, and so on. Nevertheless, subjects assigned to the imaginary creation condition believed less strongly in the reality of these identities than did those who were told that reincarnation was scientifically credible. In short, prior information from authority figures influences not only the characteristics that people attribute to their multiple identities but also the degree to which they come to believe in the reality of these identities.

Taken together, the available experimental data indicate that multiple identities are social creations that can easily be elicited from many normal people, and that are determined by the understandings that subjects develop about multiple identities from the information to which they are exposed. When the identity to be constructed is relatively complex, such as in past-life regression cases, subjects draw on information from many sources outside of the immediate situation (e.g., television shows, historical novels, aspects of their own past, wish-fulfilling daydreams) to flesh out the newly constructed identity and to provide it with the history and characteristics that are called for by how subjects understand current task demands. It is clear from these studies that the development of multiple identities is not related to psychopathology, and that males are as adept as females at creating such identities. Although none of these studies obtained information about whether subjects had been abused as children, the fact that psychopathology failed to predict either the development of these identities or the extent to which subjects construed them as real rather than imagined, makes it unlikely that early abuse played any role in their formation.

The Clinical Creation of Alter Identities

Proponents of the MPD diagnosis have described a very large and diverse number of signs that supposedly indicate the presence of this disorder, and that can be used to justify probing for confirmation of this diagnosis (e.g., headaches, depression, somatophorm symptoms, impaired concentration, drug abuse; see, e.g., Ross, Norton, & Wozney, 1989). Once the diagnosis is suspected, it is common practice to use leading and suggestive procedures in order to confirm it. Merskey (1992), recently reviewed a large number of MPD cases from the 20th century and earlier and found that highly leading and suggestive procedures have long been routinely used in the diagnosis of MPD. In some cases, therapists insisted to doubting patients that they had MPD and supplied the patients with names for their alters. In fact, Allison and Schwarz (1980) contend that patients are frequently reluctant to accept that they are multiples and, due to this circumstance, are actively persuaded by their therapists to accept the diagnosis.

The most common procedure used to elicit evidence of multiplicity involves highly leading hypnotic interviews, during which the existence of alter personalities is explicitly suggested, and the alters are explicitly asked to "come forth" and talk with the therapist (Allison & Schwarz, 1980; Bliss, 1980, 1986). Wilbur (1984) described this process as follows: "The patient is hypnotized and each alternate, in turn, is asked to tell what precipitated it into the life of the birth personality" (p. 28). The following verbatim excerpt from a hypnotic interview with a suspected multiple named Ken Bianchi demonstrates the leading nature of these procedures. Bianchi had been charged with murder and was interviewed in a forensic context. Following a hypnotic induction procedure, the clinician proceeded as follows:

> I've talked a bit to Ken but I think that perhaps there might be another part of Ken that I haven't talked to. And I would like to communicate with that part. And I would like that other part to come and talk to me . . . And when you are here, lift the left hand off the chair to signal to me that you are here. (Schwarz, 1981, pp. 142–143)

During this interview, Bianchi displayed an alter personality that confessed to the murders with which he had been charged. Importantly, the clinician who conducted this hypnotic interview pointed out that he employed such interview procedures regularly when diagnosing MPD (Watkins, 1984). In other words, leading hypnotic interviews in which the patient is repeatedly informed that he or she has other parts that can be addressed and communicated with as if they were separate people are employed routinely when diagnosing MPD.

Spanos, Weekes, and Bertrand (1985) used the hypnotic interview techniques employed with Bianchi to examine whether such procedures can provide naive subjects with the information required to enact multiple identities. The subjects were college students, who were asked to pretend that they had been accused of committing a series of murders. As in the Bianchi case, they were also informed that the evidence against them was strong and that they had been remanded for a psychiatric interview. Subjects were instructed to use whatever background information they possessed and whatever they could glean from their interview to behave the way they believed an accused in that situation would behave. However, they were told nothing about MPD. Subjects in one group were administered an interview modeled closely on the one used with Bianchi. Role-playing control subjects were also interviewed, but were never informed by the interviewing "psychiatrist" that they possessed another part that could be communicated with directly.

Most of the role players given the Bianchi hypnotic interview enacted MPD symptoms by adopting a different name, referring to their primary personality in the third person, and displaying amnesia for their alter personalities after termination of the interview. None of the role-playing controls displayed any of these symptoms. Role-playing multiples developed in the first session maintained their roles successfully in the second session by exhibiting marked and consistent differences from the primary personality on a variety of psychological tests. Role-playing controls performed similarly on the two administrations of the test. A replication of this study by Rabinowitz (1989) yielded similar findings.

Spanos, Weekes, Menary, and Bertrand (1986) extended these findings by again exposing role players to the Bianchi interview, in addition to an interview that focused on their childhood experiences. The task of the role players was to use cues gleaned from the interviews to present a childhood history that was consistent with the role called for by the interviews. Like the histories given by actual MPD patients, the role-playing multiples reported unhappy childhoods, described their parents as punitive and rejecting, described an early onset (before age 10) for their alter personalities, and described their alters as "taking over" in order to handle difficult situations and express strong emotions. The findings of these studies demonstrate that the interviewing procedures used routinely to diagnose MPD convey all of the information required to allow even psychiatrically unsophisticated subjects to enact the cardinal symptoms of multiplicity.

Because the subjects in these studies had been explicitly asked to fake their responses, it can be argued that people who were not told to do so would be unlikely to develop multiple identities following exposure to even leading hypnotic interviews. This argument is contradicted by the ample evidence described earlier, which demonstrated that hypnotic procedures that were even less leading than the one used with Bianchi regularly led to enactments of hidden selves and past-life personalities in normal non-simulating college students (Spanos & Hewitt, 1980; Spanos, Menary, et al., 1991).

Given that knowledge of MPD is widespread in our culture, it is not surprising that patients sometimes present with MPD symptoms in the absence of cuing from therapists. Nevertheless, people are unlikely to sustain the enactment of such a role in the absence of legitimation. For instance, Fahy, Abas, and Brown (1988) described a patient who had read a popular book about MPD, seen the movie *The Three Faces of Eve*, and presented herself to her therapist as having alter personalities. The therapist, however, directed attention away from the patient's alters and focused on her other problems in living. In the absence of the therapist's legitimation, the patient's MPD enactments went into sharp decline.

Kohlenberg (1973) also demonstrated the importance of interpersonal legitimation in the maintenance of alter identity enactments. Baseline rates of occurrence were obtained for the behaviors associated with each of an MPD patient's three personalities. When the behaviors associated with only one of the alters were selectively reinforced, those behaviors showed a dramatic increase in frequency. In later extinction trials, the frequency of occurrence of these behaviors decreased to baseline levels.

Currently, the legitimation of MPD often involved a broad social dimension. For instance, many MPD patients and therapists participate regularly in MPD workshops and conferences, and have access to national newsletters that provide updated information about the syndrome. Along with their individual therapy, many patients participate in MPD self-help and therapy groups that provide ongoing legitimation for their multiple self enactments (Mulhern, 1991b, 1994).

In summary, psychotherapy and therapy-related social supports appear to play a central role in the production and maintenance of MPD. Therapists are typically viewed by their patients as competent experts, whose suggestions are treated seriously. Further, patients are often insecure, unhappy people with a strong investment in winning the concern, interest, and approval of their therapist. Consequently, mutual shaping between therapists looking for signs of MPD and patients involved in creating an impression that will elicit approval is likely to lead to enactments of MPD that confirm the initial suspicions of the therapist and, in turn, lead the therapist to encourage and validate more elaborate displays of the disorder (Ganaway,

1992; Sutcliffe & Jones, 1962). In addition, the newsletters, therapy groups, workshops, and informal interactions with other multiples that have become an important part of the social life of many MPD patients serve to continually shape and legitimate multiple self enactments.

This analysis suggests that MPD patients come view themselves as they are viewed by their therapists. Adopting the view that they suffer from MPD involves patients coming to construe their various "symptoms" (e.g., mood swings, shameful and/or unrepresentative behaviors, ambivalent feelings, hostile fantasies, forgetfulness, guilt-inducing sexual feelings, bad habits) as the results of personified alter selves. In our culture, it is common for people to describe uncharacteristic or ambivalent feelings and behaviors metaphorically, wherein different parts of themselves are held accountable (e.g., "One part of me wanted to do it but another part said no," "I'm of two minds about the issue"). In conclusion, a sociocognitive analysis suggests that the development of MPD involves a therapist-supported reification of such metaphors wherein both the patient and the therapist come to construe the client as possessing multiple selves.

HYPNOTIC AND MPD AMNESIA

During the 19th century, hypnotic amnesia was thought to occur spontaneously as a function of the transition from being "hypnotized" to being awake (Sarbin & Coe, 1972). Similarly, MPD patients frequently behave as if some of their alters are amnesic for the actions and thoughts of other alters. Such amnesia is typically described as an involuntary and spontaneous occurrence akin to hypnotic amnesia (Bliss, 1986; Ross, 1989). Contrary to these descriptions, however, spontaneous amnesia is rare even among highly hypnotizable subjects, and when it does occur, it may simply reflect subjects' implicit understandings of the hypnotic role (Coe, 1989).

MPD patients are frequently described as living for years with alter personalities of which they are totally unaware (Kluft, 1985). However, hypnotic amnesia is rarely complete even amongst highly hypnotizable subjects. Moreover, among those few subjects who do exhibit total amnesia, more than half report postexperimentally that, during the amnesia test period, they consciously remembered but failed to report at least some of the target information (Spanos & Bodorik, 1977).

While subjects offer widely different descriptions of hypnotic amnesia, many describe their forgetting as an active process, which involves self-distraction and other conscious strategies aimed at inhibiting recall (Spanos & Bodorik, 1977). Some subjects do report that they were unable to recall target material, and that their amnesia felt involuntary. Nevertheless, the available experimental data indicate that even these subjects retain rather than lose control of memory processes (Coe, 1989; Spanos & Coe, 1992).

As an example of the above, Spanos, Radtke, and Bertrand (1984) convinced highly hypnotizable hypnotic subjects that concrete and abstract words were stored in different brain hemispheres, and that each hemisphere was associated with its own hidden self, which remained aware of everything that occurred in "its" hemisphere. Subjects were then taught a list of concrete and abstract words and given an amnesia suggestion for the list. Although subjects exhibited high levels of amnesia, they recalled all of the concrete words but none of the abstract words when the "hidden self" for their concrete hemisphere was contacted, and the opposite pattern of recall when the "hidden self" for their abstract hemisphere was contacted. In other words, instead of losing control over memory processes, all of these highly hypnotizable subjects behaved according to the expectations conveyed to them. Specifically, they acted as if they possessed hidden selves and recalled and failed to recall "forgotten" material in the appropriate sequences. Relatedly, Coe and Sluis (1989) exposed highly hypnotizable subjects who exhibited posthypnotic amnesia to strong and repeated demands to remember. Under these circumstances, even subjects who had insisted that their amnesia was involuntary showed very substantial recovery of the "forgotten" memories.

The "memory deficits" displayed by hypnotically amnesic subjects vary dramatically as a function of the expectations transmitted to them. Thus, depending upon the suggestions they are given, these subjects will behave as if they have forgotten an entire list, or only a subset of the list, the number 4, while recalling all remaining numbers, and so on (Coe, 1989). In one study, hypnotic subjects showed deficits on episodic memory tasks but not on semantic memory tasks (thus exhibiting dissociation between memory systems) or on both episodic and semantic tasks (i.e., no dissociation) as a function of subtle experimental demands (Spanos, Radtke, & Dubreuil, 1982). In order to exhibit the very wide range of memory "deficits" called for in these different experiments, hypnotic subjects must retain rather than lose control of memory processes, and guide their amnesic displays in terms of their understanding of what is called for by the amnesia test situation.

MPD patients also exhibit a wide range of amnesic deficits that are difficult to explain in terms of involuntary memory dysfunction. Some of these patients show a one-way amnesia between alter identities, while others show a two-way amnesia. When switching alter identities, most of these patients retain basic skills like reading and writing. In some early cases, however, these abilities were supposedly lost and had to be relearned by the new identity (Hacking, 1991; Kenny, 1986). In many modern cases,

MPD patients switch back and forth between alters (and thereby between sets of supposedly segregated memories) very quickly following a cue from their therapist. However, with a series of 19th-century British cases described by Hacking (1991) these kinds of switches between alters frequently involved a period of transitional sleep. Nineteenth- and early 20th-century MPD patients rarely displayed more than two or three alter identities (Bowman, 1990). Modern patients, on the other hand, display an average of 15 or more alters, and some of these patients exhibit over 100 alters (Ross, Norton, & Fraser, 1989). In other words, the number of "dissociated memory systems" supposedly possessed by MPD patients has grown dramatically since the beginning of the present century. These kinds of differences in amnesic displays over time and across MPD populations suggest that these patients, like hypnotically amnesic subjects, alter their patterns of recall as a function of their understanding of what is expected. As the expectations of therapists concerning the amnesia of their patients change, patients change their amnesic displays to meet the new expectations.

CHILD ABUSE MEMORIES AND
MULTIPLE PERSONALITY DISORDER

Most studies find that MPD patients report extremely high rates of childhood sexual and/or physical abuse (e.g., Ross, Norton, & Fraser, 1989; Ross et al., 1991). Nevertheless, these findings do not demonstrate that child abuse causes MPD. At least three noncausal factors probably influence the high rates of child abuse reported by these patients: (1) high base rates of child abuse in the samples from which those who will be given MPD diagnoses are drawn, (2) the use of a child abuse history to justify using leading hypnotic interviews that produce enactments of alter identities, and (3) confabulation of abuse in patients who generate such "memories" only after being exposed to interviews in which such reports are suggested and legitimated (Spanos, 1993).

The role of leading interviews in the confabulation of abuse histories was assessed experimentally by Spanos, Menary, and colleagues (1991; Experiment 2) in the context of their past-life regression research. Before past-life regression was enacted, subjects were informed that questions would be asked about the childhoods of their past-life identities in order to obtain information about how children were reared in earlier historical times. Subjects in one condition were further told that children in past eras had frequently been abused, while those in the other condition were given no information about abuse. When enacting their past-life identities, subjects given abuse information reported significantly higher levels of abuse during childhood than did the past-life identities of control subjects. Thus, subjects shaped the biographies attributed to their past-life identities by "remembering" the early abuse that they expected their past-life identities had experienced.

Early cases of MPD (pre-1920) were much less likely than modern ones to be associated with child abuse (Bowman, 1990; Kenny, 1986), and one modern study (Ross, Norton, & Fraser, 1989) found that American MPD patients were much more likely to report early abuse than were Canadian MPD patients. Although the relationship between MPD and child abuse was well established by 1980, patients' reports of abuse before this time did not include the ritualistic satanic elements that are now becoming increasingly prominent. Taken together, these cross-cultural and transhistorical differences in the early abuse reports of MPD patients suggest that abuse memories that are first recalled in adulthood may frequently be inaccurate and shaped by expectations created by their therapists about what must have happened to them as children.

Although it is often impossible to confirm or disconfirm the validity of child abuse memories that are recalled for the first time during adulthood, memories of ritual satanic abuse are an exception. The available evidence indicates that such reports are fantasies rather than memories of actual events (Mulhern, 1991b; Spanos, 1994). Consequently, the huge increase in the frequency of these memory reports in the last 10 years suggests that confabulation plays a prominent role in the abuse memories reported by MPD patients.

In 1980, Smith and Pazder reported on ritual satanic tortures that a young woman named "Michelle" had supposedly experienced during childhood and then forgotten until they were recovered during therapy (1980). Michelle's story was then used as propaganda by the Christian fundamentalist movement, which became increasingly prominent in many facets of American life during the 1980s. This movement helped to reinvigorate the Medieval mythology of Satanism. One aspect of this reinvigorated mythology is the belief in a powerful but secret international satanic conspiracy that carries out the kidnapping, torture, and sexual abuse of countless children, as well as engages in murder, forced pregnancies, and cannibalism (Hicks, 1991).

Therapists who were involved in the Christian network frequently joined the MPD movement in the 1980s (Mulhern, 1994), and, soon, memories like those Michelle related began to be reported by the alters of many MPD patients during therapy (Fraser, 1990; Young, Sachs, Braun, & Watkins, 1991). According to Mulhern (1994), by the mid-1980s, 25% of MPD patients had recovered memories of ritual satanic abuse, and, by 1992, the percentage who recovered such memories was as high as 80% in some treatment facilities.

If the ritual satanic memories of MPD patients were indeed accurate, there would have to exist a monumental criminal conspiracy that has been operating for at least 50 years and that has been responsible for the murder of thousands of people (Hicks, 1991). Law enforcement agencies throughout North America have investigated numerous allegations of satanic abuse made by MPD patients but have failed to substantiate the existence of the requisite criminal conspiracy (Lanning, 1989). The consistent failure of law enforcement agencies to uncover objective evidence (e.g., sacrificed bodies) that would support the satanic abuse allegations of MPD patients is very strong evidence that the vast majority of these allegations are false, and that the memories on which they are based are fantasies rather than remembrances of actual events (Hicks, 1991).

A recent survey of clinical psychologists in the United States indicated that 70% of the respondents had never seen patients who reported ritual abuse memories. A small minority, however, had seen large numbers of patients who reported ritual abuse (Bottoms, Shaver, & Goodman, 1991). These findings suggest that therapists who regularly obtain such reports may play a role in shaping the ritual abuse "memories" of their patients.

Satanic abuse memories are frequently elicited during hypnotic interviews that explicitly suggest such abuse took place. During these interviews, therapists sometimes describe satanic rituals and show the patients pictures of them or photographs of possible cult leaders. The therapist then addresses the patient's alters and asks if any of them remember such experiences or recognize the material (Mulhern, 1991a). Given the ease with which normal college students were induced to enact past-life personalities who "remembered" suffering abuse as children (Spanos, Menary, et al., 1991), it is hardly surprising that hypnotic interviews that strongly suggest satanic abuse lead MPD patients to "remember" such abuse.

Some patients report memory fragments or dreams with satanic content, and afterward are exposed to hypnotic interviews aimed at confirming such abuse. Since many MPD patients are enmeshed in a social network wherein they hear about satanic abuse from other patients, therapists, and MPD newsletters, and wherein they or their fellow patients attend workshops devoted to such abuse, "spontaneous" dreams and memories of this kind are hardly surprising and do not provide serious evidence of actual ritual abuse.

No doubt many people who become MPD patients were abused during childhood. Nevertheless, most people who suffer even severe child abuse do not exhibit MPD, and many people who have not been abused can easily and quickly be induced to display multiplicity (e.g., college students given past-life regression suggestions). Taken together, these findings argue against a causal relationship between child abuse and later displays of multiplicity.

MULTIPLE PERSONALITY DISORDER
AND HYPNOTIZABILITY

MPD patients frequently attain high scores on standardized hypnotizability scales (Bliss, 1980, 1986; Bliss & Larson, 1985). This finding is usually interpreted to mean that hypnotizability scores reflect individual differences in the capacity for dissociation (e.g., Bliss, 1986). According to this hypothesis, a substantial correlation between hypnotizability and independent measures of dissociation can be predicted. Stava and Jaffa (1988) developed several objective measures of dissociative capacity (e.g., degree of success at dividing attention and performing two tasks simultaneously). None of these dissociative measures correlated significantly with hypnotizability. Bernstein and Putnam (1986) developed a questionnaire that measures dissociation, and Putnam (1989) reported that it correlated significantly with hypnotizability. However, Spanos, Arango, and deGroot (1993) found that dissociation scores correlated significantly with hypnotizability only when both indices were assessed in the same context. When dissociation was assessed in a context that subjects did not connect with their hypnotizability testing, it failed to correlate significantly with hypnotizability. Even when tested in the same context, correlations between dissociation scores and hypnotizability were weak. For instance, in the Spanos et al. (1993) study the in-context correlation between dissociation and a behavioral index of hypnotizability was only $r = .23$. These findings indicate a lack of any intrinsic relationship between dissociation scores and hypnotizability. In short, whether or not these dimensions are found to be related seems to be dependent upon expectations generated by testing both dimensions in the same context.

Several studies indicate that the relationship between hypnotizability and the degree to which subjects respond to nonhypnotic suggestions is context-dependent (Spanos, Kennedy, & Gwynn, 1984; Spanos, Quigley, Gwynn, Glatt, & Perlini, 1991). In these studies, hypnotizability correlated significantly with suggestibility and with response to leading questions only when subjects connected their hypnotizability with their performance in these other suggestibility test situations.

The leading questions and leading interviews used to diagnose MPD are very frequently conducted in a hypnotic context, and the psychotherapeutic procedures employed with these patients almost always make use of hypnotic procedures. In other words, almost all MPD patients have been repeatedly administered hypnotic procedures, and have responded repeatedly to these procedures by displaying alter personalities. Given this fact, it follows that MPD patients would be very likely to construe themselves as highly hypnotizable subjects, who are motivated to respond as directed to communications delivered in an hypnotic context, and who expect to respond in this manner. Consequently, when they are tested on standardized hypnotizability scales, they are likely to respond in terms of the motivations and expectations derived from their earlier hypnotic experiences and, therefore, attain high hypnotizability scores.

This contextualist hypothesis does not deny that individual differences on some cognitive or interactional style dimensions may influence the ease with which people carry out multiple identity enactments. However, motivational and contextual demand variables are likely to interact with and may at times even override the effects of such individual variables (see Spanos, 1994, for fuller discussion of this point).

CONCLUSION

The theory of MPD propounded by the investigators who support this diagnosis is based on the idea that unhappiness and/or behavioral deviance in adulthood stems from particular traumatic events occurring in childhood. The particular childhood traumas focused upon by modern MPD proponents are physical abuse and, especially, sexual abuse. Because of its emphasis on childhood antecedents and on the notion that "symptoms" reflect unconscious defenses, this approach tends to greatly deemphasize the social nature of multiple identity enactments and the roles played by the institutionalized contexts, wherein these enactments are encouraged, shaped, and legitimated. In particular, this emphasis deflects attention away from the role played by clinicians themselves in cuing and legitimating manifestations of multiplicity. It also deflects attention away from the marked charges that have occurred over the years in MPD symptomatology. These changes clearly illustrate the role of social factors in shaping MPD displays. Since the 19th century, for example, the number of personalities per patient has jumped from two or three to frequently over twenty, and sometimes into the hundreds. Many early cases were marked by displays of catalepsy, transitional periods of sleep between the appearance of alters, and often convulsions, which are all uncommon today. The alter personalities of early patients were human, whereas recently scholarly articles have focused on animal alters (e.g., Hendrickson, McCarty, & Goodwin, 1990). While child abuse was reported to have occasionally accompanied early MPD cases, now we have the ritual satanic abuse of today.

Historical changes in the manifestations of MPD are difficult to deal with from a perspective that explains alter identity enactments as "symptoms" caused by past traumas rather than as expectancy guided goal-directed displays that change as a function of new information concerning role demands. Hence, we suggest that the phenomenon of multiplicity can be better understood when viewed from a sociocognitive and historical perspective.

ACKNOWLEDGMENT

Preparation of this chapter was supported by a grant from the Social Sciences and Humanities Research Council of Canada.

REFERENCES

Aldridge-Morris, R. (1989). *Multiple personality: An exercise in deception.* Hove, England: Lawrence Erlbaum.

Allison, R. B. (1978). On discovering multiplicity. *Swedish Journal of Hypnosis, 2,* 4–8.

Allison, R. B., & Schwarz, T. (1980). *Minds in many pieces.* New York: Rawson Wade.

Baker, R. A. (1992). *Hidden memories.* Buffalo, New York: Prometheus.

Barber, T. X. (1979). Suggested ("hypnotic") behavior: The trance paradigm versus an alternative paradigm. In E. Fromm & R. E. Shor (Eds.), *Hypnosis: Developments in research and new perspectives* (pp. 217–271). New York: Aldine.

Bernstein, E. M., & Putnam, F. W. (1986). Development, reliability, and validity of a dissociation scale. *Journal of Nervous and Mental Disease, 174,* 727–735.

Bliss, E. L. (1980). Multiple personalities: A report of 14 cases with implications for schizophrenia and hysteria. *Archives of General Psychiatry, 37,* 1388–1397.

Bliss, E. L. (1986). *Multiple personality, allied disorders and hypnosis.* New York: Oxford University Press.

Bliss, E. L., & Larson, E. M. (1985). Sexual criminality and hypnotizability. *Journal of Nervous and Mental Diseases, 173,* 522–526.

Bottoms, B. L., Shaver, P. R., & Goodman, G. S. (1991). *Profile of ritual and religion related abuse allegations reported to clinical psychologists in the United States.* Paper presented at the 99th annual convention of the American Psychological Association, San Francisco.

Bowman, E. S. (1990). Adolescent multiple personality disorder in the nineteenth and early twentieth centuries. *Dissociation, 3,* 179–187.

Braun, B. G. (1990). Multiple personality disorder: An overview. *American Journal of Occupational Therapy, 44,* 971–976.

Burgess, C. A., Spanos, N. P., Ritt, J., Hordy, T., & Brooks, S. (1993). *Compliant responding among high hypnotizables: An experimental demonstration.* Unpublished manuscript, Carleton University, Northfield, MN.

Coe, W. C. (1989). Posthypnotic amnesia: Theory and research. In N. P. Spanos & J. F. Chaves (Eds.), *Hypnosis: The cognitive-behavioral perspective* (pp. 418–436). Buffalo, NY: Prometheus.

Coe, W. C., & Sarbin, T. R. (1977). Hypnosis from the standpoint of a contextualist. *Annals of the New York Academy of Sciences, 295,* 2–13.

Coe, W. C., & Sluis, A. S. E. (1989). Increasing contextual pressures to breach posthypnotic amnesia. *Journal of Personality and Social Psychology, 57,* 885–894.

Fahy, T. A., Abas, M., & Brown, J. C. (1989). Multiple personality. A symptom of psychiatric disorder. *British Journal of Psychiatry, 154,* 99–101.

Fraser, G. A. (1990). Satanic ritual abuse: A cause of multiple personality disorder. *Journal of Child and Youth Care,* [Special issue], 55–66.

Ganaway, G. K. (1992). Some additional questions: A response to Shaffert Cozolino, to Gould & Cozolino, and Friesen. *Journal of Psychology and Theology, 20*, 201–205.

Hacking, I. (1986). The invention of split personalities. In A. Donagan, A. N. Perovich Jr., & M. V. Wedin (Eds.), *Human nature and natural knowledge* (pp. 63–85). New York: D. Reidel.

Hacking, I. (1991). Double consciousness in Britain 1815–1875. *Dissociation, 4*, 134–146.

Hendrickson, K. M., McCarty, T., & Goodwin, J. M. (1990). Animal alters: Case reports. *Dissociation, 4*, 218–221.

Hicks, R. D. (1991). *In pursuit of Satan*. Buffalo, NY: Prometheus.

Hilgard, E. R. (1979). Divided consciousness in hypnosis: The implications of the hidden observer. In E. Fromm & R. E. Shor (Eds.), *Hypnosis: Developments in research and new perspectives* (pp. 45–79). New York: Aldine.

Hilgard, E. R. (1991). A neodissociation interpretation of hypnosis. In S. J. Lynn & J. Rhue (Eds.), *Theories of hypnosis: Current models and perspectives* (pp. 83–104). New York: Guilford Press.

Kampman, R. (1976). Hypnotically induced multiple personality: An experimental study. *International Journal of Clinical and Experimental Hypnosis, 24*, 215–227.

Kenny, M. G. (1986). *The passion of Ansel Bourne: Multiple personality and American culture*. Washington, DC: Smithsonian Institution Press.

Kluft, R. P. (1985). The natural history of multiple personality disorder. In R. P. Kluft (Ed.), *Childhood antecedents of multiple personality* (pp. 197–238). Washington, DC: American Psychiatric Press.

Kohlenberg, R. J. (1973). Behavioristic approach to multiple personality: A case study. *Behavior Therapy, 4*, 137–140.

Lanning, K. V. (1989). Satanic, occult and ritualistic crime: A law enforcement perspective. *Police Chief, 56*, 62–85.

Merskey, H. (1992). The manufacture of personalities: The production of multiple personality disorder. *British Journal of Psychiatry, 160*, 327–340.

Mulhern, S. (1991a). Letter to the editor. *Child Abuse and Neglect, 15*, 609–611.

Mulhern, S. (1991b). Satanism and psychotherapy: A rumor in search of an inquisition. In J. T. Richardson, J. Best, & D. G. Bromley (Eds.), *The satanism scare* (pp. 145–172). New York: Aldine.

Mulhern, S. (1994). *Le trouble de la personnalité multiple à la recherche du trauma perdu*. Unpublished manuscript, Laboratorie des Rumeurs des Mythes du Futur et des Sectes, U.F.R. Anthropologie, Ethnologie, Science des Religions, Université de Paris, France.

Orne, M. T. (1979). On the simulating subject as a quasi-control group in hypnosis research: What, why and how. In E. Fromm & R. E. Shor (Eds.), *Hypnosis: Developments in research and new perspectives* (pp. 519–566). New York: Aldine.

Putnam, F. W. (1989). *Diagnosis and treatment of multiple personality disorder*. New York: Guilford Press.

Putnam, F. W., Guroff, J. J., Silberman, E. K., Barban, L., & Post, R. M. (1986). The clinical phenomenology of multiple personality disorder: A review of 100 recent cases. *Journal of Clinical Psychiatry, 47*, 285–293.

Rabinowitz, F. E. (1989). Creating the multiple personality: An experimental demonstration for an undergraduate abnormal psychology class. *Teaching of psychology, 16*, 69–71.

Ross, C. A. (1989). *Multiple personality disorder: Diagnosis, clinical features and treatment.* New York: John Wiley.

Ross, C. A., Miller, S. D., Bjornson, L., Reagor, P., & Fraser, G. A. (1991). Abuse histories in 102 cases of multiple personality disorder. *Canadian Journal of Psychiatry, 36*, 97–101.

Ross, C. A., Norton, C. R., & Fraser, G. A. (1989). Evidence against the iatrogenesis of multiple personality disorder. *Dissociation, 2*, 61–65.

Ross, C. A., Norton, R., & Wozney, K. (1989). Multiple personality disorder: An analysis of 236 cases. *Canadian Journal of Psychiatry, 34*, 414–418.

Sarbin, T. R., & Coe, W. C. (1972). *Hypnosis: A social-psychological analysis of influence communication.* New York: Holt, Rinehart & Winston.

Schwarz, T. (1981). *The hillside strangler: A murderer's mind.* New York: New American Library.

Smith, M., & Pazder, L. (1980). *Michelle remembers.* New York: Pocket Books.

Smith, M. C. (1983). Hypnotic memory enhancement of witnesses: Does it work? *Psychological Bulletin, 94*, 387–407.

Spanos, N. P. (1982). A social psychological approach to hypnotic behavior. In G. Weary & H. L. Mirels (Eds.), *Integrations of clinical and social psychology* (pp. 231–271). New York: Oxford University Press.

Spanos, N. P. (1986). Hypnotic behavior: A social-psychological interpretation of amnesia, analgesia and "trance logic." *Behavioral and Brain Sciences, 9*, 449–502.

Spanos, N. P. (1989). Hypnosis, demonic possession and multiple personality: Strategic enactments and disavowals of responsibility for actions. In C. A. Ward (Ed.), *Altered states of consciousness and mental health: Theoretical and methodological issues* (pp. 96–124). Newbury Park, CA: Sage.

Spanos, N. P. (1994). Multiple identity enactments and multiple personality disorder: A sociocognitive perspective. *Psychological Bulletin, 116*.

Spanos, N. P., Arango, M., & de Groot, H. P. (1993). Context as a moderator in relationships between attribute variables and hypnotizability. *Personality and Social Psychology Bulletin, 19*, 71–77.

Spanos, N. P., & Bodorik, H. L. (1977). Suggested amnesia and disorganized recall in hypnotic and task-motivated subjects. *Journal of Abnormal Psychology, 86*, 295–305.

Spanos, N. P., & Chaves, J. F. (Eds.). (1989). *Hypnosis: The cognitive-behavioral perspective.* Buffalo, NY: Prometheus.

Spanos, N. P., & Coe, W. C. (1992). A social psychological approach to hypnosis. In E. Fromm & M. R. Nash (Eds.), *Contemporary hypnosis research* (pp. 102–130). New York: Guilford Press.

Spanos, N. P., Flynn, D. M., & Gabora, N. J. (1989). Suggested negative visual hallucinations in hypnotic subjects: When no means yes. *British Journal of Experimental and Clinical Hypnosis, 6*, 63–67.

Spanos, N. P., Flynn, D. M., & Gwynn, M. I. (1988). Contextual demands, negative hallucinations and hidden observer responding: Three hidden observers observed. *British Journal of Experimental and Clinical Hypnosis, 5*, 5–10.

Spanos, N. P., Gwynn, M. I., & Stam, H. J. (1983). Instructional demands and ratings of overt and hidden pain during hypnotic analgesia. *Journal of Abnormal Psychology, 92*, 479–488.

Spanos, N. P., & Hewitt, E. C. (1980). The hidden observer in hypnotic analgesia: Discovery or experimental creation? *Journal of Personality and Social Psychology, 39*, 1201–1214.

Spanos, N. P., Kennedy, S. K., & Gwynn, M. I. (1984). The moderating effect of contextual variables on the relationship between hypnotic susceptibility and suggested analgesia. *Journal of Abnormal Psychology, 93*, 285–294.

Spanos, N. P., Menary, E., Gabora, N. J., DuBreuil, S. C., & Dewhirst, B. (1991). Secondary identity enactments during hypnotic past-life regression: A sociocognitive perspective. *Journal of Personality and Social Psychology, 61*, 308–320.

Spanos, N. P., Quigley, C. A., Gwynn, M. I., Glatt, R. L., & Perlini, A. H. (1991). Hypnotic interrogation, pretrial preparation, and witness testimony during direct and cross-examination. *Law and Human Behavior, 15*, 639–653.

Spanos, N. P., Radtke, H. L., & Bertrand, L. D. (1984). Hypnotic amnesia as a strategic enactment: Breaching amnesia in highly hypnotizable subjects. *Journal of Personality and Social Psychology, 47*, 1155–1169.

Spanos, N. P., Radtke, H. L., & Dubreuil, D. L. (1982). Episodic and semantic memory in posthypnotic amnesia: A reevaluation. *Journal of Personality and Social Psychology, 43*, 565–573.

Spanos, N. P., Rivers, S. M., & Ross, S. (1977). Experienced involuntariness and response to hypnotic suggestions. *Annals of the New York Academy of Sciences, 296*, 208–221.

Spanos, N. P., Weekes, J. R., & Bertrand, L. D. (1985). Multiple personality: A social psychological perspective. *Journal of Abnormal Psychology, 94*, 362–376.

Spanos, N. P., Weekes, J. R., Menary, E., & Bertrand, L. D. (1986). Hypnotic interview and age regression procedures in the elicitation of multiple personality symptoms: A simulation study. *Psychiatry, 49*, 298–311.

Stava, L. J., & Jaffa, M. (1988). Some operationalizations of the neodissociation concept and their relationship to hypnotic susceptibility. *Journal of Personality and Social Psychology, 54*, 989–996.

Sutcliffe, J. P., & Jones, J. (1962). Personal identity, multiple personality and hypnosis. *International Journal of Clinical and Experimental Hypnosis, 10*, 231–269.

Wagstaff, G. F. (1981). *Hypnosis, compliance and belief.* New York: St. Martin's Press.

Wagstaff, G. F. (1989). Forensic aspects of hypnosis. In N. P. Spanos & J. F. Chaves (Eds.), *Hypnosis: The cognitive-behavioral perspective* (pp. 340–357). Buffalo, NY: Prometheus.

Wambaugh, H. (1979). *Life before life.* New York: Bantam.

Watkins, J. G. (1984). The Bianchi (L.A. Hillside Strangler) case: Sociopath or multiple personality. *International Journal of Clinical and Experimental Hypnosis, 32*, 67–101.

Wilbur, C. B. (1984). Treatment of multiple personality. *Psychiatric Annals, 14*, 27–31.

Young, W. C., Sachs, R. G., Braun, B. G., & Watkins, R. T. (1991). Patients reporting ritual abuse in childhood: A clinical syndrome. Report of 37 cases. *Child Abuse and Neglect, 15*, 181–189.

II

DIAGNOSIS, ASSESSMENT, AND TREATMENT PERSPECTIVES

8

The Diagnosis and Assessment of Dissociative Disorders

Eve B. Carlson
Judith Armstrong

In recent years, a burgeoning awareness of the prevalence of trauma-related disorders has motivated researchers and clinicians to study effective methods for diagnosing dissociative disorders. Recent estimates of the rate of the most severe dissociative disorder, multiple personality disorder (MPD), in the inpatient psychiatric population have ranged from 2.4% to 11.3% (Bliss & Jeppsen, 1985; Graves, 1989; Ross, Anderson, Fleisher, & Norton, 1991), while prevalence rates for other dissociative disorders have not yet been estimated. While these estimates indicate that patients with dissociative disorders make up a relatively small minority of psychiatric patients, the rates are higher than most clinicians were trained to expect. Unfortunately, few mental health professionals have received any formal training in the diagnosis and assessment of dissociative disorders. It is not surprising, then, that those with dissociative disorders are frequently misdiagnosed and typically spend many years in the mental health system before receiving an accurate diagnosis (Putnam, Guroff, Silberman, Barban, & Post, 1986).

Several measures have proved promising in accurately identifying and assessing patients with dissociative disorders. Some of these are new instruments, developed specifically for this purpose, and some are standard psychological tests that have been recently applied to this diagnostic problem. We have divided our discussion into four sections which focus on the following: (1) some special issues involved in assessing dissociative-disordered patients, (2) the use of self-report measures of dissociation, (3) the use of structured clinical interviews with dissociative-disordered patients, and (4) the use of standard psychological tests in diagnosis and assessment.

CONSIDERATIONS IN ASSESSING
DISSOCIATIVE-DISORDERED PATIENTS

As of the writing of this chapter, the controversies surrounding the dissociative disorders, and, in particular, MPD, have not abated. The meaning and usefulness of the concepts of dissociation and self-multiplicity, the role of suggestion and clinical bias in diagnosing or failing to diagnose dissociative syndromes, the validity of patients' reports of childhood abuse or their amnesia for such experiences, are all concerns that are likely to complicate the referral for a dissociative disorder assessment. In a treatment atmosphere of dissension and confusion, a careful, detailed evaluation of the existence, nature, and importance of the patients' dissociative behaviors and experiences can play an educative and supportive role for all involved. The measures that will be discussed in this chapter are designed to provide systematic, standardized methods for gathering information about patients' dissociative symptomatology, so that leading questions, the suggestion of responses, and biased interpretations are minimized. Such concrete, objective data can be enormously helpful in refocusing the treatment team away from polemic to the therapy task at hand.

Assessors new to the field of dissociation will be reassured to learn that the general rules for good assessment hold true for dissociative disorders as well. They include the importance of establishing good rapport, of maintaining a neutral stance, of following standardized procedures, and of observing and documenting notable extra-test behaviors. What follows is a brief introduction to some special issues that must be considered when evaluating dissociative-disordered patients.

Gaining rapport with a patient suspected of having a dissociative disorder can be challenging. Issues of privacy, control, and trust that are often raised by the assessment process can be particularly intense for a traumatized patient who has experienced physical or sexual abuse, helplessness, and betrayal. Structured interviews and tests that assess dissociation may even exacerbate these sensitivities. The patient is specifically being asked to report on severe and quite unusual symptoms such as "losing" time, hearing internal conversations, and feeling bodily invaded by alien forces. While it may be a relief to find oneself mirrored in a test, the patient is likely to feel ambivalent about the experience. The dissociative-disordered person has often learned to keep his or her experiences secret in order to avoid experiencing disbelief from friends and family members, as well as to avoid being labeled an attention-getting fraud, or even worse, a psychotic.

Anxieties about maintaining one's privacy, power, and self-protection cannot be eliminated in the face of a procedure that, by its very nature, is designed to examine symptoms and conflicts that may be outside of awareness. However, it is helpful for the examiner to address these issues at the outset of the evaluation in order to minimize the patient's fear of the procedure and encourage his or her active participation in the assessment.

One can begin by inquiring about earlier assessment experiences (which have often been quite negative for these long-misdiagnosed people), responding to any questions and concerns about the present evaluation, and, most importantly, helping the patient to define a personal goal for the assessment (e.g., an area about his or her life that he or she would like to better understand). Procedures that make the test situation a reasonable and predictable process also serve to maximize active cooperation and control. Thus, the tester can briefly describe the measures, their general purpose, and the order in which tests will be given. It is also helpful to make it clear that the patient has a right to withhold information if it feels unsafe to respond, and that this will not ruin the assessment process or displease the examiner. Indeed, such reactions give helpful information about areas in which the patient may require special self-protection and support.

For dissociative-disordered patients who are assessed during times when their adjustment is fragile or deteriorating, concerns about safety, and of not precipitating further disorganization, should be paramount to the therapist. One difficulty with severe dissociation is that it blocks awareness of unpleasant affects until they reach intolerable levels. Thus, the vulnerable, dissociative-disordered patient can be quite susceptible to having startlingly abrupt and explosive, as well as delayed reactions, to anxiety-provoking material in the assessment. Such experiences of dyscontrol can be minimized by helping the patient to focus, in an anticipatory fashion, on his or her affective style. During the pretest interview, one can inquire about the ways in which the patient typically experiences feelings and shows distress and then discuss the most effective methods for calming him- or herself down, should the need arise. This approach has the additional benefit of giving early clues about the nature and extent of the patient's affective dissociation, his or her capacity to reflect on this, and associated coping strategies.

In planning for the safety of the patient, it cannot be emphasized too strongly that dissociation is a psychological defense; that is, by not integrating intolerable experiences into awareness, the patient is engaging in a self-protective activity. Therefore, probes for details of traumatic experiences and hazy memories must be approached with caution and with the patient's clear permission, lest one upset a fragile equilibrium. (See Herman, 1992, and Kluft, 1992, for discussions of this important issue.)

The measures to be described below assess observable dissociative and post-traumatic behaviors such as ongoing amnesia, disjunctive state changes, hyperarousal, and self-hypnotic behaviors. When a patient is asked to rate past symptoms and experiences, the questions remain at a purely descriptive level. The most defensible evidence for dissociative and post-traumatic phenomena does not lie in recollections of experiences from long ago, but in the patient's ongoing dissociative and post-traumatic behaviors, which, because they occur in the present, can be observed and documented by others.

USE OF SELF-REPORT MEASURES OF DISSOCIATION FOR DIAGNOSIS AND ASSESSMENT

Since the mid-1980s, several new self-report instruments have appeared that were designed to measure dissociation (Bernstein & Putnam, 1986; Briere & Runtz, 1990; Riley, 1988; Sanders, 1986; Wogan, 1992). All of these measures have potential as screening instruments for identifying patients with dissociative disorders and for assessing patients with dissociative disorders. To date, however, only the Dissociative Experiences Scale (DES) has been the subject of published research beyond an initial appearance in the literature. By the spring of 1994, the DES had been used as a measure in over 100 published studies. We will focus our discussion, then, on this self-report measure of dissociation.

The DES is a 28-item self-report measure of dissociation, that inquires about the frequency of amnestic experiences, gaps in awareness, depersonalization (distortions in perceptions of oneself), derealization (distortions in perceptions of one's environment), absorption, and imaginative involvement (Bernstein & Putnam, 1986). Examples of experiences described in the items include finding evidence of having done things that you do not remember doing (amnesia), listening to someone talk and suddenly realizing that you did not hear part or all of what was said (a gap in awareness), looking in a mirror and not recognizing yourself (depersonalization), being in a familiar place and finding it strange and unfamiliar (derealization), becoming so absorbed in watching television or a movie that you are unaware of what is happening around you (absorption), and not being sure whether things that you remember really did happen or whether you just dreamed them (imaginative involvement). Directions on the cover sheet specify that subjects should report only those experiences that occur when they *are not* under the influence of alcohol or drugs. The scale takes about 10 minutes to complete and yields item and total scores that range from 0 to 100. The original version of the scale required subjects to answer each question by marking a line (with anchor points of 0 and 100) to show what percentage of the time they have the experience. A second version of the scale requires subjects to circle a number from 0 to 100 (0, 10, 20, 30, etc.) to show what percentage of the time they have the experience. For both versions, total scores are calculated by averaging the 28 item scores.

Studies of the scale's reliability showed that the scale has good internal consistency and that scores on the scale are consistent over time. Studies of the internal consistency of scores have yielded split-half reliability correlation coefficients ranging from .83 to .93 (Bernstein & Putnam, 1986; Pitblado & Sanders, 1991). Another study of internal consistency of scores yielded a Cronbach's alpha of .95 (Frischholz, et al., 1990). Test–retest reliability for the scale has been studied by administering the measure to subjects on two different occasions (about 4 weeks apart). Correlations between scores on the first and second administrations have ranged from .84 to .96 in various studies (Bernstein & Putnam, 1986; Carlson & Rosser-Hogan, 1991; Frischholz et al., 1990; Pitblado & Sanders, 1991). Studies of both internal and test–retest reliability have included subjects from clinical populations that show high levels of dissociation.

Results from studies on the use of the DES as a clinical tool have been promising as they show high levels of dissociation in conditions related to dissociative disorders. For instance, elevated levels of dissociation were found in adult survivors of child abuse (Chu & Dill, 1990; Coons, Bowman, Pellow, & Schneider, 1989; Goodwin, Cheeves, & Connell, 1990; Herman, Perry, & van der Kolk, 1989; Sandberg & Lynn, 1992; Sanders & Giolas, 1991; Strick & Wilcoxon, 1991; van der Kolk, Perry, & Herman, 1991), in subjects with post-traumatic stress disorder (PTSD) (Branscomb, 1991; Bremner, et al., 1992; Carlson & Rosser-Hogan, 1991), and in subjects with dissociative disorders (Armstrong & Loewenstein, 1990; Carlson et al., 1993; Coons, Bowman, & Milstein, 1988; Coons et al., 1989; Frischholz et al., 1990; Loewenstein & Putnam, 1990; Ross, Norton, & Anderson, 1988; Ross, Norton, & Wozney, 1989).

The next step was to directly investigate the capacity of the DES to accurately predict a dissociative diagnosis. The DES should be able to accurately identify subjects with dissociative disorders if it is to be useful as a screening tool. Three recent studies have tested the scale's ability to correctly classify dissociative and nondissociative subjects. In two of these studies, the DES performed well in distinguishing between dissociative and normal subjects (Frischholz et al., 1990; Steinberg, Rounsaville, & Cicchetti, 1991). Distinguishing between these two types of subjects, however, is not the kind of clinical decision that is normally necessary. Typically, clinicians (and scales) must distinguish between dissociative patients and patients with other disorders. This task is made increasingly difficult because of the fact that subjects who have one fairly common disorder (PTSD) often have substantial dissociative symptoms. This more difficult classification decision was explored in the Steinberg et al. (1991) study, and the DES performed well in distinguishing dissociative patients from patients with other disorders, but a much larger study was needed before those results could be considered conclusive.

In a large, multicenter study described in detail elsewhere (Carlson et al., 1993), a cutoff score of 30 or above on the DES was used to classify a pool of 1,051 general psychiatric inpatients as either having MPD or not. Those with scores of 30 or more were classified as having MPD and those with scores below 30 were classified as not having the disorder. The results of this analysis were that 74% of those with MPD were correctly identified (sensitivity), and 80% of those who did not have MPD were correctly identified (specificity). In addition, 61% of the false positive identifications (those who scored 30 or above who did not have MPD) had post-traumatic stress disorder or a dissociative disorder other than MPD. Further analysis indicated that the cutoff score of 30 was optimal for maximizing the accuracy of classification decisions.

This picture is complicated a bit by application of Bayes's theorem, which enables us to take into account base rates for disorders to determine what proportion of those who score negative for a disorder are true negatives and what proportion of those who score positive are true positives. These are usually the questions we really want answered when we use scales to make classification decisions. In the case of an MPD screening tool, how many of the "low" scorers will actually have MPD, and how many of the "high" scorers will really have MPD? If the analysis of the multicenter study is representative, in psychiatric samples only 1% of those scoring under 30 will have MPD, and about 17% of those scoring 30 or over will really have MPD (though many of these will have PTSD or a dissociative disorder other than MPD). In other words, in actual practice, using a cutoff score of 30 to identify MPD patients will rarely result in classifying someone with MPD incorrectly, but it will frequently result in classifying someone who does not have MPD incorrectly. This curious result occurs because of the very low base rate of MPD in the psychiatric population (estimated in this study to be at 5%). Since MPD is such a relatively "unlikely" event, most of those with high DES scores will be "false positives," that is, people who are identified as having MPD, but actually do not. For this reason, it is advisable to consider a cutoff score of 30 or over as identifying those with a "possible dissociative disorder." Those with high DES scores should certainly be interviewed further to determine whether or not a dissociative diagnosis is accurate.

It is also important to note that *for each individual classification decision* the classification of MPD is either right or wrong. This implies that the DES is useful for screening large numbers of psychiatric patients to "flag" those with high levels of dissociation, but that its ability to correctly diagnose any one individual is not at all certain. The DES should never be used, by itself, to make a dissociative disorder diagnosis.

Several factor analytic studies have found a trifactorial structure for the DES and have suggested that subscale scores might be used to measure these factors in clinical and research settings (Carlson et al.,1991; Frischholz, Schwartz, Braun, & Sachs, 1992; Ross, Joshi, & Currie, 1991). The three factors identified have been thought to measure amnestic dissociation, depersonalization and derealization, and absorption and imaginative involvement. However, a subsequent analysis of the Carlson et al. (1991) data has revealed that the factors are confounded with frequency of item endorsement (Waller, in press). Waller's reanalysis controlled for skewness of item scores and found only one general dissociation factor that could be reliably measured. Hence, the three factors described above may measure high, medium, and low endorsement frequency (respectively) in addition to measuring subtypes of dissociation. Consequently, for any particular subject or for any group of subjects, it is impossible to tell whether the subscales accurately measure subtypes of dissociation. Clinicians may still find the subscales useful, but they should be cautious in interpreting them, given their ambiguous nature.

In addition to helping quantify the level of dissociation a person is experiencing, the DES can be used to qualitatively assess dissociative experiences. With patients who have high scores, it is often useful to go through the DES with them and inquire about items that they endorsed at high rates. The clinician can ask them to describe in detail examples of experiences they have had for each "high" item. This method is effective in confirming that patients understood the questions well and are indeed having the dissociative experiences described in the items.

DIAGNOSING DISSOCIATIVE DISORDERS
WITH STRUCTURED CLINICAL INTERVIEWS

There are two major structured interviews and one semistructured interview now available to clinicians and researchers for diagnosing dissociative disorders.

In 1985, Steinberg developed the Structured Clinical Interview for DSM-III Dissociative Disorders (SCID-D). It has since been updated to correspond to DSM-III-R and DSM-IV diagnostic criteria. The full interview and an interviewer's guide are now available through the American Psychiatric Press (Steinberg, 1992a; Steinberg, 1992b). On field testing with a variety of psychiatric disorders, the SCID-D has shown good to excellent reliability and ability to discriminate dissociative disorders from other clinical disorders (Goff, Olin, Jenike, Baer, & Buttolph, 1992; Steinberg, Cicchetti, Buchanan, Hall, & Rounsaville, 1993; Steinberg, Rounsaville, & Cicchetti, 1990). Specifically, reliability rates for symptom scales have ranged from .60 to .95, with a .96 agreement between interviewers for the presence or absence of a dissociative disorder. The SCID-D was able to distinguish dissociative-disordered from nondissociative-disordered patients and from normal controls at better than the .0001 confidence level, with almost no overlap of scores between the three groups. The Dutch translation of the SCID-D (Boon & Draijer, 1991) has yielded nearly identical symptom profiles for the Dutch subjects, suggesting some degree of universality in the expression of dissociative symptoms.

This more than 250-item interview takes from 10 to 90 minutes to administer, depending upon the number and complexity of dissociative symptoms observed. The procedure enables the trained clinician to use the interviewee's verbal and nonverbal responses to rate the existence and severity of five dissociative symptoms; amnesia, depersonalization, derealization, identity confusion, and identity alteration. The SCID-D also can be used to diagnose the five DSM dissociative disorders: Psychogenic Amnesia, Psychogenic Fugue, Depersonalization Disorder, Multiple Personality Disorder, and Dissociative Disorder Not Otherwise Specified. While scoring criteria are clearly defined, the format does require some diagnostic sophistication, since it includes branching options that allow the clinician to do an in-depth exploration of specific dissociative symptomatology. In other words, the SCID-D has been designed to capture an expert clinical interview about dissociation within a standardized format. A screening variant of the SCID-D, the Mini-SCID-D (Steinberg, Rounsaville, & Cicchetti, 1992) is capable of rapidly assessing the presence or absence of significant dissociative pathology. It may prove to be a cost-effective method of identifying patients in need of the more extensive SCID-D evaluation.

The Dissociative Disorders Interview Schedule (DDIS) was developed by Ross, Heber, Norton, and Anderson in 1989. The full interview is now available in two publications (Ross, 1989; Ross, Joshi, & Currie, 1990). In several epidemiological studies, the DDIS has shown an overall interrater reliability of .68; it also demonstrated a low false positive rate for MPD in a clinical population of less than 1% (Ross, 1991; Ross et al., 1990).

The 131-item measure involves a straightforward "yes/no" format, which simplifies the training and administration process. The full interview takes an average of 40 minutes to complete. In addition to questions about dissociation, the DDIS includes an evaluation of childhood physical and sexual abuse, as well as other trauma-related features such as Schneiderian first-rank symptoms, somatic complaints, and paranormal experiences. The DDIS also yields DSM-III-R diagnoses for Borderline Personality Disorder, Somatization Disorder, and Major Depression episodes. Regarding this latter feature, it should be kept in mind that severe dissociative disorders typically involve a plethora of symptoms that mimic an array of Axis I and II disorders. For example, Ross, Ellason, and Fuchs (1992) found that their MPD sample met SCID I and II criteria for approximately 8 Axis I disorders and 4.5 Axis II disorders. Since it is implausible that patients could have this many concomitant disorders, a DDIS diagnosis of MPD probably obviates the need for additional diagnoses.

Loewenstein's (1991) semistructured Office Mental Status Examination for Complex Dissociative Symptoms and Multiple Personality Disorder provides a set of questions as well as typical patient responses that illustrate the range of dissociative presentations. The interview questions are grouped into the following symptom clusters: affective symptoms, somatoform symptoms, amnesia symptoms, autohypnotic symptoms (e.g., spontaneous trances), and process symptoms (i.e., signs of state and identity changes). Surprisingly, in view of the fact that dissociative disorders are generally understood as trauma-based pathologies, this is the only interview to systematically assess the presence and severity of PTSD symptoms, such as hyperarousal and numbing.

Unlike the SCID-D and DDIS, the Loewenstein interview is not meant to offer structured guidelines for diagnosis. Rather, this clinical procedure organizes the process of surveying the patient's dissociative symptoms and then relies upon the interviewer's clinical judgment for a diagnostic decision. While the reliability for the Loewenstein interview has not yet been established and while it is a much less structured method of assessment than the SCID-D and DDIS, it may prove to be a valid measure of dissociative psychopathology.

The decision of which measure to utilize will depend on the particular needs and resources of the clinician or researcher. As can be seen, the three instruments measure a somewhat different range of symptoms and associated experiences. They also differ in length and complexity. Ross's DDIS has a clarity, simplicity, and brevity that makes it ideal for large-scale epidemiological studies (it can even be administered by telephone), and for settings where time and/or scarcity of trained interviewers are factors. Both the Steinberg and Loewenstein interviews require greater clinical expertise and investment of time. Steinberg's SCID-D combines a standardized format with a thorough examination of the patient's dissociative symptoms. Its excellent reliability for diagnosing both dissociative symptoms and dissociative disorders makes it the tool of choice for studying dissociative processes in a range of dissociative disorders, as well as other psychopathologies. If interrater reliability can be established, the Loewenstein interview will be useful for clinical studies on the phenomenology of dissociative disorders, and for clarifying complex clinical cases. As it stands, the interview can be used as a tool for clinical training in the diagnosis of severe dissociative disorders.

ASSESSING DISSOCIATIVE DISORDERS WITH STANDARD TEST BATTERIES

Research with standard test batteries to date has been limited because of the prevalence of single case studies and studies with very few subjects which are not necessarily generalizable. Nonetheless, psychological testing has played an important role in establishing MPD as a valid diagnostic entity. Studies using psychological test batteries have substantiated the unusual variability of cognitive and emotional functioning across alter personalities (e.g., Alpher, 1991; Ludwig, Brandsma, Wilbur, Bendfeldt, & Douglas, 1972). Unfortunately, use of test batteries across alter personalities is rare because it is so time consuming.

When alter personalities are carefully evaluated, the results can be quite useful and can lead to advances in our understanding of dissociative disorders. One example of such a comprehensive evaluation of alter personalities is Erickson and Rapaport's early single case study of an MPD subject, which was republished in Erickson's collected papers (1980). Using a standard test battery, these researchers documented an obsessive compulsive personality style that was expressed across the alter personalities of their subject. Notably, this finding contradicted the prevailing assumption of the time that dissociative disorders were simply variants of "hysteria." Recent research of Armstrong (1991), and Armstrong and Loewenstein (1990), has replicated Erickson and Rapaport's findings. These researchers found that the Rorschach responses of their dissociative-disordered inpatient sample were characterized by an obsessive compulsive coping style, involving behavioral delay, internalization, distancing, and avoidance of affect.

Other studies using traditional tests have examined either the Rorschach or the Minnesota Multiphasic Personality Inventory (MMPI) alone, searching for diagnostic signs specific to MPD. Wagner and Heise (1974) and Wagner, Allison, and Wagner (1983) studied several MPD subjects with the Rorschach. Their scoring rules, however, have not been supported by later research (e.g., Lovitt & Lefkof, 1985). One useful outcome of this Rorschach research has been the growing evidence that traumatic responses to the inkblots are characteristic of MPD subjects. Wagner and coworkers first noted the tendency of MPD patients to react to the inkblots with the generally rare blood and aggression responses. Armstrong and Loewenstein (1990) developed a Traumatic Content Index (which represents the sum of the Exner anatomy, blood, aggression, and morbid responses) to examine this hypothesis. They found that, on average, half of each test protocol completed by their dissociative-disordered sample contained traumatic material. Similar indications of elevated morbid and aggressive content have been found in Rorschach studies of traumatized subjects with a variety of clinical diagnoses (see, e.g., Saunders, 1991; van der Kolk & Ducey, 1989). Such findings suggest that these responses are not indicators of psychotic or regressed function, as they have been traditionally interpreted to be. Rather, the responses appear to represent expressions of traumatic memories evoked by the test stimuli. In other words, for traumatized patients, tests like the Rorschach can cease to be projective measures, and become instead traumatic triggers. Unless the assessor is conversant with the PTSD literature, including the signs of flashback, traumatic reactions are likely to be misdiagnosed as indicators of psychotic or characterologically primitive functioning.

While traumatic content may indeed be one indicator of dissociation, the search for Rorschach markers of dissociative disorders has generally been limited by a number of methodological problems. Scoring systems and the establishment of scorer reliability have not been uniform across studies. Procedures and hypotheses have usually not been guided by clear decisions about how to test (e.g., which personalities to assess in MPD patients), or by explicit theory (e.g., which test variables signal dissociation, trauma, and state changes). Most importantly, substantial numbers of dissociative-disordered patients must first be assessed before we can have a clear understanding of what this group "looks like" on tests and how they can be expected to differ from other diagnostic groups. For example, we do not yet know whether dissociative-disordered patients all have the same personality style, whether their styles are completely heterogeneous, or whether there are several different personality subgroups in this group of patients. Until larger descriptive studies are done, significant Rorschach findings may reflect a variety of sampling errors and demographic correlates rather than the personality characteristics of dissociative patients.

Studies that use the MMPI (e.g., Coons, 1986; Bliss, 1984) tend to have the same strengths and weaknesses as those that employ the Rorschach. These studies have revealed that the MMPI does not produce markers that can distinguish MPD from borderline personality disorder or from a spectrum of psychotic disorders. However, the data collected have been very useful from a clinical standpoint.

One of the most consistent findings is the frequent elevation of the MMPI "F" scale in dissociative-disordered patients. In the general test literature, this scale is often interpreted as an indicator of an "invalid" or histrionically exaggerated symptom profile. However, an examination of the items in the "F" scale shows that, rather than measuring exaggerated reporting or deception, the questions included survey a variety of atypical experiences common to dissociation and dissociative disorders. Indeed, dissociative-like items are scattered throughout subscales of the MMPI, the Millon Clinical Multiaxial Inventory (MCMI), and other structured tests. Since none of these tests have been standardized with dissociative-disordered subjects, the interpretation of all scale elevations remains unknown for this clinical group. As with the Rorschach, test interpretations that do not take into account dissociative and PTSD phenomena, and which are faulty because of our present state of knowledge about these phenomena, are likely to lead to misdiagnoses and misinterpretations of the actual functioning of dissociative-disordered patients.

For example, Coons (1986) found that his MPD treatment sample showed high elevations on the "Schizophrenia" scale (Scale 8) of the MMPI, a scale that also contains items related to dissociative phenomena. Such an elevation might indicate these MPD subjects are prone to severe psychological disorganization. On the other hand, it could signal that these treatment-sophisticated subjects are able to admit and work on dissociative experiences, such as the hearing of voices (of alter personalities). In other words, we do not know whether the elevation on the "Schizophrenia" scale reflects a serious ego weakness or a valuable ego strength in this group. Clearly, making diagnostic judgments about dissociative-disordered patients on the basis of structured measures such as the MMPI is, at this point in our knowledge, premature.

A promising approach to the use of standard test batteries can be seen in Ross, Ellason, and Fuchs's recent work (1992). They are employing the MMPI and MCMI to look at the within-group variability of MPD patients. These researchers have isolated several different scale patterns shown by subgroups within their larger sample. Examination of the relationship between these different test patterns and behavioral and treatment variables may prove of considerable practical use.

In conclusion, from both a clinical and methodological standpoint, insufficient attention has been paid to the problem of how to reliably assess dissociative patients who, by their very nature, are hidden, divided, and unusually variable persons. Armstrong (1991, in press) has discussed the test implications of such issues. She presents an approach to establishing good rapport with patients suspected of having dissociative disorders, as well as a checklist for identifying and recording dissociative, state change, hypnotic, and traumatic reactions during testing. Allen and Smith (1993), utilizing Armstrong's approach, were able to show improved IQ functioning in a dyslexic MPD patient through eliciting a cognitively compensating alter. They discuss the effects of this on the patient's move toward integration.

CONCLUSION

In a brief period of years, a number of tests that diagnose and assess for dissociative disorders have become available to the clinician and researcher. These developments should shorten the excessive amount of time dissociative-disordered patients spend in the health system before they receive the correct diagnosis and treatment. The extensively researched and validated DES can be successfully used by clinicians to identify patients needing further evaluation for dissociative disorders. A structured or semistructured interview (e.g., SCID-D, DDIS, or Loewenstein interview) can then be given to clarify the diagnosis for clinical and/or research purposes. Judiciously interpreted psychological testing can supplement this process by clarifying the presence and severity of PTSD and determining the coping style and the personality strengths and weaknesses the patient brings to treatment. One positive outcome of the validity controversy surrounding the dissociative disorders has been that it has encouraged researchers to move quickly to develop measures that allow us to objectively diagnose and evaluate the treatment progress of these patients.

REFERENCES

Allen, J. G., & Smith, W. H. (1993). Diagnosing dissociative disorders. *Bulletin of the Menninger Clinic, 57*, 328–343.

Alpher, V. S. (1991). Assessment of ego functioning in multiple personality disorder. *Journal of Personality Assessment, 56*, 373–387.

Armstrong, J. G. (1991). The psychological organization of multiple personality disordered patients as revealed in psychological testing. *Psychiatric Clinics of North America, 14*, 533–546.

Armstrong, J. G. (in press). A method of assessing multiple personality disorder through psychological testing. In B. M. Cohen & J. A. Turkus (Eds.), *Multiple personality: Continuum of care*. New York: Jason Aronson.

Armstrong, J. G., & Loewenstein, R. J. (1990). Characteristics of patients with multiple personality and dissociative disorders on psychological testing. *Journal of Nervous and Mental Disease, 178*, 448–454.

Bernstein, E. M., & Putnam, F. W. (1986). Development, reliability, and validity of a dissociation scale. *Journal of Nervous and Mental Disease, 174*, 727–735.

Bliss, E. (1984). A symptom profile of patients with multiple personality disorder, including MMPI results. *Journal of Nervous and Mental Disease, 174*, 197–202.

Bliss, E. L., & Jeppsen, E. A. (1985). Prevalence of multiple personality among inpatients and outpatients. *American Journal of Psychiatry, 142*, 250–251.

Boon, S., & Draijer, N. (1991). Diagnosing dissociative disorders in the Netherlands. *American Journal of Psychiatry, 148*, 458–462.

Branscomb, L. (1991). Dissociation in combat-related post-traumatic stress disorder. *Dissociation, 4*(1), 13–20.

Briere, J., & Runtz, M. (1990). Augmenting Hopkins SCL scales to measure dissociative symptoms: Data from two nonclinical samples. *Journal of Personality Assessment, 55*, 376–379.

Carlson, E. B., Putnam, F. W., Ross, C. A., Anderson, G., Clark, P., Torem, M., Coons, P., Bowman, E., Chu, J. A., Dill, D., Loewenstein, R. J., & Braun, B. G. (1991). Factor analysis of the Dissociative Experiences Scale: A multicenter study. In B. G. Braun & E. B. Carlson (Eds.), *Proceedings of the Eighth International Conference on Multiple Personality and Dissociative States*. Chicago: Rush–Presbyterian.

Carlson, E. B., Putnam, F. W., Ross, C. A., Torem, M., Coons, P., Dill, D., Loewenstein, R. J., & Braun, B. G. (1993). Validity of the Dissociative Experiences Scale in screening for multiple personality disorder: A multicenter study. *American Journal of Psychiatry, 150,* 1030–1036.

Carlson, E. B., & Rosser-Hogan, R. (1991). Trauma experiences, posttraumatic stress, dissociation, and depression in Cambodian refugees. *American Journal of Psychiatry, 148,* 1548–1551.

Chu, J. A., & Dill, D. L. (1990). Dissociative symptoms in relation to childhood physical and sexual abuse. *American Journal of Psychiatry, 147,* 887–892.

Coons, P., Bowman, E., & Milstein, V. (1988). Multiple personality disorder: A clinical investigation of 50 cases. *Journal of Nervous and Mental Disease, 176,* 519–527.

Coons, P. M. (1986). Treatment progress in 20 patients with multiple personality disorder. *Journal of Nervous and Mental Disease, 174,* 715–721.

Coons, P. M., Bowman, E., Pellow, T. A., & Schneider, P. (1989). Post-traumatic aspects of the treatment of victims of sexual abuse and incest. *Psychiatric Clinics of North America, 12,* 325–335.

Erickson, M. H., & Rapaport, D. (1980). Findings on the nature of the personality structures in two different dual personalities by means of projective and psychometric tests. In E. L. Rossi (Ed.), *The collected papers of Milton Erickson* (Vol. 3, pp. 271–291). New York: Irvington.

Frischholz, E. J., Braun, B. G., Sachs, R. G., Hopkins, L., Shaeffer, D. M., Lewis, J., Leavitt, F., Pasquotto, M. A., & Schwartz, D. R. (1990). The Dissociative Experiences Scale: Further replication and validation. *Dissociation, 3*(3), 151–153.

Frischholz, E. J., Schwartz, D. R., Braun, B. G., & Sachs, R. G. (1992). *Factor analytic studies of dissociative experiences in normal and abnormal populations.* Unpublished manuscript.

Goff, D. C., Olin, J. A., Jenike, M. A., Baer, L., & Buttolph, M. L. (1992). Dissociative symptoms in patients with obsessive compulsive disorder. *Journal of Nervous and Mental Disease, 180,* 332–337.

Goodwin, J. M., Cheeves, K., & Connell, V. (1990). Borderline and other severe symptoms in adult survivors of incestuous abuse. *Psychiatric Annals, 20,* 22–32.

Graves, S. M. (1989). Dissociative disorders and dissociative symptoms at a community health center. *Dissociation, 2,* 119–127.

Herman, J. L. (1992). *Trauma and recovery.* New York: Basic Books.

Herman, J. L., Perry, J. C., & van der Kolk, B. A. (1989). Childhood trauma in borderline personality disorder. *American Journal of Psychiatry, 146,* 490–495.

Kluft, R. P. (1992). Discussion: A specialist's perspective on multiple personality disorder. *Psychoanalytic Inquiry, 12,* 139–171.

Loewenstein, R., & Putnam, F. W. (1990). The clinical phenomenology of males with multiple personality disorder. *Dissociation, 3*(3), 135–143.

Lovitt, R., &. Lefkof, G. (1985). Understanding multiple personality disorder with the Comprehensive Rorschach System. *Journal of Personality Assessment, 59,* 289–294.

Ludwig, A. M., Brandsma, J. M., Wilbur, C. B., Bendfeldt, F., & Douglas, J. H. (1972). The objective study of a multiple personality. *Archives of General Psychiatry, 26,* 298–310.

Pitblado, C. B., & Sanders, B. (1991). Reliability and short-term stability of scores on the Dissociative Experiences Scale. In B. G. Braun & E. B. Carlson (Eds.),

Proceedings of the Eighth International Conference on Multiple Personality and Dissociative States. Chicago: Rush–Presbyterian.

Putnam, F. W., Guroff, J. J., Silberman, E. K., Barban, L., & Post, R. M. (1986). The clinical phenomenology of multiple personality disorder: Review of 100 recent cases. *Journal of Clinical Psychiatry, 47,* 285–293.

Riley, K. C. (1988). Measurement of dissociation. *Journal of Nervous and Mental Disease, 176,* 449–450.

Ross, C. A. (1989). *Multiple personality disorder: Diagnosis, clinical features, and treatment.* New York: John Wiley.

Ross, C. A. (1991). Epidemiology of multiple personality disorder and dissociation. *Psychiatric Clinics of North America, 14,* 503–517.

Ross, C. A., Ellason, B. A., & Fuchs, D. (1992). Axis I and Axis II comorbidity of multiple personality disorder. In B. G. Braun & E. B. Carlson (Eds.), *Proceedings of the Ninth International Conference on Multiple Personality and Dissociative States.* Chicago: Rush–Presbyterian.

Ross, C. A., Anderson, G., Fleisher, W. P., & Norton, G. R. (1991). The frequency of multiple personality disorder among psychiatric inpatients. *American Journal of Psychiatry, 148,* 1717–1720.

Ross, C. A., Joshi, S., & Currie, R. (1991). Dissociative experiences in the general population: Identification of three factors. *Hospital and Community Psychiatry, 42,* 297–301.

Ross, C. A., Joshi, S., & Currie, R. (1990). Dissociative experiences in the general population. *American Journal of Psychiatry, 147,* 1547–1552.

Ross, C. A., Norton, G. R., & Anderson, G. (1988). The Dissociative Experiences Scale: A replication study. *Dissociation, 1*(3), 21–22.

Ross, C. A., Norton, G. R., & Wozney, K. (1989). Multiple personality disorder: An analysis of 236 cases. *Canadian Journal of Psychiatry, 34,* 413–418.

Sandberg, D. A., & Lynn, S. J. (1992). Dissociative experiences, psychopathology and adjustment, and child and adolescent maltreatment in female college students. *Journal of Abnormal Psychology, 101,* 717–723.

Sanders, B., & Giolas, M. H. (1991). Dissociation and childhood trauma in psychologically disturbed adolescents. *American Journal of Psychiatry, 148,* 50–54.

Sanders, S. (1986). The perceptual alteration scale: A scale measuring dissociation. *American Journal of Clinical Hypnosis, 29,* 95–102.

Saunders, E. A. (1991). Rorschach indicators of chronic childhood sexual abuse in female borderline inpatients. *Bulletin of the Menninger Clinic, 55,* 48–70.

Steinberg, M. (1992a). *The interviewer's guide to the structured clinical interview for DSM-IV dissociative disorders.* Washington, DC: American Psychiatric Press.

Steinberg, M. (1992b). *The structured clinical interview for DSM-IV disorders.* Washington, DC: American Psychiatric Press.

Steinberg, M., Cicchetti, D., Buchanan, J., Hall, P., & Rounsaville, B. (1993). Clinical assessment of dissociative symptoms and disorders: The structured clinical interview for DSM-IV dissociative disorders (SCID-D). *Dissociation, 6,* 3–15.

Steinberg, M., Rounsaville, B., & Cicchetti, D. (1991). Detection of dissociative disorders in psychiatric patients by a screening instrument and a structured diagnostic interview. *American Journal of Psychiatry, 148,* 1050–1054.

Steinberg, M., Rounsaville, B., & Cicchetti, D. V. (1992). New research findings on a screening instrument for DSM-IV dissociative disorders. In B. G. Braun & E. B. Carlson (Eds.), *Proceedings of the Ninth International Conference on Multiple Personality and Dissociative States*. Chicago: Rush–Presbyterian.

Steinberg, M., Rounsaville, B., & Cicchetti, D. (1990). The structured clinical interview for DSM-III-R dissociative disorders: Preliminary report on a new diagnostic instrument. *American Journal of Psychiatry, 147*, 76–82.

Strick, F. L., & Wilcoxon, S. A. (1991). A comparison of dissociative experiences in adult female outpatients with and without histories of early incestuous abuse. *Dissociation, 4*(4), 193–199.

van der Kolk, B. A., Perry, J. C., & Herman, J. L. (1991). Childhood origins of self-destructive behavior. *American Journal of Psychiatry, 148*, 1665–1671.

van der Kolk, B. A., &. Ducey, C. P. (1989). The psychological processing of traumatic experience: Rorschach patterns in PTSD. *Journal of Traumatic Stress, 2*, 259–263.

Wagner, E. E., Allison, R. B., & Wagner, C. F. (1983). Diagnosing multiple personalities with the Rorschach. *Journal of Personality Assessment, 47*, 143–149.

Wagner, E. E., &. Heise, M. R. (1974). A comparison of Rorschach protocols of three multiple personalities. *Journal of Personality Assessment, 38*, 308–331.

Waller, N. G. (in press). The Dissociative Experiences Scale. In *Twelfth mental measurements yearbook*. Lincoln, NE: Buros Institute of Mental Measurement.

Wogan, M. (1992). *The Bliss Scale: Development, reliability, and validity*. Unpublished manuscript.

9

Dissociative Disorders
in Children and Adolescents

Frank W. Putnam

This chapter provides an overview of child and adolescent dissociative disorders with regard to their clinical phenomenology, diagnosis, and treatment. Although recent work has significantly increased our knowledge of these disorders, our understanding of them in children and adolescents is still at a very early stage. Hence, it is important to remain aware of how very little we really know about normal and pathological dissociation in youth. A number of factors complicate the assessment of dissociation in children and adolescents, particularly the high background levels of "normal" dissociation manifest across this developmental epoch. Scales and diagnostic interviews are just appearing for the detection and quantification of dissociation in children and adolescents, thus systematic data are sparse. Debate about the suitability of the current adult diagnostic criteria, given the existence of childhood dissociative-disorder variants, is gathering momentum and likely to become a focus of considerable attention in the years ahead. This makes for an exciting field, which will generate its own share of controversy and points of contention with the field of adult dissociative disorders.

DEFINITIONS AND DIMENSIONS OF DISSOCIATION

Dissociation is a complex psychophysiological process that produces alterations in sense of self, accessibility of memory and knowledge, and integration of behavior (Putnam, 1991a). Dissociation exists on a continuum, with most individuals manifesting short, often situation-dependent, episodes of normative dissociation such as daydreaming (Putnam, 1991a). Some individuals may experience prolonged or frequent episodes of dissociation that interfere with their functioning and significantly alter their sense of self. In extreme cases, individuals may develop a dissociative disorder, such as multiple personality disorder (MPD), that produces profound disturbances in self and availability of information and memories. Although most definitions of dissociation focus on the failure of the individual to integrate information in a normal way, research suggests that dissociation has several underlying dimensions. These include alterations in memory, disturbances of identity, passive influence experiences, and trance/absorption phenomena.

Clinically, the memory dysfunctions are quite complicated and interconnected, but they can be experimentally dissected to some degree in laboratory studies (Putnam, 1991b). Memory dysfunctions include: (1) deficits in retrieval of implicit knowledge across behavioral states; (2) deficits in retrieval of autobiographical material; (3) deficits in retrieval of explicit information on free-recall tests across behavioral states (cued-recall appears to be less disrupted by dissociation—at least in laboratory settings); (4) intermittent and disruptive intrusions of traumatic memories into awareness; and (5) difficulties in determining whether a given memory reflects an actual event or information acquired through a nonexperiential source (e.g., reading or hearing about the event).

Disturbances of identity found in a dissociative-disordered patient include: (1) the existence of alter "personalities" that exchange control over the individual's behavior and express a sense of individuality and separateness; (2) depersonalization, wherein the individual feels as if he or she is dead, unreal, or detached from his or her surroundings and situation; and (3) psychogenic amnesia in which the individual forgets important highly personal information, for example, his or her name. The alter personality states of MPD patients are often incorrectly portrayed as if they were separate and distinct individuals. In actuality, these entities exhibit narrow ranges of functioning and affect and are best conceptualized as discrete behavioral states (Putnam, 1991b).

Passive influence experience, especially prominent in MPD, refers to a situation wherein an individual feels as if he or she were controlled by a force from within (Kluft, 1987). Intensely dysphoric, passive influence experiences may include a sense that one is being made to do something against one's will that is loathsome or harmful to oneself or others. At times, the dissociating individual may feel as if he or she has lost control over part of his or her body, so that it has "a mind of its own." For example, patients with MPD may experience "automatic writing," in which they subjectively do not feel as if they are in control of the writing hand and are surprised by what they write.

Auditory hallucinations, another kind of a dissociative passive influence experience, take a distinct form in the dissociative disorders, which helps to differentiate them from hallucinations found with the psychotic disorders (Putnam, 1989). Dissociative hallucinations are most likely to be experienced as internalized voices rather than externalized voices. The voices are heard distinctly, often have distinctive attributes such as gender, age, and affect, and may be pejorative and berating or supportive and comforting (Putnam, 1989). Hallucinated voices are frequently associated with specific situations or experiences, for example, when a depressed, dissociative adolescent hallucinates the voice of her stepfather commanding her to commit suicide. The dissociating individual is generally aware that the voices are hallucinations, but for fear of being labeled "crazy" may not report the hallucinations until a secure therapeutic alliance is established.

The fourth dimension of dissociation involves the experiencing of intense absorption or enthrallment and spontaneous trance states. Spontaneous trance states, common in children and adolescents, occur frequently with adult dissociative-disordered patients and interfere with the ongoing processing of information. The trance and absorption experiences and symptoms in dissociative patients resemble phenomena seen in hypnosis and in individuals labeled as "fantasy-prone." Unfortunately, the interrelationships amongst hypnosis, fantasy, absorption, and dissociation are poorly understood at present.

A HISTORICAL OVERVIEW OF CHILD AND ADOLESCENT DISSOCIATION

The unfolding history of child and adolescent dissociative disorders parallels that of the adult dissociative disorders in many respects. Like the adult disorders, child dissociative disorders were described in the 18th and 19th centuries and then forgotten. Recent scholarship by Fine (1988), Bowman (1990), Hacking (1991), and others has uncovered a number of these lost cases. In general, historical cases closely resemble their modern counterparts and serve as examples of syndromic continuity over time, a form of diagnostic validity.

The modern era of interest in childhood dissociative disorders began with a series of articles and chapters by Richard Kluft published in the mid 1980s. (Kluft, 1984, 1985a, 1985b, 1986). These first cases, together with the reports of a few other therapists working independently (Fagan & McMahon, 1984; Putnam, 1985b), initiated the current clinical interest in child and adolescent dissociative disorders. Like the adult dissociative disorders, initial child and adolescent reports were confined to a single case or a small series, generally fewer than five patients. Beyond clinical description, little analysis was, then, possible. Recently published reports involve larger numbers of cases, often ten or more (see, e.g., Dell & Eisenhower,

1990; Hornstein & Putnam, 1992; Hornstein & Tyson, 1992). Even larger samples are known to be under investigation, which should provide us with even more comprehensive and representative descriptions.

The advent of child dissociation measures has facilitated the investigation of the spectrum of dissociation in normal children, in maltreated children, and in other clinical samples. Developmental psychologists are studying the relationship of dissociation to critical developmental processes such as attachment and the consolidation of self. These studies provide us with rich additional sources of scientific data and new perspectives on dissociation in children. The study of dissociation in children may well provide an extremely important focus around which to integrate our clinical knowledge of dissociative disorders with the emerging science of developmental psychopathology.

DIAGNOSTIC ISSUES

The Suitability of Adult DSM Dissociative Disorders Criteria

During the drafting of the fourth edition of the *Diagnostic and Statistical Manual of Mental Disorders* (DSM-IV; American Psychiatric Association, 1993) many child psychiatrists pressed for the inclusion of developmentally appropriate diagnostic criteria for those adult disorders shared by children and adolescents. In the area of the dissociative disorders, this effort was partially successful in that these conditions were included under the differential diagnoses of Attention-Deficit Disorder and Schizophrenia. A note was also placed in the MPD (now controversially renamed Dissociative Identity Disorder) text section excluding as criteria for the disease imaginary companionship and fantasy phenomena in children. However, the DSM operates under the misguided principle that whenever possible, adult criteria should be applied to children and adolescents. In general, in making a diagnosis, the DSM ignores all contextual information about a child's developmental history, capacities, strengths, and life circumstances (Richters & Cicchetti, 1993). With a number of conditions, such as the affective disorders, the somatoform disorders, and the dissociative disorders, adult diagnostic criteria are grossly inappropriate and misleading. Furthermore, current and proposed DSM-IV dissociative disorders criteria are based on nonrepresentative adult studies. Published adult samples are strongly skewed toward Caucasian, middle-class (often professional), and female subjects (Coons, Bowman, & Milstein, 1988; Putnam, Guroff, Silberman, Barban, & Post, 1986; Putnam & Loewenstein, 1993). Most were seen in private practice settings (Putnam & Loewenstein, 1993). Hence, it is likely that access to health insurance and other factors bias these findings.

The unsuitability of adult criteria for children and adolescents is further complicated by the question of the existence of child "variants" and "incipient" cases (Fagan & McMahon, 1984; Hornstein & Putnam, 1992; Kluft, 1985a; Peterson, 1991; Putnam, 1992, 1993b). Children with clear-cut MPD resemble adult MPD patients in many respects, which, in fact, is why these cases are deemed "clear-cut." However, many child clinicians report grappling with more ambiguous dissociative presentations, which involve less than fully developed MPD. These cases generally end up being labeled Dissociative Disorder Not Otherwise Specified (DDNOS), a wastebasket category, which lacks specific criteria and includes a diverse range of dissociative reactions and cultural variants. In response to these concerns, Peterson proposed a set of DSM-type criteria for a diagnosis of Dissociative Disorder of Childhood (Peterson, 1990, 1991). His criteria are currently being field tested with a questionnaire study child clinicians are completing.

Another unresolved question involves the problem of high comorbidity with other major psychiatric disorders in dissociative patients. The Dell–Eisenhower and Hornstein–Putnam samples highlight the considerable overlap and comorbidity with other mental disorders in child and adolescent dissociative patients (Dell & Eisenhower, 1990; Hornstein & Putnam, 1992). These studies found that the average dissociative-disordered patient had received several prior diagnoses and had numerous major symptoms or behavioral problems. However, high rates of comorbidity are not unique to the dissociative disorders. Indeed, high rates of comorbidity are the norm for child and adolescent psychiatric inpatients and reflect the larger set of problems produced by the DSM approach toward child and adolescent diagnosis (Richters & Cicchetti, 1993).

Normative Dissociation

Dissociative experiences and behaviors occur along a continuum and, at times, can be very difficult to determine if a given individual has crossed over into the region deemed pathological. This is especially true for children and adolescents who exhibit an array of dissociative behaviors that often would be considered pathological in adults. In normal, nontraumatized children many of these behaviors are commonly associated with make-believe and fantasy phenomena and are generally viewed as positive, creative expressions of the child's imagination. In adults, many of these same behaviors would be considered evidence of a gross loss of contact with reality.

Imaginary companionship is an excellent example of a phenomena that children normally engage in, but that would be considered abnormal for adults. Traditionally, an imaginary companion is defined as "an invisible character, named and referred to in conversation with other persons or played with directly for a period of time, at least several months, having an air of reality for the child but no apparent objective basis" (Svendsen, 1934, p. 988). Imaginary companionship is common in children, peaking around the ages of 5–6 years. Between 30% and 60% of normal children have imaginary companions, and they are more prevalent in girls (Sanders, 1992). While studies differ on whether normal children with imaginary companions are significantly more creative or better adjusted, no study suggests that imaginary companionship is a pathological process. However, between 50% to 80% of children with dissociative disorders are reported to have vivid imaginery companions (Bliss, 1984; Hornstein & Putnam, 1992; Peterson, 1991; Sanders, 1992; Vincent & Pickering, 1988). The question exists as to whether the imaginary companions reported in dissociative-disordered children represent the same imaginary/dissociative process as those found in normal children. Studies of adults with dissociative disorders suggest that, as reported retrospectively, imaginary companions in the childhoods of these individuals were more vivid than those reported by normal adults. Further, studies of normal adults reporting histories of childhood imaginary companions indicate that those who report vivid imaginary companions also have significantly higher Dissociative Experiences Scale (DES) scores (Sanders, 1992).

Spontaneous trancelike states and staring spells, which are very common in child dissociative disorders, are not at all uncommon in normal children. There is a subgroup of normal children and adolescents who have vivid, serialized daydreams in which they progressively construct and inhabit extensive fantasy worlds, which are populated by imaginary characters with strong personality attributes. Shared imaginary games such as "Dungeons and Dragons" tap these adolescent fantasy capacities. In addition, many children and adolescents spend long periods immersed in "trance"-inducing activities, such as watching television or listening to loud throbbing music through earphones. They also practice "tuning out" parents and other challenging authority figures. Transient episodes of depersonalization, a form of dissociative-identity alteration, is also very common during normal adolescence (Putnam, 1985a; Steinberg, 1991).

Development of self and identity is a lifelong task, but much of the formative work occurs during childhood and adolescence. Children exhibit a developmental progression of self-elaboration, which involves the creation and integration of different aspects of the self, as well as perspective taking. The edited book *The Self in Transition: Infancy to Childhood* (Cicchetti & Beeghly, 1990) is an excellent introduction to the extraordinary complexity and multiplicity of a child's development of his or her sense of self and theory of mind. The chapter on the multiple voices and versions of the self in early childhood is a sensitive discussion of the role of emerging selves in a normal child's course of development (Wolf, 1990). Adolescents, in particular, may undergo abrupt alterations in their sense of self and identity, and are prone to strong identifications with public figures such as sports, music, or television stars. The work of Susan Harter and others on the development of identity during adolescence indicates that there is frequently a period around the age of 14 when the adolescent feels divided into different selves that are contextually activated (e.g., by being with different groups of friends) (Harter, 1983). These different versions of the self are often in psychological conflict with one another.

All of the above examples indicate that at different times during normal development, a number of dissociative and developmental phenomena occur that could be mistaken for pathological dissociation by clinicians unaware of the normal developmental aspects of identity formation. Hence, therapists assuming the responsibility of diagnosing dissociative disorders in youth should familiarize themselves with the spectrum of normal dissociation and imaginative behavior in children and adolescents.

Diagnostic Scales and Interviews

A number of child and adolescent dissociation checklists and self-report measures have recently appeared in the literature (Evers-Szostak & Sanders, 1992; Putnam, Helmers, & Trickett, 1993; Reagor, Kasten, & Morelli, 1992; Tyson, 1992). Of these, the Child Dissociative Checklist (CDC) has been the most extensively validated and most widely used research measure (Hornstein & Putnam, 1992; Putnam, Helmers, Horowitz, & Trickett, 1994; Putnam, Helmers, & Trickett, 1993). The CDC is a 20-item, parent/observer checklist with a 3-point report format (0 = not true, 1 = sometimes true, 2 = frequently true) that asks about observed dissociative behaviors. The CDC was normed on samples of normal children, sexually abused girls, and 64 boys and girls who met DSM-III-R and the National Institute of Mental Health (NIMH) dissociative-disorder criteria (Putnam et al., 1993). The 1 year test–retest reliability is r = .654, (with p = .0001, N = 91, and Cronbach's alpha = .95). A score of 12 or above on the CDC is considered evidence of significantly elevated dissociation. Children and adolescents with a diagnosis of DDNOS averaged 16.8 ± 4.8, while those with MPD averaged 25.16 ± 4.3 (Hornstein & Putnam, 1992). CDC scores are negatively correlated with age so that higher scores in younger children are generally less indicative of psychopathology. The decline of dissociative behavior with age continues throughout life (Putnam, 1991a).

Clinically, the CDC is useful as a screening instrument, but should not be regarded as diagnostic by itself. It is particularly useful as a serial measure, completed periodically on a child suspected of having dissociative psychopathology. When evaluating a child for a possible dissociative disorder, I often have teachers, parents/foster parents, and therapists collect weekly CDCs for several months. The CDC is also proving useful as a research measure, showing interesting relationships with a variety of other social, psychological, and biological measures (Putnam, 1993c).

As of this time, there are no validated structured interviews that can yield DSM-III-R/IV dissociative disorder diagnoses in children and adolescents. There are several interviews in the process of being developed including a dissociative disorder module of the Diagnostic Interview for Children and Adolescents (DICA), which Wendy Reich and David Corwin are authoring. Dorothy O. Lewis is developing a promising semi-structured dissociative-disorder interview, organized around the metaphor of television, to examine experiences such as the switching of alter personality states (personal communication, March 1993). There is also a dissociative module under consideration for the Diagnostic Interview Schedule for Children (DISC). Unfortunately, all of these interviews are handicapped by the unsuitability of the DSM dissociative disorder criteria for children and adolescents. However, DSM diagnoses and structured interviews are currently a requisite part of research and, increasingly, a part of clinical practice. Hence, one or more of these interviews will hopefully, provide us with a useful tool.

CLINICAL ISSUES

The clinical description of child and adolescent dissociative disorders has progressed from individual case studies (see, e.g., Bowman, Blix, & Coons, 1985; Congdon, Hain, & Stevenson, 1961; Fagan & McMahon, 1984; Kluft, 1984; Malenbaum & Russell, 1987; Putnam, 1993a; Riley & Mead, 1988; Weiss, Sutton, & Utecht, 1985) to statistical samples (Dell & Eisenhower, 1990; Hornstein & Putnam, 1992; Hornstein & Tyson, 1992; Vincent & Pickering, 1988). Reviews of the literature have tabulated some of the features of the individual case reports to provide an overview of these newly prominent disorders (Peterson, 1990; Tyson, 1992; Vincent & Pickering, 1988). Much can be learned from an examination of both types of report. The single case study provides a memorable illustration of pathological dissociation, while statistical analyses of large case series and the tabulations of review articles provide some measure of the range and generalizability of those individual clinical images.

At present, the Hornstein and Putnam sample provides the best single look at the clinical phenomenology of child and adolescent dissociative disorders (Hornstein & Putnam, 1992). The basic design of the study involved the comparison of two independently collected samples of children and adolescents with dissociative disorder diagnoses. The first group of children was seen by Nancy Hornstein during the time that she was unit director of an inpatient children's unit at the University of California, Los Angeles. The second sample was evaluated by myself in conjunction with my work at the National Institute of Mental Health in Bethesda, Maryland, and at the Children's National Medical Center in Washington, D.C. The two samples were matched on age, race, and type of dissociative disorder, but differed in that my sample consisted of more girls. A jointly developed computerized database served to standardize information collection. The two samples were compared with each other by dissociative disorder diagnosis (MPD or DDNOS) on over one hundred individual symptoms, behaviors, and other variables, and on 16 composite factors. There were essentially no significant differences between the two samples, which were then lumped together for descriptive analyses.

Clinical Phenomenology

A very high rate of documented trauma was found in the histories of these children. Generally, they were exposed to physical and sexual abuse, neglect, abandonment, and domestic and community violence. On average, each child received three major psychiatric diagnoses, most commonly depression, post-traumatic stress disorder, oppositional defiant disorder, conduct disorder and attention-deficit hyperactivity disorder. Affective symptoms, particularly depression and suicidal ideation, were a prominent feature of many clinical presentations, although not uncommonly the question of psychosis or schizophrenia was raised by referring clinicians (Putnam, 1993b). Rapid mood swings and marked irritability were almost universally present. Other affective features included high rates of crying and agitation, poor self-esteem, hopelessness, and self-blame.

Conduct problems, especially aggression, lying, and disruptive, oppositional, and explosive behaviors, were commonly found. Inappropriate sexual behavior, including promiscuity, compulsive masturbation, and aggressive sexual play were present in about half of the children. Interestingly, the classic antisocial triad of enuresis, cruelty to animals, and fire setting was seldom found. School reports indicated that many of these children had significant classroom behavior problems, although some were unremarkable. A few of the children were even considered to be good students. Truancy was a problem for the adolescents and learning problems and "hyperactivity" in school settings were reported for about 60% of the children.

Despite their polysymptomatic clinical presentations, these children's core problems had to do with dissociative and post-traumatic symptoms and behaviors. Pathological dissociation is a complex psychophysiological process, which involves memory impairment; identity disturbance; dissociative process symptoms, such as hallucinations and passive influence experiences, and extreme absorption or enthrallment. The basic symptoms children and adolescents express resemble those found in the adult disorders but their symptomatic expression varies over the course of development.

Amnesias and state-dependent memory retrieval phenomena central to the dissociative disorders commonly manifest themselves in children by perplexing forgetfulness and erratic variation in skills, knowledge, preferences, and habits. The children themselves rarely remark on the discrepancies and discontinuities in their behavior. Adolescents may have more classic adult amnesic symptoms, such as noticing gaps in the continuity of time or having the experience of "coming to" in the middle of some activity. Unfortunately, they are not usually troubled by these experiences to the same degree as adults, and hence might not seek help right away. Many have egosyntonic ways of explaining amnesic experiences to themselves and others (see, e.g., Reginald's concept of "flicking," which is described in relation to one adolescent MPD case study [Putnam, 1993a]). Pathological "lying" is commonly reported by adults working with these children and usually reflects the disavowal of behavior they do not remember rather than deliberate deception.

Depersonalization and derealization are probably common experiences but are rarely described by children or younger adolescents who have a dissociative disorder. Pathological identity disturbances can be very difficult to differentiate from developmentally normative phenomena, particularly in younger children. MPD alter personality-like systems may be subjectively experienced by the dissociative child as externalized imaginary companions. In young children, the "personalities" may be named and/or patterned after superheroes, or animal, cartoon, or children's fiction characters and may be very difficult to distinguish from normative imaginary companionship in younger children. One distinguishing feature is the degree to which the child feels controlled or tormented by his or her "companions." Although normal children may blame imaginary companions for their own misbehaviors, they rarely feel controlled or frightened by their imaginary companion. Normal children often boss their imaginary companions around, intercede with others on their imaginary companion's behalf, and generally feel in control of the situation. Dissociative-disordered children are often frightened by some of their externalized entities, complain that they get them in trouble, or engage in struggles with them. On occasion, a child might report that the entity "made" him or her engage in risk-taking behavior or self-mutilation, against his or her will.

High rates of auditory hallucinations are reported in child and adolescent dissociative-disordered patients (Hornstein & Putnam, 1992; Peterson, 1990; Putnam, 1993b; Vincent & Pickering, 1988). These voices are usually experienced as having distinct age, gender, and personal attributes, and are most commonly heard from within the head as opposed to coming from outside of it. As with adult dissociative patients, these voices may be pejorative or supportive. Visual hallucinations are also not uncommon. The child may report seeing ghosts or spirits, particularly at night. Tactile and olfactory hallucinations have been noted in a few cases. The effects of dissociative and post-traumatic events on cognition include various kinds of memory disturbances and impairments, such as state-dependent recall, intrusive memories and imagery, poor concentration, problems with autobiographical memory, and difficulty in determining the veracity and source of memories (e.g., Did the child experience a "remembered" event or just hear about someone else's experience?).

Passive influence phenomena, such as experiencing involuntary and complex body movements, were commonly found in the Hornstein and Putnam sample. Not infrequently, passive influence experiences occur around aggressive or risk-taking behavior. Thought insertion and thought withdrawal or blocking commonly occur as well, as do periods of confusion or disorientation. However, none of the children was thought to suffer from a formal thought disorder. Quasidelusional material organized around passive influence experiences and hallucinations occurred in about one-fifth of the sample. Rapid age regression, behaviorally more apparent in older children, was virtually universal in the Putnam and Hornstein sample.

Trancelike states, manifested by spacing out or unresponsive episodes, are extremely common in dissociative-disordered children. Trancelike states also occur in normal children, particularly during periods of low stimulation, but at much lower rates. In contrast, the trancelike states in dissociative-disordered children often appear precipitated by stress or threatening stimuli and spontaneously occur at much higher frequencies. Children who exhibit trancelike behaviors or staring spells should be evaluated for a seizure disorder before their symptoms are attributed to dissociation. Drug abuse, particularly with phencyclidine (PCP), can produce organic dissociative reactions, and should be considered when diagnosing older children and adolescents who appear in trancelike or "spacey" states.

As would be expected with such a traumatized group of children, symptoms associated with post-traumatic stress responses are very common and overlap considerably with dissociative behaviors. Avoidant behaviors triggered by traumatic stimuli; a variety of fears, anxieties, and phobias; exaggerated startle behaviors; an array of flashback phenomena; traumatic nightmares, and hypervigilance were found in 60 to 90% of Hornstein and Putnams subjects. These behaviors, together with the dissociative amnesias, identity alterations, passive influence experiences, hallucinations, abrupt age behavioral regressions, and related symptoms strongly impact on the child's coping capacities, and social and psychological development (Putnam, 1993c).

Treatment

Very little information exists on the treatment and outcome of the child and adolescent dissociative disorders. A few case reports describe individual therapies (see, e.g., Bowman et al., 1985; Fagan & McMahon, 1984; Kluft, 1984, 1985a, 1985b; Malenbaum & Russell, 1987; McMahon & Fagan, 1993; Putnam, 1993a; Riley & Mead, 1988; Weiss et al., 1985). These reports suggest that child cases respond favorably to treatments patterned along adult models. Experience with adolescent cases, particularly older adolescents, however, suggests that once established, dissociative disorders can be very problematic to manage and treat (Dell & Eisenhower, 1990; Hornstein & Putnam, 1992; Putnam, 1992, 1993b). Current child and adolescent therapeutic approaches resemble those developed with adult dissociative cases, probably in large part because these approaches constitute the best models presently available (see, e.g., Kluft, 1986; McMahon & Fagan, 1993). However, in many cases, the application of adult dissociative-disorder treatment models to children may be inappropriate. In particular, the question of the desirability of pursuing intense individual work with the alter personalities of child MPD cases, as one would do when working with adult MPD patients, remains to be critically examined. Developmental considerations suggest that children would be especially susceptible to shaping and reinforcing influences during treatment.

The development of rapport and trust are critical therapeutic issues with these cases, as they are with victimized individuals of all ages. It is important to ensure that the child is in a safe living situation and is not being maltreated, nor fearful that he or she could be maltreated in the future. Until the child or adolescent feels safe and secure, he or she will not be able to effectively engage in therapy. In short, the creation of a familiar and consistent therapeutic space along the lines described by Donovan and McIntyre is an important therapeutic intervention (Donovan & McIntyre, 1990). Hypnotic techniques may be useful in addressing behavioral problems and impaired self-esteem, and in promoting a sense of well-being and health (Kluft, 1991; Rhue & Lynn, 1991).

The absence of proven efficacy for any treatment model for the child and adolescent dissociative disorders has created a vacuum, which is unfortunately being filled by numerous "Continuing Medical Education" (CME) workshops on the subject. Clinicians working with child and adolescent dissociative disorders should be very skeptical about these workshops, and should demand a full accounting of the experience of CME presenters, as well as examine the treatment approaches they use and their results. In my opinion, there is a great deal of misinformation being promulgated on the treatment of children and adolescents with dissociative disorders. It would be tragic to repeat in this arena the considerable confusion and prolifera-

tion of inappropriate treatment models that has plagued the adult dissociative disorders.

REFERENCES

American Psychiatric Association. (1993). *DSM-IV draft criteria*. Washington, DC:
American Psychiatric Association.

Bliss, E. L. (1984). Spontaneous self-hypnosis in multiple personality disorder. *Psy-chiatric Clinics of North America, 7*, 135–148.

Bowman, E. S. (1990). Adolescent multiple personality disorder in the nineteenth
and early twentieth centuries. *Dissociation, 3*, 179–187.

Bowman, E. S., Blix, S., & Coons, P. M. (1985). Multiple personality in adolescence:
Relationship to incestual experiences. *Journal of the American Academy of Child
and Adolescent Psychiatry, 24*, 109–114.

Cicchetti, D., & Beeghly, M. (Eds.). (1990). *The self in transition*. Chicago: University
of Chicago Press.

Congdon, M. H., Hain, J., & Stevenson, I. (1961). A case of multiple personality illustrating the transition from role-playing. *Journal of Nervous and Mental Disease,
132*, 497–504.

Coons, P. M., Bowman, E. S., & Milstein, V. (1988). Multiple personality disorder:
A clinical investigation of 50 cases. *Journal of Nervous and Mental Disease, 176*,
519–527.

Dell, P. F., & Eisenhower, J. W. (1990). Adolescent multiple personality disorder.
Journal of the American Academy of Child and Adolescent Psychiatry, 29, 359–366.

Donovan, D. M., & McIntyre, D. (1990). *Healing the hurt child*. New York: W. W.
Norton.

Evers-Szostak, M., & Sanders, S. (1992). The children's perceptual alteration scale
(CPAS): A measure of children's dissociation. *Dissociation, 5*, 87–97.

Fagan, J., & McMahon, P. P. (1984). Incipent multiple personality in children: Four
cases. *Journal of Nervous and Mental Disease, 172*, 26–36.

Fine, C. G. (1988). The work of Antoine Despine: The first scientific report on the
diagnosis and treatment of a child with multiple personality disorder. *American
Journal of Clinical Hypnosis, 31*, 33–39.

Hacking, I. (1991). Double consciousness in Britian 1815–1875. *Dissociation, 4*,
134–146.

Harter, S. (1983). Developmental perspectives on the self system. In E. M. Hethering-
ton (Ed.), *Handbook of child psychology* (pp. 327–349). New York: John Wiley.

Hornstein, N., & Putnam, F. W. (1992). Clinical phenomenology of child and adolescent dissociative disorders. *Journal of the American Academy of Child and Adolescent Psychiatry, 31*, 1077–1085.

Hornstein, N. L., & Tyson, S. (1992). Inpatient treatment of children with multiple
personality/dissociative disorders and their families. *Psychiatric Clinics of North
America, 14*, 631–648.

Kluft, R. P. (1984). Multiple personality in childhood. *Psychiatric Clinics of North
America, 7*, 121–134.

Kluft, R. P. (1985a). Childhood multiple personality disorder: Predictors, clinical findings, and treatment results. In R. P. Kluft (Ed.), *Childhood antecedents of multiple personality* (pp. 167–196). Washington, DC: American Psychiatric Press.

Kluft, R. P. (1985b). Hypnotherapy of childhood multiple personality disorder. *American Journal of Clinical Hypnosis, 27,* 201–210.

Kluft, R. P. (1986). Treating children who have multiple personality disorder. In B. G. Braun (Ed.), *Treatment of multiple personality disorder* (pp. 81–105). Washington, DC: American Psychiatric Press.

Kluft, R. P. (1987). First-rank symptoms as a diagnostic clue to multiple personality disorder. *American Journal of Psychiatry, 144,* 293–298.

Kluft, R. P. (1991). Hypnosis in childhood trauma. In W. C. Wester & D. J. O'Grady (Eds.), *Clinical hypnosis with children* (pp. 53–68). New York: Brunner/Mazel.

Malenbaum, R., & Russell, A. T. (1987). Multiple personality disorder in an 11-year-old boy and his mother. *Journal of the American Academy of Child and Adolescent Psychiatry, 24,* 495–501.

McMahon, P. P., & Fagan, J. (1993). Play therapy with children with multiple personality disorder. In R. P. Kluft & C. G. Fine (Eds.), *Clinical perspectives on multiple personality disorder* (pp. 253–276). Washington, DC: American Psychiatric Press.

Peterson, G. (1990). Diagnosis of childhood multiple personality. *Dissociation, 3,* 3–9.

Peterson, G. (1991). Children coping with trauma: Diagnosis of "Dissociation Identity Disorder." *Dissociation, 4,* 152–164.

Putnam, F. W. (1985a). Dissociation as a response to extreme trauma. In R. P. Kluft (Ed.), *Childhood antecedents of multiple personality* (pp. 66–97). Washington, DC: American Psychiatric Press.

Putnam, F. W. (1985b). Pieces of the mind: Recognizing the psychological effects of abuse. *Justice for Children, 1,* 6–7.

Putnam, F. W. (1989). *Diagnosis and treatment of multiple personality disorder.* New York: Guilford Press.

Putnam, F. W. (1991a). Dissociative phenomena. In A. Tasman & S. M. Goldfinger (Eds.), *American Psychiatric Press review of psychiatry* (pp. 145–160). Washington, DC: American Psychiatric Press.

Putnam, F. W. (1991b). Recent research on multiple personality disorder. *Psychiatric Clinics of North America, 14,* 489–502.

Putnam, F. W. (1992). Dissociative disorders in children and adolescents: A developmental perspective. *Psychiatric Clinics of North America, 14,* 519–532.

Putnam, F. W. (1993a). Dissociation in the inner city. In R. P. Kluft & C. G. Fine (Eds.), *Clinical perspectives on multiple personality disorder* (pp. 179–200). Washington, DC: American Psychiatric Press.

Putnam, F. W. (1993b). Dissociative disorders in children: Behavioral profiles and problems. *Child Abuse and Neglect, 17,* 39–45.

Putnam, F. W. (1993c). Dissociative disturbances of self. In D. Cicchetti & S. Tothe (Eds.), *The self and its disorders* (pp. 283–299). Cambridge: Cambridge University Press.

Putnam, F. W., Guroff, J. J., Silberman, E. K., Barban, L., & Post, R. M. (1986). The clinical phenomenology of multiple personality disorder: Review of 100 recent cases. *Journal of Clinical Psychiatry, 47,* 285–293.

Putnam, F. W., Helmers, K., Horowitz, L. A., & Trickett, P. K. (1994). Hypnotizability and dissociativity in sexually abused girls. *Child Abuse and Neglect.*

Putnam, F. W., Helmers, K., & Trickett, P. K. (1993). Development, reliability and validity of a child dissociation scale. *Child Abuse and Neglect, 17*, 731–741.

Putnam, F. W., & Loewenstein, R. L. (1993). Treatment of multiple personality disorder: A survey of current practices. *American Journal of Psychiatry, 150*, 1048–1052.

Reagor, P. A., Kasten, J. D., & Morelli, N. (1992). A checklist for screening dissociative disorders in children and adolescents. *Dissociation, 5*, 4–19.

Rhue, J. W., & Lynn, S. J. (1991). The use of hypnotic techniques with sexually abused children. In W. C. Wester & D. J. O'Grady (Eds.), *Clinical hypnosis with children* (pp. 69–84). New York: Brunner/Mazel.

Richters, J. E., & Cicchetti, D. (1993). Mark Twain meets DSM-III-R: Conduct disorder, development, and the concept of harmful dysfunction. *Development and Psychopathology, 5*, 5–29.

Riley, R. L., & Mead, J. (1988). The development of symptoms of multiple personality disorder in a child of three. *Dissociation, 1*, 41–46.

Sanders, B. (1992). The imaginary companion experience in multiple personality disorder. *Dissociation, 5*, 159–162.

Steinberg, M. (1991). The spectrum of depersonalization: Assessment and treatment. In A. Tasman & S. M. Goldfinger (Eds.), *American Psychiatric Press review of psychiatry* (pp. 223–247). Washington, DC: American Psychiatric Press.

Svendsen, M. (1934). Children's imaginary companions. *Archives of Neurology and Psychiatry, 2*, 985–999.

Tyson, G. M. (1992). Childhood MPD dissociation identity disorder: Applying and extending current diagnostic checklists. *Dissociation, 5*, 20–27.

Vincent, M., & Pickering, M. R. (1988). Multiple personality disorder in childhood. *Canadian Journal of Psychiatry, 33*, 524–529.

Weiss, M., Sutton, P. J., & Utecht, A. J. (1985). Multiple personality in a 10-year-old girl. *Journal of the American Academy of Child and Adolescent Psychiatry, 24*, 495–501.

Wolf, D. P. (1990). Being of several minds: Voices and versions of the self in early childhood. In D. Cicchetti & M. Beeghly (Eds.), *The self in transition* (pp. 183–212). Chicago: University of Chicago Press.

10

The Aftereffects and Assessment of Physical and Psychological Abuse

Nataliya Zelikovsky
Steven Jay Lynn

This book documents the fact that dissociative disorders are intimately associated with physical and psychological abuse. Although controversy exists about whether dissociative symptoms are caused by physical and psychological abuse (see Chapter 18, this volume), there is a general consensus among experts that dissociative symptoms, particularly those linked with severe dissociative disorders like multiple personality disorder (MPD), are more likely to arise in the context of families in which the caretakers inflict physical and psychological abuse. A thorough assessment of a person who presents with dissociative symptoms must, of necessity, include a careful examination of the client's history, with particular attention to physical and psychological abuse. At the same time, the clinician must recognize that the consequences of abuse are not specific to dissociative phenomena and can be associated with a variety of personal and interpersonal deficits and symptoms of psychopathology.

This chapter provides clinicians with information relevant to assessing the consequences of abuse in self-reported or identified victims. To do so, we review the literature on the aftereffects of abuse and the characteristics that have been associated with physically and psychologically abused children, and describe assessment instruments that can assist clinicians in the evaluation of abused children and adult survivors of abuse.

Many of the tests we recommend have normative data available; all can be used to supplement the diagnostic/assessment interview, which is indispensable when working with children and adults who have been physically and/or psychologically abused. Psychological testing may need to be deferred immediately following a traumatic incident of abuse, and sometimes for many months afterward, until the client's condition is sufficiently stabilized to obtain valid test data. Perhaps more often than not, part of the trauma of child abuse is the burden of secrecy, shame, and guilt that attends the abuse. It is therefore imperative that the therapist or assessor cultivate a positive rapport and a robust working alliance with the abused child or adult survivor of abuse and carefully consider the timing of test administration and data gathering.

When administered with skill and sensitivity, psychological tests can assist the clinician in learning more about the abused person and the challenges that will confront their work together. The use of tests with established psychometric properties can also be useful in forensic cases where documentation of the aftereffects or correlates of abuse is essential. We begin with a brief discussion of definitions of physical and psychological abuse, and then consider the ramifications of these forms of abuse.

THE INCIDENCE AND DEFINITIONS OF ABUSE

Child abuse has existed for centuries. In 1874, the case of Mary Ellen, an 8-year-old girl who was chained, beaten, and starved by her adoptive parents, marked the real beginning of recognition of child maltreatment in the United States. However, it is only within recent years that it has become a focal point of social concern. This is not surprising when we consider the available statistics regarding the incidence of abuse in our society. The National Center on Child Abuse and Neglect (NCCAN; 1991) reported 838,232 substantiated cases of child abuse (e.g., physical, psychological, sexual) and neglect. Nearly a quarter (24.4% or 204,404) of these cases were classified as involving physical abuse. The Clearinghouse on Child Abuse and Neglect Information (1989) reported that physical child abuse is associated with high morbidity (psychological distress) and a mortality rate of 10–15% (cited in Kolko, 1992).

Of course, incidence figures vary widely due to definitional differences and the various criteria used for reporting such cases. In this chapter, we use a definition of childhood physical abuse adapted from Brown and Anderson (1991): Physical abuse consists of any self-reported assault during or before the age of 14 that was perpetrated by a family member in charge of the child. The physically abusive behaviors include, but are not limited to, slapping, hitting really hard, beating, punching, kicking, and any injuries resulting in bruises, broken bones, scars, or bleeding. This definition is consistent with the conception of physical abuse forwarded by the NCCAN (1988), which described physical abuse as acts of commission that involve either demonstrable harm or endangerment to the child (see also Malinosky-Rummell & Hansen, 1993; Peterson, 1993).

As alarming as the statistics are regarding the incidence of physical abuse, psychological abuse is even more prevalent and may well be at the core of all forms of child abuse and neglect. In 1991, 5.9% (49,124) of all reported cases of abuse were regarded as involving psychological abuse, which is discussed in terms of "emotional maltreatment." Rates of this type of abuse vary widely because different standards are used in reporting incidents of psychological abuse, and clinicians have different views as to whether psychological abuse co-occurs with physical abuse. In fact, cases of physical abuse that occur in the absence of any psychological abuse are the exception rather than the norm (Gross & Keller, 1992; Hart & Brassard, 1987; Hart, Germain, & Brassard, 1987). Claussen and Crittenden (1991) found that about 90% of a group of children who were physically abused also experienced psychological abuse, whereas only 25–45% of those who were psychologically abused also were physically abused.

In this chapter, we define childhood psychological abuse as involving verbal arguments and the punishing of children (younger than 14 years of age) by parents or stepparents. These behaviors include, but are not limited to, yelling, insulting, and/or criticizing the child, making him or her feel guilty or like a bad person, humiliating the child in front of others and/or embarrassing him or her. In the sections that follow we first consider the aftereffects of physical abuse and pertinent assessment instruments, followed by a discussion of psychological abuse.

PHYSICAL ABUSE AND ITS CONSEQUENCES

Consensus exists (Augoustinos, 1987; Gross & Keller, 1992; Kolko, 1992; Steele, 1986; Wolfe & Jaffe, 1991) that physical abuse represents a major disruption in a child's development, and has a pervasive influence on his or her future relationships with peers, partners, and, even, offspring. Abused children come to embrace distorted and maladaptive beliefs about themselves, the people around them, and the world at large.

The effects of physical abuse on children may range from passive and withdrawn behavior to provocative, impulsive, and aggressive behavior (Ammerman, Cassisi, Hersen, & Van Hasselt, 1986). Physically abused children are more alert and hypervigilant due to the unpredictable circumstances in which they grow up (Martin & Beezley, 1977). Sometimes they exhibit "pseudomature" behavior (i.e., the false appearance of independence and being excessively "good"), which results from the high expectations set by their parents and the need to take care of themselves when others fail to do so (Martin & Beezley, 1977). They also tend to exhibit diminished social sensitivity and have trouble discriminating emotions in others (Camras, Grow, & Ribordy, 1983). They may also have poor self-esteem, an inability to enjoy life, and be more depressed than nonabused children (Martin & Beezley, 1977). In school, they may be more aggressive, oppositional, and compulsive, and have more problems with peers (George & Main, 1979; Kent, 1976). They may also have poor concentration, more learning problems, and lower IQ scores (Toro, 1982). In the sections that follow, we consider deficits in these and other areas in more detail.

Physical and Intellectual Development

Most of the early studies (see Toro, 1982, for a review) on the developmental effects of child abuse concluded that physically abused children exhibit deficits in physical, neurological, and intellectual development. More specifically, they tended to weigh less, have speech problems, and have poorer impulse control and poorer self-concepts than nonabused children. Their language development was delayed and their ability to learn and achieve in school was degraded (Elmer & Gregg, 1967; Elmer, 1978). Controlled research (Elmer, 1977), however, suggests that although physically abused children developmentally lag traumatized but nonabused children, the differences are not apparent when socioeconomic status (SES) is taken into account. In short, SES may be more important than the presence of abuse in determining the course of certain developmental characteristics.

Although the research we reviewed makes it clear that clinicians need to be cautious with respect to attributing developmental delays in low SES children to physical abuse, severely abused children often do suffer from deficits in intellectual and language development. These deficits may be particularly significant and warrant remediation when the child's developmental lag cannot be attributed to SES and other demographic factors. To assess intellectual development, a wide range of standardized tests can be used with children. These tests include the Wechsler Preschool and Primary Scale of Intelligence for ages 4–6 ½ (WPPSI; Wechsler, 1967), the Wechsler Intelligence Scale for Children—Revised for ages 6–11 (WAIS-R; Wechsler, 1974), the Stanford–Binet Intelligence Scale—Revised (SBIS-R; Thorndike, Hagan, & Sattler, 1986), the Peabody Picture Vocabulary Test (PPVT; Dunn & Dunn, 1981), the Goodenough–Harris Drawing Test (Harris, 1963), and the Wide Range Achievement Test—Revised (WRAT-R; Jastak & Wilkinson, 1984).

Ability to Attach

Early patterns of caregiver–infant interaction may have a great impact on the quality of the child's attachments to parents and other significant figures in his or her life (Ainsworth, Blehar, Waters, & Wall, 1978). In order to develop healthy relationships with and empathy toward others, the child needs to form a secure bond or identify with a caring adult. Abusive parents are unable to provide a secure base from which the child can venture out and explore his or her environment. Because they never learned to trust adults, abused children's ability to relate to others and enjoy relationships is compromised (Jacobson & Straker, 1982; Straker & Jacobson, 1981).

A few empirical studies have examined the relationship between abuse and neglect and interaction patterns between abused children and adults (Aber & Allen, 1987; Egeland & Stroufe, 1981). In a prospective study, Egeland and Stroufe (1981) found that low SES physically abused infants at 12 months were more avoidant than low SES neglected infants (i.e., they avoided contact with their mother after separation or ignored her when she tried to interact with them) while low SES neglected infants appeared more resistant (i.e., they did not experience comfort at the mother's hands after separation) than the physically abused infants. The nonabused control group was securely attached; that is, they explored the room in the presence of the mother, and the presence of the mother reduced distress. The results indicate that physical rejection and abuse leads to avoidant behavior while insensitive and inconsistent parenting leads to resistance on the part of the child. However, at the 18-month follow-up, many of the abused infants were reclassified as securely attached while the neglected children's behavior changed from resistant to avoidant. This suggests that attachment patterns change over time. Yet, even with the passage of time, neglected children, in particular, do not form adaptive attachment bonds.

In another study (Aber & Allen, 1987), physically and emotionally abused children scored lower on tasks measuring readiness to learn in the presence of strangers than nonabused welfare children and middle-class children. Overall, abused children were unable to establish a balance between secure and safe relationships with adults and the ability to explore the outside world.

As discussed above, physical abuse can compromise a child's ability to form personal attachments with parents and other significant persons. Because the formation of secure bonds is essential for the development of social relationships, abused children's attachments should be examined in the course of a psychological evaluation. Clinicians can assess children's attachment to significant adults with the Parent Attachment Structured Interview (PASI; Roll, Lockwood, & Roll, 1981). This instrument is useful not only because it identifies the attachment figures in a child's life, but also because it measures the strength of important attachments. The interview consists of 50 questions that deal with four aspects of attachment (i.e., "Responsiveness," "Confidence," "Security," and "Hostility"). The test has been successfully administered to children ages 6 to 12, but the questions can be modified for children younger than 6 years of age.

Self-Esteem

Research (Green, 1981; Martin & Beezley, 1977; Oates, Forrest, & Peacock, 1985; Steele, 1986) indicates that children who grow up in insecure, rejecting, abusive, and nonsupportive homes tend to have lower self-esteem. They are often baffled by unexpected events and have trouble coping in stressful situations. Their early experiences teach them that their inner feelings and desires are inconsequential. Hence, the child learns to disregard pleasure and lives a mechanical and practical life. Because the child is often scapegoated for the occurrence of stressful daily events, he or she internalizes the caretaker's verbal denigrations and accusations and comes to believe that he or she is truly "bad" and unworthy. Abused children also appear to lack goals, have lower ambitions, and look forward to the future less than nonabused children. This is probably due to the high and unrealistic expectations that abusive parents set for their children, which they are unable to meet (Oates et al., 1985; Steele, 1986). Finally, abused, compared to nonmaltreated children, have fewer friends (Oates et al., 1985).

Because poor self-esteem can have a pervasive impact on a child's life, it is often evident in the course of a clinical interview with a child. Nevertheless, self-esteem measures such as Coopersmith's Self-Esteem Inventories (CSEI; Coopersmith, 1981) can pinpoint the extent to which the child feels competent, successful, significant, and worthy in social, academic, family, and personal areas. The School Form contains 50 items, including an 8-item Lie Scale, and can be administered to individuals or groups. Because the CSEI has been adapted for use with older students and adults, it can be used with any age group.

Two other assessment instruments are useful in measuring self-esteem. The Piers–Harris Children's Self Concept Scale (Piers, 1984) is an 80-item self-concept scale that gauges children's self-perceptions of their behavior, intellectual and school status, physical appearance and attributes, anxiety, and personal satisfaction. Hoffmeister's (1971) Self-Esteem Questionnaire (SEQ-3) is a shorter, 21-item self-report inventory that measures feelings of competence, worth, success, and importance to others, as well as the degree of satisfaction with the level of self-esteem achieved.

Emotional Development

The development of self-esteem can be intimately related to emotional development. Research (Allen & Tarnowski, 1989) shows that physically abused and neglected children are more depressed and have an external locus of control (i.e., they attribute negative outcomes in their life to internal, global, and stable causes, which results in feelings of helplessness), experience anhedonia, and exhibit inconsistent and unpredictable affective communication. Specifically, they tend to be either emotionally withdrawn or exhibit abrupt changes in mood (Kinard, 1982). Physically abused children report symptoms of dysphoria, including sadness, an inability to enjoy life, and low self-esteem (Green, 1981; Kinard, 1982). Abused children who were followed up 4 ½ years after the abuse (Martin & Beezley, 1977) lacked the capacity to play freely, laugh, and enjoy themselves in an uninhibited manner. Self-deprecation and lack of confidence were conveyed by such comments as "I can't do it" and "I'm bad." Their vigilance and heightened alertness to their environment appeared to reflect a heightened sensitivity to external threat. The repeated physical pain and discomfort that abused children experience fosters frustration, learned helplessness, and concomitant negative affective states (Green, 1981).

The data, however, are not entirely consistent with regard to abused children's emotional and cognitive development. Kazdin, Moser, Colbus, and Bell (1985) found that while children with both past and current histories of physical abuse self-reported lower self-esteem and higher levels of hopelessness and depression than children whose abuse was limited to their current situation, children who were abused in the past but not currently abused were indistinguishable from the nonabused group. Unfortunately, the frequency and severity of the abuse was not taken into account in this research. Furthermore, since only an inpatient sample was used, it is unclear whether the depression was associated with preexisting psychopathology that led to hospitalization in the first place.

Taken together, the studies reviewed indicate that depression can be a prominent part of the symptom picture the clinician observes with physically abused children. Hence, it is important that he or she assess for depression. The clinician will find that a number of assessment instruments provide information that is pertinent to the child's affect and the diagnosis of depression. Several semistructured and structured interviews have been developed to assess for depression. The Kiddie–SADS (Puig-Antich, Blau, Marx, Greenhill, & Chambers, 1978) is a semistructured interview for both parents and children, which is applicable to children ages 6–17. The Kiddie–SADS—P (Present version) provides severity ratings for affective symptoms, whereas the Kiddie–SADS—E (Epidemiological version) allows for the assessment of past chronic or episodic illness. The Interview Schedule for Children (ISC; Kovacs, Feinberg, Crouse-Novak, Paulauskas, & Finkelstein, 1984) is a structured interview, which can be used with children ages 8–17. It can be invaluable in arriving at a diagnosis insofar as it addresses not only the symptoms of depression but also all relevant DSM-III-R diagnoses. Although it requires the careful training of the interviewer, the instrument has good interrater reliability.

The Children's Affective Rating Scale (CARS; Cytryn & McKnew, 1974) measures mood, behavior, and fantasy. It provides a fine-grained analysis of depressive symptoms with respect to ten categories of depressive symptomatology (e.g., dysphoric mood, self-deprecatory ideation, somatic complaints, change in school performance). One limitation of this instrument is its very high sensitivity to but low specificity for identifying depression. The instrument is excellent at detecting depression when depression is truly present. However, the limitation of the instrument is that it also identifies those that are nondepressed as depressed. In other words, high scores on this measure are not very specific to depression.

Self-Destructive Behavior and Suicide

The incidence of self-destructive behavior (e.g., suicide attempts, self-mutilation, suicidal ideation) is higher among children who have been physically abused than for control groups of nonabused subjects. Physically abused adolescents tend to demonstrate more suicidal ideation and attempt suicide more often than comparison groups of subjects (Malinosky-Rummell & Hansen, 1993). These rates increase with combined (e.g., physical, psychological, and sexual) types of abuse. Kroll, Stock, and James (1985) found a higher incidence of suicide attempts among physically abused alcoholic men than among nonabused alcoholic men. With female inpatients, physical abuse accounted for a significant amount of the variance in predicting suicidal ideation, gestures, and attempts (Bryer, Nelson, Miller, & Krol, 1987). Among female college students who reported physical abuse, suicide ideation was higher than nonabused students' suicide ideation (Briere & Runtz, 1988).

Suicide potential can be assessed with interview procedures that identify those risk factors associated with suicide. However, more formal instruments may assist the clinician in making a determination of suicide potential. The Assessment of Suicide Potential (Yufit & Benzies, 1979) is a 39-item semiprojective instrument that measures the probability that a person will consciously commit an act that will end his or her life. The Suicide Probability Scale (SPS; Cull & Gill, 1982) is a self-report measure that assesses the risk of suicide in adults and adolescents aged 14 years and older. The four subscales of this measure include Suicide Ideation, Hopelessness, Negative Self-Evaluation, and Hostility. Finally, the Suicide Ideation Questionnaire (SIQ; Reynolds, 1988) consists of declarative statements that reflect thoughts related to suicide. A 30-item version is appropriate for grades 10–12, whereas a 15-item version is appropriate for grades 7–9.

Post-Traumatic Stress Disorder

The literature indicates that physical abuse can be associated with the symptoms of post-traumatic stress disorder (PTSD). Deblinger, McLeer, Atkins, Ralphe, and Foa (1989) found that 6.9% of physically abused children (ages 3–13) met the diagnostic criteria for PTSD, whereas Adam, Everett, and

O'Neal (1992), using a prospective research design, found that 20% of physically abused children (ages 4–12) met the criteria for PTSD symptomatology. Hillary and Schare (1993), however, reported that abused adolescents (ages 13–18) did not meet PTSD diagnoses when adult measures such as the Minnesota Multiphasic Personality Inventory (MMPI) were used. Apart from the problems associated with the use of the adult-normed MMPI with adolescents, the disparity between and among studies may be due to the fact that PTSD symptoms dissipate with age.

Green (1981, 1983) argues that there may be two types of abuse-related disorders. The first type of disorder is associated with acute physical assault and encompasses certain symptoms that are linked with PTSD. In response to an acute physical assault, the child reacts with painful affect, anxious and agitated behavior, hypervigilance, and attempts to achieve mastery by reenacting the trauma. In contrast, long-term traumatic experiences following exposure to repeated abuse result in a second type of disorder, marked by poor impulse control, a proclivity to engage in violence, helplessness, depressive affect, poor attachment, self-destructive behavior, and separation problems. In a recent study, Kiser and his colleagues (Kiser, Heston, Millsap, & Pruitt, 1991) confirmed that children who experience a single abusive event exhibit more behavioral disorders, whereas those who experience ongoing abuse have more depressive and psychotic symptoms. His research also indicated that PTSD symptomatology was related to the severity of abuse and the number of perpetrators of the abuse.

Chandler (1983) has developed a 40-item Stress Response Scale (SRS), which measures the impact of stressful and traumatic events on a child's behavioral adjustment with respect to five subscales (i.e., Acting Out, Passive Aggressive, Overactive, Dependent, and Repressed). This measure, which may be administered to children ages 5–18, is typically filled out by a parent or teacher. An alternative measure, the Children's Life Events Inventory—Revised (CLEI-R; Chandler, 1985), contains 37 parent-rated events in the family, home, and school that are potentially distressing for young children. This measure provides an estimate of the child's level of risk and vulnerability to post-traumatic complications. This information may be useful to the clinician who is prone to focus on abuse-related trauma and ignore or minimize other events and their repercussions, which also need to be addressed in treatment.

Behavioral and Interpersonal Difficulties

Physical aggression and antisocial behavior are the most prevalent sequelae of physical child maltreatment. In general, abused children are more aggressive than neglected children (Ammerman et al., 1986). Even when matched for low SES, Kent (1976) found that physically abused children were consistently rated as more aggressive and as having more problems with peer relationships than nonabused and neglected children, while the latter were rated as showing more withdrawal symptoms and intellectual and developmental delays. George and Main (1979) matched physically abused and nonabused children experiencing family stress (ages 1–3) on demographic variables. The authors found that the abused children were more aggressive, responded more negatively to friendly overtures, avoided caregivers three times as often, and assaulted other children twice as often as the nonabused children. In short, the effects of abuse on aggression in children cannot be explained by SES and family stress alone.

One explanation of the relative preponderance of aggressive behavior in abused children is that they tend to imitate the aggressive behavior modeled in the home. They learn to use aggressive behavior as a means of controlling others' behavior and accept it as an appropriate way with which to deal with unpleasant situations. This in turn is generalized to other relationships (Patterson, 1982). Indeed, the available evidence suggests that physically abused children are more at risk for developing poor peer relations in school, for having lower social status among friends, for being rejected by peers, for more easily experiencing frustration and distractibility, and for being less persistent in school than nonabused children (Egeland & Sroufe, 1981; Egeland, Sroufe, & Erickson, 1983; Martin & Beezley, 1977).

In a particularly well-designed longitudinal research program, Egeland and his colleagues (Egeland & Sroufe, 1981; Egeland, Sroufe, & Erickson, 1983) compared infants whose mothers were verbally abusive, physically abusive, psychologically unavailable, or neglectful, with a control group wherein the mothers were currently "adequate" but considered to be "at risk" for being abusive due to poverty, limited education, and their young age. At 12 and 18 months, most of the maltreated infants were found to be anxiously attached to their mothers, and their problem-solving abilities were found to be poor at the age of 2. At 42- and 56-month follow-ups, in which a problem-solving task and observations in a preschool situation were conducted, the physically abused children were "distractible, lacked persistence, ego control and enthusiasm, and experienced considerable negative emotion" (Egeland et al., 1983, p. 459). The children of psychologically unavailable mothers were avoidant of their mother, angry, noncompliant, and highly dependent.

One explanation of the relationship problems found in children who do not form secure attachments with their parents is that they have trouble forming close bonds with other people and coping with frustrating experiences. Another explanation is that abusive parents may be socially isolated, which denies the child formative social experiences (Howes & Espinosa, 1985; Salzinger, Feldman, Hammer, & Rosario, 1993).

When the behavior of physically abused and neglected children is compared to nonabused children in unstructured environments, such as those involving fantasy and free play, as assessed by the Thematic Apperception Test (TAT; Reidy, 1977) and the Rosenzweig Picture–Frustration Test (Kinard, 1982), abused children have been found to exhibit more aggression than nonabused normal children in their fantasies, in a free play environment, and in a school environment. Although neglected children appeared to be nonaggressive in unstructured environments such as fantasy or free play situations, they became more aggressive and frustrated in structured environments. Overall, maltreated children appear to engage more in fantasized aggression than their nonabused peers.

A number of studies stand as exceptions to these findings. For example, Straker and Jacobson (1981) found no differences between abused and control children ages 5–10 on measures of aggression in fantasy, and Mash, Johnson, and Kovitz (1983) did not find any observed behavioral differences between abused and nonabused children when they were interacting with their mothers in structured and unstructured environments. Unfortunately, in the latter study, subjects were not matched on SES and the observation time was very short (15–20 minutes), limiting the conclusions that can be drawn from the study's results.

Despite these contradictory findings, the general conclusion of the literature is that abused children experience a wide range of behavioral and interpersonal problems. Because parents and children's self-reports are limited and can be biased, it is important for clinicians to have at their disposal a number of different methods of gauging behavioral and interpersonal problems. Fortunately, multiple assessment methods have been devised including semistructured interviews, behavioral ratings, and role-play tests.

The Children's Assessment Schedule (Hodges, McKnew, Cytryn, Stern, & Kline, 1982) is a semistructured interview that assesses a broad spectrum of psychological disorders and areas of adjustment difficulty in children ages 7–12. The interview examines the onset and duration of problems in areas that include school, friends, activities, family, fears, self-image, mood, somatic concerns, anger, and symptoms of thought disorders.

The Revised Behavior Problem Checklist (RBPC; Quay, 1983) consists of 89 items that are rated according to level of severity. The RBPC measures the following problems: undersocialized conduct disorder, socialized conduct disorder, attention difficulties, anxiety–withdrawal symptoms, psychotic disorders, and motor excesses. The Child Behavior Checklist (CBCL; Achenbach & Edelbrock, 1983) consists of 118 items pertinent to internalizing and externalizing behaviors, which are rated according to the severity of the child's behavior. There is a version of this checklist for teachers (Teacher Report Form) as well as a self-report version for children ages 11–18 (Youth Report Form).

Aggressive behaviors may be particularly difficult to assess because they occur on an infrequent basis, and may only be observed in natural settings. To address this difficulty, the Behavioral Assertiveness Test for Children (BAT-C; Borenstein, Bellack, & Hersen, 1980) assesses the social skills of aggressive children in natural settings. The test requires that the clinician reads scenes to the child that are representative of situations involving positive and negative responses. The child is then prompted to interact with a confederate, and the clinician observes the child's behaviors in response to the confederate.

Delinquency, Criminality, and Substance Abuse

Most children who have been physically abused do not become violent delinquents. In fact, only about 20% of physically abused children become delinquent (Cicchetti & Carlson, 1989). A high proportion of delinquents, however, have been abused. Lewis and Shanok (1977) found that 8.6% of delinquents were physically abused, as compared to 1% of the control subjects. In a sample of 97 adolescent delinquent males, 75% of the more violent youths had been abused, as compared to 33% of the less violent youths.

McCord (1983) maintains that whereas abuse and neglect may lead to juvenile delinquency, parental rejection appears to be an even more powerful indicator of criminality. Nevertheless, children who have been physically abused have a higher likelihood of arrests for delinquency, violent behavior, and criminality in adulthood than nonabused children. Abused children tend to be suspicious, aloof, guarded, have trouble answering to authority, and are at risk for alcohol and drug abuse (Cicchetti & Carlson, 1989).

Substance abusers report a higher incidence of childhood physical abuse (13–15%) than that reported in the general population (Kroll et al., 1985). Brown and Anderson (1991) found higher rates of alcohol and drug use among physically abused inpatients. In one study, alcoholic men who had been physically abused also demonstrated a high rate of "suicidal drinking" (Kroll et al., 1985). However, the use of drugs other than alcohol has not been consistently associated with physical abuse. For instance, a prospective study (Dembro et al., 1992) did not show that physical abuse accounted for a significant amount of variance in the marijuana use of adolescents. Taken together, the reviewed evidence indicates that a reliance on chemical substances, particularly alcohol, may be a way of coping with painful emotions associated with a history of physical abuse.

When assessing for a history of delinquent behavior, the clinician needs to consider a variety of problem areas and deficits, including poor social skills, poor problem solving, lack of impulse control, poor academic performance, and hyperactivity. Although there is no well-established measure of juvenile delinquency per se, broad-based measures of problem areas and deficits such as the Child Behavior Checklist (Achenbach & Edelbrock, 1983) and the Revised Behavior Problem Checklist (Quay, 1983) can provide relevant information. In order to obtain information regarding the adolescent's offense patterns, family history, and previous treatment, information sources such as the juvenile's parents and probation officer can be consulted, and, if available, state child welfare department records can be examined.

All too often, clinicians perform a cursory evaluation of a youth's substance abuse history. Several assessment devices can provide systematic information about the consumption of legal and illicit substances. The Drug Use Index (DUI; Douglass & Khavari, 1987) surveys adolescents and adults with an eighth-grade education level with respect to whether they have consumed 19 legal and illicit drugs, along with the frequency of use of each substance. The Assessment of Chemical Health Inventory (ACHI; Krotz, 1988) is a 128-item instrument that profiles chemical/substance use and associated problems. This measure includes a validity scale, a chemical use score, and scores on indices of Family Estrangement, Use Involvement, Personal Consequences, Alienation, Depression, Family Support, Social Impact, Family Chemical Use, and Self-Regard/Abuse. This instrument is particularly useful in assessing the implications of physical abuse because it contains items pertinent to physical and sexual abuse, suicidal ideation, legal problems, family secrets, and eating concerns. The ACHI may be used with both adolescents and adults.

ADULT PSYCHOPATHOLOGY

General Psychopathology

In general, victims of physical and/or psychological abuse report higher levels of psychopathology in adulthood than those who have not been abused. Estimates of inpatients who report a history of physical abuse vary from 18% (Margo & McLees, 1991) to 28% (Chu & Dill, 1990). The literature suggests that the symptoms tend to be exacerbated when individuals are exposed to more than one type of abuse (Surrey, Swett, Michaels, & Levin, 1990), and that physical abuse is more reliably associated with psychopathology than sexual abuse (Chu & Dill, 1990).

Adult victims of childhood physical abuse are more likely than non-abused individuals to report symptoms of general psychopathology (Chu & Dill, 1990; Margo & McLees, 1991; Surrey et al., 1990), as measured by the Symptom Checklist—90 (SCL-90). Adults who report a history of abuse are likely to report more depressive symptoms (Brown & Anderson, 1991; Bryer et al., 1987; Margo & McLees, 1991; Rhue et al., 1994; Surrey et al., 1990), anxiety (Rhue et al., 1994; Surrey et al., 1990), aggression and anger

(Briere & Runtz, 1990; Rhue et al., 1994), and trouble with their inter-personal relationships (Rhue et al., 1994; Surrey et al., 1990) than nonabused persons. Abused individuals are often diagnosed with depression (Brown & Anderson, 1991; Margo & McLees, 1991), dissociative disorders (see Putnam, 1989), substance abuse (Brown & Anderson, 1991), and person-ality disorders, with antisocial and borderline personality disorders being the most frequent (Brown & Anderson, 1991; Bryer et al., 1987; Margo & McLees, 1991; Ogata, Silk, Goodrich, Lohr, Westen, & Hill, 1990; Pol-lock et al., 1990; Raczek, 1992; Shearer, Peters, Quaytman, & Ogden, 1990). No specific symptom profile has been discerned across studies, perhaps due to the fact that a standardized symptom protocol has not been adopted by different investigators. Nevertheless, the link between abuse and psycho-pathology has been established in numerous studies, including studies of women inpatients (Bryer et al., 1987; Margo & McLees, 1991), women outpatients (Surrey et al., 1990), and male and female college students (Briere & Runz, 1990; Rhue et al., 1994).

Well-established omnibus psychopathology measures such as the MMPI (Hathaway & McKinley, 1983) and the SCL-90-R (Derogatis, Lipman, & Covi, 1973) are, obviously, of great value in assessing adult psychopa-thology. Projective tests (e.g., the Rorschach, the TAT) can be useful as well, particularly when supplemented by more precise structured diagnos-tic interviews such as the Structured Clinical Interview for DSM-III-R for Axis I and II disorders (Spitzer, Williams, Gibbon, & First, 1990). Because depression is probably the most common diagnosis of abuse survivors, clinicians may wish to administer tests that measure depressive sympto-matology such as the Beck Depression Inventory (BDI; Beck, Steer, & Garbin, 1988).

Dissociation

Theoretically at least, dissociation serves a protective, defensive function by helping a person to separate or detach from the potentially overwhelm-ing experience of abuse, thereby reducing concomitant physical pain, fear, and anxiety (Spiegel, 1986; Spiegel & Cardeña, 1991; van der Kolk & van der Hart, 1989). This hypothesis is buttressed by studies that document an association between abuse and dissociative phenomena.

In an adult female inpatient population, reports of childhood physical (28%) and sexual abuse (12%) were associated with higher levels of disso-ciative symptoms in adulthood (Chu & Dill, 1990). Scores on the Disso-ciative Experiences Scale (DES; Bernstein & Putnam, 1986) were higher in cases of physical abuse when the perpetrator was a family member than when the perpetrator was not a family member. Furthermore, subjects who ex-perienced both physical and sexual abuse had higher DES scores than subjects who experienced a single type of abuse. Sanders and Giolas (1991) essentially replicated this association between dissociation and abuse, through using trauma and abuse questionnaires, with both adolescent psychiatric inpatients and a college student sample (Sanders, McRoberts, & Tollefson, 1989). In the latter study, the highest dissociation scores, as indexed by both the DES and the Bliss Dissociation Scale (Wogan, 1987), were found among students who experienced both physical and psychological abuse. Finally, Sandberg and Lynn's (1992) research indicated that dissociation was related to the subjects' retrospective reports of physical and psychological abuse and general psychopathology.

Even though findings converge on the fact that dissociation and a number of different types of abuse are related, the studies to date do not effectively rule out the hypothesis that the association between dissociation and physical abuse can be accounted for by elevations in general psychopathology that are not specific or limited to dissociation. The assessment of dissociation in children (see Chapter 9) and in adults (see Chapter 8) is discussed elsewhere in this book, and thus will not be addressed here.

PSYCHOLOGICAL ABUSE

Psychopathology

Many negative child characteristics have been associated with psychological abuse: poor appetite, lying and stealing, enuresis and encopresis, low self-esteem, emotional instability, dependency, incompetence or underachievement, inability to trust others, depression, suicide, withdrawal, and aggression (Hart et al., 1987). Of course, these resemble the previously discussed characteristics of physically abused children. Hence, sequelae discussed previously will not be reiterated here.

Because psychological abuse often accompanies physical abuse, it is difficult to discriminate the specific role of psychological abuse from that of physical abuse. Nevertheless, according to empirical studies (Briere & Runtz, 1990) and reviews (Gross & Keller 1992), there appears to be a unique relation between retrospective reports of psychological abuse in childhood and low self-esteem when other forms of abuse are statistically controlled for. Furthermore, psychological abuse is a much stronger predictor of depression, poor self-esteem, and attributional style than physical abuse. The child internalizes the criticisms and statements made by parents and blames him- or herself for negative events later in life. When the effects of psychological abuse are controlled for statistically, physical abuse does not significantly contribute to the variance in the variables mentioned above.

Although few studies have examined the independent effects of psychological abuse in the adult population, it is clear that physical and psychological abuse tend to occur together and, in combination, have a greater influence on later symptomatology than when only one type of abuse takes place (see Briere & Runtz, 1988). Briere and Runtz (1988) found that children who experience both types of abuse tend to have low self-esteem, anger, aggression, and dysfunctional sexual behavior. A multivariate analysis suggested that various types of abuse have both specific and overlapping effects on later psychosocial functioning.

Role of Family Environment

Interactions in Abusive Families

Any complete discussion of the effects of psychological abuse, and physical abuse for that matter, must include a consideration of the role of social interactions within the family context. It is unclear whether the personal and interpersonal problems of abuse survivors result from physical punishment in childhood, the psychological and verbal abuse that often accompanies physical abuse, or some other aspect of early family interactions. Nash, Hulsey, Sexton, Harralson, and Lambert (1993) concluded that how a person perceives his or her family environment appears to be an important variable in determining adult psychological functioning. In fact, they found no effect for abuse per se on psychological impairment when they statistically controlled for familial factors.

A series of studies by Burgess and Conger (1977, 1978) investigated abuse in the context of the family environment by studying mother and child interactions in abusive and nonabusive families. They observed mothers and their children perform tasks that encouraged interaction and cooperation and increased physical contact and discussion. In the initial study, Burgess and Conger (1977) concluded that the abusive and neglectful families exhibited the same behaviors as other problem families. Both initiated less contact, and when they did use physical contact, they did so excessively and inappropriately. In a second study, the authors (Burgess & Conger, 1978) found that abusive mothers were less verbal and had fewer positive interactions with their children than nonabusive mothers did; they also tended to emphasize the negative aspects of the relationship. In fact, the frequency of the abusive mothers' negative behaviors was 77% greater than that of the nonabusive controls.

Relatedly, a recent study (Silber, Bermann, Henderson, & Lehman, 1993) found that abusive fathers displayed more controlling and coercive behaviors and were more critical of their children than nonabusive fathers.

It is important to note that while nonabusing families criticize the child at certain times, they are also likely to be accepting of the child at other times. In abusive families, however, the frequency of negative responses is much higher than the frequency of positive ones.

Although Mash, Johnson, and Kovitz (1983) found that abused children are as responsive and compliant with their mothers as nonabused children and interact with them as adaptively, when greater demands were placed on the mother and the child during a task, the abusive mothers tended to be more directive and controlling than the nonabusive mothers, and failed to interact with their children in a reciprocal manner.

Inconsistent interaction patterns associated with abuse may have a negative impact on children's development (Steele, 1986). In the absence of consistency, the child fails to develop a reliable sense of the relationship between his or her actions and their outcome. Hence, the child must look for cues in the environment indicative of threatening situations. In the process, the child becomes hypervigilant and comes to rely on the external environment for information.

Family Environment, Psychological Functioning, and Axis I Pathology

Wolfe and Mosk (1983) controlled for family dysfunction by comparing psychologically abused children, children from distressed homes, and non-abused children from distressed homes. Abused children displayed poorer school performance and less competent social behaviors than nonabused children. Nonabused children from dysfunctional homes (no physical abuse or neglect were reported, but there was parent–child conflict in the home and the child was often out of parental control) displayed slightly higher rates of problem behaviors (hyperactivity, internalizing symptoms, delinquency) than abused children. Overall, the researchers found that abused children's behavior and social competence did not differ significantly from that of children from distressed families. Unfortunately, the investigation relied primarily on the mothers' perceptions of their children's behaviors, which has frequently been shown to be an inaccurate indicator (Burgess & Conger, 1977). Moreover, the fact that the nonabused children were referred from social service agencies suggests that they may have had other difficulties that may have confounded the results.

It has been hypothesized (Burgess & Conger, 1978; Kazdin, Moser, Colbus, & Bell, 1985) that parents who are emotionally unresponsive, rejecting, and do not interact positively with their children might predispose them toward depression in later life. Studies have attempted to identify aspects of the early parent–child relationship that can lead to the development of depressive symptoms in adulthood. Depressed individuals describe their mothers and fathers as rejecting and report that they used aversive techniques to control behavior, such as derision, debasement, withdrawal of affection, and manipulation through guilt and anxiety (Crook & Raskin, 1981). Lefkowitz and Tesiny (1984) concluded that depression may result from such family factors as parental disharmony, inconsistent parental rearing practices, dominance of the father in the home, separation from the mother, death of one of the parents, inability to control the environment, and the inability to live up to parental expectations.

In conclusion, feelings of self-worthlessness and depression may originate in the early parent–child relationship. Higher levels of self-criticism in adulthood seem to be related to perceptions of the parents as lacking in warmth, nurturance, and affection. The association between self-criticism in adulthood and recall of poor parenting does not seem to result from present mood state or a social desirability response set (Brewin, Firth-Cozens, Furnham, & McManus, 1992).

What our brief review suggests is that disturbances in children's social and behavioral development, as well as negative affective states, may be a function of the family environment and interaction patterns rather than, or in addition to, isolated episodes of psychological abuse. Because abusive parental behaviors may interact with other aspects of a child's environment, a comprehensive examination of abusive incidents in the context of an analysis of more global family interactions and the family environment is a prerequisite to a complete understanding of the abused child.

To accomplish this more comprehensive assessment, it is particularly important to observe children's interactions with abusive parents. Inasmuch as the behavioral consequences of abuse vary greatly from child to child, it is worthwhile to assess the frequency, intensity, and duration of coercive interactions with coding systems that have been devised for this purpose (Reid, 1978). Furthermore, the Child Abuse Potential Inventory (Milner, 1986) and the Parenting Stress Index (Abidin, 1983) can be used to examine parents' responsiveness to the child, attitudes about child rearing, and use of corporeal punishment. It is also important to evaluate parents' expectations of their children and their problem-solving abilities.

Several instruments can be used to evaluate the suitability of the child-rearing environment to the specific needs of the child. The Child Neglect Severity Scale (Hall, DeLaCruz, & Russell, 1982) measures nine categories of child neglect: abandonment, health care, nutrition, supervision, personal hygiene, clothing, shelter, emotional neglect, and education. The Home Observation for the Measurement of the Environment Scale (Caldwell & Bradley, 1985) and the Childhood Level of Living Scale (Polansky, Chalmers, Buttenweiser, & Williams, 1981) can assist in measuring the quality of parent–child interactions, the availability of play and stimulation in the environment, health care, and discipline practices in the home.

CONCLUSION

Information regarding the characteristics frequently displayed by physically and psychologically abused children can be used to anticipate areas in which they might encounter difficulties in childhood and in later life. The research presented indicates that maltreated children are at a higher risk for developing a deficit or disorder in one or more of the areas of functioning discussed. Because multiple types of abuse often occur in the same family, clinicians and researchers need to consider the effects of each type of abuse as well as the combined influence they have on the child. Moreover, insofar as aversive family interactions may have a great impact on the child, independent of physical abuse that may occur (Conway & Hansen, 1989; Malinosky-Rummel & Hansen, 1993), it is incumbent on the clinician to assess parent–child interactions, parental discord, and parental psychiatric disorders when comprehensively evaluating a child. Whereas a causal relation cannot be assumed between childhood abuse and adulthood psychopathology, evidence suggests that clinicians need to conduct a careful assessment of psychopathology and dissociation with respect to clients who report a history of physical or psychological abuse.

REFERENCES

Aber, J. L., & Allen, J. P. (1987). Effects of maltreatment on young children's socioemotional development: An attachment theory perspective. *Developmental Psychology, 23*(3), 406–414.

Abidin, R. (1983). *Parenting Stress Index—Manual*. Charlottesville, VA: Pediatric Psychiatry Press.

Achenbach, T. M., & Edelbrock, C. S. (1983). *Manual for the Child Behavior Checklist and the Revised Child Behavior Profile*. Burlington, VA: University Associates in Psychiatry.

Adam, B. S., Everett, B. L., & O'Neal, E. (1992). PTSD in physically and sexually abused psychiatrically hospitalized children. *Child Psychiatry and Human Development, 23*(1), 3–8.

Ainsworth, M. D. S., Blehar, M., Waters, E., & Wall, S. (1978). *Patterns of attachment: Observations in the strange situation at home*. Hillsdale, NJ: Lawrence Erlbaum.

Allen, D. M., & Tarnowski, K. J. (1989). Depressive characteristics of physically abused children. *Journal of Abnormal Child Psychology, 17*(1), 1–11.

American Humane Association. (1992). *National analysis of official child neglect and abuse reporting*. Denver, CO: Author.

Ammerman, R. T., Cassisi, J. E., Hersen, M., & Van Hasselt, V. B. (1986). Consequences of physical abuse and neglect in children. *Clinical Psychology Review, 6*, 291–310.

Augoustinos, M. (1987). Developmental effects of child abuse: Recent findings. *Child Abuse and Neglect, 11*, 15–27.

Beck, A. T., Steer, R. A., & Garbin, M. G. (1988). Psychometric properties of the Beck Depression Inventory: Twenty five years of evaluation. *Clinical Psychology Review, 8,* 77–100.

Bernstein, E. M., & Putnam, F. W. (1986). Development, reliability, and validity of a dissociation scale. *Journal of Nervous and Mental Disease, 174,* 727–735.

Borenstein, M. R., Bellack, A. S., & Hersen, M. (1980). Social skills training for highly aggressive children: Treatment in an inpatient setting. *Behavior Modification, 4,* 173–186.

Brewin, C. R., Firth-Cozens, J., Furnham, A., & McManus, C. (1992). Self-criticism in adulthood and recalled childhood experience. *Journal of Abnormal Psychology, 101*(3), 561–566.

Briere, J., & Runtz, M. (1988). Multivariate correlates of childhood psychological and physical maltreatment among university women. *Child Abuse and Neglect, 12,* 331–341.

Briere, J., & Runtz, M. (1990). Differential adult symptomatology associated with three types of child abuse histories. *Child Abuse and Neglect, 14,* 357–364.

Brown, G. R., & Anderson, B. (1991). Psychiatric morbidity in adult inpatients with histories of sexual and physical abuse. *American Journal of Psychiatry, 148,* 55–61.

Bryer, J. B., Nelson, B., Miller, J. B., & Krol, P. A. (1987). Childhood sexual and physical abuse as factors in adult psychiatric illness. *American Journal of Psychiatry, 144,* 1426–1430.

Burgess, R. L., & Conger, R. D. (1977). Family interaction patterns related to child abuse and neglect: Some primary findings. *Child Abuse and Neglect, 1,* 269–277.

Burgess, R. L., & Conger, R. D. (1978). Family interaction in abusive, neglectful and normal families. *Child Development, 49,* 1163–1173.

Caldwell, B., & Bradley, R. (1985). *Home observation for measurement of the environment.* New York: Dorsey Press.

Camras, L. A., Grow, G., & Ribordy, S. C. (1983). Recognition of emotional expression by abused children. *Journal of Clinical Child Psychology, 2*(3), 325–328.

Chandler, L. A. (1983). The Stress Response Scale: An instrument for use in assessing emotional adjustment reactions. *School Psychology Review, 12,* 260–265.

Chandler, L. A. (1985). *The Children's Life Events Inventory: Instructions for use.* Unpublished mimeograph, The Psychoeducational Clinic, University of Pittsburgh, Pittsburgh, PA.

Chu, J. A., & Dill, D. L. (1990). Dissociative symptoms in relation to childhood physical and sexual abuse. *American Journal of Psychiatry, 147,* 887–892.

Cicchetti, D., & Carlson, V. (Eds.). (1989). *Child maltreatment: Theory and research on the causes and consequences of child abuse and neglect.* Cambridge, MA: Cambridge University Press.

Claussen, A. H., & Crittenden, P. M. (1991). Physical and psychological maltreatment: Relations among types of maltreatment. *Child Abuse and Neglect, 15,* 5–18.

The Clearinghouse on Child Abuse and Neglect Information. (1989). *Child abuse and neglect: A shared community concern.* Washington, DC: National Center on Child Abuse and Neglect.

Conway, L. P., & Hansen, D. J. (1989). Social behavior of physically abused and neglected children: A critical review. *Clinical Psychology Review, 9,* 627–652.

Coopersmith, S. (1981). *Self-Esteem Inventories.* Palo Alto, CA: Consulting Psychologists Press.

Crook, T., Raskin, A., & Eliot, J. (1981). Parent–child relationships and adult depression. *Child Development, 52,* 950–957.

Cull, J. G., & Gill, W. S. (1982). *Suicide Probability Scale.* Los Angeles: Western Psychological Services.

Cytryn, L., & McKnew, D. H. Jr. (1974). Factors influencing the changing clinical expression of the depressive process in children. *American Journal of Psychiatry, 131,* 879–881.

Deblinger, E., McLeer, S. V., Atkins, M. S., Ralphe, D., & Foa, E. (1989). Posttraumatic stress in sexually, physically and nonabused children. *Child Abuse and Neglect, 13,* 403–408.

Dembro, R., Williams, L., Schmeidler, J., Berry, E., Wothke, W., Getreu, A., Wish, E. D., & Christensen, C. (1992). A structural model examining the relationship between physical child abuse, sexual victimization, and marijuana/hashish use in delinquent youth: A longitudinal study. *Violence and Victims, 7*(1), 41–62.

Derogatis, L. R., Lipman, R. S., & Covi, L. (1973). The SCL—90: An outpatient psychiatric rating scale. *Psychopharmacology Bulletin, 9,* 13–28.

Douglass, E. M., & Khavari, K. A. (1978). The Drug Use Index: A measure of the extent of polydrug usage. *International Journal of Addiction, 13,* 981–993.

Dunn, L. M., & Dunn, L. M. (1981). *Peabody Picture Vocabulary Test—Revised.* Circle Pines, MN: American Guidance Service.

Egeland, B., & Stroufe, L. A. (1981). Attachment and early maltreatment. *Child Development, 52,* 44–52.

Egeland, B., Stroufe, L. A., & Erickson, M. (1983). The developmental consequences of different patterns of maltreatment. *Child Abuse and Neglect, 7,* 459–469.

Elmer, E., & Gregg, G. S. (1967). Developmental characteristics of abused children. *Pediatrics, 40,* 596–602.

Elmer, E. (1977). A follow-up study of traumatized children. *Pediatrics, 59,* 273–279.

Elmer, E. (1978). Effects of early neglect and abuse on latency age children. *Journal of Pediatric Psychology, 3*(1), 14–19.

George, C., & Main, M. (1979). Social interactions of young abused chidren: Approach, avoidance and aggression. *Child Development, 50,* 306–318.

Green, A. H. (1981). Core affective disturbance in abused children. *Journal of the American Academy of Psychoanalysis, 9*(3), 435–446.

Green, A. H. (1983). Dimension of psychological trauma in abused children. *Journal of the American Academy of Child Psychiatry, 22*(3), 231–237.

Gross, A. B., & Keller, H. R. (1992). Long-term consequences of childhood physical and psychological maltreatment. *Aggressive Behavior, 18,* 171–185.

Hall, M., DeLaCruz, A., & Russell, P. (1982). Working with neglecting families. *Children Today, 36,* 6–9.

Harris, D. B. (1963). *Children's drawings as measures of intellectual maturity: A revision and extension of the Goodenough Draw-a-Man Test.* New York: Harcourt, Brace & World.

Hart, S. N., & Brassard, M. R. (1987). A major threat to children's mental health: Psychological maltreatment. *American Psychologist, 42*(2), 160–165.

Hart, S. N., Germain, R. B., & Brassard, M. R. (1987). The challenge: To better understand and combat psychological maltreatment of children and youth. In M. R. Brassard, R. Germain, & S. N. Hart (Eds.), *Psychological maltreatment of children and youth* (pp. 3–24). New York: Pergamon Press.

Hathaway, S. R., & McKinley, J. C. (1983). *Minnesota Multiphasic Personality Inventory manual*. New York: Psychological Corporation.

Hillary, B. E., & Schare, M. L. (1993). Sexually and physically abused adolescents: An empirical search for PTSD. *Journal of Clinical Psychology, 49*(2), 161–165.

Hodges, K., McKnew, D., Cytryn, L., Stern, L., & Kline, J. (1982). The Child Assessment Schedule (CAS) diagnostic interview: A report of reliability and validity. *Journal of the American Academy of Child Psychiatry, 21*, 468–473.

Hoffmeister, J. K. (1971). *Self-Esteem Questionnaire*. Boulder, CO: Test Analysis and Development Corporation.

Howes, C., & Espinosa, M. P. (1985). The consequences of child abuse for the formation of relationships with peers. *Child Abuse and Neglect, 9*, 397–404.

Jacobson, R. S., & Straker, G. (1982). Peer group interaction of physically abused children. *Child Abuse and Neglect, 6*, 321–327.

Jastak, S., & Wilkinson, G. S. (1984). *Wide Range Achievement Test—Revised*. Wilmington, DE: Jastak Associates.

Kazdin, A. E., Moser, J., Colbus, D., & Bell, R. (1985). Depressive symptoms among physically abused psychiatrically disturbed children. *Journal of Abnormal Psychology, 94*(3), 298–307.

Kent, J. (1976). A follow-up study of abused children. *Journal of Pediatric Psychology, 1*, 5–31.

Kinard, E. M. (1982). Experiencing child abuse: Effects on emotional adjustment. *American Journal of Orthopsychiatry, 52*(1), 82–91.

Kiser, L., Heston, J., Millsap, P., & Pruitt, D. B. (1991). Physical and sexual abuse in childhood: Relationship with post-traumatic stress disorder. *Journal of American Academy of Child and Adolescent Psychiatry, 30*(5), 776–783.

Kolko, D. J. (1992). Characteristics of child victims of physical violence: Research findings and clinical implications. *Journal of Interpersonal Violence, 7*(2), 244–276.

Kovacs, M., Feinberg, T. L., Crouse-Novak, M. A., Paulauskas, S. L., & Finkelstein, R. (1984). Depressive disorders in childhood: 1. A longitudinal prospective study of characteristics and recovery. *Archives of General Psychiatry, 41*, 229–237.

Kroll, P. D., Stock, D. F., & James, M. E. (1985). The behavior of adult alcoholic men abused as children. *Journal of Nervous and Mental Disease, 173*, 689–693.

Krotz, D. (1988). *Assessment of Chemical Health Inventory*. Minneapolis, MN: Renovex.

Lefkowitz, M. M., & Tesiny, E. P. (1984). Rejection and depression: Prospective and contemporaneous analyses. *Developmental Psychology, 20*(5), 776-785.

Lewis, D. O., & Shanok, S. S. (1977). Medical histories of delinquent and nondelinquent children: An epidemiological study. *American Journal of Psychiatry, 134*, 1020–1025.

Malinosky-Rummell, R., & Hansen, D. J. (1993). Long-term consequences of childhood physical abuse. *Psychological Bulletin, 114*(1), 68–79.

Margo, G. M., & McLees, E. M. (1991). Further evidence for the significance of childhood abuse history in psychiatric inpatients. *Comprehensive Psychiatry, 32*(4), 362–366.

Martin, H. P., & Beezley, P. (1977). Behavioral observations of abused children. *Developmental Medicine and Child Neurology, 19*, 373–387.

Mash, E. J., Johnson, C., & Kovitz, K. (1983). A comparison of mother–child interactions of physically abused and nonabused children during play and task situations. *Journal of Clinical Child Psychology, 12*(3), 337–346.

McCord, J. (1983). A forty year perspective on effects of child abuse and neglect. *Child Abuse and Neglect, 7*, 265–270.

Milner, J. S. (1986). *The Child Abuse Potential Inventory: Manual* (2nd ed.). Webster, NC: Psytec, Inc.

Nash, M. R., Hulsey, T. L., Sexton, M. C., Harralson, T. L., & Lambert, W. (1993). Long-term sequelae of childhood sexual abuse: Perceived family environment, psychopathology, and dissociation. *Journal of Consulting and Clinical Psychology, 61*(2), 276–283.

National Center on Child Abuse and Neglect. (1988). *Study of national incidence and prevalence of child abuse and neglect: 1988*. Washington, DC: U.S. Department of Health and Human Services.

National Center on Child Abuse and Neglect. (1991). *National child abuse and neglect data system* (Working Paper No. 2). Washington, DC: U.S. Department of Health and Human Services.

Oates, R. K., Forrest, D., & Peacock, A. (1985). Self-esteem of abused children. *Child Abuse and Neglect, 9*, 159–163.

Ogata, S. N., Silk, K. R., Goodrich, S., Lohr, N. E., Westen, D., & Hill, E. M. (1990). Childhood sexual and physical abuse in adult patients with borderline personality disorder. *American Journal of Psychiatry, 147*, 1008–1013.

Patterson, G. R. (1982). *Coercive family processes*. Eugene, Oregon: Castalia.

Peterson, M. P. (1993). Physical and sexual abuse among school children: Prevalence and prevention. *Educational Psychology Review, 5*(1), 63–87.

Piers, E. V. (1984). *Revised manual for the Piers–Harris Children's Self-Concept Scale*. Los Angeles, CA: Western Psychological Services.

Polansky, N. A., Chalmers, M., Buttenwieser, E., & Williams, D. (1981). *Damaged parents: An anatomy of child neglect*. Chicago: University of Chicago Press.

Pollock, V. E., Briere, J., Schneider, L., Knop, J., Mednick, S. A., & Goodwin, D. W. (1990). Childhood antecedents of antisocial behavior: Parental alcoholism and physical abusiveness. *American Journal of Psychiatry, 147*, 1290–1293.

Puig-Antich, J., Blau, S., Marx, N., Greenhill, L., & Chambers, W. (1978). Prepubertal major depressive disorder: A pilot study. *Journal of the American Academy of Child Psychiatry, 17*, 695–707.

Putnam, F. W. (1989). *Diagnosis and treatment of multiple personality disorder*. New York: Guilford Press.

Quay, H. C. (1983). A dimensional approach to behavior disorder: The Revised Behavior Problem Checklist. *School Psychology Review, 12*, 244–249.

Raczek, S. W. (1992). Childhood abuse and personality. *Journal of Personality Disorders, 6*(2), 109–116.

Reid, J. B. (Ed.). (1978). *A social learning approach to family intervention: Observation in home settings* (Vol. 2). Eugene, OR: Castalia.

Reidy, T. J. (1977). The aggressive characteristics of abused and neglected children. *Journal of Clinical Psychology, 33*(4), 1140–1145.

Reynolds, W. M. (1988). *Suicidal Ideation Questionnaire: Professional manual.* Odessa, FL: Psychological Assessment Resources.

Rhue, J. W., Lynn, S. J., Green, J., Buhk, K., Henry, S., & Boyd, P. (1994). *Child abuse and psychopathology in college students: A controlled study.* Unpublished manuscript, Ohio University, Athens, OH.

Roll, S., Lockwood, J., & Roll, S. (1981). *Preliminary manual: Parent Attachment Structured Interview.* Albuquerque, NM: Author.

Salzinger, S., Feldman, R. S., Hammer, M., & Rosario, M. (1993). The effects of physical abuse on children's social relationships. *Child Development, 64*(1), 169-187.

Sandberg, D. A., & Lynn, S. J. (1992). Dissociative experiences, psychopathology and adjustment, and child and adolescent maltreatment in female college students. *Journal of Abnormal Psychology, 101*(4), 1–7.

Sanders, B., McRoberts, G., & Tollefson, C. (1989). Childhood stress and dissociation in a college population. *Dissociation, 2*(1), 17–23.

Sanders, B., & Giolas, M. H. (1991). Dissociation and childhood trauma in psychologically disturbed adolescents. *American Journal of Psychiatry, 148*, 50–54.

Shearer, S. L., Peters, C. P., Quaytman, M. S., & Ogden, R. (1990). Frequency and correlates of childhood sexual and physical abuse histories in adult female borderline patients. *American Journal of Psychiatry, 147*, 214–216.

Silber, S., Bermann, E., Henderson, M., & Lehman, A. (1993). Patterns of influence and response in abusing and nonabusing families. *Journal of Family Violence, 8*(1), 27–37.

Spiegel, D. (1986). Dissociative damage. *American Journal of Clinical Hypnosis, 29*(2), 123–131.

Spiegel, D. & Cardeña, E. (1991). Disintegrated experience: The dissociative disorders revisited. *Journal of Abnormal Psychology, 100*(3), 366–378.

Spitzer, R. L, Williams, J. B. W., Gibbon, M., & First, M. B. (1990). *SCID: User's guide for the structured clinical interview for DSM-III-R.* Washington, DC: American Psychiatric Press.

Steele, B. (1986). Notes on the lasting effects of early child abuse throughout the life cycle. *Child Abuse and Neglect, 11*, 371–383.

Straker, G., & Jacobson, R. S. (1981). Aggression, emotional maladjustment, and empathy in the abused child. *Developmental Psychology, 17*(6), 762–765.

Surrey, J., Swett, C., Michaels, A., & Levin, S. (1990). Reported history of physical and sexual abuse and severity of symptomatology in women psychiatric outpatients. *American Journal of Orthopsychiatry, 60*(3), 412–417.

Thorndike, R. L., Hagan, E. P., & Sattler, J. M. (1986). *Guide for administering and scoring, the Stanford–Binet Intelligence Scale* (4th ed.). Chicago: Riverside Publishing.

Toro, P. A. (1982). Developmental effects of child abuse: A review. *Child Abuse and Neglect, 6*, 423–431.

van der Kolk, B. A. & van der Hart, O. (1989). Pierre Janet and the breakdown of adaptation in psychological trauma. *American Journal of Psychiatry, 146*(12), 1530–1540.

Wechsler, D. (1967). *Manual for the Wechsler Preschool and Primary Scale of Intelligence.* San Antonio: The Psychological Corporation.

Wechsler, D. (1974). *Manual for the Wechsler Intelligence Scale for Children—Revised.* San Antonio: Psychological Corporation.

Wogan, M. (1987). *The Bliss Dissociation Scale.* Unpublished manuscript, Rutgers University, Camden, NJ.

Wolfe, D. A., & Jaffe, P. (1991). Child abuse and family violence as determinants of child psychopathology. *Canadian Journal of Behavioral Science, 23*(3), 282–299.

Wolfe, D. A., & Mosk, M. D. (1983). Behavioral comparisons of children from abused and distressed families. *Journal of Consulting and Clinical Psychology, 51*, 702–708.

Yufit, R. I., & Benzies, B. (1979). *Preliminary manual: Time Questionnaire: Assessing suicide potential.* Palo Alto, CA: Consulting Psychologists Press.

11

The Treatment of
Post-Traumatic Stress Disorder

Jose R. Maldonado
David Spiegel

Trauma constitutes a sudden discontinuity in both physical and mental experience, an unwelcome intrusion of external forces on our control of our bodies and environment. The effect of a natural disaster, assault, combat, or torture is to force the victim to reorganize mental and psychophysiological processes to initially buffer the immediate impact of the trauma. This process often represents an adaptive means of maintaining psychological control during a time of enormous stress. However, a substantial minority of trauma victims go on to suffer acute or chronic symptoms, such as dissociation, intrusive thoughts, anxiety, withdrawal, and hyperarousal, leading to a diagnosis of acute stress disorder or post-traumatic stress disorder (PTSD). In this chapter, we will define the phenomenology of these disorders, and review pharmacotherapeutic and psychotherapeutic treatments, with an emphasis on the use of hypnosis.

PHENOMENOLOGY OF ACUTE AND POST-TRAUMATIC STRESS DISORDERS

The stressors that can lead to the development of post-traumatic stress disorder and acute stress disorder are quite varied. In most instances, they involve some form of physical trauma (i.e., an accident) to self or a loved one, combat experience, natural and man-made disasters, and deliberate violence (i.e., rape, assault) (American Psychiatric Association, 1987, 1993. In the new edition of the *Diagnostic and Statistical Manual of Mental Disorders* (DSM-IV; American Psychiatric Association, 1994) the psychological impact of the stressor (Criterion A) is defined as involving "intense fear, helplessness or horror."

The diagnosis of Acute Stress Disorder was added to the DSM in its fourth edition because of the growth in literature documenting that there is a substantial prevalence of serious dissociative and anxiety symptoms in the month following trauma (Classen, Koopman, & Spiegel, 1993; Koopman, Classen, Spiegel, & Cardeña, 1994). This is too short a time for the individual to qualify for a diagnosis of PTSD. Trauma researchers investigating disasters such as the Hyatt Regency Skywalk collapse (Wilkinson, 1983), the Ash Wednesday bush fires (McFarlane, 1986, 1988), Israeli combat stress response (Solomon, Mikulincer, & Benbenishty, 1989), and the Loma Prieta earthquake (Cardeña & Spiegel, 1993) documented a substantial prevalence of acute symptomatology, including numbing, depersonalization, and amnesia.

Indeed, Solomon and colleagues (Solomon et al., 1989) found numbing to be the single best predictor of a later diagnosis of PTSD. Similarly, Koopman et al. (1994) found that a combination of acute dissociative and anxiety symptoms were significant predictors of PTSD 7 months later among victims of the Oakland–Berkeley fires. Weiss and colleagues found a similar connection between dissociation and later PTSD among rescue workers after the Loma Prieta earthquake (Weiss, Marmar, Metzler, & Ronfeldt, 1993).

Criterion A for the diagnosis of Acute Stress Disorder is basically the same as it is for PTSD; it requires the patient to have been exposed to a traumatic event in which he or she was confronted with actual or threatened death or serious injury. In addition, he or she must respond with intense fear, helplessness, or horror. The rest of the criteria for Acute Stress Disorder is slightly different. To receive the diagnosis, an individual must have 3 of 5 dissociative symptoms: amnesia, depersonalization, derealization, numbing, and lack of responsiveness. In addition, he or she must have at least one intrusive, avoidance, and hyperarousal symptom, occurring within 1 month of the trauma (American Psychiatric Association, 1994).

In contrast, DSM-IV diagnostic criteria for PTSD include three symptom categories, besides the initial stressor (Criterion A), and require that the symptoms last for over 1 month (American Psychiatric Association, 1987, 1994; Brett, Spitzer, & Williams, 1988).

The first category includes the reexperiencing of the traumatic event, which can occur in a variety of ways. The patient might experience recurrent and intrusive recollections in the form of thoughts or dreams that are perceived as distressing (Marshall, 1975; van der Kolk, Blitz, Burr, Sherry, & Hartmann, 1984; Ziarnowski & Broida, 1984); sudden episodes during which he or she acts or feels as if the events were recurring; or, finally, a sense of intense psychological distress when exposed to events that resemble or symbolize an aspect of the original trauma.

The second category includes a tendency to persistently avoid all stimuli associated with the trauma. It also includes the numbing of general responsiveness, or "psychic numbing." This can be seen in the form of conscious efforts to avoid thoughts, feelings, situations, or activities associated with the trauma; amnesia to important aspects of the trauma; diminished interest in significant activities; restricted range of affect; feelings of detachment from others; anhedonia; and a sense of a foreshortened future.

Finally, the third category includes the persistence of symptoms associated with an increased level of arousal. This is usually associated with recurrent nightmares, which are commonly accompanied by alterations in the sleep pattern (Greenberg, Pearlman, & Gampel, 1972; Horowitz, Wilner, Kaltreider, & Alvarez, 1980; Kramer, Schoen, & Kinnie, 1984; Lavie, Hefez, Halperin, & Enoch, 1979; Marshall, 1975; Ross, Ball, Sullivan, & Caroff, 1989; van der Kolk et al., 1984; Ziarnoswki & Broida, 1984) irritability; outbursts of anger; difficulty concentrating; a state of hypervigilance, which is often associated with the presence of an exaggerated startle response; and physiological reactivity when reexposed to situations that symbolize an aspect of the original trauma.

ETIOLOGICAL FACTORS

While severity of the traumatic stressor is a significant variable in the production of acute and chronic symptoms, not everyone exposed to trauma will develop these symptoms. Indeed, Keane and Fairbank (1983) reported that only about 25% of soldiers exposed to combat go on to develop PTSD. Therefore, there must be something else that renders certain individuals vulnerable to the disorder.

There are multiple factors that must also be considered besides the initial stressor. Indeed, the different premorbid factors must be analyzed independently since they may directly affect the treatment of the condition.

Social Factors

Given a specific event, the way it is handled by society as a whole will have a significant impact in terms of the intensity and degree to which it will affect the individual(s) involved. For example, a major man-made (e.g., a gas leak) or natural (e.g., floods) disaster that affects a large portion of the community and their social environment may impair emotional recovery more than a disaster that affects a smaller portion of the community, due to the fact demoralization will be more widespread and there will be a decreased availability of social support for the victims. On the other hand, a common community experience of stress may enhance social support for the victims, since there will be considerable mutual discussion about the event(s) and help in the immediate aftermath. Contrast this with the sense of isolation and shame that is often the lot of rape victims.

Societal attitudes can also exert a great influence on the way a trauma is perceived. For example, in the case of a hostage situation there will likely be public manifestations of sorrow, compassion, and support for the victim and his or her family. On the other hand, a woman victim of sexual assault is usually victimized even further by societal prejudice. The event tends to be kept secret, which decreases the possibility for the expression of emotions and the acquisition of support. Often such victims are considered "contaminated" by the assault, even when its occurrence is widespread, as in the case of the tragic mass rapes in the former Yugoslavia.

Finally, the media can play an important role in the case of trauma. On the one hand, media coverage can prolong and even deepen the effects of the trauma by providing unbidden reminders of the event. On the other hand, it may mobilize sympathy and public support.

Personal Factors

The stage of life in which the trauma occurs is an important factor in the amount and type of psychological damage it produces. The earlier in life the trauma occurs, the greater the chance that it will cause major psychic harm. This is due in part to the maturational level and the defense mechanisms and coping styles that the person has had an opportunity to develop prior to the occurrence of the trauma. This in turn will modulate the way in which the victim perceives the experience.

In particular, trauma suffered in childhood is more likely to influence cognitive development and self-organization. Children have difficulty understanding independent causation, and thus are even more inclined than adults to blame themselves for trauma inflicted upon them, leading to a pervasive sense of unworthiness, which might be labeled "survivor shame" rather than "survivor guilt." The victimization comes to seem justified rather than unwarranted, and anger that might appropriately be directed at abusive caretakers is instead directed at the self, resulting in various post-traumatic stress, dissociative, and depressive symptoms (Spiegel & Cardeña, 1991; Kluft, 1985, 1990).

Psychological Factors

Although a thorough discussion of psychological factors is beyond the scope of this chapter, some points are worth clarifying. As discussed above, the traumatic experience needs to be understood not only from the point of view of the type of stressor, but more importantly from the perspective of the victim's own reality. The impact conveyed by the traumatic stressor will depend on the way in which the victim interprets the experience, and his or her subsequent reaction to it.

More work needs to be done to elucidate the possible relationship between a patient's premorbid personality style and the type and degree of impairment generated by a traumatic stressor. Anecdotal evidence from our clinic suggests that characterological structure may correlate with factors such as type, duration, and severity of PTSD symptoms and the patient's ability to generate adaptive coping behaviors.

For example, a 59-year-old widowed female, diagnosed with Schizoid Personality Disorder (DSM-III-R), sought treatment for PTSD symptoms following an incident in which she was assaulted in her automobile. During treatment, it became evident that aspects of the patient's personality were influencing her adjustment to the trauma. For instance, the patient displayed the typical schizoid restricted range of emotional responsiveness. Her lack of adeptness at managing strong emotions, coupled with her fears of experiencing the physiological arousal associated with them, made it extremely difficult for her to address the persistent symptoms of increased arousal (e.g., insomnia, anger, irritability, and hypervigilance) that were generated by the assault. This characterological tendency to repress emotions caused her to initially delay seeking psychiatric care, which increased the severity of symptoms that she presented for treatment with and also lengthened the course of therapy.

Moreover, the patient's ability to generate other adaptive coping behaviors, such as seeking appropriate social support in the form of friends or community resources, was severely limited by her characteristic proclivity to withdraw from interpersonal contact in times of stress. Even in less stressful times the patient's style was to avoid confronting the vulnerability she felt in interpersonal contexts by avoiding them altogether.

Her tendency to retreat from both her emotions and interpersonal situations during times of stress seemed to be related to the development of a preponderance of phobic features after the trauma. More than any of the other symptoms usually associated to PTSD, phobic-like behaviors were a real problem for this woman. The patient engaged in frantic efforts to avoid thoughts, feelings, and situations reminiscent of the trauma. She was unable to drive or even sit in an automobile. Her fears of assault generalized to the point that she was afraid of going into her garage to do laundry due to fears of being attacked. In other words, her personality style seemed to be influencing the relative severity of psychological symptoms generated by the initial trauma.

Finally, the course of treatment was also influenced by the need to focus a great deal of attention on integrating her emotional and behavioral responses to the trauma with her identity. Since the patient's view of herself was based primarily on the notion that she was an "independent, emotionally and behaviorally controlled, respectable individual," she was particularly shaken by the emotional extremes she experienced and her inability to manage them on her own. The need to address these fundamental deficits in interpersonal functioning extended the duration of treatment and the expected natural course of the illness.

Biological Factors

When a person is subjected to a traumatic experience, his or her initial reaction to it will involve activating the sympathetic component of the autonomic nervous system. This will be displayed through both physical symptoms (e.g., tachycardia, hyperventilation, increased muscle tension, hyperactivity, sweating), as well as subjective experiences (e.g., anxiety, hypervigilance, increased startle response).

If patients suffering from PTSD are subjected to situations that symbolize the initial trauma, or in some cases even the recollection of the events, a number of physiological responses can be objectively measured. Among them are the changes in vital signs discussed above, as well as dramatic increases in peripheral measurements of autonomic function that are often used in biofeedback, such as baseline heart rates, systolic blood pressure, electroencephalographic (EEG) alpha rhythms, and electromyographic (EMG) readings (Blanchard, Kolb, Pallmeyer, & Gerardi, 1982; McFarlane, 1986, 1988; Solomon et al., 1989; Wilkinson, 1983).

Based on the above observations, a number of investigators have proposed several models that link the clinical symptoms of PTSD with hyperarousal of the central noradrenergic system (Friedman, 1988, 1991; Kosten & Krystal, 1988; Kosten, Giller, & Mason, 1988; Kosten, Mason, Giller, Ostroff, & Harkness, 1987). Since the locus coeruleus plays a central role in the production of arousal, anxiety, and panic, chemical manipulation of this system should play a role in the biological treatment of PTSD. Even the principle of "kindling" has been proposed as a way of explaining some of the clinical manifestations of PTSD (Friedman, 1988, 1991; van der Kolk, 1983). Kindling refers to increased behavioral and electrophysiological responsivity to repeated intermittent low level electrical stimulation of the brain. Because of this, antikindling anticonvulsants (e.g., carbamazepine, valproate) have been proposed for the treatment of the condition (Fesler, 1991; Lipper, 1988).

Alterations in sleep patterns and the quality of dreams are common symptoms of PTSD. Most patients exhibit difficulty initiating and maintaining sleep. Some of the changes reported in the sleep architecture include increased Stages 1 and 2 sleep, decreased delta (deep) sleep, decreased REM latency, and an increased percentage of REM sleep (Friedman, 1991; Ross et al., 1989).

The qualitative changes in dreams are equally important. Disturbed dreaming is a common and prominent abnormality seen with PTSD. What is particularly interesting is that the traumatic dreams experienced by trauma victims occur during either REM and non-REM (NREM) sleep (Kramer et al., 1984; Ross et al., 1989; van der Kolk et al., 1984; Ziarnowski & Broida, 1984). These nightmares are unique to PTSD patients because they are neither anxiety attacks ocurring during REM sleep, nor NREM night terrors (Kramer, 1979; Kramer & Kinney, 1988; Ross et al., 1989). Hence, PTSD might involve either an inappropriate recruitment of essentially normal REM sleep processes or a coming into play of inherently dysfunctional REM sleep mechanisms (Ross et al., 1989). Whichever the case, it is not unusual to find patients who are experiencing active dreaming accompanied by gross body movements, instead of the usual atonia that normally accompanies REM sleep dreaming.

Most authors argue that the dreams of PTSD patients are replicative in quality, meaning that they are exact replicas or "instant replays" of the actual events or trauma (Friedman, 1991; Kinzie, 1991). The patients usually report awakening from a distressing dream that contains images associated with the initial trauma, as well as strong emotions in congruence with the original event. These authors postulate that those dreams that most closely resemble exact memories of the incident tend to correlate with a definite and more severe diagnosis of PTSD (Hartmann, 1984; Ross et al., 1989).

In our experience, some of the dreams may not be so obvious in content. In many instances, patients will report having had "disturbing dreams" that they cannot remember. Sometimes they only know about the presence of these nightmares through accounts from their bed partners, who are awakened in the middle of the night by the patients' screams and body movements. When awakened, many of these patients will have no clear recollection of the nightmares. Or, it may be that such patients can remember that their nightmares have a recurrent theme (e.g., being chased or followed) but they cannot recall the specific details of the dreams. These dreams represent the door to repressed traumatic memories for which the patient in question has no conscious recollection.

For example, one of Maldonado's patients, a 24-year-old, married woman, used to report a repetitive theme from her nightmares. In them, she saw herself as a child, playing on her living room or bedroom floor. After a while, a man came into the room and attempted to attack her. Initially, she was able to escape, but after a while he caught up. She remembered running through a complicated labyrinth of hallways, doors, and windows. On many occasions, the windows had bars on them or there was a brick wall waiting for her once the door opened. In either case, there was no escape. Finally, the attacker would grab her. She then felt like she was floating, and suddenly, while looking down, she witnessed him either shooting or stabbing her to death. At that point, her "soul" would float over the man and her own dead body. She then woke up in a panic. It is notable that at the time she reported the dream she had no recollection of physical or sexual abuse. Later, during the course of therapy, the meaning of her nightmares became more clear as memories of sexual abuse by a paternal uncle emerged.

Multiple neuroendocrinological changes have also been noted in the victims of PTSD (Friedman, 1991; Kosten et al., 1987, 1988). As a result of the initial traumatic experience (both psychological and physical), the body generates high amounts of endogenous opioid peptides, resulting in the reduction of physical pain, aggression, and anxiety. Upon reexposure to stimuli or events that recall the initial trauma, the body responds with a similar burst of endogenous opioid peptides, which provide the patient with an artificial sense of calmness (Friedman, 1991; Kinzie, 1991).

Similarly, Kosten and Krystal (1988) described the alterations in the endogenous opioid system as a state of chronic deficiency resulting from excessive sympathetic arousal. The rationale is that, as described above, PTSD is associated with increased central noradrenergic activity. In turn, high levels of norepinephrine will inhibit the release of corticotropin-releasing hormone (CRH; Price, Charney, Rubin, & Heninger, 1986). Therefore, Kosten and Krystal (1988) postulate that the abnormally high levels of norepinephrine found in patients suffering of PTSD may cause inhibition of the entire hypothalamic–pituitary–adrenocortical axis (HPA), which will produce a state of endogenous opioid deficiency. This view might explain clinical reports of lowered pain thresholds in PTSD patients (Perry, Cella, Falkenberg, Heidrich, & Goodwin, 1987), as well as provide a possible explanation for the prevalence of chronic pain in the PTSD population (Benedikt & Kolb, 1986).

The above changes may possibly represent the biological basis for the phenomenon known as "repetition compulsion," in which victims repeatedly seek out situations that remind them of the trauma. Every reexposure to the trauma will trigger the production and liberation of endogenous opioids. To some extent the numbing of responsiveness and stress-induced analgesia observed in PTSD may be related to elevated endogenous opiate secretion in response to a situation that resembles the initial trauma, and the repetition of exposure to traumatic circumstances may be an attempt to overcome this state of chronic adrenergic hyperarousal.

If the above theory is indeed correct, these patients may be experiencing the symptoms of opioid withdrawal every time the reminding stimulus is stopped and the opioid levels are reduced. Unfortunately, the symptoms of opioid withdrawal are strikingly similar to those of the acute reaction phase of PTSD (i.e., anxiety, startle response, tachycardia, irritability, insomnia, and hyperalertness). We will return to the significance of these findings when we discuss the use of alpha-adrenergic agonists in the treatment of PTSD.

COMORBIDITY

In considering a particular treatment strategy, one must also consider possible comorbid conditions since they will have a direct impact on the patient's response to treatment. Several studies have shown the high prevalence (up to 80%) of at least a second concurrent psychiatric diagnosis (Keane & Wolfe, 1990; Kinzie, 1991; Solomon, Gerrity, & Muff, 1992).

A concomitant episode of major depression is an important Axis I diagnosis to keep in mind. There is a great overlap between the symptoms of these two diagnoses. DSM-IV allows for the dual diagnosis of an affective disorder, with PTSD if the patient fits the criteria for both (American Psychiatric Association, 1994). Indeed, Kling and colleagues have hypothesized that depression represents a state of chronic neuro-endocrine arousal (Kling et al., 1989). The vegetative symptoms, especially loss of appetite and sleep, are consistent with the adaptive pattern of acute stress response arousal and inhibition of digestion made chronic and maladaptive.

Victims of intense trauma may also develop another anxiety disorder concomitant with or subsequent to the development of PTSD. Again, DSM-IV allows for the concurrent diagnosis of either Generalized Anxiety Disorder or a phobic disorder, if the patient was to meet the diagnostic criteria for both (American Psychiatric Association, 1994).

A concomitant Axis I diagnosis of alcohol or drug abuse is also not uncommon. The abuse of alcohol or illegal substances may be a way of self-medicating (Branchey, Davis, & Lieber, 1984; Jelinek & Williams, 1984; Kosten & Krystal, 1988; Sapol & Roffman, 1969; Schnitt & Nocks, 1984; Wedding, 1987). It is also important to consider the possibility of abuse of the medication used to treat the primary diagnosis. Whenever there is physical trauma, especially if accompanied by head injury, the possibility of an organic mental disorder, such as Organic Anxiety Disorder or Organic Personality Disorder should also be considered.

Finally, the presence of a concomitant dissociative disorder should be considered. As we will describe later in this chapter, and as already expressed by other authors, chronic exposure to trauma can lead not only to anxiety disorders like PTSD, but to dissociative disorders such as Dissociative Identity Disorder (DID; referred to as Multiple Personality Disorder [MPD] in DSM-III-R) (Coons, Bowman, & Pellow, 1989; Kluft, 1984; Spiegel, 1984, 1986; Spiegel & Cardeña, 1991). It is very uncommon to see a patient suffering from DID who has not been exposed to intense trauma, usually physical (or sexual) abuse, to the point of also fulfilling the Criterion A (DSM-IV) for the diagnosis of PTSD (American Psychiatric Association, 1994).

As with any other diagnostic population we must consider that there may be considerable secondary gain to the patient in the form of both financial and legal benefits, following the diagnosis of PTSD. Therefore, we must always consider in the differential diagnosis the possibility of a Factitious Disorder or Malingering (American Psychiatric Association, 1994), since the presence of either will have a major impact on the patient's treatment (Lynn & Belza, 1984).

TREATMENT OPTIONS

Pharmacotherapy

The diagnosis of PTSD was introduced in the DSM-III in 1980. By 1984, there were many articles suggesting a number of different psychopharmacological approaches to treating the disorder, with most of them based on either case reports or open trials. No systematically controlled studies had been undertaken. All of them operated according to the premise that in order for a drug to be of benefit in the treatment of PTSD it must somehow dampen the excessive activity of the noradrenergic system centrally. However, control of all of the symptoms of PTSD was also desired.

In order for a drug to effectively treat PTSD, it must perform an extraordinary number of functions. It must balance the dysregulation of the sympathetic nervous system, regulate the sleep pattern, and diminish the presence of disturbing nightmares. It must stop recurrent and intrusive thoughts, as well as flashbacks. It should be able to improve interpersonal problems associated with PTSD such as psychic numbing, decreased interest in other people and activities, avoidance, and the sense of detachment so frequently encountered in this population. It should facilitate the recovery and integration of memories. It should have antidepressant as well as anti-anxiety properties, and, putatively, antikindling ones as well.

The above is a tall order, and no definitive pharmacological treatment has been discovered to fulfill it. A controlled study was not published until 1988. To date, only five controlled, double-blind drug therapy trials have been reported (Kudler, Davidson, Stein, & Erickson, 1989; Solomon et al., 1992). Four of them included antidepressants (Davidson et al., 1990; Frank, Kosten, Giller, & Dan, 1988; Reist, Kauffman, & Haier, 1976; Shestatzky, Greenberg, & Lerer, 1988), while the fifth involved the benzodiazepine alprazolam (Braun, Greenberg, Dasberg, & Lerer, 1990). A full discussion is beyond the scope of this chapter and has already been published elsewhere (Braun et al., 1990; Davidson et al., 1990; Friedman, 1988, 1991; Frank et al., 1988; Kinzie, 1991; Kitchner & Greenstein, 1985; Kolb, Burris, & Griffiths, 1984; McFarlane, 1986, 1988; Reist et al., 1976; Shestatzkzy et al., 1988; Solomon et al., 1992; van der Kolk, 1983, 1987), but we will summarize the findings here.

Antidepressant medications were found to be somewhat helpful in treating the intrusive symptoms associated with PTSD (i.e., nightmares, flashbacks), but they did little for the avoidance symptoms (Friedman, 1991). Antidepressants were also found to be effective in treating some of the depressive symptoms, such as insomnia and nightmares, and some of the anxiety associated with these phenomena probably because of their sedative effect (Kudler et al., 1989; Solomon et al., 1992). On the other hand, benzodiazepines were found to be effective only in the reduction of anxiety symptoms, with little, if any, effect on the avoidant or intrusive symptoms (Braun et al., 1990; Solomon et al., 1992).

Other medications have also been proposed. The rationale behind using them has mostly been anecdotal in nature, as there have been no controlled trials that prove their efficacy. The anticonvulsant medication carbamazepine has been proposed due to its antikindling effects (Fesler, 1991; Friedman, 1988, 1991; Lipper, 1988). Lithium has also been used to lessen the negative affective components of PTSD, as well as to control aggression (Kitchner & Greenstein, 1985). Beta-blockers (e.g., propranolol) and alpha-adrenergic agonists (e.g., clonidine) have been used with some success in open trials, supporting the notion of noradrenergic hyperactivity in PTSD (Kolb et al., 1984; Kosten et al., 1987, 1988). Beta-adrenergic blockers antagonize the peripheral sympathetic hyperarousal that results from anxiety and some of the other symptoms of PTSD. The alpha-adrenergic agonists reduce central adrenergic activity. The advantage offered by these two classes of medication is that because they are not primarily CNS depressants, they do not foster the addiction or chemical dependence associated with benzodiazepines.

At this point, there is little reason to expect medications to provide definitive treatment for PTSD, although they can be helpful adjuvants to other treatment modalities. The specific choice of medication should then be directed toward target symptoms that impair the patient's ability to participate in other treatment modalities.

Psychotherapy

As with pharmacotherapy, almost every kind of psychotherapy has been applied to this diagnostic problem.

Behavioral Therapy

The behavioral therapies are probably the most studied of all the psychotherapeutic approaches (Solomon et al., 1992; Wolpe, 1973). Most of these include either relaxation techniques (Bernstein & Borkovec, 1973; Jacobson, 1938), systematic desensitization, biofeedback (Peniston, 1986), implosion (flooding) (Cooper & Clum, 1989; Keane, Fairbank, Caddell, & Zimering, 1989; Pitman et al., 1991), or direct therapeutic exposure (DTE; Boudewyns & Hyer, 1990). Overall it appears that all of these techniques are superior to no treatment. The improvement produced by behavioral techniques has been more noticeable in symptoms related to depression, anxiety, fear, and the intrusive symptoms of PTSD. The techniques produce little or no improvement in the symptoms related to avoidance behavior and emotional numbing. Of them all, flooding has been found to be the most effective for anxiety symptoms (Cooper & Clum, 1989; Keane et al., 1989; Pitman et al., 1991). Unfortunately, flooding also has the highest rate of complications, namely the exacerbation of depression, relapse of alcoholic behavior, and precipitation of panic episodes (Pitman et al., 1991).

Cognitive Therapy

Because the symptoms of PTSD are so frequently associated with depression (i.e., sadness, anger, low self-esteem, shame, and guilt), it makes sense to consider other treatment modalities instead of, or as an adjuvant to, behavioral techniques. Stress-inoculation training (SIT) is the only form of cognitive therapy that has been studied in a controlled fashion for the treatment of PTSD (Foa, Steketee, & Rothbaum, 1989; Meichenbaum, 1974; Solomon et al., 1992). This technique actually consists of a combination of a number of techniques, wherein behavioral approaches are integrated with cognitive restructuring.

The only study published thus far that addresses the use of various treatment modalities compared SIT to flooding (Frank et al., 1988; Solomon et al., 1992). It showed that both are superior to supportive counseling or no treatment. Patients in the SIT group showed greater improvement in the acute posttreatment period, but in long-term (3 months) follow-up the patients treated with flooding did better.

Group Therapy

This treatment modality is used as an adjuvant to either behavioral therapy or psychoanalytically oriented psychotherapy. It is commonly used in the Veteran's Administration (VA) system, but probably not so commonly in other therapy settings. The benefits include providing a structure of support and stability for these patients. Also, it may help to promote socialization, therefore helping to decrease the intensity of the avoidant symptoms. It is recommended for patients suffering from chronic PTSD.

Psychoanalytically Oriented Psychotherapy and Hypnosis

Any psychotherapeutic approach to PTSD must be directed at helping the victim acknowledge and bear the extent of the psychic damage caused by the trauma and then to develop adequate coping mechanisms so that it can be put into perspective. The goal is, therefore, to allow the patient to adapt to a new life that includes memories of the traumatic experience, worked through in a way that they interfere as little as possible with his or her daily living activities.

Unfortunately, the effects of most traumatic experiences are not simple to deal with. Overwhelming trauma, such as that resulting from assault, sexual abuse, and natural disasters, disrupts many aspects of the victim's life; for example, one's sense of control over one's body and actions; one's sense of security; and the predictability of the future. In effect, the traumatic experience makes the victim feel like an object of the perpetrator's rage, or of nature's indifference (Spiegel & Cardeña, 1990).

Defense mechanisms play a special role in the management of reactions to overwhelming trauma. While Freud described defenses as mechanisms that serve to ward off unacceptable wishes (Freud, 1946), the psychiatric literature contains reports that describe the use of defenses such as dissociation to help people cope with traumatic events as they are occurring (Spiegel, 1986, 1988, 1990; Spiegel, Hunt, & Dondershine, 1988; van der Kolk & van der Hart, 1989). Recent reports suggest that major stress and trauma are common antecedents of dissociative phenomena, including some of the symptoms observed in PTSD victims (Cardeña & Spiegel, 1993; Classen et al., 1993; Coons et al., 1989; Keane & Wolfe, 1990; McFarlane, 1986, 1988; Solomon et al., 1989; Spiegel, 1984, 1986, 1990; Wilkinson, 1983; van der Kolk & van der Hart, 1989). Let us focus first on the use of defenses like dissociation for protection against traumatic experiences as they are occurring.

The phenomenon of dissociation has been previously reported as a response to traumatic events (Coons et al., 1989; Freud, 1946; Kihlstrom, 1984, 1990; Kluft, 1985, 1990, 1991; Nash & Lynn, 1986; Spiegel, 1984, 1988; Spiegel & Cardeña, 1990, 1991; Spiegel & Fink, 1979; Spiegel & Spiegel, 1987; Spiegel et al., 1988). It is not uncommon for individuals undergoing severe stress (e.g., rape, assault) to report the occurrence of spontaneous dissociative experiences at the time of the trauma. These experiences take the form of depersonalization (e.g., "out-of-body experiences"), derealization (feeling as if one is "in a dream"), difficulty concentrating, or amnesia. This memory loss may be for part, or all of the traumatic experience, and may develop gradually over the days and weeks after the trauma.

Dissociation, then, can be seen as serving a dual purpose. Dissociative states can be viewed as efforts to preserve some form of control, comfort, safety, and identity when faced with overwhelming stress. They give the victim a false sense of control and relief from the experience, so that it is as if the event is not happening and, later, as if it had never happened. In short, victims use dissociative states in an attempt to separate themselves from the full impact of the trauma.

Unfortunately, such victims pay a high price for their behavior. They are unable to work through, in a conscious way, the meaning of the stressful event and to put into perspective the facts surrounding the traumatic experience. This adds to the trauma by creating more anxiety. The dissociated feelings of fear and shame can leak into the conscious mind without the associated memories, and thereby create a state of panic since the patient feels that the content of these memories is so terrible it cannot be faced. Eventually, many trauma victims with PTSD isolate themselves from others based on the shame they feel in relation to the trauma. Furthermore, they become unable to enjoy personal pleasure or intimate relationships, because of a numbing of feelings.

Trauma victims often come to feel as if they were to start with the object that the trauma temporarily made them into. For example, they believe they were somehow deserving of the assailant's rage. Research on the phenomenon of state-dependent memory (Bower, 1981) shows that memory retrieval is associated with activating the affect that was linked with the memory as it was stored. Thus, when memories of a traumatic experience are elicited, the painful affect associated with them will also be reactivated. If the individual wants to keep the painful affects associated with a traumatic experience out of awareness, he must also keep the associated cognitions out of consciousness. In order to do so, the person may treat these memories as if they belong to someone else (e.g., "not mine" = dissociation) or as if the event had never occurred (e.g., "not to me" = amnesia). For trauma victims, dissociation is a useful defense, since it allows for a discontinuity of mental processes that would ordinarily be integrated in consciousness (Hilgard, 1977; Spiegel & Cardeña, 1991).

While dissociated memories may be out of conscious awareness, this does not prevent them from affecting mood, behavior, and cognitive processes. Indeed, recent experimental data (Kihlstrom, 1984, 1990) suggest that dissociated information does affect current life events.

For example, one of Maldonado's patients, a 52-year-old married woman, was sexually abused by her father between the ages of 2 and 6. At the time when she presented for therapy, due to feelings of depression and marital problems, she had no recollection of the abuse. Even though she was "able to completely dissociate" the memories of the incest from consciousness, she did report that her behavior was subsequently affected indicating not only that everything had not been completely forgotten, but that somehow the knowledge she had subsequently influenced her behavior. She continued to "love" her father, indeed, she was able to talk about how he taught her to appreciate opera, classical music, and ballet. She felt a high regard for him, too, but also remembered always "feeling funny when I was around him, especially when he hugged me." Sometimes, she described this as "the silly feeling of fear of being in his presence, or being touched by him," even though she could not recall why she felt this way. Probably even more remarkable was the fact that the patient always felt "as if my mother never loved me. She was never cruel or anything, but I always have had a very resentful feeling toward her." This patient eventually dissociated in her therapist's office while discussing a recurring dream. She spontaneously regressed to the age of 7 and remained in that state for 12 days. She was admitted to the inpatient unit in which we used hypnosis to elucidate the memories that triggered the dissociation. Under hypnosis, we discovered that she had not only been sexually molested by her father, but that her mother had known all along. She actually described how "mom used to dress me up for him."

Why Use Hypnosis?

It is our experience that some trauma victims may accidentally learn how to use hypnotic-like techniques in order to avoid the full impact of a traumatic experience.

A patient seen by Maldonado was sexually abused as a child by a neighbor. The abuse took place over a number of years, during which time her imagination was her only source of help or escape. As a child the patient was actually able to enter a self-hypnotic trance and mentally transport herself to a beautiful and tranquil spot in a meadow. In this trance, she would entertain herself with scenes in which she played on the grass, ran after butterflies, and picked up flowers by a nearby pond, while her body was being brutally violated. As an adult the patient continued this once useful, but now pathological use of dissociative behavior. Not knowing what she was doing, but knowing it would prevent further suffering, she would induce a self-hypnotic/dissociated state whenever an emotionally charged experience elicited feelings that resembled those she experienced during the initial trauma.

Exposure to stressful events may be one of the paths that naturally leads toward the development of high hypnotizability. This idea is supported by reports of a positive correlation between severity of punishment during childhood and hypnotizability (Nash & Lynn, 1986; Spiegel & Cardeña,

1991). It is conceivable that the impact of the stress suffered by the victim of early physical or sexual abuse encourages a more effective use of self-hypnosis. Spiegel and Spiegel (1987) have reported that young children are more highly hypnotizable than adults, with a peak in hypnotic capacity around age 12 and a moderate decline thereafter. The need for and frequent use of self-hypnosis (whether conscious or not) due to repeated exposure to abuse may prevent its extinction later in life (as normally happens during late adolescence in many individuals [Morgan & Hilgard, 1973]), which accounts in part, for the high level of hypnotizability seen in adults who were once victims of abuse (Kluft, 1984, 1992; Spiegel, Detrick, & Frischholz, 1982).

Hypnosis can be defined as a psychophysiological state of aroused, attentive, and receptive focal concentration, with a corresponding relative suspension of (or diminution in) peripheral awareness (Spiegel & Spiegel, 1987). The phenomenon known as hypnosis can be conceptualized as having three main components: absorption, dissociation, and suggestibility (Spiegel, 1990). Absorption refers to the tendency to engage in self-altering and highly focused attention (Tellegen & Atkinson, 1974). Dissociation can be considered complementary to absorption (Spiegel, 1990), which allows us to carry on more than one complex task or action simultaneously (e.g., driving a car while holding a conversation). Suggestibility can be defined as a heightened responsiveness to social cues. Hypnotized individuals are not deprived of their will but rather are less likely to judge instructions critically and therefore more likely to act upon them (Spiegel & Cardeña, 1990).

These components of hypnotic phenomena are similar to the major categories of PTSD symptoms in DSM-IV (American Psychiatric Association, 1994). There is a resemblance between absorption and the intrusive reliving of traumatic events. When doing so, trauma victims become so absorbed in the memories of the trauma they lose touch with their present surroundings and even forget that the events took place in the past. One can observe an almost identical effect when hypnotized individuals, while intensely absorbed in the hypnotic trance, are able to reenact previous life events using hypnotic age regression.

Individuals experiencing trance phenomena may be able to completely separate from or dissociate an emotion or a somatic sensation. Some subjects can achieve this to the extent that they do not recognize a body part as belonging to their own body, or they remember an emotionally charged event with no emotions attached. Similarly, PTSD patients experience so-called "psychic numbing." By virtue of this mechanism, some individuals are able to isolate or disconnect relevant affect from their current experience. In this way, they can prevent feelings in the present from triggering past memories. Unfortunately, as they separate feelings from actions, they also dissociate relevant affect in the present, resulting in the loss of enjoyment and interest in previously pleasurable activities.

Finally, the principle of suggestibility is comparable to hyperarousal, the heightened sensitivity to environmental cues observed in those patients suffering from PTSD. Just as hypnotized individuals may "become drunk" after the suggestion that they have consumed several glasses of wine, so the PTSD patient acts as if he were back in combat after hearing the sound of a helicopter.

Patients with PTSD tend to experience a polarization, wherein they alternate between the intense, vivid, and painful memories and images associated with a traumatic event and a kind of artificial normality in which these painful experiences are avoided by a dissociative process that might have begun at the time of the trauma itself. There is ample evidence linking the dissociative processes of PTSD to hypnotic responsiveness. Several papers have reported that Vietnam veterans who score high in PTSD symptomatology also have higher scores on a number of hypnotic scales (Spiegel, 1988; Spiegel et al., 1988; Stuntman & Bliss, 1985).

Because many patients suffering from PTSD are highly hypnotizable and because of the remarkable resemblance between the symptoms of the disorder and hypnotic phenomena, it makes sense to study the usefulness of hypnosis in the treatment of PTSD.

Hypnosis as a Treatment Tool in Psychotherapy

Several principles provide guidance as to the use of hypnosis in psychotherapy. The first is that all hypnosis is self-hypnosis. The psychotherapist using hypnosis acts as a guide to patients, seeking to help them use their own capacity to undergo trances. The second principle is that there is nothing you can do with hypnosis that you can not do without it. It is a state of heightened concentration and focused attention that may facilitate and speed treatment, but it is not in and of itself a therapy. Thirdly, it is very likely that patients suffering from PTSD are highly hypnotizable (Kluft, 1984; Spiegel, 1988, 1989; Spiegel et al., 1982, 1988; Stuntman & Bliss, 1985).

If indeed patients suffering from PTSD are unknowingly using their own hypnotic capacities (Kluft, 1991, 1992; Spiegel, 1986, 1989; Spiegel et al., 1988), it makes sense to teach them, during the course of psychotherapy, how to enter, access, and control their trance potential. Hypnosis then becomes a tool to access previously dissociated material. It is the spontaneous mobilization of these dissociative mechanisms at the time of trauma that makes the use of hypnosis especially relevant in the treatment of PTSD.

The purpose of hypnotic techniques is not simply to help the patient remember the trauma. The old concept of abreaction has proven to be insufficient. In a way, what the patient goes through with each flashback is an uncontrolled abreaction. Indeed, some authors (Kluft, 1992, 1993; Spiegel, 1981) state that when abreaction is not done within the context of cognitive restructuring and before new defenses are in place it can lead to the further retraumatization of the patient. Therefore, hypnosis should be used in the course of psychotherapy to facilitate the controlled remembering of traumatic memories.

Since a hypnotic-like state is elicited spontaneously during traumatic experiences, it makes sense that the very entry into this same state may well lead to a retrieval of memories and affects associated with the original trauma (state-dependent memory theory; see Bower, 1981). This means that the transition into the hypnotic trance alone can facilitate access to memories related to a dissociated state, as might have happened at the time of the trauma. One should keep in mind that hypnosis is in itself a controlled form of dissociation. Hence, the hypnotic process may increase the likelihood of retrieving strong emotional reactions and previously unavailable memories associated with the trauma.

Many patients fear that if they allow memories associated with the trauma to surface, they will loose control over their lives once more. This is partly due to the fact that they have a difficult time separating themselves from their memories. It is the therapist's role to help the patient by structuring the retrieval and expression of these painful memories and feelings associated with them.

By means of hypnotic techniques, patients can slowly remember pieces of the traumatic experience at a pace they can tolerate. To achieve this, they are taught to enter a relaxing, peaceful state. This can easily be achieved by imagining oneself physically floating. Images of floating in a hot tub, a river, a pool, or any other scene that they associate with physical relaxation can be used. Patients are instructed to maintain this image even when they are facing emotionally charged traumatic memories. Each new bit of information can then be processed within the context of therapy.

Another technique consists of having patients project images or thoughts onto an imaginary screen. This activity facilitates the process of separating the memories ("facts") from the physically painful sensations (in order to minimize retraumatization). Then they are requested to divide the screen in half. The condensed image of the trauma is pushed to the left. On the right, they try to picture something they did in order to protect themselves. This might have been something like fighting back, screaming, or just lying still in order to avoid further abuse.

The above process causes the memory of the trauma to become more bearable since the patients can see the part of themselves that attempted to provide protection, maintain dignity, or protect others. Thus, the two images serve to restructure the memory of the trauma. The images on the right help patients to realize that while they were indeed victimized, they were also attempting to master the situation, and displayed courage or compassion in the process. These images also encourage them to realize that the humiliation of the trauma is only one aspect of the experience.

Another technique is age regression. With this technique, patients can be helped to recall dissociated memories. Also, it allows for the recovery of long-forgotten memories such as what he or she did, as a child, in order to survive; the paralyzing fear that did not allow for flight; the awful feeling that if he or she were not "to do as told something horrible would happen"; or being told by the perpetrator that their parents would not believe them, or would punish them further if they were to tell the truth.

The acquisition of this knowledge allows the patient to reassess the situation both from the point of view at the time (i.e., when he or she was a child) and from his or her current perspective (i.e., distanced from the threat, with more information and more control). In most cases, this knowledge helps patients to see themselves in a new light. Before acquiring it, patients frequently blame themselves for not having done something differently, for "allowing" the trauma to happen, or even for provoking it. After these memories have been retrieved through the use of hypnosis and the facts analyzed from a different perspective, patients realize that they actually did the best they could under the circumstances and with the knowledge they had.

Following this stage of memory retrieval and understanding, trauma patients can be guided through an exercise in which they can allow themselves to accept the victimized self. They can learn to acknowledge and even thank themselves for what they did as a child in order to survive—thus changing their self-image from that of a victim to that of a survivor. Then, through the use of hypnotic imagery, a scene in which the patient joins the "victimized" memory with the current perception of self may be facilitated. Thus, the intense concentration of the hypnotic state may serve to reverse the fragmentation of the mind that was elicited by the trauma. Teaching patients that they can control the access and retrieval of traumatic memories, and then later reconsolidate themselves from a new point of view will give them an enhanced sense of control. It also provides them with a therapeutic method for managing the memories.

In many instances, patients can learn that the intrusive memories and other bodily symptoms (commonly present in PTSD) are the way the unconscious attempts to communicate and express painful and overwhelming memories. They can also learn that if they are able to find a controlled method (i.e., self-hypnosis) to access the memories, the frequency of their spontaneous intrusion will often decrease.

Hypnosis involves a suspension of critical judgment, and therefore a state of heightened suggestibility, or responsivity, to social cues. Because of the memories can be created during this state, it is important that the interview be conducted with a minimum of inserted information, and that open-ended questions are used such as, "What happens next?" rather than "How did he sexually abuse you?" Also, the use of hypnosis may compromise a witness's ability to testify in court. Hence, legal ramifications should be explored before hypnosis is used in the elicitation of memories (Scheflin & Shapiro, 1989).

Hypnosis Applied

The use of self-hypnosis as an adjuvant to psychotherapy in the treatment of PTSD can be summarized as having two major goals, that can be achieved by the use of six different techniques (adapted from Spiegel, 1992).

The goals are to *bring into conscious awareness* previously repressed memories and to *develop a sense of congruence* between past memories and current self-images. Bringing previously repressed memories into consciousness gives the patient the opportunity to understand, accept, and restructure them. And if congruence is achieved among the content and feelings associated with the trauma and the patients' ongoing feelings and views of self, there will no longer be a need to dissociate memories. In short, "there will no longer be a need for secrets." The result is a diminution of symptoms (i.e., flashbacks, intrusive recollections, nightmares, anxiety) that were initially associated to the threat posed by the presence of traumatic memories.

The above goals can be achieved by the use of six different techniques or treatment stages: confrontation, condensation, confession, consolation, concentration, and control. The patient must first *confront the trauma*. The therapist's role is to help the patient recognize that there were important factors in the development of the symptoms for which he or she now seeks help. It is important to keep in mind that the patients may have been told on many occasions, "forget it . . . it is all in the past . . . there is nothing you can do about it, just let go of it. . . ." Comments like these only add to the guilt and the sense that there must be something wrong with oneself. Hence, these should be eliminated.

Hypnosis becomes extremely helpful in the process of *condensation* of the traumatic experience. This is done when the patient defines a particularly frightening segment during the revisiting of traumatic memories that summarizes (i.e., condenses) a series of conflicts with which the patient is struggling. As mentioned before, the intense focus of the hypnotic state can be used to place boundaries around traumatic memories and restructure them. A woman who was forced to have oral sex at age 12 by a drunken stepfather recalled in hypnosis that she "gagged and threw up all over him. He threw me against a wall, but I spoiled his fun." She was thus able to compare her traumatic memory with her recognition that she had foiled his efforts to further abuse her.

After condensing the traumatic material the patient usually feels the need to *confess* the feelings and/or experiences that he or she is profoundly ashamed of and that he or she may have told no one else of before. During this stage, the therapist's task is to dispel all judgments that the patient attributes to the actions he or she is able to recall. These are usually cognitions that the patient has integrated from external sources (e.g., parents, church). This confession of shameful memories is no easy task and requires the "presence" of the therapist. At this point, the task of *consolation* takes place. During this stage, it is extremely important that the therapist be emotionally available to the patient and console him or her in a professionally appropriate manner.

A note of warning is in order at this time. The presence and strength of transference during the psychotherapy of trauma victims is enormous, and the use of hypnosis does not prevent the development of a transference reaction. Indeed, it actually may facilitate its emergence earlier than in regular therapy due to the intensity with which the material is expressed and the memories are recovered. The kind of transference elicited during the psychotherapy of trauma victims is different in the sense that the feelings that are being transferred are not so much related to early object relationships as to the abuser or circumstances associated with the trauma (Spiegel, 1992).

Hypnosis allows the patient to turn on the memories during the psychotherapeutic session, and then shut them off once the work has been done. This promotes *concentration* on a desired goal, under the guidance of the therapist. A common fear of the trauma patient is that if he or she allows him or herself to remember, the memories will take over and he or she will be rendered defenseless once more. Using the structured experience of the hypnotic trance, the patient learns that rather than not think about the trauma, he or she can learn how to think about it in a constructive fashion.

Finally, *control* must be given back to the patient. The core conflict of the trauma experience lies in the patient's sense of helplessness and loss of physical and emotional control. Hence, it is critical that the therapist guide the therapeutic interaction in such a way that the patient's sense of control over his or her memories is enhanced. Since all hypnosis is self-hypnosis, it can be usefully employed by the patient to master his or her past experiences, as well as current symptoms (e.g., flashbacks, anxiety, nightmares). The therapist should convey to the patient the sense he or she has self-control by not "pushing him or her to remember," but rather by instructing the patient to "remember as much as can safely be remembered now."

The therapist should also reinforce the notion that hypnosis is a collaborative enterprise, not something done to a patient by a therapist. Indeed, the metaphor of the athlete and the coach often comes in handy: The coach (therapist) may design a strategy and suggest alternatives, but eventually it is up to the athlete (patient) to implement them and, even more, to decide when it is appropriate to use them. Of equal importance, the patient must not only learn how to be independent, but also to know when to call for help.

SUMMARY

The phenomenon known as post-traumatic stress disorder is a very complicated one. In studying its etiology, one must consider social, personal, biological, and psychological factors. Multiple biological and psychotherapeutic approaches have been studied, which have all been found to have variable impact on the condition. In this chapter, we have acknowledged the contribution and value of treatment modalities such as pharmacotherapy, behavioral and group therapy, and psychoanalytically oriented psychotherapy.

The challenge in treating victims of overwhelming trauma is to help them achieve a new sense of unity within themselves after the initial fragmentation caused by the traumatic experience. The trauma itself tends to cause sudden and radical discontinuities in consciousness, due to the nature of the assault itself. This leaves victims with a polarized view of themselves, involving, on the one hand, the old self (prior to the trauma) and, on the other, the helpless, defenseless, soiled victim.

The goal of therapy involves finding a way to integrate these two aspects of the self. The purpose is not to deny that victimization did indeed happen once, but to do so while enabling patients to develop some restructured self-image that provides for the recognition of the victimization, but does not allow it to dominate the overall view of the self.

In effect, this approach can be seen as a form of grief work. Here, the patients' task is to acknowledge, bear, and put into perspective painful life events, thereby making them acceptable to conscious awareness. The shift in concentration elicited in hypnosis, which is so useful in defending against the immediate impact of trauma as it is occurring and so problematic in the aftermath of trauma, can be quite helpful in mobilizing and putting into perspective traumatic memories and in reducing the symptoms of PTSD.

The controlled experience of the hypnotic abreaction itself provides boundaries around the psychotherapeutic mourning process. Instead of telling patients not to ruminate over the details of a traumatic experience, the therapist does the opposite. He or she instructs the patient how to think about the experience. The inferred message is that once this piece of therapeutic work has been accomplished, he or she can go on to work on other things. Thus, patients are slowly separated from the victim role as they see themselves from a different perspective and step into the role of survivor, which involves mastering rather than being mastered by their dissociative defenses.

REFERENCES

American Psychiatric Association. (1987). *Diagnostic and statistical manual of mental disorders* (3rd ed., rev.). Washington, DC: Author.

American Psychiatric Association. (1994). *Diagnostic and statistical manual of mental disorders* (4th ed.). Washington, DC: Author.

Benedikt, R., & Kolb, L. (1986). Preliminary findings on chronic pain and posttraumatic stress disorder. *American Journal of Psychiatry, 143*, 908–910.

Bernstein, D. A., & Borkovec, T. D. (1973). *Progressive relaxation training.* Champaign, IL: Research Press.

Blanchard, E. B., Kolb, L. C., Pallmeyer, T. P., & Gerardi, R. J. (1982). A psychophysiological study of post-traumatic stress disorder in Vietnam veterans. *Psychiatric Quarterly, 54*, 220–229.

Boudewyns, P. A., & Hyer, L. (1990). Physiological response to combat memories and preliminary treatment outcome in Vietnam veterans PTSD patients treated with direct therapeutic exposure. *Behavior Therapy, 21*, 63–87.

Bower, G. H. (1981). Mood and memory. *American Psychology, 36*, 129–148.

Branchey, L., Davis, W., & Lieber, C. S. (1984). Alcoholism in Vietnam and Korea veterans: A long term follow-up. *Alcoholism: Clinical and Experimental Research, 8*, 572–575.

Braun, P., Greenberg, D., Dasberg, H., & Lerer, B. (1990). Core symptoms of posttraumatic stress disorder unimproved by alprazolam treatment. *Journal of Clinical Psychiatry, 51*, 236–238.

Brett, E., Spitzer, R., & Williams, J. B. W. (1988). DSM-III-R criteria for posttraumatic stress disorder. *American Journal of Psychiatry, 145*(10), 1232–1236.

Cardeña, E., & Spiegel, D. (1993). Dissociative reactions to the San Francisco Bay Area earthquake of 1989. *American Journal of Psychiatry, 150*, 474–478.

Classen, C., Koopman, C., & Spiegel, D. (1993). Trauma and dissociation. *Bulletin of the Menninger Clinic, 2*, 179–194.

Coons, P. M., Bowman, E. S., & Pellow, T. A. (1989). Post-traumatic aspects of the treatment of victims of sexual abuse and incest. *Psychiatric Clinics of North America, 12*, 325–337.

Cooper, N. A., & Clum, G. A. (1989). Imaginal flooding as a supplementary treatment for PTSD in combat veterans: A controlled study. *Behavior Therapy, 20*, 381–391.

Davidson, J., Kudler, H., Smith, R., Mahorney, S. L., Lipper, S., Hammett, E., Saunders, W. B., & Cavenar, J. O. (1990). Treatment of posttraumatic stress disorder with amitriptyline and placebo. *Archives of General Psychiatry, 47*, 259–266.

Fesler, F. A. (1991). Valproate in combat-related posttraumatic stress disorder. *Journal of Clinical Psychiatry, 52*, 361–364.

Foa, E. B., Steketee, G., & Rothbaum, B. O. (1989). Behavioral/cognitive conceptualizations of post-traumatic stress disorder. *Behavior Therapy, 20*, 155–176.

Frank, J. B., Kosten, T. R., Giller, E. L., & Dan, E. (1988). A randomized clinical trial of phenelzine and imipramine for posttraumatic stress disorder. *American Journal of Psychiatry, 145,* 1289–1291.

Freud, A. (1946). *The ego and mechanisms of defense.* New York: International Universities Press.

Friedman, M. (1988). Toward rational pharmacotherapy for post-traumatic stress disorder. *American Journal of Psychiatry, 145*, 281–285.

Friedman, M. (1991). Biological approaches to the diagnosis and treatment of post-traumatic stress disorder. *Journal of Traumatic Stress, 4*, 67–91.

Greenberg, R., Pearlman, C. A., & Gampel, D. (1972). War neuroses and the adaptive function of REM sleep. *British Journal of Medical Psychology, 45*, 27–33.

Hartmann, E. (1984). *The nightmare: The psychology and biology of terrifying dreams.* New York: Basic Books.

Hilgard, E. R. (1977). *Divided consciousness: Multiple controls in human thoughts and action.* New York: John Wiley.

Horowitz, M., Wilner, N., Kaltreider, N. & Alvarez, W. (1980). Signs and symptoms of post-traumatic stress disorder. *Archives of General Psychiatry, 37*, 85–92.

Jacobson, E. (1938). *Progressive relaxation.* Chicago: University of Chicago Press.

Jelinek, J. M., & Williams, T. (1984). Post-traumatic stress disorder and substance abuse in Vietnam combat veterans: Treatment problems, strategies and recommendations. *Journal of Substance Abuse Treatment, 1*, 87–97.

Keane, T. M., & Fairbank, J. A. (1983). Survey analysis of combat-related stress disorders in Viet Nam veterans. *American Journal of Psychiatry, 140*, 348–350.

Keane, T. M., Fairbank, J. A., Caddell, J. M., & Zimering, R. T. (1989). Implosive (flooding) therapy reduces symptoms of PTSD in Vietnam combat veterans. *Behavior Therapy, 20*, 245–260.

Keane, T. M., & Wolfe, J. (1990). Comorbidity in post-traumatic stress disorder: An analysis of community and clinical studies. *Journal of Applied Social Psychology, 20*, 1776–1788.

Kihlstrom, J. F. (1984). Conscious, subconscious, unconscious: A cognitive perspective. In K. S. Bowers & D. Meichenbaum (Eds.), *The unconscious reconsidered* (pp. 149–211). New York: John Wiley.

Kihlstrom, J. F. (1990). Repression, dissociation and hypnosis. In J. L. Singer (Ed.), *Repression and dissociation* (pp. 180–208). Chicago: University of Chicago Press.

Kinzie, J. D. (1991). Post-traumatic stress disorder. In H. I. Kaplan & B. J. Sadock (Eds.), *Comprehensive textbook of psychiatry* (Vol. 6, pp. 1000–1008). Baltimore: Williams and Wilkins.

Kitchner, L., & Greenstein, R. (1985). Low dose lithium carbonate in the treatment of post-traumatic stress disorder. *Military Medicine, 150*, 378–381.

Kling, M. A., Perini, G. I., Demitrack, M. A., Geracioti, T. D., Linnoila, M., Chrousos, G. P., & Gold, P.W. (1989). Stress-responsive neurohormonal systems and the symptom complex of affective illness. *Psychopharmacology Bulletin, 25*(3), 312–318.

Kluft, R. P. (1984). Treatment of multiple personality disorder. *Psychiatric Clinics of North America, 7*, 9–29.

Kluft, R. P. (Ed.). (1985). *Childhood antecedents of multiple personality.* Washington, DC: American Psychiatric Press.

Kluft, R. P. (Ed.). (1990). *Incest-related syndromes of adult psychopathology.* Washington, DC: American Psychiatric Press.

Kluft, R. P. (1991). Clinical presentations of multiple personality disorder. *Psychiatric Clinics of North America, 14*(3), 605–629.

Kluft, R. P. (1992). The use of hypnosis with dissociative disorders. *Psychiatric Medicine, 10*(4), 31–46.

Kluft, R. P. (1993). The physician as perpetrator of the abuse. *Primary Care; Clinics in Office Practice, 20*, 459–480.

Kolb, L., Burris, B., & Griffiths, S. (1984). Propranolol and clonidine in the treatment of the chronic post traumatic stress disorder of war. In B. A. van der Kolk (Ed.), *Post-traumatic stress disorder: Psychological and biological sequelae* (pp. 97–107). Washington, DC: American Psychiatric Press.

Koopman, C., Classen, C., Spiegel, D., & Cardeña, E. (1994). When disaster strikes, acute stress disorder may follow. *Journal of Traumatic Stress.*

Kosten, T. R., & Krystal, J. (1988). Biological mechanisms in post-traumatic stress disorder: Relevance for substance abuse. *Recent Developments in Alcoholism, 6,* 49–68.

Kosten, T. R., Giller, E. L., & Mason, J. W. (1988, May). *Psychoendocrine assessment of PTSD.* Paper presented at the 141st annual meeting of the American Psychiatric Association, Montreal, Quebec.

Kosten, T. R., Mason, J. W., Giller, E. L., Ostroff, R. B., & Harkness L. (1987). Sustained urinary norepinephrine and epinephrine elevation in post-traumatic stress disorder. *Psychoneuroendocrinology, 12,* 13–30.

Kramer, M. (1979). Dream disturbance. *Psychiatric Annals, 9,* 50–60.

Kramer, M., & Kinney, L. (1988). Sleep patterns in trauma victims with disturbed dreaming. *Psychiatric Journal of the University of Ottawa, 13,* 12–16.

Kramer, M., Schoen, L., & Kinney, L. (1984). The dream experience in dream disturbed Vietnam veterans. In B. A. van der Kolk (Ed.), *Post-traumatic stress disorder: Psychological and biological sequelae.* Washington, DC: American Psychiatric Press.

Kudler, H. S., Davidson, J. R. T., Stein, R., & Erickson, L. (1989). Measuring results of treatment of PTSD. *American Journal of Psychiatry, 146,* 1645–1646.

Lavie, P., Hefez, A., Halperin, G., & Enoch, D. (1979). Long-term effects of traumatic war-related events on sleep. *American Journal of Psychiatry, 136,* 175–178.

Lipper, S. (1988). PTSD and carbamazepine. *American Journal of Psychiatry, 145,* 1322–1323.

Lynn, E. J., & Belza, M. (1984). Factitious posttraumatic stress disorder: The veteran who never got to Vietnam. *Hospital and Community Psychiatry, 35,* 697–701.

Marshall, J. R. (1975). The treatment of night terrors associated with the posttraumatic syndrome. *American Journal of Psychiatry, 132,* 293–295.

McFarlane, A. C. (1986). Posttraumatic morbidity of a disaster: A study of cases presenting for psychiatric treatment. *Journal of Nervous and Mental Disease, 174,* 4–13.

McFarlane, A. C. (1988). The longitudinal course of posttraumatic morbidity: The range of outcomes and their predictors. *Journal of Nervous and Mental Disease, 176,* 30–39.

Meichenbaum, D. (1974). *Cognitive behavior modification.* Morristown, NJ: General Learning Press.

Morgan, A. H., & Hilgard, E. R. (1973). Age differences in susceptibility to hypnosis. *International Journal of Clinical and Experimental Hypnosis, 21,* 78–85.

Nash, M. R., & Lynn, S. J. (1986). Child abuse and hypnotic ability: *Imagination, Cognition and Personality, 5*, 211–218.

Peniston, E. G. (1986). EMG biofeedback-assisted desensitization treatment for Vietnam combat veterans' post-traumatic stress disorder. *Clinical Biofeedback Health, 9*, 35–41.

Perry, S. W., Cella, D. E., Falkenberg, J., Heidrich, G., & Goodwin, C. (1987). Pain perception in burn patients with stress disorders. *Journal of Pain and Symptom Management, 2*, 29–33.

Pitman, R. K., Altman, B., Greenwald, E., Longpre, R. E., Macklin, M. L., Poire, R. E., & Steketee, G. S. (1991). Psychiatric complications during flooding therapy for posttraumatic stress disorder. *Journal of Clinical Psychiatry, 52*, 17–20.

Price, L. H., Charney, I. D. S., Rubin, A. L., & Heninger, G. R. (1986). Alpha-2 adrenergic receptor function in depression: The cortisol response to yohimbine. *Archives of General Psychiatry, 43*, 849–858.

Reist, C., Kauffman, C. D., & Haier, R. J. (1976). A controlled trial of desipramine in 18 men with post-traumatic stress disorder. *American Journal of Psychiatry, 146*, 513–516.

Ross, R., Ball, W., Sullivan, K., & Caroff, S. (1989). Sleep disturbance as the hallmark of posttraumatic stress disorder. *American Journal of Psychiatry, 146(6)*, 697–707.

Sapol, E., & Roffman, R. A. (1969). Marijuana in Vietnam. *Journal of the American Pharmaceutical Association, 9*, 615–618.

Scheflin, A. W., & Shapiro, J. L. (1989). *Trance on trial.* New York: Guilford Press.

Schnitt, J. M., & Nocks, J. J. (1984). Alcoholism treatment of Vietnam veterans with post-traumatic stress disorder. *Journal of Substance Abuse Treatment, 1*, 179–189.

Shestatzky, M., Greenberg, D., & Lerer, B. (1988). A controlled trial of phenelzine in posttraumatic stress disorder. *Psychiatry Research, 24*, 149–155.

Solomon, S. D., Gerrity, E. T., & Muff, A. M. (1992). Efficacy of treatments for posttraumatic stress disorder. *Journal of the American Medical Association, 268*, 633–638.

Solomon, Z., Mikulincer, M., & Benbenishty, R. (1989). Combat stress reaction: Clinical manifestations and correlates. *Military Psychology, 1*, 35–47.

Spiegel, D. (1981). Vietnam grief work using hypnosis. *American Journal of Clinical Hypnosis, 24*, 33–40.

Spiegel, D. (1984). Multiple personality as a post-traumatic stress disorder. *Psychiatric Clinics of North America, 7*, 101–110.

Spiegel, D. (1986). Dissociating damage. *American Journal of Clinical Hypnosis, 29*, 123–131.

Spiegel, D. (1988). Dissociation and hypnosis in posttraumatic stress disorder. *Journal of Traumatic Stress, 1*, 17–33.

Spiegel, D. (1989). Hypnosis in the treatment of victims of sexual abuse. *Psychiatric Clinics of North America, 12*, 295–305.

Spiegel, D. (1990). Hypnosis, dissociation and trauma: Hidden and overt observers. In J. L. Singer (Ed.), *Repression and dissociation* (pp. 121–142). Chicago: University of Chicago Press.

Spiegel, D. (1992). The use of hypnosis in the treatment of PTSD. *Psychiatric Medicine, 10*, 21–30.

Spiegel, D., & Cardeña, E. (1990). New uses of hypnosis in the treatment of post-traumatic stress disorder. *Journal of Clinical Psychiatry, 51*(Suppl. 10), 39–43.

Spiegel, D., & Cardeña, E. (1991). Disintegrated experience: The dissociative disorders revisited. *Journal of Abnormal Psychology, 100*(3), 366–378.

Spiegel, D., Detrick, D., & Frischholz, E. (1982). Hypnotizability and psychopathology. *American Journal of Psychiatry, 139*, 431–437.

Spiegel, D., & Fink, R. (1979). Hysterical psychosis and hypnotizability. *American Journal of Psychiatry, 136*, 777–781.

Spiegel, D., Hunt, T., & Dondershine, H. E. (1988). Dissociation and hypnotizability in posttraumatic stress disorder. *American Journal of Psychiatry, 145*, 301–305.

Spiegel, H., & Spiegel, D. (1987). *Trance and treatment.* New York: Basic Books.

Stuntman, R. K., & Bliss, E. L. (1985). Posttraumatic stress disorder, hypnotizability and imagery. *American Journal of Psychiatry, 142*, 741–743.

Tellegen, A., & Atkinson, G. (1974). Openness to absorbing and self-altering experiences ("absorption"), a trait related to hypnotic susceptibility. *Journal of Abnormal Psychology, 83*, 268–277.

van der Kolk, B. A. (1983). Psychopharmacological issues in post-traumatic stress disorder. *Hospital and Community Psychiatry, 34*, 683–691.

van der Kolk, B. A. (1987). The drug treatment of post-traumatic stress disorder. *Journal of Affective Disorder, 13*, 203–213.

van der Kolk, B. A., Blitz, R., Burr, W., Sherry, S., & Hartmann, E. (1984). Nightmares and trauma: A comparison of nightmares after combat with lifelong nightmares in veterans. *American Journal of Psychiatry, 141*, 187–190.

van der Kolk, B. A., & van der Hart, O. (1989). Pierre Janet and the breakdown of adaptation in psychological trauma. *American Journal of Psychiatry, 146*, 1530–1540.

Wedding, D. (1987). Substance abuse in the Vietnam veteran. *AAOHN Journal, 35*, 74–76.

Weiss, D. S., Marmar, C. R., Metzler, T., & Ronfeldt, H. (1993). *Predicting symptomatic distress in emergency services personnel.* Unpublished manuscript, University of California, San Francisco.

Wilkinson, C. B. (1983). Aftermath of a disaster: The collapse of the Hyatt Regency Hotel skywalks. *American Journal of Psychiatry, 140*, 1134–1139.

Wolpe, J. (1973). *The practice of behavior therapy.* New York: Pergamon Press.

Ziarnowski, A. P., & Broida, D. C. (1984). Therapeutic implications of the nightmares of Vietnam combat veterans. *VA Practitioner, 1*, 63–68.

12

Sexual Abuse and Revictimization: Mastery, Dysfunctional Learning, and Dissociation

David Sandberg
Steven Jay Lynn
Joseph P. Green

The incidence and prevalence of sexual assault in the United States is disturbingly high. Researchers (Kilpatrick et al., 1985; Russell, 1986; Sorenson, Stein, Siegel, Golding, & Burnam, 1987) now estimate that as many as 20–40% of all women in our society will experience some form of sexual assault during their lifetime.

Two studies illustrate the magnitude of the problem. One study, conducted by Russell (1984, 1986), involved a large-scale investigation of 930 women living in the San Francisco area. Her study pioneered the use of personal interviews to identify victims of sexual assault. Further, her sample of subjects was designed to represent the demographic characteristics (e.g., age, ethnicity, and marital status) of the population at large as gauged by the 1980 Census. Russell's research was also exemplary in that trained female interviewers were employed to question subjects about sexual victimization, whenever possible, in the subject's home. Of the total sample, 24% reported that they had experienced forced intercourse or intercourse without consent (i.e., "when drugged, unconscious, asleep, or otherwise totally helpless and unable to consent" [Russell, 1984, p. 35]).

In what is one of the most ambitious studies of sexual victimization to date, Koss and her colleagues (see Koss, Gidycz, & Wisniewski, 1987) administered a self-report measure of sexual victimization (Sexual Experiences Survey; Koss & Oros, 1982) to a national sample of 6,159 male and female students. Of the 3,187 female subjects, 53.7% reported experiencing some form of sexual victimization after the age of 14. Approximately 12% of the women in the sample reported attempted rape, and 15.4% reported completed rape. These statistics are consistent with results of previous research (e.g., Kanin & Parcell, 1977; Muehlenhard & Linton, 1987).

These studies underline the fact that sexual abuse has reached near epidemic proportions in America. Just as shocking as the scope of sexual victimization is the rate at which women suffer repeated victimization. It is well documented (e.g., see Kluft, 1990a, 1990b; van der Kolk, 1989; Chu, 1992) that many women are repeatedly victimized throughout their lives. In this chapter, we examine the evidence that sexual victimization increases the risk of subsequent victimization.

Numerous explanations have been offered to account for repeated victimization, including repetition compulsion, post-traumatic symptomatology, relational disturbances, inappropriate state-dependent learning, physiological addiction to trauma, and cognitive distortions (Chu, 1992; van der Kolk, 1989; Kluft, 1989, 1990a, 1990b; Koss & Dinero, 1989; Finkelhor & Browne, 1985). In this chapter, we place a variety of explanations of revictimization in three categories, which can be thought of as representing different factors that can operate independently or in concert with one another to increase the risk of revictimization: (1) the search for meaning and mastery, (2) dysfunctional learning, (3) dissociation and coping strategies. In presenting this conceptual scheme, we discuss the strengths and limitations of the research conducted to date and draw out some of the clinical implications of the extant literature.

REVICTIMIZATION: IS THERE A VICIOUS CYCLE?

The fact that some individuals are subject to "multiple victimization" has long been documented by sociology and criminology research (see Becker-Lausen, Sanders, & Chinksy, 1992; Mandoki & Burkhart, 1989; Walklate, 1989). As part of a national survey of violent crime victims, Ziegenhagen (1976) reported that 28% of the victims were prior victims of a similar crime. Similar rates have been reported with respect to sexual assault. Miller and colleagues (1978) reported that of the 341 victims seen by the University of New Mexico Medical School's Sexual Response Team, 24% were "recidivist" victims of sexual assault. Similarly, Ellis, Atkeson, and Calhoun (1982) found that 21% of 117 rape victims who sought treatment at a rape crisis center reported that they had been previously victimized. Because these statistics were based on informants' reports at crisis settings, which are not conducive to gathering sensitive historical information, the data may underestimate the actual occurrence of revictimization (see Miller et al., 1978).

Childhood Sexual Victimization
as a Precursor to Adult Victimization

When defined as sexual contact ranging from fondling to intercourse between a child or adolescent and a person at least 5 years older, the childhood sexual victimization rate generally hovers around 20% (see Briere, 1992; Finkelhor, 1979; Finkelhor, Hotaling, Lewis, & Smith, 1989). The available evidence suggests that women with histories of childhood sexual abuse are more likely than nonvictims to be sexually assaulted in adulthood.

Of Russell's (1986) sample of 930 women, 28% reported that they had been sexually abused before the age of 14. With Miller et al.'s (1978) study, in which 24% (82 of 341) of rape victims seen in an emergency setting were found to have been previously victimized, 18% of the recidivist victims were incestuously abused. In her study, Russell (1986) confirmed that incest may be an important risk factor for subsequent victimization. She found that 65% of the identified incest victims were also victims of rape or attempted rape by a nonrelative at or after the age of 14, compared to only 36% of the women in the study who had never experienced incest.

In Briere and Runtz's (1987) study of 152 adult women presenting to a community counseling center, approximately 44% reported a history of childhood sexual victimization. In addition to reporting greater symptomatology than nonabused clients, women who related a history of childhood sexual abuse were more than twice as likely as nonvictims to report having been both battered and raped in adulthood.

In examining the relationship between childhood sexual abuse and later psychological and sexual adjustment in 383 female college students, Fromuth (1986) found a significant relationship between sexual abuse in childhood and subsequent rape. This relationship remained significant even when Fromuth statistically controlled for the effects of parental supportiveness (see Fromuth, 1986). Childhood sexual abuse also predicted less severe forms of subsequent sexual victimization, defined as any nonconsensual experience that involves threat or use of force.

Based on a representative national sample of 2,723 college women, Koss and Dinero (1989) determined that a history of childhood sexual abuse was one of four key variables that significantly predicted adult sexual victimization. Similarly, in a community sample of 248 women between the ages of 18 and 36, Wyatt, Guthrie, and Notgrass (1992) found that subjects who reported being sexually abused in childhood were 2.4 times more likely than women who did not report childhood sexual abuse to be revictimized in adulthood.

A relation between childhood sexual abuse and later sexual victimization has also been documented in samples of psychiatric inpatients. Bryer,

Nelson, Miller, and Krol (1987) reported that 52% of a group of 29 patients who reported early sexual abuse also reported sexual abuse in adulthood. Based on a much larger sample (105 female state hospital patients), Craine, Henson, Colliver, and MacLean (1988) found that 41% of the 54 patients who reported a history of childhood sexual abuse also reported a history of rape after the age of 18, compared to 20% of the 51 patients who did not report a history of childhood sexual abuse. Similarly, in a study of 98 female psychiatric inpatients, Chu and Dill (1990) concluded that having a history of childhood sexual abuse nearly doubles a woman's risk of being sexually victimized in adulthood.

It is important to note that childhood sexual abuse appears to place a woman at risk for numerous other forms of maltreatment. Russell (1986) for example, discovered that incest victims (compared to nonvictims) were more likely to report being physically abused by their husbands, experiencing unwanted sexual advances from an authority figure, receiving obscene phone calls, being pinched or rubbed against in a public place, and being asked to pose for pornographic materials. Similarly, in a nonclinical sample of 301 female college students, Sedney and Brooks (1984) found that subjects who reported childhood sexual abuse were more likely than nonabused subjects to report being a victim of crime in adulthood.

Childhood Sexual Victimization and Involvement in Prostitution

As pointed out by Finkelhor and Browne (1985), child sexual abuse victims appear to be at risk for becoming involved in prostitution. Of course, disparate motives may be at play in a person's decision to embark on a career as a prostitute; however, several authors (Finkelhor & Browne, 1985; Chu, 1992; van der Kolk, 1989) consider prostitution to be a variant of sexual victimization.

In 1977, James and Meyerding conducted two self-report questionnaire studies of adult and adolescent prostitutes in a large western city. All together, the authors were able to solicit the participation of 228 subjects. In one study, 46% of the subjects reported that prior to experiencing intercourse for the first time, someone at least 10 years older attempted to engage in sexual play or intercourse with them. The rate of occurrence of this type of victimization for women in the general population has been estimated at 28% (Gagnon, 1965). Thirty-seven percent of James and Meyerding's sample (Study 1) reported that they had engaged in incestuous activities, as compared to 15% (Gagnon, 1965) of women from the general population. In their second study, James and Meyerding found that 13 of 20 adolescent prostitutes reported having experienced forced sex, with the great majority of instances occurring before the age of 15.

Silbert and Pines (1981) conducted a study of 200 juvenile and adult street prostitutes in the San Francisco Bay area. Their subjects' mean age was 22, with some being as young as 10 years old. Subjects were interviewed by former prostitutes who took part in a 3-week intensive training program to learn interviewing techniques and basic research methodology. The authors found that, as reported, 60% of the sample had been sexually exploited by an average of two people each, over an average period of 20 months prior to the age of 16.

Not only are childhood sexual abuse victims more likely than nonvictims to enter prostitution, they also are overrepresented among exotic dancers. When studying dissociative phenomena among various groups of individuals, Ross, Anderson, Heber, and Norton (1990) found that 11 of 20 prostitutes, and 13 of 20 exotic dancers, reported a history of sexual abuse.

Childhood Sexual Victimization and Therapist–Patient Sexual Exploitation

Kluft (Kluft, 1989, 1990a, 1990b) has suggested that therapist–patient sexual exploitation can be thought of as a specific type of revictimization (see Kluft, 1989, 1990a). According to Kluft (1990), incest survivors in particular are overrepresented among those patients who are sexually abused by their therapists. In studying the prevalence of therapist–patient misadventures, Pope and Bouhoutsos (1986) concluded that incest victims were at high risk for therapist–patient sexual exploitation. Similarly, DeYoung (1981) noted that 3 members of a 10-women incest support group reported that they had had sexual liaisons with their therapists.

In summary, the available evidence suggests that women who are sexually abused in childhood have an increased likelihood of being sexually victimized in adulthood. Women who are raped in adulthood report increased levels of previous sexual victimization, prostitutes and exotic dancers frequently report histories of childhood sexual abuse, and women sexually exploited by their therapists report histories of incest.

There are, however, certain limitations in the research and conclusions that can be drawn that should be duly noted. Unfortunately, the majority of evidence gathered thus far has been retrospective in nature. Furthermore, when sexual assault victims are interviewed by individuals who are themselves former prostitutes (e.g., Silbert & Pines, 1981) or abuse victims, it is possible that demand characteristics and reconstructive memory processes lead to biased recall and inaccurate reporting.

Clearly, prospective studies are needed before firm conclusions can be drawn about a link between childhood sexual abuse and subsequent victimization. On a positive note, researchers at Ohio University (e.g., Gidycz, Nelson, & Latham, 1992) have initiated a series of prospective analyses of the impact of childhood sexual victimization on subsequent sexual assault. So far, the data gathered from 927 female college students indicate that sexual victimization early in life acts as a risk factor for adult sexual victimization. For example, women who reported a history of childhood sexual abuse were more likely than women who did not report abuse to be sexually victimized over the course of one academic quarter (approximately 9 weeks). However, Gidycz et al.'s findings are not definitive in that it is unclear whether other forms of childhood maltreatment (e.g., physical or emotional abuse) lead to comparable base rates of sexual victimization.

As alluded to above, another problem in interpreting the data is that it is unclear what role sexual victimization plays apart from dysfunctional family dynamics. Whereas it is widely acknowledged that sexual abuse occurs in the context of a disturbed family unit, research efforts have not discriminated the effects of dysfunctional family relationships from the effects of sexual victimization. Prospective studies, which control for the effects of various forms of child maltreatment and dysfunctional family dynamics, are obviously a priority.

The literature contains dozens of explanations for why women are repeatedly victimized (see Chu, 1992; Kluft, 1990a, 1990b; van der Kolk, 1989; Koss & Dinero, 1989; Finkelhor & Browne, 1985). While disagreeing about which factors are the most important, clinicians generally concur that revictimization is a complex, overdetermined process. In other words, there appears to be no *single* reason why a woman who has been previously victimized is at risk for further victimization.

THE SEARCH FOR MASTERY AND MEANING

In this section, we review theories that suggest that persons who have been sexually victimized are motivated to repeat the experience in order to gain a sense of mastery over their initial experience of victimization, as well as to be able to attach meaning to it. Numerous authors (e.g., Chu, 1992; van der Kolk, 1989) have argued that the "repetition compulsion" is an integral part of understanding revictimization. In *Beyond the Pleasure Principle* (1920/1954), Freud related his observations of his 18-month-old grandson, Ernst, who had experienced repeated separations from his mother. Freud noted that the child had a wooden reel with a piece of string wound around it, which he would repeatedly throw over the side of his cot, making the reel disappear from view. Immediately after throwing the reel, Ernst would draw it back and greet it. Freud interpreted the meaning of the game to be connected to the child's repeated separations from his mother. In essence, the child was repeating the stressful loss experience, but in a way that allowed him to master, or control, it. As Freud observed, "children repeat in their play everything that has made a great impression on them in actual life," thereby abreacting the strength of the impression and making themselves masters of the situation (p. 18).

In her article on psychic trauma in children and adolescents, Terr (1985) provides a more contemporary description of the same phenomenon. She presents the case of a girl named Leslie who was a victim of the Chowchilla bus kidnapping at the age of 7. After the experience, Leslie would repetitively play a game she called "bus driver." The main idea of the game was that all of the passengers in a certain bus would get off of it safely. Four years after the kidnapping, Leslie was still reenacting the event through a game called "traveling Barbies," wherein a Barbie doll would attend some function and safely come back home.

The most upsetting manifestation of her repetition compulsion occurred when Leslie ran away from home at the age of 10. Unbeknownst to her parents, she hitchhiked a ride from a stranger in the middle of the night. Although Leslie's parents told the police a kidnapping had occurred, Leslie insisted the event was something completely different. In her mind, she had gone away—not been taken. Consistent with Freud's observations, there was a distinct element of mastery in Leslie's reenactments, although it was overshadowed by the alarming dangerousness of her behavior.

Freud's notion of the repetition compulsion provides a theoretical explanation for why some women are sexually revictimized at such astounding rates. As Freud pointed out, "We all know people with whom every human relationship ends in the same way" (1920/1954, p. 18). For some women who have been sexually victimized, their fate seems to be revictimization.

According to Freud, the initial traumatic experience, although repressed, returns and influences the victim's capacity to deal with current challenges: "The patient is obliged . . . to *repeat* as a current experience what is repressed, instead of . . . *recollecting* it as a fragment of the past" (1920/1954, p. 18). Until the person is capable of "working through" the original trauma, repressed elements will continue to compel him or her to repeat the experience, despite the harm it may cause. Working through can be conceptualized as remembering and reexperiencing repressed memories, usually in the context of a therapeutic relationship. Because the process occurs at the unconscious level, the person is unaware of the connection between the initial traumatic experience and current life situations.

As noted previously, many prostitutes are victims of child sexual abuse. Regarding this fact from the perspective of Freud's theory of the repetition compulsion, one can conclude that many of these women are unconsciously compelled to place themselves in sexual situations to work through, or master, the original traumatic experience. As a prostitute, the abuse victim will continually reenact the abuse scenario, and on some level take charge of, control, or alter the situation and/or her reaction to it. For instance, rather than being forced to have intercourse with a perpetrator, the prostitute is in charge of administering sex.

Because childhood sexual abuse is fundamentally interpersonal in nature, object relations theory can be used to broaden our understanding of revictimization. The theory itself is a dynamic one, and focuses on human relationships and attachment. As opposed to classical Freudian theory, which emphasizes the importance of sex and aggression as underlying drives, object relations theory focuses on the way the developing child creates mental representations of the self and others (e.g., Fairbairn, 1954; Cashdan, 1988; Masterson & Klein, 1989). Through a process known as "introjection," the child comes to view him- or herself in the same way he or she is treated by significant others. Thus, if the child is subjected to severe abuse, he or she will form a negative view of the self. Furthermore, because it would be too threatening to view the parent (object) as bad or evil, since the child must depend upon him or her for survival, the child is likely to blame him- or herself for being maltreated, thus preserving the "all good" view of the needed object.

Over time, the abused child will tend to reenact the perpetrator–victim dynamic with others. Based on the mental representation he or she has developed of the self, he or she will tend to allow, or even elicit, abusive interchanges with others (see Gelinas, 1983). According to object relations theory, she will recapitulate such relationships via projective identification. Because the victim views herself as bad, and therefore worthy of punishment, she will tend to act in ways that induce mistreatment. She may also punish the "bad part" of herself through self-mutilation (Buchele, 1993; Gelinas, 1983).

Object relations theory, like Freudian theory, postulates that attempts at mastery occur at an unconscious level, so that the victim is unaware of what he or she is doing, and why. Even when an abusive pattern is identified, these individuals have tremendous difficulty changing their behavior. In the words of one adult female incest victim, "I have a pattern of getting attached to assholes. My current lover is a xerox copy of my [abusive] stepfather" (Tsai & Wagner, 1978, p. 422). As pointed out by van der Kolk (1989), abuse victims rarely succeed in gaining a sense of control or mastery. Because the search for mastery is fruitless, they continue to be victimized repeatedly without a clear understanding of why this occurs.

In line with the current zeitgeist, some contemporary authors have conceptualized the repetition compulsion phenomenon in terms of information processing. Horowitz (1975), for example, has argued that the "instinctual" properties of Freud's original theorizing "can best be restated in terms of cognitive operations" (p. 1461). According to Horowitz, repetition is a normal response to stress and is manifested by way of intrusive and repetitive thoughts.

Active memory storage has an intrinsic tendency to engage in repetition, and memories of a stressful stimulus will continue to be processed indefinitely until cognitive processing has been completed. Memories will return to awareness, and be experienced as intrusive, if they have not yet been fully integrated into the person's cognitive schema. Cognitive processing is conceptualized in terms of Piaget's work on assimilation and accommodation wherein new information is matched with and integrated into preexisting schemas. With integration comes diminished repetition; the stressful event becomes like other memories—available for recall but no longer intrusive and disturbing. The successful processing and integration of the traumatic experience into schematic representation is thus fundamental to the eradication of post-traumatic reactions.

Importantly, Horowitz (1976) did not limit the scope of the repetition compulsion to thoughts, but argued that the phenomenon may occur at the emotional or behavioral level as well. For example, a trauma victim might exhibit panic attacks or crying spells, or even engage in repeated behavioral reenactments of the event. Gelinas (1983), Chu (1992), and van der Kolk (1989) all provided clinical examples of child sexual abuse victims who engaged in "behavioral reenactments" of traumatic events. All three authors consider sexual revictimization to be a specific form of behavioral reenactment, and cite evidence indicating that childhood abuse victims are at risk for revictimization in adulthood, and for becoming involved in prostitution.

Horowitz's model differs from Freud's repetition compulsion model in one important respect: Whereas Freud argued that traumatic memories are repressed (i.e., out of conscious awareness), Horowitz claimed that trauma-related memories continue to be consciously processed. Although it is certainly possible that repressed memories and unconscious motivation to experience mastery can increase vulnerability to revictimization, many victims of sexual abuse are in touch with their motivation to participate in sexual situations. What these persons may not be aware of, or what may not be particularly salient to them, is the idea that they are involved in activities or situations associated with a high risk of revictimization.

In providing a clinical example of the repetition compulsion, Chu (1992) quoted a prostitute who was victimized as a child as saying: "When I do it, I'm in control. I can control them [men] through sex" (p. 261). The woman's explanation for why she was involved in prostitution clearly conveys the message that her action was intentional, and that she was keenly aware of what she was doing.

It is perhaps ironic that the authors (Silbert & Pines, 1981) of an article frequently cited to support a link between childhood sexual abuse and subsequent involvement in prostitution discuss at length how entrance into the profession is largely a matter of survival, not a compulsion. Indeed, 96% of Silbert and Pine's juvenile sample had run away from home to avoid intolerable abuse, and had no way of surviving in the streets besides becoming involved in prostitution. When asked why they became involved, 89% of the sample reported that they "needed money" or "were hungry" (p. 410). Moreover, Silbert and Pines noted that the majority of sexually abused children do not become prostitutes, casting doubt on the causal nature of the trauma–sexual revictimization connection.

Although evidence suggests that certain women are repeatedly victimized, no data exist to support the notion that mere repetition, or repeated occurrence, can be equated with truly compulsive activity, wherein feelings of anxiety emerge if the compulsive action is not completed or prevented from occurring. Although van der Kolk (1989) conducted research that suggests that exposure to stressful stimuli can have the same effect as taking exogenous opioids, the hypothesis that victims of assault neutralize a hyperaroused state via compulsive reexposure to victimization, remains speculative. Although reexposure may result in numbness and a reduction of pain, it has not been established that victims seek out further abuse to modulate their physiological systems.

In summary, certain abuse victims may be motivated to master and understand traumatic or overwhelming experiences. One way they can do so is to engage in high-risk situations resembling or reminiscent of an earlier abuse experience, wherein they can master and control themselves and others. This may lend a compulsive appearance to their actions. While by repeatedly placing themselves in high-risk situations these women no doubt increase their vulnerability to revictimization; however, repetitive activity or behavioral consistency cannot be equated with truly compulsive activity. Due to the pejorative connotations associated with the term "repetition compulsion," and the potential implication that the woman is responsible for her sexual victimization, it is advisable to refrain from equating repetitive sexual victimization with "compulsion."

It is important to keep in mind that sexual abuse victims do not want to be revictimized. Like others with no history of sexual abuse, they are motivated to establish caring and nurturing interpersonal relationships—something many victims never had. Unfortunately, because of their dysfunctional upbringings, victims of childhood sexual abuse may have tremendous difficulty in establishing and maintaining nonabusive relationships. Indeed, childhood sexual victimization, rather than engendering a drive for mastery, may lead to a sense of powerlessness and helplessness in interpersonal situations. In the next section, we examine the dysfunctional learning that takes place in the context of childhood sexual abuse and its relation to risk for subsequent victimization.

DYSFUNCTIONAL LEARNING

We refer to dysfunctional learning as the constellation of maladaptive attitudes and beliefs about the self, others, and the world in general. Typically, dysfunctional learning is acquired in the context of interpersonal relationships and has a profound impact on how people interact with, and are treated by, others.

As pointed out by some researchers (Chu, 1992; McCann, Sakheim, & Abrahamson, 1988; Gelinas, 1983; Briere, 1992), many victims of sexual abuse (particularly childhood sexual abuse) demonstrate significant relational disturbances. Rather than developing a capacity to form healthy relationships, they appear to have problems relating to others. Unfortunately, the relational disturbances thought to arise as a consequence of childhood sexual abuse may play a role in subsequent victimization (Chu, 1992; van der Kolk, 1989).

In discussing the traumatic impact of child sexual abuse, Finkelhor and Browne (1985) identified four primary interpersonal problems that result from the psychological injury inflicted by abuse: traumatic sexualization, betrayal, powerlessness, and stigmatization. Traumatic sexualization refers to when a child's sexuality is shaped in developmentally inappropriate and interpersonally dysfunctional ways. The child who is rewarded for her sexual behavior learns that she can exchange sex for affection, attention, privileges, or love—"commodities" that are unconditionally provided in a healthy parent–child relationship. In other words, the child is socialized to view sex as a tool for manipulating others.

Childhood sexual abuse can have a profound influence on the child's developing sense of self. The child who has experienced traumatic sexualization will likely emerge from the experience with "inappropriate repertoires of sexual behavior . . . confusions about [his or her] sexual self-concept, and . . . unusual emotional associations to sexual activities" (Finkelhor & Browne, 1985, p. 531).

One common clinical observation is that child sexual abuse victims frequently engage in inappropriate, repetitive sex play with adults or peers (Kendall-Tackett, Williams, & Finkelhor, 1993; Finkelhor & Browne, 1985; Yates, 1983). Some child victims have been observed attempting to engage others in intercourse or oral–genital contact. Unfortunately, victims who engage in such behavior place themselves at great risk for revictimization. As recent studies have shown, childhood sexual victimization is related to a high number of reported consensual partners in adulthood (Mandoki & Burkhart, 1989), which is a significant predictor of sexual victimization in adulthood (Koss & Dinero, 1989; Mandoki & Burkhart, 1989). In other words, child sexual abuse is associated with a greater number of subsequent sexual partners which, in turn, increases a woman's chances of encountering a perpetrator of assault.

Koss and Dinero (1989) identified a high-risk profile for sexual assault in a sample of 2,723 female college students. While the profile characterized only 10% of the sample, risk for rape was twice as high as expected for women in this group (37% as opposed to 14%). The profile consisted of four variables: (1) child sexual abuse, (2) sexual attitudes, (3) alcohol use, and (4) sexual activity. Specifically, the women in this study who were most likely to report having been sexually victimized were those who reported having a history of childhood sexual abuse, liberal attitudes about sex, above average sexual activity, and higher than average alcohol use.

Child sexual abuse victims feel betrayed when they discover that the people they depended on to protect and nurture them (i.e., their parent or caretaker) caused them harm. This breech of trust obviously carries with it a tremendous sense of anger, sadness, and loss, along with grave disenchantment and disillusionment. Consequently, many victims develop an intense need to regain a sense of trust and security in interpersonal relationships.

In childhood, this dynamic frequently manifests itself in extreme dependency and clinging. In adulthood, the same unresolved issue may result in "impaired judgment about the trustworthiness of other people" (Finkelhor & Browne, 1985, p. 535; see also McCann, Sakheim, & Abrahamson, 1988). It has been found, for example, that adult female incest victims appear to have marked difficulty in processing danger cues in their environment (see Kluft, 1990a, 1990b). A high level of sexual activity, combined with a diminished capacity to detect threat, places a woman at risk for subsequent victimization.

Powerlessness and attendant feelings of impotence, depression, and despair, commonly result from the feelings of entrapment and disempowerment an abusive experience elicits. Due to the abuse, the child's feelings of self-efficacy and his or her coping skills are greatly diminished. When confronted with threatening interpersonal situations (e.g., a potential assault), the victim is likely to feel powerless and ineffective. She may succumb to a feeling of "learned helplessness" (Seligman, 1975) and no longer try to control noxious events. According to Briere (1992), childhood maltreatment encourages passivity, helplessness, and dependency, and teaches the victim to tolerate, if not accept, violence in intimate relationships. In other words, victims are socialized to be subordinate to perpetrators of maltreatment.

Stigmatization occurs when, as a result of the abuse, the victim comes to see herself as bad. The pressure for secrecy, the knowledge of incest taboos, and the demeaning comments made by the perpetrator can all lead to overwhelming feelings of shame and guilt on the part of the victim. When people react to news of the abuse with shock or hysteria, or if they blame the victim for "seducing" the perpetrator, the situation is further exacerbated. Child victims may also be stigmatized by people who view them as "spoiled goods" (Finkelhor & Browne, 1985, p. 533). Unfortunately, in many cases, the victim comes to internalize this negative view of herself.

Indeed, Cole and Putnam (1992) have traced the effects of child sexual abuse (specifically father–daughter incest) on the victim's developing sense of self. By the time the incest victim reaches adulthood, cumulative impairments to her sense of self and social functioning are evident in problems that increase the probability of revictimization, such as difficulty in communicating limits, impulsivity, lack of insight, and diminished self-respect. After all, if a woman does not recognize her own worth and respect herself, she may fail to protect herself from the abuse she feels she deserves. As Herman (1981) has observed, "a history of incest is associated with some impairment of the normal adult mechanisms of self-protection, and hence with a higher than average rate for rape" (p. 30).

Herman's (1981) description of the effects of father–daughter incest touches on all four aspects of Finkelhor and Browne's model. In attempting to explain how the incestuous experiences continue to shape the victim's relations with others and her image of herself, Herman noted that they (incest victims) desperately longed for the nurturance they did not receive while growing up, were keenly aware that they could use sex to gain the attention of others, and had developed a repertoire of sexually stylized behavior (traumatic sexualization). In addition to feeling lonely and depressed much of the time, victims also experienced profound betrayal by both parents (betrayal). Furthermore, they felt different, unusual, bad, or dirty (stigmatization), and many thought that they had deserved to be abused or that they had somehow asked for it. As a result of their experiences, victims ultimately came to expect abuse and disappointment in all intimate relationships (powerlessness).

Adopting a biopsychosocial view of attachment, van der Kolk (1987, 1989) contended that early parent–child interactions have a profound influence on the child's later social attachments and his or her capacity to mentally process stressful experiences. Healthy, secure attachments, he argued, help the child learn to modulate physiological arousal. If a child has come to depend on more primitive coping styles (i.e., dissociation), he or she will tend to experience later stresses "as somatic states, rather than as specific events that require specific means of coping" (van der Kolk, 1989, p. 405). Furthermore, the child is likely to have difficulties with impulse control, which can be an antecedent to substance abuse, sexual acting out, and running away—three factors that have been shown to be associated with victimization (Koss & Dinero, 1989; Silbert & Pines, 1981).

To support his notion of attachment, van der Kolk (1987, 1989) reviewed a series of studies conducted with nonhuman primates. In one study (Suomi, 1984), rhesus monkeys that were subjected to early abuse and deprivation were found to function appropriately with peers under normal circumstances. However, when confronted with stress, mistreated male monkeys became hyperaggressive, whereas mistreated females failed to protect themselves and their offspring from danger.

With regard to revictimization in humans, it seems plausible that females who have experienced child sexual abuse would be at risk for failing to protect themselves at times of stress. Because they have not been able to successfully integrate past traumatic experiences (see section on the repetition compulsion), they are prone to reexperience heightened arousal in response to environmental stimuli that trigger memories of dissociated traumatic events. Furthermore, in order to rid themselves of overwhelming anxiety, they might unknowingly engage in behaviors that place them at risk for subsequent victimization, the most dangerous of which appears to be heavy alcohol consumption and drug use (Koss & Dinero, 1989).

Briere (1992) has noted that victims of childhood abuse tend to engage in "tension-reducing behaviors" (p. 64), in order to cope with stressors that occur as a result of unresolved childhood abuse issues. These unresolved issues restimulate or exacerbate strong feelings of rage, anxiety, helplessness, self-loathing, and/or emptiness. As a result, behaviors that serve to distract, calm, or anesthetize are used to vitiate the unbearable internal state.

People who have suffered severe abuse often engage in self-mutilating or self-destructive behaviors (Green, 1978; Shapiro, 1987; van der Kolk, Herman, & Perry, 1988). According to some researchers (e.g., van der Kolk, 1989), the self-mutilating behavior is accompanied by analgesia and an "altered state of consciousness. The pain, cutting, and burning are apparent attempts at 'repairing the cohesiveness of the self in the face of overwhelming anxiety'" (p. 402). As previously mentioned, other self-destructive behaviors include heavy alcohol consumption and drug use (van der Kolk, 1989). In short, a variety of activities and behaviors can be initiated to cope with the aftereffects of abuse that, although effective in the short run in reducing anxiety and altering mental states, are unproductive and self-destructive in the long run.

In summary, children raised in an abusive environment are at risk for acquiring dysfunctional beliefs about themselves, those around them, and the world in general. As a function of their upbringing, they may be deprived of basic social skills and coping strategies, which may put them at risk for further maltreatment. The very activities that are of limited effectiveness in coping with the aftermath of abuse in the short run, may be self-destructive in the long run.

The way that dysfunctional learning, personality characteristics, and situational factors interact to produce revictimization is in need of further investigation. Specifying the role of situational factors in revictimization and their interaction with other factors is particularly important because situational factors play a prominent role in predicting sexual assault. Risk of revictimization may increase in direct proportion to the extent to which victims repeatedly involve themselves with the following high-risk situations: alcohol consumption (Koss & Dinero, 1989; Miller & Marshall, 1987; Muehlenhard & Linton, 1987), dates wherein the man is always the initiator and pays all the expenses (Muehlenhard & Linton, 1987), secluded dating locations (Muehlenhard & Linton, 1987), and poor communication about sex (Muehlenhard & Linton, 1987; Byers, Giles, & Price, 1987).

The research in this area is hampered by the lack of adequate measures of constructs such as traumatic sexualization. Furthermore, prospective studies of revictimization are needed to determine just which aspects of interpersonal relationships are the most compromised by sexual abuse. Research is also needed to examine the role of social support in buffering the effects of abuse on the risk of revictimization.

In the previous section, we noted how certain behaviors can mitigate stress reactions, at least in the short-term; in the next section, we discuss some of the cognitive defenses used by victims of severe child abuse. Analogous to the use of drugs or alcohol as a way of escaping from painful internal states, defenses such as dissociation, repression, and denial are employed to block or distort painful experiences. Unfortunately, defenses that were once adaptive in childhood often become maladaptive in adulthood. In some cases, defenses may even increase the risk of subsequent victimization.

COGNITIVE DEFENSES

When exposed to overwhelming trauma, individuals tend to protect themselves by relying on cognitive defenses. These defenses serve to distort, block, or prevent threatening material from entering conscious awareness, or to minimize its impact. A variety of mechanisms have been identified over the years, including repression, denial, suppression, and dissociation.

Until recently, Freud's concept of repression had received more attention than all of the other cognitive defenses combined. However, over the past 10 years, there has been a resurgence of interest in Pierre Janet's concept of dissociation. van der Kolk and van der Hart (1991) suggest that it is reasonable to use the concept of repression for the defense against primitive, forbidden, that is, id-impulses. The concept of dissociation, they argue, "is best suited for application with regard to traumatic memories . . . [as] there is little evidence for an active process of [the] pushing away of the overwhelming experience" (p. 437).

Investigators have found that dissociative pathology is associated with a variety of traumatic experiences, including severe childhood sexual and physical abuse (see Putnam, 1989; Briere, 1992), combat exposure (Brende, 1986), witnessing a violent death during childhood (Putnam, Guroff, Silberman, Barbau, & Post, 1986), and rape in adolescence or adulthood (Coons & Milstein, 1986). In turn, it has been hypothesized that dissociation is a normal defensive process that is employed to cope with traumatic experiences (Evans, 1988; Terr, 1991; Spiegel, 1986; Beahrs, 1990). Putnam (1989), for example, argued that dissociation can be functional since it provides: "(1) escape from the constraints of reality; (2) [the] compartmentalization of traumatic memories and affect outside of conscious awareness; (3) alteration or detachment from the trauma (so that the trauma happens to someone else or the depersonalized self); and (4) analgesia" (p. 53).

Spiegel (1986) presented a similar view: "Dissociation is a defense often mobilized against the pain and helplessness engendered by traumatic experiences" (p. 123). Serving to block the immediate experience of a painful event from awareness, dissociative processes allow the individual to go about his or her life as if nothing traumatic had happened, and this can be viewed as adaptive. With regard to incest victims, Evans (1988) described how dissociation represents a survival tool. Dissociation protects the ego by keeping traumatic experiences from conscious awareness, since affect and memory are encapsulated and split off from the self.

Although dissociation may represent an adaptive coping strategy in the short run, continual reliance on the phenomena can become maladaptive and place the individual at risk for subsequent victimization. Indeed, many believe that the more dissociation is used to defend against repeated childhood trauma, the greater the chances the individual will employ dissociation as a primary method of defense in adulthood (Braun & Sachs, 1985; Putnam, 1989). Chu (1992) postulated that adult women with histories of childhood sexual abuse, who rely heavily on cognitive defenses such as dissociation, frequently lack the anticipatory anxiety that would normally signal the presence of danger, and thus are at substantial risk for revictimization.

Other researchers in the field have endorsed similar views on the topic. Kluft (1990b) studied 18 incest victims (17 females and 1 male) who had developed dissociative disorders and had been sexually exploited by at least one psychotherapist. Of this group, 78% had been raped as adults. With regard to their adult victimization experiences, Kluft found that the patients experienced "extreme difficulty in perceiving and reacting to danger signals appropriately" (p. 169).

Many of the individuals in Kluft's sample blocked out or minimized information that might have given them reason for caution. For example, one woman was unable to perceive sexual advances by her therapist as inappropriate or wrong. Specifically, she failed to integrate this information into conscious awareness, which prevented her from perceiving the situation accurately and from taking action to avoid further victimization. In another case, a woman allowed her victimizer to babysit her own children. According to Kluft, the woman was "decatastrophizing," or minimizing the seriousness of the situation, and in effect denying, or demonstrating an inability to see, the potential danger involved.

Kluft (1990b) explained that "the exclusion of subsets of material from conscious awareness sets the stage for the development of faulty cognitions that, by failing to alert the sufferer of possible dangers, facilitate subsequent revictimization" (p. 171). In other words, dissociation excludes from awareness unsettling information that could prevent the formation of inaccurate or distorted views of the situation. With regard to relationships, some patients even demonstrate confabulation or outright distortion (Kluft, 1990b, p. 171). They fill in the gaps of dissociated material with more acceptable or pleasurable information, thereby making the situation seem more tolerable.

It should be noted that Kluft's work has all the limitations that anecdotal clinical reports contain. For example, although Kluft (1990b) reported that a high percentage of his subjects experienced such abstract phenomena as "selective abstraction," "arbitrary inference," and "distortion of self-perception" (p. 170), his data came from personal impressions rather than reliable, well-validated measures. Clearly, controlled studies are needed to elucidate the role of cognitive defenses in the revictimization cycle.

Despite the fact that many clinicians have hypothesized that certain cognitive defenses place a woman at risk for revictimization, only a few empirical studies have been conducted on this topic. When investigating the psychological aftermath of sexual assault in a sample of university students ($N = 502$) and university employees ($N = 503$), Roth, Wayland, and Woolsey (1990) found that subjects who reported repeated incestuous sexual victimization had elevated scores on the Denial subscale of the Impact of Events Scale. The authors argue that a primitive defense mechanism (denial) is needed to protect ego integrity in the face of massive or repeated trauma, and that avoidant defense strategies such as repression, denial, and dissociation place a woman at risk for further victimization. However, because Roth et al.'s study was not prospective in nature, their data cannot be used to establish a definitive link between denial and subsequent victimization.

The first large-scale study designed to examine whether dissociation might be a risk factor for victimization was conducted by Becker-Lausen, Sanders, and Chinsky (1992). Noting that child abuse frequently seems to be related to depression (see also Finkelhor & Browne, 1985; Gidycz, Nelson, & Latham, in press; Goldston, Turnquist, & Knutson, 1989; Herman, 1981; Mannarino & Cohen, 1986) and dissociation (Briere & Runtz, 1987, 1988a, 1988b; Chu & Dill, 1990; Sanders & Giolas, 1991; Sanders, McRoberts, & Tollefson, 1989), and that increased levels of general symptomatology are associated with a variety of negative life events (see Sarason, Johnson, & Siegel, 1978), the authors tested the assumption that dissociation and depression mediate the process of revictimization by performing a structural analysis on data obtained from 299 undergraduate college students.

In the study, subjects were asked to fill out a series of questionnaires, including the Dissociative Experiences Scale (DES), the Child Abuse and Trauma (CAT) Scale (Sanders & Giolas, 1991), the Beck Depression Inventory (BDI), an object relations measure of interpersonal relationship impairment, the Life Experiences Survey (LES), and a negative events checklist. All data were gathered during one session; the study was not prospective.

Based on the results of a series of path analyses, the authors concluded that child maltreatment was significantly related to depression, dissociation, and negative life outcomes, and that both dissociation and depression mediated the effects of child maltreatment. In other words, subjects who were maltreated experienced both depressive and dissociative symptoms, which in turn led to negative life events. Interestingly, there seemed to be two distinct mediational effects. Whereas both depression and dissociation mediated the connection between child maltreatment and negative life events, dissociation, but not depression, was related to later victimization. Victimization was defined liberally, and included such experiences as rape, robbery, or being involved with an alcoholic or drug addict. On the other hand, depression, but not dissociation, was responsible for interpersonal difficulties.

Becker-Lausen et al.'s findings (1992) are consistent with previous research in the areas of depression and dissociation. The "gloom-and-doom" outlook characteristic of depressed individuals is likely to lead to interpersonal rejection. Friends who are potential sources of nurturance and support quickly tire of a pessimistic outlook and pull away from the depressed individual. This retreat only confirms the depressed person's negative world view, and he or she falls prey to a self-fulfilling prophecy (Coyne, 1976; Yapko, 1988).

Dissociative symptomatology, on the other hand, was not found to be related to self-reported interpersonal difficulties. Becker-Lausen et al. (1992) suggest that one possible explanation for the absence of such a relation is that individuals who dissociate lack awareness of the nuances of interpersonal interactions. In other words, their relationships are, in fact, poor, although they are not perceived that way, because these individuals have learned to tune out, or block from conscious awareness, potentially painful information in their environment. This detachment allows dissociators, compared to depressed subjects, to be less sensitive to interpersonal hurt and rejection.

Unfortunately, when people are detached from hurt and rejection, they are also increasingly at risk for subsequent victimization. In Kluft's words, dissociators become "sitting ducks." They detach from reality and disregard cues that lead nondissociators to use caution when entering into interpersonal relationships. Dissociative patients seem to have extreme difficulty in perceiving and reacting to danger signals appropriately. As Becker-Lausen et al. (1992) noted, high dissociators might have difficulty learning from their experiences to avoid danger because they tend to detach themselves from those experiences, and in the process compartmentalize rather than integrate important information.

Becker-Lausen et al.'s (1992) findings are extremely interesting to researchers studying dissociation and revictimization. As previously mentioned, their study is the first of its kind to examine whether dissociation might play a role in the process of revictimization. One overriding limitation of their study, however, is that Becker-Lausen et al. did not gather their data prospectively. Because dissociation scores were obtained at the same time that victimization status was determined, directionality is unclear. Becker-Lausen et al.'s findings could simply reflect the fact that subjects who have endured a greater number of traumatic or aversive experiences have higher dissociation scores than other subjects.

The authors use the term "causal" when reporting their findings, claiming that their research extends previous findings by establishing a causal relationship between dissociation and victimization, as opposed to one that simply involves a correlation between the two factors. (Becker-Lausen et al., 1992, p. 1). Yet researchers should not make definitive causal statements simply because of the appearance of causal modeling, particularly when data are not collected prospectively. Although Becker-Lausen et al.'s (1992) findings are intriguing, their study needs to be replicated with prospective data.

Cognitive defenses are mechanisms that are hypothesized to distort, block, or prevent threatening material from entering conscious awareness. However, very little is known about how dissociation affects the way information is processed in actual situations where a high risk for abuse and victimization exists. To address this issue, we are presently conducting a study to determine whether subjects who score high on the DES (Bernstein & Putnam, 1986) are less able to detect danger cues in a videotape of events culminating in a date rape than subjects who score in the midrange of the scale.

Furthermore, because dissociation is a multidimensional construct, with components of amnesia, fantasy/absorption, and depersonalization emerging from factor analytic studies (see Ross, Joshi, & Currie, 1991); Lynn, Newfeld, Green, Sandberg, & Rhue, in press), it would be interesting to determine which of these factors, in combination with measures of general psychopathology (e.g., depression, anxiety), post-traumatic symptoms, and situational factors, predict revictimization.

CLINICAL IMPLICATIONS

Clinicians need to be aware of the fact that a history of abuse places the client at risk for revictimization. At the very least, it is wise for clinicians to apprise clients of their high-risk status and evaluate the degree to which one or more specific risk factors are evident in the clinical picture. All of the factors we have discussed may influence the lives of various people, at various times, and under various conditions. For instance, certain clients might be motivated to master or control their behaviors and feelings (and that of others) in sexual situations that are somehow associated with or reminiscent of sexual situations in which abuse occurred in the past; other clients might lack social skills, have poor self-esteem, or be willing to accept a high level of aggression or interpersonal violence; while still other clients might repeatedly ignore or minimize danger cues or alter their level of psychophysiological stress by consuming alcohol in high-risk situations. Of course, certain clients might be particularly prone to revictimization in that they exhibit multiple motives, behavior patterns, and cognitive coping strategies that place them at high risk.

Ultimately, the therapist's responsibility is to carefully examine the repercussions of earlier abuse-related experiences in light of the clients' post-traumatic symptoms, current behaviors and involvement in high-risk situations, representations of the self and others, and coping mechanisms. Of course, this must be done in a caring, empathic manner to avoid retraumatizing the client and provoking a negative transference reaction. The clinical implications of, and useful directions for, working with high-risk clients can be derived from each of the three categories we discussed.

Theories that emphasize the client's need to master and control situations suggest that insight can be an important therapeutic mechanism. Helping the client to draw a connection between his or her earlier traumatic experiences and current life situations, behavioral reenactments, and cognitive patterns of intrusion and avoidance is integral to minimizing the risk of revictimization. Insight into the ways in which the client's current representations of others are related to earlier abusive relationships is necessary to free the client of his or her need to recapitulate earlier dysfunctional relationships and master the unresolved feelings associated with them.

Information processing theory also suggests that clients need to place abuse-related experiences into an acceptable cognitive frame or "perspective on life" in order to break the cycle of intrusion and avoidance of abuse-related thoughts and experiences. For instance, the abuse victim can come to view the world as "basically good," but the perpetrator as psychologically disturbed, while he or she recognizes the need to take due caution in his or her relationships with others.

Understanding the various abuse-related manifestations of dysfunctional learning can assist the clinician in tailoring specific treatment interventions. These can be targeted at altering faulty views of the self and others, modifying inappropriate sexual behaviors, mitigating extreme dependency, improving interpersonal judgment, and minimizing feelings of passivity, helplessness, and excessive impulsivity. Helping clients gain self-respect, learn to accept and communicate the idea that violence is unacceptable in intimate relationships, and learn that it is imperative to establish appropriate limits in such relationships, will, in all likelihood, minimize the risk of revictimization.

Some clients who present with a history of abuse will, no doubt, also present with dissociative symptoms. Rather than retreating, avoiding, or detaching from threatening or conflict-laden situations in a dysfunctional, passive manner, dissociative clients can profit from learning behavioral and cognitive coping strategies that might involve rehearsing more adaptive self-talk and assertive behaviors. Behavioral techniques such as systematic desensitization, directed imagery, and cue-controlled relaxation, could also be used to reduce anxiety symptoms that, hypothetically, contribute to dissociative reactions. With dissociative clients, it may be particularly important for therapists to learn about their perceptions of relationships and their ability to perceive and react to danger signals appropriately. For example, certain clients may need to be alerted and sensitized to high-risk situations to minimize their tendency to compartmentalize, deny, or distort their perceptions of "dangerous" situations to make them palatable or acceptable.

In fact, for all clients at high risk for revictimization, education is a crucial component of psychotherapy. Hence, therapists must assess the degree to which clients engage in high-risk behaviors and deal in a direct and forthright way with clients' substance abuse problems and poor communication techniques about such matters as sexual feelings and limit setting. Each client will present a unique blend of challenges for the therapist to struggle with. Hence, a knowledge of the personal and behavioral dynamics associated with increased risk for victimization is essential in order for the therapist to convert the challenges the client presents into opportunities for the client's growth and development.

REFERENCES

Beahrs, J. O. (1990). The evolution of post-traumatic behavior: Three hypotheses. *Dissociation, 3*, 15–21.

Becker-Lausen, E., Sanders, B., & Chinsky, J. M. (1992). *A structural analysis of child abuse and negative life experiences.* Paper presented at the 100th annual convention of the American Psychological Association, Washington, DC.

Bernstein, E. M., & Putnam, F. W. (1986). Development, reliability, and validity of a dissociation scale. *Journal of Nervous and Mental Disease, 174*, 727–735.

Braun, B. G., & Sachs, R. G. (1985). The development of multiple personality disorder: Predisposing, precipitating, and perpetuating factors. In R. P. Kluft (Ed.), *Childhood antecedents of multiple personality* (pp. 37–64). Washington, DC: American Psychiatric Press.

Brende, J. O. (1986, September). *Dissociative disorders in Vietnam combat veterans.* Paper presented at the conference for Multiple Personality Disorder and Dissociative States, Chicago, IL.

Briere, J. N. (1992). *Child abuse trauma: Theory and treatment of the lasting effects.* Newbury Park, CA: Sage.

Briere, J., & Runtz, M. (1987). Post sexual abuse trauma: Data and implications for clinical practice. *Journal of Interpersonal Violence, 2*, 367–379.

Briere, J., & Runtz, M. (1988a). Symptomatology associated with childhood sexual victimization in a nonclinical adult sample. *Child Abuse and Neglect, 12*, 51–59.

Briere, J., & Runtz, M. (1988b). Multivariate correlates of childhood psychological and physical maltreatment among university women. *Child Abuse and Neglect, 12*, 331–341.

Bryer, J. B., Nelson, B. A., Miller, J. B., & Krol, P. A. (1987). Childhood sexual and physical abuse as factors in adult psychiatric illness. *American Journal of Psychiatry, 144*, 1426–1430.

Buchele, B. J. (1993, Spring). *Object-relations theory and the treatment of sexual abuse victims.* Paper presented at the symposium on the Treatment of Sexual Abuse, Harding Hospital, Colombus, Ohio.

Byers, E. S., Giles, B. L., & Price, D. L. (1987). Definiteness and effectiveness of women's responses to unwanted sexual advances: A laboratory investigation. *Basic and Applied Social Psychology, 8*, 321–338.

Cashdan, S. (1988). *Object relations therapy: Using the relationship.* New York: W. W. Norton.

Chu, J. A. (1992). The revictimization of adult women with histories of childhood abuse. *Journal of Psychotherapy Practice and Research, 1*, 259–269.

Chu, J. A., & Dill, D. L. (1990). Dissociative symptoms in relation to childhood physical and sexual abuse. *American Journal of Psychiatry, 147*, 887–892.

Cole, P. M., & Putnam, F. W. (1992). Effect of incest on self and social functioning:

A developmental psychopathology perspective. *Journal of Consulting and Clinical Psychology, 60*, 174–183.

Coons, P. M., & Milstein, V. (1986). Psychosexual disturbances in multiple personality: Characteristics, etiology, and treatment. *Journal of Clinical Psychiatry, 47*, 106–110.

Coyne, J. C. (1976). Depression and the responses of others. *Journal of Abnormal Psychology, 85*, 186–193.

Craine, L. S., Henson, C. E., Colliver, J. A., & MacLean, D. G. (1988). Prevalence of a history of sexual abuse among female psychiatric patients in a state hospital system. *Hospital and Community Psychiatry, 39*, 300–304.

DeYoung, M. (1981). Case reports: The sexual exploitation of incest victims by health professionals. *Victimology, 6*, 92–101.

Ellis, E. M., Atkeson, B. M., & Calhoun, K. S. (1982). An examination of differences between multiple- and single-incident victims of sexual assault. *Journal of Abnormal Psychology, 91*, 221–224.

Evans, S. (1988). *The treatment of shame and guilt.* Minneapolis: Haworth Press.

Fairbairn, W. R. D. (1954). Observations on the nature of hysterical states. *British Journal of Medical Psychology, 27*, 105–125.

Finkelhor, D. (1979). *Sexually victimized children.* New York: The Free Press.

Finkelhor, D., & Browne, A. (1985). The traumatic impact of child sexual abuse: A conceptualization. *Americal Journal of Orthopsychiatry, 55*, 530–541.

Finkelhor, D., Hotaling, G., Lewis, I. A., & Smith, C. (1990). Sexual abuse in a national survey of adult men and women: Prevalence, characteristics, and risk factors. *Child Abuse and Neglect, 14*, 19–28.

Freud, S. (1954). *Beyond the pleasure principle.* In J. Strachey (Ed. and Trans.), *The standard edition of the complete psychological works of Sigmund Freud* (Vol. 18, pp. 7–64). London: Hogarth Press. (Original work published 1920)

Fromuth, M. E. (1986). The relationship of childhood sexual abuse with later psychological and sexual adjustment in a sample of college women. *Child Abuse and Neglect, 10*, 5–15.

Gagnon, J. (1965). Female child victims of sex offenses. *Social Problems, 13*, 176–192.

Gelinas, D. J. (1983). The persistent negative effects of incest. *Psychiatry, 46*, 312–332.

Gidycz, C. A., Nelson, C. L., & Latham, L. (1992). *Relation of a sexual assault experience in adulthood to prior victimization experiences: A prospective analysis.* Unpublished manuscript, Ohio University.

Green, A. (1978). Self-destructive behavior in battered children. *American Journal of Psychiatry, 135*, 579–582.

Herman, J. L. (1981). *Father–daughter incest.* Cambridge, MA: Harvard University Press.

Horowitz, M. J. (1975). Intrusive and repetitive thoughts after experimental stress. *Archives of General Psychiatry, 32*, 1457–1463.

James, J., & Meyerding, J. (1977). Early sexual experience and prostitution. *American Journal of Psychiatry, 134*, 1381–1385.

Kanin, E. J., & Parcell, S. R. (1977). Sexual aggression: A second look at the offended female. *Archives of Sexual Behavior, 6*, 67–76.

Kendall-Tackett, K. A., Williams, L. M., & Finkelhor, D. (1993). Impact of sexual abuse on children: A review and synthesis of recent empirical studies. *Psychological Bulletin, 113*, 164–180.

Kilpatrick, D. G., Best, C. L., Veronen, L. J., Amick, A. E., Villeponteaux, L. A., & Ruff, G. A. (1985). Mental health correlates of criminal victimization: A random community survey. *Journal of Consulting and Clinical Psychology, 53*, 866–873.

Kluft, R. P. (1989). Treating patients sexually exploited by a previous therapist. *Psychiatric Clinics of North America, 12*, 483–500.

Kluft, R. P. (1990a). Incest and subsequent revictimization: The case of therapist–patient sexual exploitation, with a description of the sitting duck syndrome. In R. P. Kluft (Ed.), *Incest-related syndromes of adult psychopathology* (pp. 263–287). Washington, DC: American Psychiatric Press.

Kluft, R. P. (1990b). Dissociation and subsequent vulnerability: A preliminary study. *Dissociation, 3*, 167–173.

Koss, M. P., & Dinero, T. E. (1989). Discriminant analysis of risk factors for sexual victimization among a national sample of college women. *Journal of Consulting and Clinical Psychology, 57*, 242–250.

Koss, M. P., Gidycz, C. A., & Wisniewski, N. (1987). The scope of rape: Incidence and prevalence of sexual aggression and victimization in a national sample of higher education students. *Journal of Consulting and Clinical Therapy, 55*, 162–170.

Koss, M. P., & Oros, C. J. (1982). Sexual Experiences Survey: A research instrument investigating sexual aggression and victimization. *Journal of Consulting and Clinical Psychology, 50*, 455–457.

Lynn, S. J., Newfeld, V., Green, J., Sandberg, D., & Rhue, J. (in press). Daydreaming, fantasy and psychopathology. In R. Kunzendorf, N. Spanos, & B. Wallace (Eds.), *Hypnosis and imagination*. Amityville, NY: Baywood.

Mannarino, A. P., & Cohen, J. A. (1986). A clinical-demographic study of sexually abused children. *Child Abuse and Neglect, 10*, 17–23.

Mandoki, C. A., & Burkhart, B. R. (1989). Sexual victimization: Is there a vicious cycle? *Violence and Victims, 4*, 179–190.

Masterson, J. F., & Klein, R. (1989). *Psychotherapy of the disorders of the self: The Masterson approach*. New York: Brunner/Mazel.

McCann, I. L., Sakheim, D. K., & Abrahamson, D. J. (1988). Trauma and victimization: A model of psychological adaptation. *The Counseling Psychologist, 16*, 531–549.

Miller, B., & Marshall, J. C. (1987). Coercive sex on the university campus. *Journal of College Student Personnel, 28*, 38–47.

Miller, J., Moeller, D., Kaufman, A., Divasto, P., Pathak, D., & Christy, J. (1978). Recidivism among sex assault victims. *American Journal of Psychiatry, 135*, 1103–1104.

Muehlenhard, C. L., & Linton, M.A. (1987). Date rape and sexual aggression in the dating situation: Incidence and risk factors. *Journal of Counseling Psychology, 34*, 186–196.

Pope, K. S., & Bouhoutsos, J. C. (1986). *Sexual intimacy between therapists and patients*. New York: Praeger.

Putnam, F. W. (1989). *Diagnosis and treatment of multiple personality disorder*. New York: Guilford Press.

Putnam, F. W., Guroff, J. J., Silberman, E. K., Barban, L., & Post, R. M. (1986). The clinical phenomenology of multiple personality disorder: Review of 100 recent cases. *Journal of Clinical Psychiatry, 47*, 285–293.

Ross, C. A., Anderson, G., Heber, S., & Norton, G. R. (1990). Dissociation and abuse among multiple personality patients, prostitutes, and exotic dancers. *Hospital and Community Psychiatry, 41*, 328–330.

Ross, C. A., Joshi, S., & Currie, R. (1991). Dissociative experiences in the general population. *American Journal of Psychiatry, 147*, 1547–1552.

Roth, S., Wayland, K., & Woolsey, M. (1990). Victimization history and victim–assailant relationship as factors in recovery from sexual assault. *Journal of Traumatic Stress, 3*, 169–180.

Russell, D. (1984). *Sexual exploitation: Rape, child sexual abuse, and workplace harassment*. Beverly Hills, CA: Sage.

Russell, D. (1986). *The secret trauma: Incest in the lives of girls and women*. New York: Basic Books.

Sanders, B., & Giolas, M. H. (1991). Dissociation and childhood trauma in psychologically disturbed adolescents. *American Journal of Psychiatry, 148*, 50–54.

Sanders, B., McRoberts, G., & Tollefson, C. (1989). Childhood stress and dissociation in a college population. *Dissociation, 2*, 17–23.

Sarason, I. G., Johnson, J. H., & Siegel, J. M., (1978). Assessing the impact of life changes: Development of the Life Experiences Survey. *Journal of Consulting and Clinical Psychology, 46*, 932–946.

Sedney, M. A., & Brooks, B. (1984). Factors associated with a history of childhood sexual experience in a nonclinical female population. *Journal of the American Academy of Child Psychiatry, 23*, 215–218.

Seligman, M. E. P. (1975). *Helplessness: On depression, development, and death*. New York: W. H. Freeman.

Shapiro, S. (1987). Self-mutilation and self-blame in incest victims. *American Journal of Psychotherapy, 41*, 46–54.

Silbert, M. H., & Pines, A. M. (1981). Sexual child abuse as an antecedent to prostitution. *Child Abuse and Neglect, 5*, 407–411.

Sorensen, S. B., Stein, J. A., Siegel, J. M., Golding, J. M., & Burnam, M. A. (1987). Prevalence of adult sexual assault: The Los Angeles epidemiologic catchment area study. *American Journal of Epidemiology, 126*, 1141–1164.

Spiegel, D. (1986). Dissociating damage. *American Journal of Clinical Hypnosis, 29*, 123–131.

Suomi, S. J. (1984). The development of affect in Rhesus monkeys. In N. Fox & R. Davidson (Eds), *The psychobiology of affective development* (pp. 119–159). Hillsdale, NJ: Lawrence Erlbaum.

Terr, L. C. (1985). Psychic trauma in children and adolescents. *Psychiatric Clinics of North America, 8*, 815–835.

Terr, L. C. (1991). Childhood traumas: An outline and overview. *American Journal of Psychiatry, 148*, 10–20.

Tsai, M., & Wagner, N. (1978). Therapy groups for women sexually molested as children. *Archives of Sexual Behavior, 7*, 417–427.

van der Kolk, B. A. (1987). *Psychological trauma*. Washington, DC: American Psychiatric Press.

van der Kolk, B. A. (1989). The compulsion to repeat the trauma: Re-enactment, revictimization, and masochism. *Psychiatric Clinics of North America, 12*, 389–411.

van der Kolk, B. A., Herman, J., & Perry, J. (1988). *Childhood trauma and self-destructive behavior in adulthood*. Unpublished data.

van der Kolk, B. A., & van der Hart, O. (1991). The intrusive past: The flexibility of memory and the engraving of trauma. *American Imago, 48*, 425–454.

Walklate, S. (1989). *Victimology*. Boston: Unwin Hyman.

Wyatt, G. E., Guthrie, D., & Notgrass, C. M. (1992). Differential effects of women's child sexual abuse and subsequent sexual revictimization. *Journal of Consulting and Clinical Psychology, 60*, 167–173.

Yapko, M. D. (1988). *When living hurts: Directives for treating depression*. New York: Brunner/Mazel.

Yates, A. (1983). Children eroticized by incest. *American Journal of Psychiatry, 139*, 482–485.

Ziegenhagen, E. A. (1976). The recidivist victim of violent crime. *Victimology, 1*, 538–550.

13

Pseudo-Identity and the Treatment of Personality Change in Victims of Captivity and Cults

Louis Jolyon West
Paul R. Martin

Dissociative phenomena are not necessarily symptomatic of illness, and probably represent a continuum beginning with normal psychobiological modulation of information—incoming, stored, and outgoing—by the brain (West, 1967). In recent years there has been a sharp increase of interest in dissociative phenomena accompanying psychiatric disorders, especially multiple personality and related disorders of identity, including states of possession (Bliss, 1986; Kluft, 1991; Suryani & Jensen, 1993). Dissociative *symptoms* also are important in many other types of psychopathology, and commonly accompany a range of psychiatric disorder from schizophrenic illnesses to severe stress reactions. Still, the distortion or alteration of a person's identity and the appearance of a new and different persona remains one of the most interesting manifestations of dissociation.

Prolonged environmental stress, or life situations profoundly different from the usual, can disrupt the normally integrative functions of personality. Individuals subjected to such forces may adapt through dissociation by generating an altered persona, or pseudo-identity (West, 1994). Such a pseudo-identity enables the subject better to cope with the extraordinary situation in which he finds himself, regardless of how he got there.[1] Parents and others close to individuals who have become members of totalist cults are often astonished at such changes, saying "He has become a different person." This article is based on observations of such changelings from a clinical point of view.

Conditions of brutal captivity, such as those experienced by prisoners of war (POWs) or civilian victims of hostage taking, in which the captor seeks to force a false confession or induce compliant behavior, can generate a type of post-traumatic stress disorder (PTSD) in which dissociative features are prominent. During the Korean war, the relative success of the Chinese communists in eliciting false confessions of war crimes (e.g., germ warfare), self-denunciations, and participation in propaganda activities was in large measure achieved because of the captors' absolute control over the environment of the prisoners. To achieve this control, the communists contrived a variety of stressors, which produced in their captives a state of debility, dependency, and chronic apprehension or dread (Farber, Harlow, & West, 1957; West, 1964).

Civilian prisoners were also subjected to prolonged manipulation by their Chinese communist captors to produce altered political convictions, as described in Lifton's discussion of thought reform (Lifton, 1961). As with the Korean War POWs, these civilian victims were subjected to prolonged stress in situations from which, at least for a time, there was no escape. Necessarily, they became dependent upon their captors for various physical and psychological needs. In response to these conditions their personalities begin to change in many cases. O'Neil and Demos (1977) have likened the first step in the thought reform process to the creation of an identity crisis. In our view, it is during such a crisis that a new pseudo-identity may begin to emerge. Once formed, it is likely to endure, and gradually grow stronger and better defined, as long as the demand characteristics of the situation require it.

Long before the term "Stockholm syndrome" was coined (see below), difficult-to-explain feelings of sympathy and even identification with one's captors were recounted by former prisoners. One of these was Hungary's late Cardinal Mindszenty, who was arrested, tried, and imprisoned from 1948 until the 1956 uprising in Budapest. In his *Memoirs* (1974), Mindszenty wrote that within 2 weeks of his arrest, under constant coercive interrogation he found himself thinking along different lines from before and seeing things from his captors' point of view. His judgment, reasoning, and sense of self became distorted. He wrote: "Without knowing what had happened to me, I had become a different person" (p. 114).

Patricia Hearst was violently abducted by members of the Symbionese Liberation Army in February of 1974, brutalized, raped, tortured, and forced to participate in illegal acts beginning with the bank robbery for which she was later (in our view wrongly) convicted. The traumatic kidnapping and subsequent 2 months of torture produced in her a state of emotional regression and fearful compliance with the demands and expectations of her captors. This was quickly followed by the coerced transformation of Patty into Tania and subsequently (less well known to the public) into Pearl, after additional trauma over a period of many months (Hearst & Moscow, 1988; *The Trial of Patty Hearst*, 1976). Tania was merely a role coerced on pain of death; it was Pearl who later represented the pseudo-identity which was found on psychiatric examination by one of us (West) shortly after Hearst's arrest by the FBI. Chronic symptoms of PTSD were also prominent in this case.

The term "Stockholm syndrome" was coined to describe a certain psychological phenomenon in hostages following a 1974 bank holdup in Sweden. Four employees were held captive by two robbers for 5½ days. During the ordeal, some hostages became sympathetic toward the robbers. In fact, one female hostage swiftly and unaccountably fell in love with one of her captors and then publicly berated the Swedish prime minister for his failure to understand the criminal's point of view. For a limited period of time after her release, the former hostage continued to express affection for her captor (Ochberg, 1978).

Other hostages have also developed sympathy for—or identified with—their captors. For example, in 1975, during the 13-day seizure of a Dutch train by South Moluccan gunmen demanding freedom for their islands in the Malay archipelago, despite the executions of 2 hostages, some of the surviving captives rapidly developed feelings of affection or sympathy for their murderous captors, along with attitudes of distrust toward the legitimate Dutch authorities. A psychiatrist might better define this phenomenon using the more psychodynamically descriptive phrase: "identification with the aggressor" (coined for a different purpose during World War II by Anna Freud). If this process is sufficiently profound and prolonged, in our view the accompanying personality change may best be understood in terms of pseudo-identity as explicated below.

Identification with the aggressor has been analyzed in relation to a variety of psychiatrically important situations, ranging from imprisonment in Nazi concentration camps, where doomed prisoners sometimes sought out discarded insignias and other shreds of SS uniforms with which to adorn their rags, to the battered children who grow up to become child-battering parents. However, some cases do not involve prisoners or captives. For example, Solomon Perel, the subject of a recent film (*Europa, Europa* [Holland, Menegoz, & Brauner, 1991]), was a German Jewish boy who assumed a non-Jewish identity in order to cope with the life-threatening conditions of the time. He transformed himself into Joseph ("Jupp") under extremely stressful circumstances.

Knowing that Jews would be killed, he got rid of all documents identifying him as a Jew and, in the chaos of war, said, "I am a patriotic German." He even served in the German army. Gradually, however, the teen-ager's role became a new identity because of the demand characteristics of his situation. For years after the war, following his emigration to Israel, Perel experienced moments when he had to ascertain whether it was Sol or Jupp who was answering a question (Williams, 1992). Like the incomprehensibly compliant Jozsef Cardinal Mindszenty and the abnormally passive Patricia/Tania/Pearl/Hearst, under stress, Solomon Perel's identity had changed. The new pseudo-identity, initially formed as a role played in response to stressful circumstances, was a different personality of sorts. This personality was superimposed upon the original which, while not completely forgotten, was enveloped within the shell of the pseudo-identity.

Through the exercise of psychosocial forces more subtle than those described above, people can be deliberately manipulated, influenced, and controlled to a considerable degree, and induced to express beliefs and exhibit behaviors far different from what their lives up to then would have logically or reasonably predicted. While the thought reform program of the Chinese communists to convert people to "right thinking" was hardly subtle, the indoctrination techniques applied to new recruits by contemporary totalist cults can be very subtle indeed (West, 1989, 1993). Subjects are forced to communicate verbally and continuously, in a strictly controlled fashion. Most of these cults rely also on the effects of structured group dynamics, environmental manipulation and control, the relationship of dominant leaders to dependent members, the relative initial isolation of recruits from previous ideas or relationships, and the evolution of a new identity with constant group pressures to bring errant individuals into line.

A totalist cult is defined as follows: "*Cult* (totalist type): a group or movement exhibiting a great or excessive devotion or dedication to some person, idea, or thing, and employing unethical, manipulative or coercive techniques of persuasion and control (e.g., isolation from former friends and family, debilitation, use of special methods to heighten suggestibility and subservience, powerful group pressure, information management, promotion of total dependency on the group and fear of leaving it, suspension of individuality and critical judgment, and so on, designed to advance the goals of the group's leaders, to the possible or actual detriment of members, their families, or the community." The basis for this definition, and a general discussion of the cult problem, is given elsewhere (West, 1989). Among various totalist cults, there may be some differences as to how intense the persuasive activities are, and in the degree to which recruits can be separated from their previous social networks. Even though he may have been attracted to the cult by elaborate and deceptive recruiting techniques, the neophyte cultist enters it "voluntarily." With rare exceptions, nobody puts a gun to his head. Yet, successful indoctrination of a cult member often includes many elements similar to the political indoctrination by such groups as the Chinese communists, which Schein (1961) described as coercive persuasion. In cults, as in the Chinese "brainwashing," "thought reform," or "coercive persuasion," people are often encouraged to criticize themselves in small-group confessionals as a means of strengthening their dependence on the group. As the process continues, members are systematically trained to relinquish independent action and thought, since only obedient behaviors and passive attitudes are rewarded, while resistance or self-assertion is punished.

Even groups that have derived from respectable religious sects (such as the Lundgren cult, a splinter of a sect of the LDS, see below) or that have evolved from therapeutic communities such as Synanon, can evolve into totalist cults if the autonomy of the members is progressively diminished, while the concentration of power in the leadership grows more and more absolute. Under these conditions usually the emphasis shifts from the members' well-being to their manipulation and exploitation. In this way, it is easy to understand how the followers of Jim Jones (People's Temple), L. Ron Hubbard (Church of Scientology), Sun Myung Moon (Unification Church), Moses David (Children of God), Elizabeth Clare Prophet (Church Universal and Triumphant), Rajneesh, and others are successfully influenced to become "different people."

Lifton (1961) describes how certain Chinese citizens and Westerners, having undergone the stressful process of "thought reform" and apparently changed their political beliefs, upon liberation continued to parrot the programmed Maoist clichés for a time until, in the new and free environment, those beliefs and the attendant formulae began to crumble away, leaving each bewildered survivor with an acute identity problem. Lifton characterizes this process as resembling death and rebirth. Former members of religious cults, or veterans of mass-marketed group therapies and self-help techniques, have called abrupt forms of such transformation "snapping" (Conway & Siegelman, 1978). This corresponds to the observations of many former cult victims, who have undergone "deprogramming" and, as a result, abruptly reverted from their cult-induced pseudo-identity to something resembling their previous or original personality. Indeed, "snapping" seems like an appropriate term when the victim, having been coerced or manipulated into his strange pseudo-identity, eventually "snaps out of it." He is again his old self, but with some serious new problems as a result of the cult-related experience and the trauma involved in relation to it. Furthermore, years may have passed since the original identity was functioning normally; meanwhile the world has become a different place.

The term pseudo-identity has only been used twice previously in the scientific literature. In 1974, Glatzel used it to describe a delusional alteration of self in cases of major depression involving cyclothymic illness (Glatzel, 1974). To the best of our knowledge this usage has not since been repeated. More recently, Girodo (1985) employed the term when describing problems experienced by certain undercover narcotics agents who, after prolonged role playing, found it difficult to discontinue assumed behaviors when an operation was finished. Employed only once or twice in Girodo's article, the term was used casually to convey the sense of a long-assumed role, not a dissociative disorder, and was limited to the highly specialized circumstances of undercover work. In fact, Girodo minimized the possibility of dissociative reactions in the subjects he studied. However, careful review of his clinical material suggests that some cases of pseudo-identity in our sense may indeed have occurred in certain cases, studied by Girodo, of law-enforcement officers who were required to play the part of criminals for months or even years. In our view some of these officers showed symptoms of PTSD as well.

Through hypnotic suggestion, it may be possible to create temporary distortions of values, viewpoints, or perceptions of reality, which are sufficient to induce in some subjects behaviors that would be otherwise unacceptable to them. Certain hypnotists (e.g., the late Harold Rosen and Milton Erickson) specialize in hypnotic induction that does not involve trance induction or the exercise of traditional techniques such as eye closure. Clinical literature is also replete with examples of increased suggestibility or controllability of individuals during altered states of consciousness, such as those induced by psychotropic substances, environmental manipulation, sensory isolation, powerful emotions elicited by group dynamics (especially in large groups), religious ceremonies, and other special circumstances. *Latah* is a special case in that hyper-suggestibility usually occurs as the consequence of the subject being taken by surprise through a harmless maneuver (e.g., an abrupt noise, tickling, etc.) (Suryani & Jensen, 1993).

Pseudo-identity is more than a temporary role assumed by a subject in a laboratory exercise or during a transient period of intoxication. It is more like an "alter" in a case of multiple personality disorder (MPD). However, pseudo-identity differs from the alter of MPD in the following important respects:

1. *Pathogenesis.* MPD is most likely a consequence of early childhood trauma, with symptoms appearing later in life as a result of inner conflicts interacting with experiential circumstances. A pseudo-identity is usually generated by external stress originating in the environment of a person who may have been previously quite free of any signs or symptoms of personality malfunction, and for whom the new persona represents a transformation required to meet the demand characteristics of a life situation markedly different from the person's previous one.

2. *Psychopathology.* The MPD patient may have more than one alter; in the case of pseudo-identity, the personality change, whether swift or gradual, usually involves the generation of a single different personality. In pseudo-identity, under certain conditions there may be abrupt switch-

ing back and forth between behaviors characteristic of the two separate personalities (a phenomenon sometimes referred to as "floating"), but without MPD's typical boundaries between the two personalities, and without the MPD patient's sense that one self is separate from the other one. In MPD, the different alters or personalities primarily reflect facets of the original character. In pseudo-identity, the new personality primarily reflects the new situational forces and requirements. In MPD, the original identity is usually unconscious of the existence of the alters as they emerge and submerge. In pseudo-identity, the original persona remains but is overlaid or enveloped by the new identity.

3. *Prognosis.* MPD is notoriously difficult to treat (Braun, 1986; Kluft, 1984b). The outlook is generally better for the patient with pseudo-identity, although the syndrome may become chronic like any dissociative disorder or (in the old terminology) monosymptomatic major hysteria. Sometimes merely returning the patient to his original life situation (or even a neutral environment where information is freely and honestly exchanged and nonexploitive people are available for support) will, in a few weeks, result in the abrupt ("snapping") or gradual disappearance of the pseudo-identity. However, the patient then faces resuming many long-neglected functions of his former personhood, and working through the complex emotional aftermath of having—for whatever period of time and to whatever degree—become a different person.

4. *Treatment.* Therapy of both syndromes requires appreciation of the mental mechanisms involved, the reality of traumata or stress—however subtle—in pathogenesis, and the technical maneuvers known to be useful in management of dissociative disorders. While in the psychotherapy of MPD the usual goal is primarily the reconciliation and integration of the alters into a new and healthier whole, the goal in therapy of the patient with pseudo-identity is restoration of the original identity. However, the patient then usually requires treatment for the residual PTSD which is the legacy of the stress that produced and maintained the pseudo-identity syndrome.

Cases of pseudo-identity observed among cult victims are often very clear-cut, classic examples of transformation through deliberately contrived situational forces of a normal individual's personality into that of "a different person." (Others are colored by certain prominent additional symptoms into types that have been described as "floaters," "contemplators," and "survivors," see below.) The following brief case description illustrates a more or less classical case of pseudo-identity in a small totalist cult.

Danny Kraft grew up in a small town in the midwest. Testimony from over 60 family members, friends, and former teachers indicated that Danny was a fairly normal young man. He appeared to be well adjusted, sociable, performed well in school, had many friends, and showed no signs of anti-social behavior. There was no evidence that Danny suffered from any mental or personality disorder. His parents were divorced, and he sometimes appeared to experience conflicted loyalties between his father and mother, but not inappropriately so.

Towards the end of his teen years, Danny became interested in religion and eventually joined a sect (by our definition a totalist cult) that was an offshoot of the Reorganized Church of Jesus Christ of Latter Day Saints (LDS). His parents grew concerned about the personality change they saw in their son. Danny's father made several trips to the town where the cult was located and talked to pastors, police officers, and the FBI. They assured him that his son was merely going through a "phase" and that he would soon grow weary of the group and return home. However, far more ominous events transpired. The cult leader, Jeffrey Lundgren, declared that God had told him that members of a certain family within the group must be judged. "Judgment" meant that blood must be shed. Danny participated in Lundgren's murder of the victimized family. He assisted the Lundgrens in killing the two parents and all three daughters, aged 7, 13, and 15. The family members were lured one by one into a barn, bound and gagged, and then taken to a large hole that had been dug in the barn floor, where Lundgren shot them with a .45 automatic pistol and buried the bodies. Lundgren, his family, and his followers then moved westward. Eventually they were apprehended in California, returned to Ohio, and tried for murder.

In subsequent interviews, Danny appeared calm and unperturbed. There was no evidence of a personality disorder, except for the appearance of high dependency elevations and high normal elevations on the narcissistic and antisocial scales of the Millon Clinical Multiaxial Inventory (MCMI). All other tests and repeated clinical interviews showed no evidence of emotional distress or thought disorder.

At first Danny denied that he had had anything to do with the murder of the family. But when he was asked about the judgment of God, he admitted that he had served as God's instrument in executing His judgment. While confessing, Danny showed no apparent remorse. In fact, there was a wooden, matter-of-fact quality in his admission and in his entire demeanor.

At the sentencing hearing, Danny's father appealed without success for professional help for his son to break the spell that Lundgren had seemingly cast over him. As one reporter observed, "the younger Kraft (Danny) only smirked and appeared indifferent as Lake County Common Pleas Judge James W. Jackson listened to witnesses in the second day of the ex-cult member's sentencing hearing" (McGillivray, 1990, p. 2). His defense lawyer, Elmer Giuliani, argued, "He (Lundgren) has divided this young man from what he was at one time to what you see today. He divided this man's mind from a free thinker to a mirror image [of Lundgren]" (McGillivray, 1990, p. 2).

Other than Lundgren's wife and son, Danny is the only person who was convicted who is apparently still under the control of Lundgren. The zealous beliefs of the other cultists eventually faded, and they now perceive Jeffrey Lundgren as anything but a prophet of God. It remains to be seen whether Danny's fairly classical case of pseudo-identity will yield to treatment (if any can be provided in prison) or to the passage of time.

Sometimes the pseudo-identity becomes destabilized. Such destabilization can occur when internal defense mechanisms break down; when changes in the group occur that cannot be explained or tolerated by the member; when information is received from outside sources that is dissonant with currently held beliefs, or otherwise anxiety provoking; when gradual fatigue and strain occur after a period of arduous work on behalf of the cult, perhaps with concomitant threats of punishment for poor performance; or when the cult member is traumatized by such events as humiliation by a superior. Destabilization may also be seen when a cult member experiences a sense of failure or impending doom for not being able to meet the group's demands or otherwise satisfactorily to conform. The three clinical pictures described below may be seen in recent converts who experience destabilization to the point that they drop out before a more fixed pseudo-identity is formed. They may also be seen after a pseudo-identity is formed but is subsequently destabilized, even after departure from the cult.

1. *The "Floater."* Nothing distresses parents and loved ones more than witnessing a recovering, former cult member begin to "float." Floating is a dissociative phenomenon that is best described as a sudden switch back to the pseudo-identity, a regression which is most commonly triggered by certain sights, sounds, touches, smells, or tastes in everyday life that were ubiquitous and salient stimuli in the cultic milieu. Characteristically, floating occurs in cult members who have left the group of their own accord, have received incomplete counseling, or are still in the beginning phases of counseling. A former member who floats after phoning a cult member may, as a result, even return to the cult.

Jennifer, a college graduate, had served as a teacher overseas for 7 years with a well-respected religious organization. She then returned to the United States and joined a different church. Gradually, she and others of the congregation became entranced by their charismatic pastor. Over time, Jennifer began to believe ideas and to practice behaviors that previously would have been unthinkable to her. Despite her previous fundamentalist Christian beliefs regarding ethics and morality, Jennifer repeatedly engaged in illicit sexual activity with her cultic pastor, who told her that it would make her "more spiritual." No amount of persuasion by friends and family could convince her that the group or its teachings and practices were unhealthy. She eventually agreed to seek counseling, but only to convince her parents and friends that the cult was in fact healthy and that their fears were unfounded.

Initially Jennifer presented a rather robotic picture to the therapist. Her affect was flat and her speech was mechanical, as were her bodily movements. She exhibited clinical signs of dependency, anxiety, and depression. After many daily sessions, one day the therapist said something that shifted Jennifer away from her pseudo-identity. In the following session her affect and bodily movements were no longer stilted, and she began to express some of the doubt and pain that were appropriate to the reality of her experiences in the cult. In short, the "old Jennifer" began to re-emerge. The change was dramatic. Needless to say, Jennifer's parents were much encouraged.

A few days later in a group therapy session another patient said something critical about Jennifer's cult leader. The therapist watched Jennifer's eyes loose their focus. She stared off into space. Suddenly the pseudo-identity was back. Criticism of the leader apparently served as a trigger for her automatically to recite the programming that she had received in the group: that is, to defend the leader against all criticism. Subsequently Jennifer required 5 to 6 hours of continuous discussion during which the therapist reviewed with her the cult leader's abusive and unethical behavior. With this cognitive exercise, Jennifer's frozen affect began to thaw again. She has since remained free from the cult, is now married with one child, and works as a school teacher.

2. The "Contemplator." Dissociated trance-like symptoms are often seen in members of cults or sects in which contemplative exercises are practiced, such as chanting or meditation. "Speaking in tongues" may also produce this effect.

Sabrina was a member of a martial arts cult for a number of years. Her parents became concerned about progressive behavioral and personality changes, together with her gradual estrangement from the family. Eventually Sabrina sought counseling when she began to experience significantly distressing symptoms. She was found to be suffering from a major depressive episode, with predisposing passive dependent and schizoid personality characteristics. Her therapist noted that sometimes Sabrina would begin to stare, her eyes would become unfocused, and she would become unaware of her surroundings. The therapist would literally have to call out her name several times in order for Sabrina to reorient herself as to time, place, person, and event. With Sabrina, there were no apparent cues or triggers for these trancelike states. When she entered these states she would find herself automatically engaging in some of the activities that had been a part of her martial arts training. Over the course of several weeks of therapy, Sabrina's episodes of contemplative dissociation diminished in frequency. In time, they disappeared entirely.

Sabrina was fortunate. In some cases, contemplative dissociation is very resistant to modification. Former cult members who have practiced chanting and meditation for hours a day over a period of many years may require special rehabilitation or extensive therapeutic measures (see "General Treatment Issues," below).

3. *The "Survivor."* Certain dissociative symptoms are frequently evident in persons who have survived severely traumatic events. Herman (1992) notes that victims of incest, rape, terrorism, concentration camps, and cults share common responses to trauma, which may include feeling disconnected or detached from their selves or their surroundings (depersonalization, derealization), psychophysiological hyperarousal, intrusive memories of the trauma, and/or emotional and behavioral constriction.

Our clinical experiences with former cultists confirm that they may develop symptoms similar to those seen in victims of imprisonment, torture, terrorism, incest, physical abuse, or rape. In about 25% of our cases, cults are found to have perpetrated sexual and physical coercion and other abuse, including the inculcation of fear, terror, or dread. Further, cults are seen to exploit group dynamics for social control, and to employ specific techniques to induce altered states of consciousness. It is interesting to note that one study of former cultists (Martin, Langone, Dole, & Wiltrout, 1992) revealed no significant differences in the MCMI between those who had been subjected to sexual and/or physical abuse, and those who did not report an abuse history. While usually the case, apparently neither brutal treatment nor confinement is necessary to produce the survivor type of clinical picture, as is illustrated in the following case.

Charles was a graduate of a large state university. His parents enjoyed a solid marriage. His father was an anesthesiologist. Charles had joined a Bible study group while at the university and after graduation he, along with many of the group's members, moved to be closer to the leader of the group. These Bible study members found themselves part of a small, cultic rural compound that advocated white supremacy, militancy, and a belief in demons as the source of virtually every personal problem. The leader advocated a series of extreme measures to rid the cultists of their demons. These measures included long and arduous fasts, beatings, physical threats of death, prolonged verbal abuse, isolation, public confession, and almost constant shaming and humiliation. Charles was subjected to all of these methods to exorcise his demons. His parents, fearing that he might be dying from the fasts, contacted local police and had their son seen by a counselor. Charles was later referred for more extensive counseling in a residential setting.

At first appearance Charles was gaunt, his eyes were sunken, and he stared into space incessantly. He was listless and passive, resembling a Holocaust survivor. Although Charles was no longer in the cult, he had apparently come to believe that he was indeed hopeless, wicked, and demonized. Clinically, Charles suffered from a depressive illness with obsessive compulsive features. He also met the criteria for the *Diagnostic and Statistical Manual of Mental Disorders,* fourth edition (DSM-IV; American Psychiatric Association, 1994) diagnosis of Acute Stress Disorder and Brief Reactive Dissociative Disorder. His dissociative symptoms included trance-like states, derealization, depersonalization, and psychic numbing: "I feel nothing; I feel dead." In addition, Charles experienced fear, intrusive recollections or flashbacks, hopelessness, and despair. Charles received daily intensive psychotherapy for more than 5 weeks. He was also prescribed fluoxetine, an antidepressive medication. By the time Charles left the treatment center he had gained weight and was no longer depersonalized, numb, or feeling a sense of despair. He continued in outpatient therapy for nearly a year. Currently, he is performing very well as a graduate student and was recently married.

GENERAL TREATMENT ISSUES

Misunderstandings about cult victims and their treatment abound (Martin, 1989; Singer & Addis, 1992). Perhaps the most disturbing myth is that only troubled individuals or those from dysfunctional homes join cults, while well-adjusted youth are immune. Although several well-designed studies and numerous clinical reports have refuted this idea, it stubbornly persists (Wright & Piper, 1986; Maron, 1988). Another common misconception about cults is that their dangers are either greatly exaggerated or are nothing more than fictitious concoctions by overcontrolling, neurotic, or ignorant parents; by misinformed religious (or antireligious) bigots; or by unscrupulous therapists bent on terrifying families, traumatizing followers of "new religions" through brutal deprogramming sessions, and collecting enormous fees (Bromley & Shupe, 1981; Bromley & Richardson, 1983; Barker, 1984; Robbins, 1988). Objective therapists will reject such viewpoints (often promulgated by nonclinicians if not armchair philosophers) and will prefer to trust the evidence of their own information as obtained from experienced colleagues, patients, family members and other reliable informants. Such therapists will quickly perceive that the cultic situation impinges upon the particularities of each member's personality and behavioral history to produce a resulting constellation of symptoms, or even to precipitate a serious psychiatric illness.

Some specific methods used in treating cult victims have been described in a number of recent books and articles (Martin, 1989; Martin, Langone, Dole & Wiltrout, 1992; Martin, 1993a; Martin, 1993b). These publications note that proper treatment can be difficult, that it is more education-oriented than many other therapies, and that it progresses through several fairly predictable phases. Following is a brief summary of some of the salient features of these treatment methods.

The goal of treating a former cultist is to relieve the patient's cult-induced psychopathology and thus to restore his pre-cult personality. This can be a daunting task. The difficult and necessary challenge of all therapy with former cult members is to carefully restructure the patient's unhealthy responses to the stressful demands made by the cult on the patient's previous sense of identity, including values, mood, thought and behavior. The therapist must also clearly define the patient's dissociative symptoms, so that treatment can be oriented toward the particular type of psychopathology that is present. For example, dissociation caused by meditative practices may require a different approach than dissociation secondary to physical trauma. Moreover, more than one dissociative symptom may be manifest in the same patient, either simultaneously or sequentially. Different types of dissociation must be identified clearly and treated appropriately for the best therapeutic results.

Classic pseudo-identity cases require treatment very much like that employed by most therapists who treat patients coming out of cults. Generally treatment of cult victims contains several elements. Some or all of the following may be required:

1. Medical care for illness, often related to malnutrition, avitaminosis, neglect of chronic disorders such as diabetes or peptic ulcer, and neglect of preventive health measures such as inoculations, proper diet, regular exercise, and the like.
2. Psychiatric treatment for mental illness, including medication to manage symptoms of depression, anxiety, panic disorder, etc., and perhaps the use of special methods such as hypnosis or narcosynthesis for resistant dissociative symptoms.
3. Individual psychotherapy.
4. Group psychotherapy.
5. Exit counseling.
6. Family therapy.
7. Educational guidance and counseling.
8. Vocational rehabilitation and training.
9. Special referrals for pastoral counseling if indicated (e.g., when the recovering patient seeks affiliation with a legitimate religious group, or wishes to return to his original family church).
10. Legal consultation, if needed, to help the patient put his affairs back in proper order if—as often happens—they have been much neglected, disrupted, or exploited during the period of cult mem-

bership. Legal action, including both punishment of offenders and recovery of damages by the victim, can be very therapeutic in many cases.

TREATMENT STRATEGIES

Patients showing clinical pictures of the subtypes described above may require special treatment strategies. Suggestions about these include the following.

1. *Treating the "Contemplator."* Dissociative and other symptoms resulting from contemplative cult practices may continue to be problematic in treatment long after other symptoms have improved. Contemplative symptoms can include inability to concentrate, relaxation-induced anxiety, and dissociative phenomena such as automatic lapsing into meditation, chanting, or trance-like states. Ryan (1993) found that one of the most effective methods to remedy "spacing out" is physical exercise. Exercise may also help to alleviate other contemplative symptoms, such as lack of awareness of bodily sensations, muscle tension, fatigue, and the association of these with emotional dysfunction or distress. Other helpful techniques include identifying aspects of the environment that create stimulus overload, slowly building up reading stamina by setting a timer and thereby gradually prolonging reading time, and learning to counter magical thinking through a specific series of reality checks.

Dissociation has been viewed as a phenomenon that is associated with subcortical areas of the brain (West, 1967; Putnam, 1989). To a certain, though lesser, degree the cognitive processing problems ex-cultists experience resemble difficulties encountered by some head trauma or stroke patients. Therefore, as with patients who have known neural lesions, selected cult victims may benefit from the employment of structured linguistic remediation. Some patients report that such methods, which focus on memory, concentration, and linguistic encoding and decoding, are very helpful in reducing various types of dissociation. Specific exercises include (1) reading several paragraphs aloud to the patient and asking him to restate the ideas expressed in the passage, (2) asking questions pertinent to the sequence of the content read to the patient, (3) asking the patient to analyze the story or to repeat it, and (4) inviting the patient to respond to sentences that require an expression of opinion relevant to the content. The clinician should note the latency of responses, the need for clarification of the task or topic, the patient's memory for details, problems in his ability to focus and concentrate on the task, and deficits in expressive verbal skills.

Since altered states may result from a narrowed focus of attention and a limiting or restricting of external stimuli (as occurs in many cultic environments), awareness training in the visual, auditory, and aesthetic modes can be helpful. For example, by encouraging clients to name all the different sounds they hear in 30 seconds, and then all the colors and shapes they see in a room, the therapist reinforces awareness of sensory stimuli that a dissociative state may have diminished or even (in the case of a trance) abolished.

Various mnemonic devices for remembering the details needed to engage in everyday activities can be taught to a former member so that he can better recall, for example, the five or six items he recently purchased at the grocery store. Daily readings of newspapers, magazines, or short stories can be useful as well, particularly when the patient interrupts the activity at regular intervals to check his recall ability and his awareness of the present environmental situation.

2. *Treating the "Floater."* Typically, a former member floats, or returns to a pseudo-identity state, as a result of a trigger that can be visual (e.g., seeing a book written by the cult leader), verbal, physical, gustatory, or even olfactory. To defuse the trigger, it must be identified and the cultic language or jargon associated with it examined. Words that are given unique or idiosyncratic meaning by the cult should be correctly redefined by showing the client the dictionary definition of the word. Sometimes merely concentrating on crossword puzzles and other word games may help a patient to diminish or prevent floating (Tobias, 1993).

The immediate or crisis treatment for floating involves orienting the patient sharply to present reality with respect to time, place, person, event, and self. It may be necessary to remind him repeatedly that he is no longer in the cult, to encourage him to engage in conversation, and to review facts that promote the experience of being himself in the here and now. Crisis treatment should also include a review of why he left the cult and the problems associated with it (e.g., exploitative or criminal behavior). Patients should be encouraged to make notes and list the reasons why they left the cult, along with the personal and social problems that ensued from their cult experience. If they cannot reach their clinicians when episodes of floating occur, they can review their notebooks until the floating stops or they receive help.

Generally, floating is diminished by a thorough and comprehensive exit counseling process. The more the former member learns about the cult, and the more he is helped to understand the negative impact the cult has had on him, the less likely he will be to experience episodes of floating. If these episodes persist, more rigorous methods—similar to those employed in treatment of major dissociative disorders—may be required.

3. *Treating the "Survivor."* People forced by manipulative cult leaders to engage in and/or witness heinous acts often manifest symptoms of PTSD. Nightmares, intrusive thoughts or images, fearfulness, and various psychosomatic malfunctions are common reactions. However, the formation of a pseudo-identity is not necessarily associated with specific traumata, and the symptoms that cult members experience after they leave the cult may not be exactly those which meet the diagnostic criteria for PTSD. Nevertheless, the cult experience itself, and the process of disengaging from the cult, inevitably involve some degree of trauma to the person. The picture of a concentration camp survivor may result. To promote a full recovery from the sequelae of cult membership, the therapist should help the former member to learn about the dynamics of cultic groups and to understand how individuals in such situations can be induced to behave in ways highly deviant from their previous patterns, or to fail to behave in ways that were previously characteristic. Therapy should focus on "detriggering" and "reframing" the traumatic incidents that continue to affect the former cult member via educative strategies, cognitive-behavioral techniques, memory work, and dynamically oriented psychotherapy, as indicated.

SPECIFIC TREATMENT ISSUES

During the course of therapy, the following issues must be addressed in treating the traumatized former cult member.

1. Formulate how the cultic trauma interacted with the unique aspects of the patient, pre-abuse factors must be evaluated including the patient's age, gender, personality, coping style, family of origin, and pre-cult personal history.

2. The specific nature of the cultic trauma must also be examined; including the following:

a. Did predisposing personality or situational factors render the cult member vulnerable to recruitment? It is important to note that most people who are recruited into cults were not seeking to become cult members, did not suffer from any significant psychosocial handicaps, and did not come from atypical family situations. Although it is important to explore the individual vulnerabilities of the patient to the recruitment process, it can also be helpful for former cult members to recognize that cult recruiters regularly play on a myriad of personal characteristics that are normal or even desirable in the general population—characteristics such as loyalty, honesty, idealism, and a trusting nature.

b. How was the cult member's pseudo-identity shaped by use of deception, guilt, coercion, conditioning techniques involving deliberate positive and negative reinforcement, group indoctrination, environmental manipulation, hypnotic methods, and other maneuvers to increase suggestibility or produce trance-like states?

c. How was the patient affected psychologically by the "thought reform" elements in the cultic environment? Specific issues and symptoms that can be addressed include denial, fragmentation of the self, depression, anxiety, phobias, dissociation, dissociation triggers, and how these various mental mechanisms and symptoms are related to the cultic milieu.

d. How were specific traumatic incidents stored? Storage could be cognitive via the doctrinal framework, sensory via visual and auditory stimuli, or interpersonal in terms of automatized behaviors, action tendencies, or group-determined roles. Further, what is the means by which this patient's trauma-related stimuli trigger memories of painful, confusing, and guilt-producing cult experiences?

e. How can painful memories of the cult experience, and the eventual disillusionment, be defused? As with victims of other types of trauma, three basic assumptions have been violated or undermined with respect to ex-cult members' view of themselves and the world: "the belief in personal invulnerability, the perception of the world as meaningful, and the perception of oneself as positive" (Janoff-Bulman, 1985, p. 15). The clinician must facilitate the former member's task of recapturing or reframing positive attitudes about life, the self, the family, society, and the like.

The consequences of pre-cult abuse (if any) and the subsequent cultic abuse are treated initially by educating the former cult member with respect to the psychological manipulation techniques that were used to deceive or mislead him. In this way, he learns that he was not solely responsible for his misfortune. (Blaming the victim is ubiquitous; even victims do it.) Some former members may say, "I'm fine," and show extreme defensiveness about the group's flagrant abuses. Such denial must be confronted by educating them about the after effects of cultic abuse in a manner analogous to the early intervention work with victims of rape, physical abuse, and other types of interpersonal trauma.

Former members can gain a sense of perspective about their cultic involvement by learning about the manipulative teaching of their particular cult, the practices of their cult leader, and the group's ethical tenets and exploitative use of personal relationships. This can be accomplished by presenting didactic material on the techniques of thought reform used; showing the ex-member testimonials of other former cult members who have made a successful post-cult recovery; encouraging the ex-member to talk to or visit with other former members; providing general readings and other educational materials about cults; and examining how a cult, if it claims to be religious, actually deviates from the main traditions of the religion from which it presumably derived (e.g., Protestant Christianity), or how a psychotherapy cult departs from the accepted standards of care and ethics practiced by reputable mental health professionals.

The educational aspects of treatment are primarily part of the first of the three stages of recovery, which overlap with each other. The three stages of recovery can generally be assessed by the type of questions the ex-cultist asks. For example, when a therapist hears the following questions and statements, he will know that the former cult member is in the first phase of recovery: "Is the group really a cult?" "Maybe I could have tried harder." "I'm so confused." "Were my needs really being met in the group?" "I'm fine. The group had some problems, but it wasn't that bad." "I know something is wrong; I just can't put my finger on it." The initial treatment goal for the patient who asks such questions is to finish the exiting process. This entails a thorough examination of the cultic milieu, the resultant trauma, and the various pre-abuse factors that may be relevant. In short, the clinician must *educate* the patient, as described above. Valuable insights may be gained at this stage by using instruments such as the MCMI and asking patients specific questions about the cult and why they left. High scores on the Dependency, Avoidant, Schizoid, Anxiety, and Dysthymia scales are typically associated with untreated former cultists. Defensive and guarded answers about the group may indicate that the patient is still processing or denying a well-documented history of abuse within the cult.

Once issues in the first stage of post-cult recovery are resolved, patients will begin to make comments along the following lines: "I miss my friends in the group." "I feel like a fool." "I want to get my things back from the cult." "I don't know what to believe anymore about God, groups, religion, or friends." "There are issues I never dealt with before joining." "I want to learn all I can about cults." "Will they try to come after me?" "I have lost all this time." Patients who express such thoughts are in the second stage of recovery. While the first stage corresponds to a focus on the past, comments made during the second stage of recovery reflect an ability to focus on the present, and to view the cult involvement as a past experience. At this point, the dissociative symptoms of floating are usually no longer evident. Likewise, the stunned and frozen affect of the post-traumatic first phase is often much diminished, although in some ex-members, contemplative dissociative states may linger and persist throughout the second and even the third stages of recovery.

Treatment issues at the second stage correspond more to those of traditional therapy. Permission to grieve is of utmost importance. Anger and rage at this stage can be intense. Agonized verbalizations such as "I feel as though I have been murdered" are not uncommon. In addition to grief work, patients are now able to examine how they were recruited. Because cults manipulate each person's strengths and weakness, it is important for the patient to realize fully how he was lured into involvement with the cult. At this stage, it is important for the ex-cultist to regain his ability to validate the pre-cult self and to learn in more detail how this self was suppressed and displaced by the pseudo-identity. Work on emotional expression and self-awareness of feeling states is essential because psychic numbing can still persist at this stage of treatment. Special exercises are necessary for patients who cannot yet normally experience emotions, or who are too guilt ridden to express rage or anger.

Stage three is more future oriented and optimistic than stage two. At this phase of treatment, patients ask questions pertinent to what they will do in the future regarding jobs, going back to school, finding careers, where they will live, whom they will date, and how they will rejoin their families. Treatment at this time is best oriented to career and guidance counseling. Family therapy, time and skills management training, and job and interview skills training may well be pursued at this juncture. Certain cult victims may require legal advice if criminal or civil charges against the cult are contemplated or pending.

Each stage of recovery can be marked not only by progressive insight but also by appropriate emotions. It is important for the clinician repeatedly to return to the source of emotional distress. For example, the early depression that a former member might feel for having "failed God," which accounts for why he is no longer in the group, is very different from the depression of a member who finally comes to the full realization that his trust fund was stolen by the cult leader or that his spouse became the cult leader's concubine. It is important for the clinician to analyze the nature of the conflicts and issues facing the patient, in addition to evaluating the patient's psychopathology, as treatment proceeds.

Natural strengths and assets can be discerned in the recovering cultist, and the clinician will be gratified to notice the accelerating momentum of improvement as he fosters the former cult member's progress from the early to the more advanced stages of recovery. In every way the clinician should strive to facilitate the recovery process and to help provide the appropriate resources, support, and tools needed by the patient along the path of recovery. Ultimately, if all goes well, the clinician who has facilitated the patient's recovery will be deeply gratified as the symptoms of the pseudo-identity syndrome progressively vanish, and the pre-cult self is restored, repaired, and returned to a more normal life.

NOTE

1. The detached masculine pronoun is used throughout in the traditional convention to designate both sexes.

REFERENCES

American Psychiatric Association. (1994). *Diagnostic and statistical manual of mental disorders* (4th ed.). Washington, DC: Author.

Barker, E. (1984). *The making of a Moonie.* New York: Basil Blackwell.

Bliss, E. L. (1986). *Multiple personality, allied disorders and hypnosis.* New York: Oxford University Press.

Bromley, D. G., & Shupe, A. D. Jr. (1981). *Strange gods: The great American cult scare.* Boston: Beacon Press

Bromley, D. G., & Richardson, J. T. (Eds.). (1983). *The brainwashing/deprogramming controversy: Sociological, psychological, legal and historical perspectives* (Studies in Religion and Society, Vol. 5). New York: Edwin Mellen Press.

Conway, F., & Siegelman, J. (1978). *Snapping: America's epidemic of sudden personality change.* Philadelphia: J. B. Lippincott.

Farber, I. E., Harlow, H. F., & West, L. J. (1957). Brainwashing, conditioning and DDD: Debility, dependency, and dread. *Sociometry, 20,* 271–285.

Girodo, M. (1985). Health and legal issues in undercover narcotics investigations: Misrepresented evidence. *Behavioral Sciences and the Law, 3,* 299–308.

Glatzel, J. (1974). Zur psychopathologie zyklothym-depressiver verlaufe. *Psychiatria Clinica, 7,* 120–128.

Hearst, P., & Moscow, A. (1988). *Patty Hearst: Her own story.* New York: Avon.

Herman, J. L. (1992). *Trauma and recovery.* New York: Basic Books.

Holland, A. (Director), Menegoz, M. (Producer), & Brauner, A. (Producer). *Europa, Europa* [Film]. Los Angeles: Orion Classics.

Janoff-Bulman, R. (1985). The aftermath of victimization: Rebuilding shattered assumptions. In C. R. Figley (Ed.), *Trauma and its wake: The study and treatment of post-traumatic stress disorder.* New York: Brunner/Mazel.

Kluft, R. P. (1991). Multiple personality disorder. In A. Tasman & S. M. Goldfinger (Eds.), *American Psychiatric Press review of psychiatry* (Vol. 10). Washington D.C.: American Psychiatric Association Press.

Lifton, R. J. (1961). *Thought reform and the psychology of totalism.* New York: W. W. Norton.

Lifton, R. J. (1986) *The Nazi doctors.* New York: Basic Books.

Maron, N. (1988). Family environment as a factor in vulnerability to cult involvement. *Cultic Studies Journal, 5,* 23–43.

Martin, P. R. (1989). Dispelling the myths: The psychological consequences of cultic involvement. *Christian Research Journal, 11,* 9–14.

Martin, P. R. (1993a). *Cult-proofing your kids.* Grand Rapids, MI: Zondervan House.

Martin, P. R. (1993b). Post-cult recovery: Assessment and rehabilitation. In M. D. Langone (Ed.), *Recovery from cults* (pp. 203–231). New York: W. W. Norton.

Martin, P. R., Langone, M. D., Dole, A. A., & Wiltrout, J. (1992). Post-cult symptoms as measured by the MCMI before and after residential treatment. *Cultic Studies Journal, 9,* 219–249.

McGillivray, M. (1990, November 7). Kraft's father pleads: Please get some help. *Lake County News-Herald,* p. 2.

Mindszenty, J. C. (1974). *Memoirs.* New York: Macmillan.

O'Neill, W. F., & Demos, G. D. (1977). The semantics of thought reform. *Etc., 34,* 413–430.

Ochberg, F. M. (1978). The victim of terrorism. *The Practitioner, 220,* 293–302.

Putnam, F. (1989). *Diagnosis and treatment of multiple personality disorder.* New York: Guilford Press.

Robbins, T. (1988). *Cults, converts and charisma.* London: Sage.

Ryan, P. L. (1993). A personal account: Eastern meditation group. In M. D. Langone (Ed.), *Recovery from cults* (pp. 129–139). New York: W. W. Norton.

Schein, E. H. (1961). *Coercive persuasion.* New York: W. W. Norton.

Singer, M. T., & Addis, M. E. (1992). Cults, coercion, and community. In A. Kales, C. M. Pierce, & M. Greenblatt (Eds.), *The mosaic of contemporary psychiatry in perspective* (pp. 130–142). New York: Springer-Verlag.

Suryani, L. K., & Jensen, G. D. (1993). *Trance and possession in Bali: A window on western multiple personality, possession disorder, and suicide.* New York: Oxford University Press.

Tobias, M. L. (1993). Guidelines for ex-members. In M. D. Langone (Ed.), *Recovery frorn cults,* (pp. 300–324). New York: W. W. Norton.

The trial of Patty Hearst. (1976). [Transcript]. San Francisco: Great Fidelity Press.

West, L. J. (1964). Psychiatry, "brainwashing," and the American character. *American Journal of Psychiatry, 120,* 842–850.

West, L. J. (1967). Dissociative reaction. In A. M. Freedman & H. I. Kaplan (Eds.), *Comprehensive textbook of psychiatry* (pp. 885–899). Baltimore: Williams and Wilkins.

West, L. J. (1989). Persuasive techniques in contemporary cults. In M. Gallanter (Ed.), *Cults and new religious movements* (pp. 165–192). Washington, DC: American Psychiatric Association Press.

West, L. J. (1993). A psychiatric overview of cult-related phenomena. *Journal of the American Academy of Psychoanalysis, 21,* 1–19.

West, L. J. (1994). The pseudo-identity syndrome. *Journal of Nervous and Mental Disorders.*

Williams, D. (1992, March 30). Mending a split personality. *Los Angeles Times,* pp. F-1, F-4.

Wright, S. A., & Piper, E. S. (1986, February). Families and cults: Familial factors related to youth leaving or remaining in deviant religious groups. *Journal of Marriage and the Family,* 15–25.

14

The Rational Treatment
of Multiple Personality Disorder

Richard Horevitz
Richard J. Loewenstein

Dissociative disorders involve chronic disturbances in the normal integrative functioning of memory, identity, or consciousness (American Psychiatric Association, 1987).[1] Multiple personality disorder (MPD) and its variants reflect specific deficits in the integration of both identity and memory. Secondary impairments of integrative function may also be evident in deficits in the ability to transfer learned knowledge, information, and skills; in characteristic behavioral patterns and interpersonal relationships; in the recognition of known individuals; and, finally, in the stability of affective processes. These disturbances in normal integrative function persist despite changing life circumstances, though they may well become "background" phenomena that have negligible impact on current functioning (Kluft 1985).

Dissociative symptoms may dominate current functioning to the point that the patient is rendered completely dysfunctional. Unfortunately, there is no evidence that MPD ever spontaneously remits (Putnam, 1989). The less serious symptoms of depersonalization and derealization, conceptualized as dissociative phenomena, are common to many psychiatric conditions ranging from schizophrenia to post-traumatic stress disorder (PTSD), depression, panic disorder, and MPD, where they may either be symptoms of anxiety or dissociation (Putnam, 1989; Steinberg, 1993). Classic "hysterical" conversion symptoms and overall patterns of somatization are also associated with MPD (Bliss, 1984; Coons, 1984; North, Ryall, Ricci, & Wetzel, 1993). In this volume, Kihlstrom (see Chapter 17) argues that conversion disorder is best understood as a dissociative disorder.

Numerous studies have reported that the childhood histories of MPD patients are marked by extreme family dysfunction. In particular, studies using questionnaires, clinical case series, and structured interview data have all shown that MPD patients report the highest rates of childhood physical, sexual, and other forms of abuse and trauma amongst those suffering from any known psychiatric disorder (Boon & Draijer, 1993; Kluft, Braun, & Sachs, 1984; Loewenstein & Putnam, 1990; Ross et al., 1990, 1991). These studies also demonstrate that most MPD patients describe repeated forms of multiple types of abuse or trauma usually beginning before the age of 5. Often the reported abuse is profound, unrelenting, and intolerably bizarre, frequently unmitigated or only unpredictably mitigated by nurturance in the environment. The literature on MPD also reports the highest rate of victimization by both male and female perpetrators (> 50%) of any known trauma-based condition (Schultz, Braun, & Kluft, 1989).

With reported abuse histories in virtually all patients, MPD has been conceptualized as a special variant of PTSD (Spiegel, 1984), that is, as a traumatically induced developmental disorder of childhood (Horevitz, 1993; Loewenstein, 1991a; Loewenstein & Ross, 1992; Putnam, 1989). While the abuse reports do not constitute an adequate basis to infer causal linkages (see Chapter 18, this volume), they are, nevertheless, consistent with the finding that 80% of MPD patients meet *Diagnostic and Statistical Manual of Mental Disorders*, third edition, revised (DSM-III-R; American Psychological Association, 1987) diagnostic criteria for PTSD at the time of diagnosis, and that post-traumatic stress symptoms affect virtually all MPD patients during the course of treatment (Armstrong & Loewenstein, 1990). These PTSD symptoms are often an integral part of the larger clinical picture that the therapist will be treating (Kluft & Fine, 1993).

A RATIONAL APPROACH TO TREATMENT

This chapter will present a rational model of the psychotherapy of MPD. A rational model of therapy requires clear and specific treatment objectives. It must also chart the course of treatment from beginning to end, recognize that MPD patients are not a homogeneous population, and specify treatment alternatives for patients who are not amenable to the treatment specified by the rational approach. The treatment model we advocate attempts to achieve these objectives. In explaining the model, we will specify the knowledge base on which recommended interventions rest. We advocate a long-term, multimodal treatment of MPD because the literature suggests that this is the most efficacious approach to this complex disorder. Although no controlled treatment outcome studies have been reported in the literature, and conclusions must therefore be tentative, a consensus exists among experienced clinicians that the treatment must be long-term and multimodal (see Putnam, 1989; Ross, 1989).

At the outset, it should be noted that the treatment of the vast majority of MPD patients does not proceed smoothly. It is, rather, punctuated by many crises and many unexpected turns. Clinicians often find themselves unable to navigate a reasonable, systematic treatment course when the interventions available do not address current crises or atypical symptom presentations. In many ways, one can say more about the handling of the unexpected than one can say about the outline of a systematic treatment model, which can never fully anticipate the vagaries in the course of treatment of MPD. Although all these problems cannot be addressed in this chapter, there are good sources of information available in both treatment-oriented textbooks (e.g., Putnam, 1989; Ross, 1989) and specialized articles on this topic (Chu, 1988; Greaves, 1988; Kluft, 1988a, 1988b, 1989, 1990, 1991a, 1991b, 1993).

Assessment and Diagnosis

The cornerstone of any rational treatment is adequate assessment. Although MPD is a coherent, definable syndrome that can be diagnosed with high reliability (Steinberg, Rounsaville, & Cicchetti, 1991; Horevitz, Chapter 20, this volume), the population of MPD patients is extremely diverse. Nevertheless, MPD patients can be readily divided into three groups that reflect important differences in treatment complexity and prognosis.

1. *High-functioning MPD patients.* Patients in this group have significant psychological, interpersonal, social, vocational, and financial resources. High-functioning patients present with little personality disorder comorbidity and significant capacity to master affect, control dysphoria, and participate in a productive therapeutic alliance. They generally experience positive outcomes in outpatient treatment and pose relatively fewer significant therapeutic management problems. Patients with these characteristics have been found to range from 30% (Horevitz & Braun, 1984) to more than 50% (Kluft, 1984) of the samples studied.

2. *Complicated cases with comorbid conditions.* The available data (Horevitz & Braun, 1984; Schultz, Braun, & Kluft, 1989) suggests that one-half to two-thirds of MPD patients present with a clinical picture complicated by the coexistence of symptoms that meet the DSM-III-R criteria for Borderline Personality Disorder. Other complicating factors may include organic brain damage, severe medical illness, severe substance abuse, and eating disorders. However, for assessment purposes, this "complicated" category should be reserved for patients who have been in treatment for a signifi-

cant period of time with little evidence of treatment gain, and who exhibit personality characteristics (i.e., dependency, low autonomy, external locus of control, blaming, and self-preoccupation) generally associated with poor therapeutic outcomes (e.g., older and more severe family, marital, and medical problems; complex PTSD symptoms refractory to treatment; severe memory problems; affect dysregulation). With this group of patients, treatment is of necessity much slower, the potential for gain is less certain, and the ideal goal of full fusion and integration may not be attainable.

3. *Enmeshed patients.* The group of patients that is the most recalcitrant to treatment tend to remain enmeshed in abusive relationships, have a "dissociative" lifestyle, and actively participate in self-destructive and/or antisocial behaviors and habits. For example, Horevitz worked with a patient who was living in three different states and was married to three different men. Enmeshed patients may function at this level of presentation or have severe schizophrenic-spectrum disorders and tend to be chronic consumers of mental health services. Not surprisingly, they have a poor therapeutic prognosis and can be treated most effectively when therapy is geared toward symptom stabilization and crisis management rather than toward the uncovering integration of alters (cf. Turkus, 1991).

During the past 10 years, reliable and valid diagnostic measures have been developed in the fields of psychiatry and psychology, paralleling important developments in the assessment and diagnosis of MPD. Recent years have witnessed the development of reliable and valid structured (Ross et al., 1989) and semistructured interviews (Steinberg, 1993), mental status interview protocols (Loewenstein, 1991a), psychometrically sound self-report measures (Bernstein & Putnam, 1986), and novel uses of hypnotizability testing for diagnostic purposes (Frischholz & Braun, 1991). Furthermore, clinicians now have at their disposal ways of detecting signs of dissociation and multiplicity using traditional psychological assessment instruments such as the Rorschach and the Minnesota Multiphasic Personality Inventory (MMPI; Armstrong & Loewenstein, 1990; Labott, Leavitt, Braun, & Sachs, 1992). Details about the diagnostic and assessment process, including the use of specific testing instruments, are presented in Chapter 8 (Carlson & Armstrong, Chapter 8, this volume).

Advances in assessment and diagnostic procedures are signficant because MPD is frequently diagnosed only after a patient has endured a long and costly history in the mental health system (Ross & Dua, 1993; Putnam, Guroff, Silberman, Barban, & Post, 1986). When diagnosed and properly treated, many MPD patients' tenure in treatment diminishes, and treatment costs may drop dramatically over time, even for those remaining in chronic care treatment settings (Ross & Dua, 1993; Fraser & Raine, 1993). Some patients encounter many therapists before a correct diagnosis is made, whereas others must wait for many years before they are diagnosed by a therapist they have been seeing for a long time. Increasingly, early detection has become of paramount importance.

Difficult Cases

False positive and false negative diagnoses of MPD constitute a significant diagnostic dilemma. Because of the inherent difficulty in making the diagnosis of MPD, and the increased popularity of the diagnosis, the occurrence of false positives is all too common. A false positive diagnosis propels the patient into a particular patient career and course of experience that may be very difficult to alter. The patient's acceptance of the diagnosis of MPD is often so agonizing and transforming in its effect on the person and the therapeutic alliance that "backtracking" is difficult, if not, occasionally, perilous. Preliminary evidence (Kluft, 1991c; Chu, 1991) suggests that, among experts, the incidence of false positives is low, but it is unclear how many false positive diagnoses are made by less well-trained clinicians. The question of false positives has been of greatest concern to critics of the renewed interest in MPD. These concerns and the evidence for them are best summarized by North and colleagues (North et al., 1993).

The evidence suggests that false negative diagnoses have equal, if not greater, consequences: Patients with significant psychological problems who are not accurately diagnosed spend fruitless years in the mental health system, often at great financial and personal cost. In a review of over 200 cases, Kluft (1985) noted that for a large percentage of cases accurate diagnoses were only possible when extreme measures were employed. Specifically, in these cases, patients were so invested in the "pathology of secrecy" that they hid all evidence of dissociation to the degree that it was impossible to accurately diagnose them. Only when interviewed in extended sessions (up to 3 hours) did their masking of symptoms crumble and dissociative symptoms become manifest in the diagnostic evaluation. Subsequent to this, these patients provided more accurate and consistent information in response to straightforward mental status questions. Thus, a wider use of standardized assessment measures may help speed correct diagnosis.

Stages of Treatment

Kluft (1993) maintained that a consensus is emerging with respect to the wisdom of using a three-stage model to treat MPD and PTSD. The three stages specified by Kluft are: (1) stabilization; (2) the working through of trauma and the resolution of dissociative defenses, culminating in integration; and (3) postintegration treatment. Our rational model is framed in terms of these three stages.

STAGE 1

The first stage, the stabilization phase, covers at a minimum the period of treatment during which the therapeutic relationship and treatment ground rules are established, trust issues are explored, data relevant to the clarification of the diagnosis are gathered, diagnostic and prognostic information is presented to the patient, and preliminary interventions are designed and implemented to stabilize the patient's affect and behavior in the face of life stressors. Most authors (see Braun, 1986; Putnam, 1989) suggest that the initial stage of treatment should include the delineation of the specific features of each patient's system of divided self-representations (i.e., the "alter" system).

We would suggest that rather than define the stages of treatment in terms of "tasks" to be accomplished, it is more useful to define the stages in terms of qualitative changes in the process of therapy. In this sense, we extend Stage 1 of treatment to cover the period during which the stabilization and temporary relief of trauma symptoms predominate. During this period, the patient often experiences herself as being haplessly tossed about by turbulent emotions, "flashbacks," and other uncontrolled dissociative phenomena (e.g., "switching," amnesias, and/or extreme depersonalization).

Often, patients make concerted and persistent efforts to flee the implications of their diagnosis, which can be both terrifying and humiliating. Some MPD patients traverse this stage relatively quickly, expressing relief that they have a diagnosis that finally makes sense. However, the majority of MPD patients have considerable difficulty with accepting the diagnosis and its implications and may require months, or even years, to negotiate this stage sufficiently to move on in treatment.

Entry into Stage 2 is marked by the establishment of an adequate therapist–patient "working alliance" that is characterized by collaborative planning around the timing and the structure of the working through of remaining therapeutic issues. During this stage, the true "working through" or resolution of both the patient's traumatic history and dissociative pathology becomes possible.

From this perspective, Stage 1 is clearly the longest stage of treatment. In many cases, particularly for less experienced clinicians, Stage 1 might more aptly be described in terms of a cycle of stabilization, crisis, and restabilization. When the treatment begins too aggressively, most typically because of the assumption that the more one uncovers the better and faster the treatment will progress, Stage 1 often consists one of downward spiraling crises with intermittent periods of restabilization.

A common assumption is that the core of treatment consists of evoking the traumatic history. A corollary assumption is that the more rapid the history is uncovered, the more rapid and effective treatment will be.

Patients often encourage, or at least do not discourage, the practice of rapid uncovering because they experience intense distress that they believe can be relieved by emotional catharsis. Although systematic research with respect to this assumption is lacking, the patient's quality of life may, in fact, deteriorate when the primary treatment focus is on emotional catharsis rather than on symptom stabilization. Indeed, catharsis may not be of particular value because the essence of the trauma response is fear rather than encapsulated pain that needs to be vented (Kolb, 1988). Unmitigated fear can lead to the destabilization of defenses rather than personality integration when it is evoked in treatment. At this point, therapy produces fear and uncertainty in the MPD patient. The perception of therapy as unsafe only amplifies rather than soothes the patient's post-traumatic reactivity and panic, usually leading to an increase in self-destructive, post-traumatic and dissociative symptoms and behaviors. Not infrequently, this leads to repeated hospitalizations and a prolonged and unsuccessful treatment course.

Putnam (1989) has noted that the treatment of MPD is inevitably punctuated by emotional crises associated with the awareness and acceptance of the diagnosis of MPD; conflicts about facing the implications of a trauma-filled history; the impact of intensive treatment on family structure, the patient's work, and social functioning; and the negative effects of physiological and mood destabilization. No matter how expert the clinician, patients may become overinvolved or invested in these inevitable crises because they can represent defense mechanisms, which help to shield them from confronting the shame and humiliation of a history of degrading trauma.

Also, living in continual crisis may represent an unconscious reenactment of the patient's reported traumatic experiences, reactions, and affects from childhood. Phenomenologically, such behavior has been termed an "unconscious flashback" by Blank (1985). The recognition that unconscious flashbacks may play a part in such difficulties can provide the clinician with useful therapeutic leverage in helping to stabilize the patient. The emotional roller coaster that many MPD patients ride during the course of treatment, necessitates that the therapist maintain a steady focus on treatment goals and objectives. In summary, when therapists encourage emotional catharsis prior to symptom stabilization, the patient's limited resources are frequently overwhelmed and crises become more prevalent, often making a goal-directed treatment impossible as the patient moves from crisis to crisis.

One of the problems that therapists frequently enounter is the unexpected abreaction of traumatic past events and/or spontaneous regression to different ages and time periods, even in the earliest stages of treatment. This may occur despite the therapist's attempts to discourage premature catharsis. At this stage of treatment, the therapist's goal is to restabilize the patient rather than to resolve the trauma.

Restabilization of the patient requires a return to the here and now. Interventions that can be of great value in achieving this can be divided into two categories: (1) symbolic manipulations, and (2) reorientation to the here and now. Symbolic manipulations involve entering into the patient's current emotional state and redirecting or transforming it to make it more tolerable. For example, if a patient was reliving a memory of being locked in a closet as a child, the therapist can temporarily ameliorate it by suggesting that the patient's adult "self" or the therapist go back in time and space and unlock the child and carry her to a safe place. Storytelling, with all of its potential to magically alter time, space, and reality, can be exploited to create a variety of scenarios and experiences that have remarkable healing potential. These techniques are limited only by the imagination of the therapist and patient, and can include imagery of safe places, magic rings, secure fortresses, and laser shields, to list just a few examples. However, some patients, particularly those that report the use of hypnosis or imagery by abusers in the past to ensure compliance, may have great difficulty in using hypnotic techniques for therapeutic benefit.

The therapist can facilitate the patient's reorientation to the here and now by using techniques that promote the physiological and cognitive control of panic states. These techniques can, for example, involve focusing on deep, diaphragmatic breathing; suggestions for deep muscular relaxation; cue-controlled relaxation; and encouraging calming self-statements that orient the patient to the present (e.g., "That was then; this is now"). It can be helpful to introduce cognitive techniques to identify physical, verbal, or interpersonal "triggers" with the goal that the patient will work actively to identify similarities and differences between current situations and past traumatic ones. MPD patients frequently need to spend considerable effort in and out of therapy on such tasks in order to feel that their perceptions of current events are freely based on contemporary information and not on peremptory post-traumatic reactions.

Introducing the Diagnosis

The specific treatment methods associated with MPD are inaugurated when the therapist introduces the diagnosis to the patient. With the possible exception of schizophrenia, no other psychiatric diagnosis can instill a comparable sense of anxiety and confusion in the patient. Therefore, the therapist must target interventions not only to the patient as a person but also to the patient as a "multiple." To provide a positive orientation to treatment, the therapist must provide a realistic appraisal of the patient's prognosis to the extent that prediction is possible; a statement regarding the relative costs (e.g., pain, distress, and temporary setbacks) and benefits of treament (i.e., financial and emotional); and an assessment of alternatives to psychological treatment (e.g., "living with it," pharmacological, focal treatment for specific symptoms [e.g., anxiety, sleep disturbance, panic, and depression]).

To reduce the internal chaos that the diagnosis provokes, the therapist provides reassurance through addressing it directly. For instance, a direct statement such as, "Everyone listen, be quiet and listen, no one has to die, everyone gets a chance, but not everyone all at once," can have an immediate calming effect and mitigate resistance against accepting the diagnosis.

At this point, catastrophic fears regarding the implications of integration or fusion often emerge. In order to reduce confusion, it is probably best to avoid technical discussions with the patient concerning how integration is accomplished, and, instead, shift the focus to the benefits of establishing an "integrated," cooperative community as the therapeutic goal. The therapist must inform the patient that one of the first steps in the treatment will be to build a strong foundation of psychological resources to cope with the challenges of recovering from MPD.

Treatment Targets

Because MPD is a complex disorder, with affective, cognitive, behavioral, and interpersonal accompaniments, each of these domains requires a separate and specific focus. Specifically, MPD patients are most likely to experience dysregulation of affect and affect instability in the following areas: (1) fear and anxiety, (2) shame and guilt, (3) anger and rage, and (4) self-hating and loathing. Loneliness, isolation, and feelings of pain and hurt also need to be addressed in treatment.

Cognitive disturbances range from functional problems with memory and identity to specific patterns of cognitive distortion that can be identified in terms of disturbed self- and other schemas, generalized negative expectancies (e.g., "I will be rejected"), and false positive expectancies (e.g., failure to attend to danger cues in interpersonal situations).

Behavioral disturbances are most notable in the form of self-harming (e.g, self-mutilation) and suicidal behaviors, drug and alcohol abuse, eating disorders, escape and avoidance behaviors (e.g., transient fugue states), destruction of property, and criminal behavior. The therapist also may find subtle manifestations of behavioral dysregulation such as exaggerated responses to threat (e.g., physically assaulting someone who raises his or her voice) or, alternately, an inability to respond to threat (e.g., "rape paralysis"). MPD patients are also at risk to abuse their own children or to enmesh them in chaotic lifestyles (Kluft, 1984).

Interpersonal and relational difficulties are frequently evidenced, in part, because of the overlap between the MPD and borderline features mentioned above (Horevitz & Braun, 1984). Therapists (see Chu, 1988) frequently encounter patients who exhibit manipulative behaviors in the therapy setting, are unable to maintain stable interpersonal relationships, have sexual difficulties, and react impulsively and angrily with others. Although not so obviously problematic, but of equal importance, are behaviors that are excessively perfectionistic and reflect a need to appear "good" and blameless. This can be seen when a patient has a strong need to be a perfect parent or caretaker, to never make mistakes that could conceivably endanger others, to constantly apologize with respect to his or her common human frailties. Many patients also function socially and economically well below their potential, or are enmeshed in destructive social environments. Occasionally, problems also arise when the patient is overidentified with the idea of "being a multiple" or a survivor of abuse.

Strategies for Building a Treatment Foundation

A treatment sensitively tuned to each individual's unique skills, deficits, and problems is required to meet the diverse needs of the MPD patient. Typically, this approach requires a well thought out integration of therapeutic strategies that targets specific problems and symptoms while providing a platform for consistent behavior and responses from the therapist (Putnam & Loewenstein, 1993; Kluft, 1993).

Pharmacological Treatments

Even before psychological interventions are implemented, it may be appropriate to consider pharmacological interventions for symptomatic relief. However, the prescription of medications must occur in the context of a total treatment approach to MPD (Loewenstein, 1991b), with the knowledge that "most problems in the treatment of MPD are not solvable with medications" (p. 727). Nevertheless, certain symptoms are valid targets for psychopharmacological interventions. To justify drug treatment, these symptoms must generally be present in the "whole person" rather than exclusively appear with a single alter personality. Symptom clusters that are obvious candidates for drug treatment include the following: (1) comorbid major depressive disorder, (2) PTSD symptoms (including panic attacks and severe generalized anxiety), (3) severe sleep disturbances, (4) obsessive compulsive symptoms, and (5) the rare occurrence of true psychotic symptoms. Some authors (e.g., Braun, 1990) have proposed using pharmacological interventions to target dissociative symptoms such as switching directly. However, these treatments remain in the experimental stage, without a systematic study as to their effectiveness. It is unclear if these interventions actually target the process of dissociation itself, or the post-traumatic symptoms of hyperarousal and reactivity that drive switching and self-mutilation.

Cognitive-Behavioral Techniques

Cognitive and cognitive-behavioral techniques can be applied to specific symptoms such as affect dysregulation, as well as to more enduring personality problems. These techniques are particularly useful in challenging persistent and often contradictory beliefs that characterize dissociative pathology. Because the rational treatment of MPD involves a process of titrating affect while exploring the patient's internal world, cognitive-behavioral techniques are useful in the early stages of treatment when the regulation of affect is paramount. Before any cognitive-behavioral interventions can be implemented, a careful assessment of the patient's assumptions, automatic thoughts, and underlying beliefs about treatment, MPD, and everyday life experiences is necessary (Fine, 1991). In addition to the cognitive-behavioral techniques mentioned above, social skills training can also be implemented, along with strategies that have proven useful in the management of borderline personality symptoms (Linehan, 1993).

The primary guide to the sequence of treatment interventions is the patient's behavior between the therapy sessions. As Linehan (1993) suggests, suicidal and parasuicidal (e.g., self-mutilation) behaviors should always be treated first. No other topics are discussed until the adequate resolution of these and related issues is achieved. If there have been any therapy-interrupting (e.g., frequent emergency calls, failure to attend sessions) or self-destructive (e.g., drug and alcohol use) behaviors, they are discussed before trauma-related issues are explored. In summary, treatment is paced by the patient's capacity to maintain behavioral self-control and to remain focused on intersession treatment goals. *Failure to maintain self-control never warrants further "depth" exploration of the historical reasons for this failure, but instead mandates close attention to the immediate precipitants of the problem and the failure to cope in everyday life.*

In some situations, it may be important to work with the patient to recognize the extent to which a failure of self-control represents a reenactment of or response to a past traumatic situation. However, this attention to historical data should not result in a complete examination of the traumatic material. Rather, it should be used to support the patient cognitively, so that he or she can separate present reality from past trauma in order adapt successfully to his or her current situation.

Dynamic Psychotherapy

Psychodynamic psychotherapy provides important guideposts to the treatment of MPD: Regardless of the therapist's preferred psychotherapeutic orientation, it is almost always helpful to create a strong therapeutic alliance and to understand the patient's reality-based and transference-based distortions of the psychotherapy relationship. In treating patients who almost always seem to deserve special consideration in light of their extensive trauma history, care is needed to prevent ethical and therapeutic boundary lapses and violations (e.g., not adhering to session time limits, befriending the patient). Attention to the dissociative and post-traumatic aspects of transference and countertransference may permit the more effective resolution of boundary difficulties, projective identification, and acting out in many MPD patients (Loewenstein, 1993; Loewenstein & Ross, 1992). Over the years, problems, such as those involving iatrogenicity treatment impasses and the behavior of delinquent therapists, have begun to receive the attention they deserve in a steadily growing literature (Fine, 1989; Greaves, 1988; Kluft, 1989).

The treatment of MPD often requires that the therapist be very active in treatment, in contrast to the therapeutic abstinence mandated by classical psychoanalytic practice. For example, it is important for the therapist to continually confront patients' refusal to deal with personal and interpersonal conflicts, as well as patients' tendency to unconsciously create crises and to provoke the therapist. Confrontation is best achieved without resorting to a confrontational style. Instead, the therapist can exhibit an openness to the patient and a high degree of curiosity about the meaning of his or her behaviors (e.g., "It is interesting that this problem is occuring right now; we'd best stop what we've been doing until we understand it better and you have it under better control").

Exploring the Patient's Internal World with Hypnosis

Hypnosis can be a very valuable tool in the treatment of MPD (Horevitz, 1993). Indeed, many of the therapists (Allison, 1974; Bowers et al., 1971; Braun, 1984; Horevitz, 1983; Kluft, 1982) who have pioneered treatment techniques for MPD have devised creative hypnotic procedures for exploring the internal world of the MPD patient. Nevertheless, many of the techniques that we describe in relation to hypnosis can also be employed in the nonhypnotic treatment of MPD.

Making "maps" of the patient's internal world if often an important component of many treatment approaches (Braun, 1986). These schematic, graphic representations lend order to a complex, often chaotic, internal world. Although the internal phenomenal world is often experienced as chaotic, the mapping of the personality system often reveals an internal world that is actually quite structured and laced with webs of interpersonal relationships, which form systems in the family or organizational systems' sense of the word. These systems may have a hierarchical organization with dominant personalities or alters playing key roles regarding the access and control of information made available to the therapist as well as the patient (cf. Horevitz, 1983, 1993). From the patient's point of view, the overarching goal of this control and regulatory function is the protection of individual personalities and the integrity of the system as a whole. Despite this, the internal relationships between and among personalities is not fixed. It changes during the course of treatment in relation to both therapeutic gains and the discovery of more deeply hidden dissociated experiences.

MPD patients vary in their ability to elicit the appearance or presence of alters. Hypnosis is useful, for example, when nonhypnotic means to elicit the appearance of an alter fail or a specific communication to a specific alter must be guaranteed to forestall a crisis. Often, there are deeply dissociated alters that do not respond or reveal themselves through ordinary means and must be searched for aggressively with hypnosis.

Since suicidal and self-destructive behavior play critical roles in MPD patients' lives, behavioral contracts of relevance to this behavior are vital. These are *internal* arrangements, not contractual agreements with the therapist (Thames, 1984). The use of hypnosis to facilitate co-consciousness helps assure the greatest degree of cooperation and compliance with contracts (cf. Putnam, 1989).

Internal communication between the alters helps to regulate crises, establish a positive therapeutic alliance, and support interventions. Formats for intervention can include indirect communication (e.g., placing a bulletin board in a safe place in the person's imagination), group communication (e.g., with adult or child alters only), nonverbal communication (e.g., having an adult alter hold a child alter), and selective communication (e.g., always having certain alters available when traumatic memories are surfacing). In many cases, however, techniques to facilitate communication and internal stabilization are thwarted by internal conflicts, mistrust, and alters sabotaging one another. Thus, techniques in and of themselves must be supplemented by interventions to enhance inter-personality empathy and collaboration. Confrontation of even subtle forms of internal abusiveness and disavowal among alters is often required to establish the basis for improved internal communication. In some cases, the MPD patient has certain basic assumptions that thwart communication, which must be challenged (e.g., "If we have any communication, then the bad people can get all of us just by getting one of us"). Others may feel so shameful and guilty that they masochistically foil helpful interventions because they feel undeserving of any relief.

One of the main tasks of the stabilization phase of treatment is to manage the inevitable crises that occur in the course of treating MPD. Certain crises, including self-mutilating urges, breakthrough memories, spontaneous abreactions, and intense loneliness, are an inherent part of treatment. Practiced responses to these crises should be developed early in therapy. Crises that arise as therapy progresses should also be dealt with immediately. Internal control techniques can include relaxation and self-hypnosis skills; audiotaped hypnotic sessions; and hypnotic interventions for symptom control or alleviation. Once internal communication is established between and among alters, more enduring patterns of communication can be developed. These enduring patterns help alters become more empathetic toward each other, thereby reducing the likelihood of self-desctructive acts and self-defeating behaviors.

Hypnotic techniques can be used to improve the communication process between and among alters. Hypnotic suggestions can be used to enhance two-way verbal communication between alters; to establish common links, interests, and goals across a variety of seemingly different alters; to promote cognitive reframing (e.g., the idea of all for one and one for all); to permit the discussion of historical events and personal perspectives; to teach models of effective communication; and to establish ground rules for effective communication. Braun (1988a, 1988b) introduced the BASK (behavior, affect, sensation, knowledge) model to describe information processing in dissociation. He described how it can be utilized clinically to enhance memory retrieval and internal communication through reassembling dissociated experience (1988b).

Hypnotic suggestions can also be employed as part of a constraint system to block the "switching process." Posed in metaphor and imagery, the suggestions can involve images of physical restraint and containment (e.g., linking arms in a circle to prevent an angry alter personality in the center from breaking out), images of "suspended animation" (e.g., floating in time and space because of cryogenic cooling), and images that empower frightened alters to restrain a dangerous or "acting out" alter.

Most therapists have techniques to "close" sessions so that upsetting material does not spill into nonsession time. Images readily accepted by many patients include: sealed boxes or chests that hold the material between sessions, books or videotapes that are placed on a library shelf, and memories captured in photographs that are placed in albums or framed and hung far away.

Existential and Experiential Treatment

Hypnosis and hypnotic-like techniques are useful in obtaining a map of the patient's inner world. However, once the dissociative defenses have been lowered to permit both internal communication between and among alters, and communication with the therapist, many suppressed issues as well as memories surface. MPD patients characteristically hold many contradictory beliefs (Fine, 1988; Ross, 1989) that create tension and emotional discomfort (e.g., they may hear contradictory internal voices, or voices that derogate present action), which prevent the patient from accepting the conclusions that would follow from holding any one set of beliefs consistently. Because childhood trauma, deprivation, and degradation play a pivotal role in the genesis of MPD, the image of self the patient sees reflected in abusive others, by virtue of their behavior, words, and facial expression, is full of horrifying contradictions, loathing, contempt, and disregard. Much of what MPD patients do behaviorally and symbolically represent attempts to nullify painful self-images either through attempting to "prove" the opposite (e.g., "I am good, not bad") or through engaging in contradictory or masochistic behaviors that relieve the burdern of self (Baumeister, 1989). In other words, behavior is used to control self-perception (Powers, 1973; Carver & Scheier, 1982). Intervention into this system precipitates the emergence of suppressed thoughts, images, and conclusions about the self, virtually all of which are charged with negative affect.

What emerges can be conceptualized as both an existential crisis and as experiential/cognitive dissonance. Existential issues that arise include profound identity questions such as the following: If I am a "multiple" and I have "alters," then what am I? Am I an "alter" too? Am I a real person? If all this really happened to me (and I did all the things I remember), how can I go on living? If I am just a psychiatric freak, who will ever want to have anything to do with me? Other existential questions related to the survival of the self include: Am I so damaged that I will never be a complete person? Am I so dirty that no one will ever want me? Can I endure all this pain and still survive? Can I view all this horror and still survive? Is there any way to live a dignified life?

In order to help the patient negotiate these crises of the "self," the therapist must have a coherent notion of what answers to these questions might be and what a pathway through these existential conundrums must look like, otherwise the therapist will be in danger of falling prey to the patient's fantasies of restitution wherein the therapist's love and caring is felt to be the basis of healing.

Who is the patient? Dissociative processes, such as those symbolized in the characters of the alter system, are best understood as ways of adapting to overwhelming stress. These characters are not autonomous individuals but discrete self-identities within a person who has one body, one set of DNA, and one life history. Patients must be encouraged to accept the fundamental unity of their personhood from the very beginning of treatment. There is little credible developmental data to support the idea often expressed in the literature that there is a "birth," or "core," personality from which others "split off" (see Putnam, 1992).

A more plausible developmental hypothesis suggests that the alters develop out of repeated experiences of extreme trauma in children before they reach an age when the capacity to maintain state stability or a sense of self across extreme state shifts has been developed (Putnam, 1992). The patient's hope for redemption from a history of intolerable pain and suffering must spring not from dependence or wishes for unity with an all powerful therapist, but instead from the patient's personal determination to create a meaningful existence. In therapy, this can be framed in terms of the idea that the patient do something to leave the world a better place than it was when he or she was born (Frankl, 1959).

Leading the patient through the most severe existential crises is part of the second stage of treatment, and will be addressed later. However, important preliminary cognitive preparatory work occurs during Stage 1 of treatment. Cognitive, paradoxical, and experiential therapeutic strategies overlap in this stage (cf. Beck, Rush, Shaw, & Emery, 1979). Encouraging each alter identity to "speak" and express core beliefs and attitudes, while reporting its experiences of trauma and its internal world, has important consequences. First, it allows hidden contradictions in attitudes, beliefs, and assumptions to emerge (e.g., the punitive angry alter that expresses hate and initiates self-harm can reveal its basic protective functions). Second, it permits the therapist to question the basis or validity of maladaptive beliefs. Third, as alters begin to confront the contradictions in their world views, the strong affect that was supported, in part, by contradictory beliefs wanes, and the ostensible differences between alters diminish, revealing an underlying unity. Contrary to the common belief that giving alters a voice tends to reify or strengthen their presentation, clinical experience suggests that while alters do become temporarily more conspicuous, encouraging each alter to "have its say" ultimately promotes the full airing of attitudes and feelings that makes integration possible.

Earlier we discussed the internal world of the MPD patient in terms of family dynamics. Thus, it is reasonable to view family therapy models as appropriate interventions in the structuring and resolving of the patient's ubiquitous internal conflicts. Not only are the rules of "good communication" required, but agreements to block violent and verbally destructive behaviors are also prerequisites to effective family therapy. MPD patients, in general, appear very willing to make and sustain internal contracts for controlling their behavior. Contracts are constructed as internal agreements that are guaranteed through the therapist. If the contract is in danger of being broken, the therapist is contacted prior to acting out (Braun, 1986).

Family therapy emphasizes the establishment and maintenance of generational boundaries (Bowen, 1966). In the treatment of MPD, as in family therapy, when adults are viewed as responsible for the well-being of their children, their role as parents and protectors is enhanced. Thus, the many caretaking tasks that child alters require should be executed by adult alters, not by the therapist. Family therapy techniques that emphasize paradoxical intervention and reframing can be utiliziled to help the patient realign his or her personality system in a healthier way and to reduce the impact of many powerful alters on the system as a whole.

Adjunctive Therapies

Many adjunctive therapies have found a place in the treatment of MPD. Art therapy (Kluft, 1984), dance and expressive therapies (E. Kluft, Poteat, & R. P. Kluft, 1986), and even body therapy (Skinner, 1990) can be useful in helping patients express, modulate, and integrate emotional experiences as well as allowing a greater freedom of expression and increased physiological capacities for the sustenance of emotion.

Family and marital therapy may also be an essential part of the patient's treatment. Occasionally, such therapy may be brief and focused on providing family members with the tools they need to cope with a family member who suffers from MPD. Often, however, serious family and marital problems have developed prior to MPD treatment and constitute yet another complication in the patient's life. Our experience suggests that when marital and family therapies are used to gain leverage or "understanding" for the MPD patient because of his or her trauma history or need for special privileges in the family due to the disorder his or her problems will very likely exacerbate. There is little warrant for violating the normative rules of family and marital therapy for MPD patients. If anything, the patient's trauma history may best be alluded to rather than reported in detail, in part because it is no easier for a spouse or family to master than for the patient to do so, although rare exceptions to this rule may exist in extremely strong marriages with high-functioning patients. However, it is important for the family/marital therapist to be familiar with the childhood abuse and trauma and with dissociative disorders in general in order to provide optimal treatment and to prevent the treatment from becoming another arena for the MPD patient's maladaptive behavior.

Group therapies and self-help support groups (Caul, Sachs, & Braun, 1986) have also been used in the treatment of MPD patients. Group treatments are best suited to the provision of emotional support and to teach psychological, social, and everyday life skills (Coons & Bradley, 1985). Linehan's (1993) well-researched and highly efficacious group treatment model for borderline patients can be adapted to treat MPD patients. Groups that specifically focus on trauma or exploring the dissociative aspects of the patients' disorders are unlikely to be successful, at least outside of a hospital setting.

MPD patients frequently start or join self-help or self-support groups. Although we would like to state otherwise, the general experience of MPD experts has been that few of these groups are helpful or long-lived. Many MPD support groups actually have been overtly destructive, especially to vulnerable MPD patients who are easily taken advantage of by more dominating, and often exploitative, group members. Therapists should be cautious before endorsing entrance into a support group for their MPD patients and should explore in depth the possible risks and benefits of doing so at their particular stage of treatment.

Many patients require hospitalization during the course of their treatment. This often presents problems when the patient is hospitalized on a general psychiatric unit with a mixed population or where the staff is hostile toward or in conflict about patients diagnosed with MPD. A number of specialized dissociative disorders units have been instituted in hospitals across the country. Nevertheless, hospitalization poses many hazards for the MPD patient, ranging from overstimulation by treatments meant to rapidly uncover trauma to exposure to highly negative environments where the patients' needs are unmet. Thus hospitalization is best reserved for severe suicidal crises, unresolved danger posed to others, overwhelming life dysfunction, severe or life-threatening eating or substance abuse disorders, or for intensive work on issues that cannot be safely addressed on an outpatient basis. When serious diagnostic confusion exists that cannot be resolved on an outpatient basis, an inpatient stay on an expert unit will often provide opportunities for systematic observation that permits the resolution of diagnostic issues (see Kluft, 1991b, for a review).

STAGE 2

During Stage 2, we address two primary goals. The overriding goal is the reduction or resolution of dissociative symptoms and defenses and the integration of dissociated aspects of the self-identity into a single functional personal identity. We refer to three distinct types of dissociative symptoms and defenses that require attention in treatment: (1) those that include amnesia and episodes of "switching" between and among alter identity states; (2) dissociative memories; and (3) dissociated, seemingly separate, identity states. Specifically, we want to minimize the use of dissociative defenses such as amnesia and "switching"; integrate dissociative memories with life events; and integrate the various identity states. As dissociative symptoms and defenses are resolved, the second goal of this stage of treatment can be realized: to resolve traumatic experience and integrate the patient's trauma history into his or her more general life history.

To be sure, work with the aftereffects of trauma is not limited to a particular stage of therapy. Indeed, it is an ongoing task of therapy and a lifelong task for the MPD patient. However, systematic efforts to resolve trauma are deferred until a strong working alliance is established, and the patient has the resources needed to cope with the intense feelings aroused by abreaction. It is very important to note that many patients may never reach this stage in their treatment. In fact, for certain patients, lifelong case management may be a preferred treatment option.

As the patient's entry into Stage 2 is marked by a strong therapeutic alliance with the therapist, a corresponding degree of internal cooperation among alters has also been achieved by this time. At this point, alters are able to freely communicate and collaborate on problem solving in relation to issues that affect the whole person. Alters who formerly demanded time for their own self-centered interests are now able to delay gratification of their own needs in favor of the interests of the whole person. Nonetheless, while they have come to share certain goals and assumptions, sufficient reasons for their continued separateness still exists. The primary remaining reasons are related not so much to differences in beliefs and assumptions, but to the need to keep painful traumatic memories encapsulated so that the person as a whole is not overwhelmed. Alters themselves will express reluctance over facing their own memories for fear of what will happen to them.

Further progress toward integration now requires obtaining each alter's agreement regarding its willingness to work with personally relevant trauma. By this point, the factual outlines of traumatic material should be apparent, and the patient should have at least some titrated exposure to the related affects.

It is necessary for the therapist and patient to plan a series of sessions designed to explore the full ramifications of the trauma in the patient's life. Part of the planning process involves discovering in advance as many of the alter identities that embody specific aspects of the trauma, and all of the historical information, beliefs, and fears patients harbor about it. A collaborative effort wherein the therapist and patient discuss safety needs, probable length of time required for the work, setting a date to commence, and all concerns about what needs to be covered are all part of the preliminary planning (cf. Steele, 1989).

Planned Abreaction

Simply stated, the working through of any material represents the symbolic transformation of traumatic experience into a verbal story that is integrated into the larger context of the personal history (Horevitz, 1993). A history consists not only of past childhood traumatic events, but also of all the events, accomplishments, behaviors, and relationships that constitute life in the present. Therefore, the working through must involve reframing the verbally transformed material into the whole of the personal history.

At the core of all traumatic memory is overwhelming terror wherein past and present cannot be differentiated, and the future does not exist. Pain and survival are the imminent realities of this experience. The grip of terror is diminished when the therapist gradually helps the patient see that history proves that he or she really did (and will) survive.

When working with memory, therapists should be less concerned with alleviating pain than with creating coping strategies that help the patient maintain personal integrity and purpose in life. Hypnotic techniques can be used to enhance this process. They can help to uncover and link current symptoms with hidden experience. Hypnosis can also be used to help identify important "personal" trauma memories of alters that are too painful to access without assistance. Age-regression techniques, common to hypnotherapy, are less commonly used in the treatment of MPD, although they can be valuable in recovering the narrative account and memories of individual traumatic events. Age regression is also utilized in reconstructing the larger picture of the relationships and events of childhood, which constitutes the patient's personal history. Hypnotic events can also be useful in localizing and identifying amnesias and their functions.

Reconstruction of fully lost, partially remembered, or missequenced events often requires the use of hypnotic techniques specifically designed to shield the patient from direct, overwhelming, or affective reactions. Patients can be encouraged first to reconstruct a memory in a detached manner. Classical hypnotic interventions such as a projective screen or stage techniques, where the patient sees the events as if on television, in the movies, or on stage, are useful here. Dissociative techniques whereby the patient envisions him- or herself as if in a depersonalized state while watching and narrating the events is another variation on this theme. While there are any number of approaches to memory reconstruction, one safe and logical approach involves beginning by first focusing on the narrative, and then repeatedly prodding with such statements as "And then what happened" or "Now what is happening," rather than by exploring meaning or feeling. As the patient discovers his or her narrative history, it can be processed in nonhypnotic sessions in terms of its meaning to the patient. When the patient has developed a cognitive framework that helps him or her to make sense of the event, hypnotic work can be reintroduced that allows the event to be relived on a more emotional basis.

Kluft's (1993) "fractionation" method involves exposure to small (ranging from seconds to a few minutes) components of a particular memory, then discussing the experience utilizing the tools of therapeutic reframing and affective processing. As the patient is able to process parts of the memory experience, increasingly large segments are covered until the entire trauma is recalled with all its intensity. This may occur in a single session or many sessions may be required to process the trauma.

The work of this stage of therapy is incomplete until an entire memory and its emotional associations is reconstructed from the combined input of all of the alters working together in harmony. Each alter eventually comes to accept the memory as valid by having the therapist help it realize that it was in fact present in the person's body at the time of the event, by the therapist's encouraging each alter to dialogue about its different perceptions of the event and its perceptions of blame and responsibility, and by discussing the impact of the experience on the whole person. This latter step is crucial to the natural process of integration, as different parts come to see themselves as increasingly similar both in terms of history and character. Even the therapist begins to have problems differentiating the previously unintegrated "parts" of the personality as shared memories become a basis for shared identity.

Frequently, even with carefully planned memory work, aspects of the original traumatic experience or its derivatives remain undiscovered. While these may be minor pieces of the story, the full existential impact of the story is not realized until they are uncovered. Working through all of the dissociated aspects of memory is critical to success. In fact, incomplete memory work is often cited as a major reason for therapeutic failure (Putnam, 1989; Kluft, 1982).

Integration and Fusion

Integration and fusion are often used as synonyms for the process by which multiple identities are reduced to a single coherent identity in MPD patients. Following Kluft's (1982) suggestion, we distinguish between *fusion*, the experience of a merging of identities, and *integration*, the more complex process of the psychological structuring of a unified individual. Thus, fusions are often symbolic events where dissociative barriers are collapsed and alters spontaneously lose a sense of separate identity. Fusions mark a particular event that is preceded by the beginning of the slow integration of memory, experiences, psychological processes, personal motives and interests, as well as functional capacities that forms the bedrock of the deeper integration of self that is the work of the third stage of treatment. Structurally, the formal fusion of alters is akin to the formal marriage ceremony—itself preceded by dating, courtship, and the negotiation of the future (engagement) and deepened through the actual years of marriage to arrive (hopefully) at a stage of mature love, marriage, and partnership. They should never be forced, except in life-threatening circumstances. Although the major work of integration and fusion is expected to occur in the latter stage of treatment, many patients present with very fragmented identity states that readily respond to suggestions for integration early in treatment, particularly if no significant reason exists for their separateness. Spontaneous integrations of this sort are not rare occurrences throughout the course of treatment. Occasionally, preliminary fusions may be attempted for protective purposes, though often they will not be permanent.

Kluft (1982) has pointed out that fusion rituals occur at the point in treatment when a group of alters has become so similar that even they have difficulty maintaining separate boundaries. Fusion rituals employ imagery in which things blend and flow together. Fusions occur throughout treatment as discrete parts of dissociative experience are worked through. Undiscovered dissociative elements, hidden trauma, or external stress may break apart a fusion. Most fusion experiences are followed by temporary periods of disorientation and physiological disequilibrium. Hypnotic interventions, similar to those traditionally used for ego strengthening or promoting general well-being (e.g., Hartland, 1971), facilitate the process of establishing inner equilibrium.

Clinicians and patients commonly anticipate that fusions will be associated with an immediate increase in subjective well-being. Although this is true in some situations, at other times, fusion may be associated with dysphoria, anxiety, a transient decrease in certain abilities, the emergence of new layers of alters, and somatic symptoms. Therapists should keep in mind that there are many potential outcomes to a fusion, even with the same patient at different times in treatment.

STAGE 3

Even after dissociative defenses and symptoms are resolved and the trauma history has been integrated into the larger personal history and is devoid of crippling anxiety, the work of therapy is not finished. The postfusion stage of treatment is sometimes long and arduous (1–2 years) and sometimes relatively brief (3 months), yet rarely crisis filled. To the disappointment of the patient, and often of the therapist, many areas of life that formerly seemed mastered by the patient are handled less well after fusion. Gaps appear in skills, knowledge, and function that had been hidden by dissociative switching. The deficits here can be a result of the inherent difficulty in maintaining consistent behavior over time when different emotions, and interpersonal and social pressures impinge on the individual who formerly mastered these pressures through dissociative stategies. Interpersonal skills are usually limited and impaired as a result of early trauma and a chaotic family life. Thus, a sense of pervasive "inner" loneliness associated with the loss of a familiar internal world is often a serious problem. For some patients, the postfusion period does not seem so problematic, although even with them, many issues that typically (e.g., career, family) had been neglected have to be attended to in this final stage of treatment.

In this stage of treatment, grief may be a particularly prominent emotion as the patient fully comprehends, without resorting to dissociative defenses, the losses that a trauma-filled dissociative life has caused. During this stage, patients must often rework significant parts of their earlier therapy from the new unified perspective they now possess. This may lead to renewed grief and confusion regarding some experiences the patient (and therapist) thought were resolved earlier in treatment. When this occurs, it should not be cause for alarm; it represents the increasing depth of meaning life has for the patient.

Before closing it is worth noting that repressed or dissociative memory recall in treatment has become an area of great controversy (Lynn & Nash, 1994; Loftus, 1993). While we cannot address this complex issue in this chapter, we believe that clinicians tend to ignore the basic findings of the cognitive sciences regarding memory, the reconstruction of memory, and the power of suggestion, context, and expectancy to affect memory recall. Thus, the probability that memory processes will be iatrogenically influenced may be high. However, to date, no one has demonstrated that significant false memory problems exist in trauma survivors (see Horevitz, Chapter 20, this volume).

In addition, memory may be distorted by a variety of patient factors, not just by injudicious therapeutic interventions or naive conceptualizations of the photographic accuracy of all trauma memories. For example, patients may report systematic efforts by perpetrators of abuse to confuse memory. Patients may also unconsciously disguise or distort aspects of memory in order to decrease their shame or horror at what they recall. Ganaway (1989) suggests that some patients may come to believe a more complex form of trauma occurred to defend against the full impact of a prosaic intrafamilial incest history. Terr (1988) noticed that documented trauma memories may be subject to the distortion of significant details, although the person recalls that the basic event occurred. It is also possible that a traumatized dissociative child may experience repeated PTSD flashbacks as additional actual events, which leads to a sense that he or she was more frequently traumatized than is actually the case.

Accordingly, some MPD patients may maintain a consistent history over treatment time and others may significantly alter their view of the past as integration proceeds. It is best for the clinician to maintain a stance of supportive neutrality concerning the accuracy of the patient's memories, thereby helping the patient to sort this out him- or herself as treatment progresses. In the course of treatment, MPD patients become far more able to consider the complex factors that may affect accurate recall, rather than focus on the question of "truth" versus "lies" or "made up." As one patient finally remarked, "I'm not asking if you believe me. I'm asking if you believe *in* me to figure it out."

The recent increase in recall of "satanic ritual abuse" has led to serious concerns regarding these patient claims. Some of these claims have not been corroborated by police investigation, although a few individuals have been convicted of crimes involving this phenomena. In light of this, perhaps the best treatment stance is not to be overinvested in the veracity of any particular memory claim and, as we suggest throughout this chapter, to attend to the core treatment issues of patient stabilization, resolution of dissociative defenses, and improved patient functioning.

NOTE

1. Multiple Personality Disorder (MPD) was renamed Dissociative Identity Disorder in DSM-IV. This change in nomenclature is a major improvement because it corrects the profound conceptual confusion that the term "multiple personalities" presents: We only poorly understand the construct of personality and the idea of multiple personalities in a single individual has seemed an oxymoron to many. Since identity represents the subjective quality of conscious experience rather than the objective pattern of traits and behaviors that characterize a person, there is no logical contradiction in either multiple and/or dissociated identities. Despite the improvement this change in nomenclature begets, it is likely that the traditional designation of MPD will endure in the literature and in both clinical and public perception. For these reasons, we have chosen to retain the traditional MPD.

Traditionally, alternate identities have been viewed as separate personalities and have frequently been treated as if they possessed separate personality organizations with unique physiological and even neurobiological substrates (Braun, 1983). Evidence for this position does not seem compelling to us; we prefer to follow Putnam (1989, 1992) and Kluft's (1991a) efforts to conceptualize these states as complex affective/cognitive processes, some of which have very stable features but great underlying plasticity. Nonetheless, subjectively, the idea of separate identities is very compelling to MPD patients, and there is little reason to invent new nomenclature to replace the term "alter," which we shall use throughout. How "alters" might become organized into a complex internal world requires a fundamental understanding of the process of the development of self, the normal and pathological patterns of cognitive and behavioral integration, the role of the imagination in the development of personal narrative, and a host of other factors that relate to the normative foundations of identity. We can only note that patients with MPD almost uniformly report organized internal worlds rather than mere collections of alter identities.

REFERENCES

Allison, R. B. (1974). A new treatment approach for multiple personalities. *American Journal of Clinical Hypnosis, 17*, 17–32.

American Psychiatric Association. (1987). *Diagnostic and statistical manual of mental disorders* (3rd ed., rev.). Washington, DC: Author.

Armstrong, J, & Loewenstein, R. J.(1990). Characteristics of patients with multiple personality and dissociative disorders on psychological testing. *Journal of Nervous and Mental Disease, 178*, 448–458.

Baumeister, R. F. (1989). *Masochism and the self.* Hillsdale, NJ: Lawrence Erlbaum.

Beck, A., Rush, J., Shaw, B., & Emery, G. (1979). *Cognitive therapy of depression.* New York: Guilford Press.

Bernstein, E. M., & Putnam, F. W. (1986). Development, reliability and validity of a dissociation scale. *Journal of Nervous and Mental Disease, 174*, 727–735.

Blank, A. S. (1985). The unconscious flashback to the war in Viet Nam veterans: Clinical mystery, legal defense, and community problem. In S. M. Sonnenberg, A. S. Blank, & J. A. Talbott (Eds.), *The trauma of war: Stress and recovery in Vietnam veterans* (pp. 293–308). Washington, DC: American Psychiatric Press.

Bliss, E. L. (1984). A symptom profile of patients with multiple personalities, including MMPI results. *Journal of Nervous and Mental Disease, 172*, 197–202.

Boon, S., & Draijer, N. (1993). Multiple personality disorder in the Netherlands: A clinical investigation of 71 patients. *American Journal of Psychiatry, 150*, 489–494.

Bowen, M. (1966). The use of family theory in clinical practices. *Comprehensive Psychiatry, 7*, 345–374.

Bowers, M. K., Brecher-Marer, S., Newton, B. W., Piotrowski, Z., Spyer, T. C., Tayler, W. S., & Watkins, J. G. (1971). Therapy of multiple personality. *International Journal of Clinical and Experimental Hypnosis, 19*, 57–65.

Braun, B. G. (1983). Neurophysiologic changes in multiple personality. *American Journal of Clinical Hypnosis, 26*, 84–92.

Braun, B. G. (1984). Uses of hypnosis with multiple personality. *Psychiatric Annals, 14*, 34–40.

Braun, B. G. (1986). Issues in the psychotherapy of multiple personality. In B. G. Braun, (Ed.), *The treatment of multiple personality disorder* (pp. 1–28). Washington, DC: American Psychiatric Press.

Braun, B. G. (1988a). The BASK (behavior, affect, sensation, knowledge) model of dissociation. *Dissociation, 1*, 4–23.

Braun, B. G. (1988b). The BASK model of dissociation: Clinical implications. *Dissociation, 1*, 16–23.

Braun, B. G. (1990). Unusual medication regimens in the treatment of dissociative disorder patients. *Dissociation, 3*, 144–150.

Braun, B. G., & Sachs, R. G. (1985). The development of multiple personality disorder: Predisposing, precipitating, and perpetuating factors. In R. P. Kluft (Ed.), *Childhood antecedents of multiple personality disorder* (pp. 37–64). Washington, DC: American Psychiatric Press.

Carver, C. S., & Scheier, M. F. (1981). *Attention and self-regulation: A control-theory approach to human behavior.* New York: Springer-Verlag.

Caul, D., Sachs, R. G., & Braun, B. G. (1986). Group therapy in the treatment of multiple personality disorder. In B. G. Braun (Ed.), *Treatment of multiple personality disorder* (pp.143–156). Washington, DC: American Psychiatric Press.

Chu, J. A. (1988). Ten traps for therapists in the treatment of trauma survivors. *Dissociation, 1*, 24–32.

Chu, J. A. (1991). On the misdiagnosis of multiple personality disorder. *Dissociation, 4*, 200–204.

Coons, P., & Bradley, K. (1985). Group psychotherapy with multiple personality patients. *Journal of Nervous and Mental Disease, 173*, 515–521.

Coons, P. M. (1984). The differential diagnosis of multiple personality disorder. *Psychiatric Clinics of North America, 7*, 51–67.

Fine, C. G. (1988). Thoughts on the cognitive perceptual substrates of multiple personality disorder. *Dissociation, 1*, 5–10.

Fine, C. G. (1989). Treatment errors and iatrogenesis across therapeutic modalities in MPD and allied dissociative disorders. *Dissociation, 2*, 77–82.

Fine, C. G. (1991). Treatment stabilization and crisis prevention: Pacing the therapy of the multiple personality disorder patient. *Psychiatric Clinics of North America, 14*, 661–675.

Frankl, V. E. (1959). *From death camp to existentialism: A psychiatrist's path to a new therapy.* Boston: Beacon Press.

Fraser, G. A., & Raine, D. A. (1993, November). *Cost analysis of the treatment of multiple personality disorders.* Paper presented at the 9th International Conference on Multiple Personality and Dissociative States, Chicago, IL.

Frischholz, E. J., & Braun, B. G. (1991, August). *Diagnosing dissociative disorders: New methods.* Paper presented at the 99th annual convention of the American Psychological Association, San Francisco, CA.

Ganaway, G. K. (1989). Historical truth versus narrative truth: Clarifying the role of exogenous trauma in the etiology of multiple personality disorder and its variants. *Dissociation, 2*, 205–220.

Greaves, G. B. (1988). Common errors in the treatment of multiple personality disorder. *Dissociation, 1*, 61–66.

Hartland, J. (1971). *Medical and dental hypnosis* (2nd ed.). London: Balliere Tindall.

Horevitz, R. (1983). Hypnosis for multiple personality disorder: A framework for beginning. *American Journal of Clinical Hypnosis, 26*, 138–145.

Horevitz, R. P., & Braun, B. G. (1984). Are multiple personalities borderline?: An analysis of 33 cases. *Psychiatric Clinics of North America, 7*, 69–88.

Horevitz, R. P. (1993). Hypnosis in the treatment of multiple personality disorder. In J. W. Rhue, S. J. Lynn, & I. Kirsch (Eds.), *Handbook of clinical hypnosis* (pp. 395–424). Washington, DC: American Psychiatric Association Press.

Kluft, E., Poteat, E., & Kluft, R. P. (1986). Movement observations in multiple personality disorder: A preliminary report. *American Journal of Dance Therapy, 9*, 31–46.

Kluft, R. P. (1982). Varieties of hypnotic intervention in the treatment of multiple personality. *American Journal of Clinical Hypnosis, 24*, 230–240.

Kluft, R. P. (1983). Hypnotherapeutic crisis intervention in multiple personality. *American Journal of Clinical Hypnosis, 26*, 73–83.

Kluft, R. P. (1984). Treatment of multiple personality disorders: A study of 33 cases. *Psychiatric Clinics of North America, 7*, 9–29.

Kluft, R. P. (1985). The natural history of multiple personality disorder. In R. P. Kluft (Ed.), *Childhood antecedents of multiple personality* (pp. 197–238). Washington, DC: American Psychiatric Press.

Kluft, R. P. (1988a). The postunification treatment of multiple personality disorder: First findings. *American Journal of Clinical Psychiatry, 42*, 212–228.

Kluft, R. P. (1988b). On giving consultations to therapists treating MPD: Fifteen years' experience. *Dissociation, 1*(1–2), 23–35.

Kluft, R. P. (1989). The rehabilitation of therapists overwhelmed by their work with multiple personality disorder patients. *Dissociation, 2*, 243–249.

Kluft, R. P. (1990). Educational domains and andragogocal approaches in teaching psychotherapists about multiple personality disorder. *Dissociation, 3*, 188–194.

Kluft, R. P. (1991a). Multiple personality disorder. In A. Tasman & S. M. Goldfinger (Eds.), *American Psychiatric Press review of psychiatry* (pp. 161–188). Washington, DC: American Psychiatric Press.

Kluft, R.P. (1991b). Hospital treatments of multiple personality disorder: An overview. *Psychiatric Clinics of North America, 14*, 695–719.

Kluft, R. P. (1991c). Clinical presentation of multiple personality disorder. *Psychiatric Clinics of North America, 14*(3), 605–629.

Kluft, R. P. (1993). Basic principles in conducting the treatment of multiple personality disorder. In R. P. Kluft & C. G. Fine (Eds.), *Clinical perspectives on multiple personality disorder* (pp. 53–73). Washington, DC: American Psychiatric Press.

Kluft, R. P., Braun, B. G., & Sachs, R. J. (1984). Multiple personality, intra-familial abuse and family psychiatry. *American Journal of Family Psychiatry, 5*.

Kluft, R. P., & Fine, C. G. (Eds.). (1993). *Clinical perspectives on multiple personality disorder*. Washington, DC: American Psychiatric Press.

Kolb, L. C. (1988). Recovery of memory and repressed fantasy in combat-induced post-traumatic stress disorder of Vietnam veterans. In H. M. Pettinati (Ed.), *Hypnosis and memory* (pp. 265–276). New York: Guilford Press.

Labott, S. M., Leavitt, F. Braun, B. G., & Sachs, R. (1992). Rorschach indicators of multiple personality disorder. *Perceptual and Motor Skills, 75*, 147–158.

Linehan, M. M. (1993). *Cognitive-behavioral treatment of borderline personality disorder*. New York: Guilford Press.

Loewenstein, R. J. (1991a). An office mental status examination for complex chronic dissociative symptoms and multiple personality disorder. *Psychiatric Clinics of North America, 14*, 567–604.

Loewenstein, R. J. (1991b). Rational psychopharmacotherapy in the treatment of multiple personality disorder. *Psychiatric Clinics of North America, 14*, 721–740.

Loewenstein, R. J. (1993). Posttraumatic and dissociative aspects of transference and countertransference in the treatment of multiple personality disorder. In R. P. Kluft & C. G. Fine (Eds.), *Clinical perspectives on multiple personality disorder* (pp. 51–85). Washington DC: American Psychiatric Press.

Loewenstein, R. J., & Putnam, F. W. (1990). The clinical phenomenology of males with multiple personality disorder. *Dissociation, 3*, 135–143.

Loewenstein, R. L., & Ross D. R. (1992). Multiple personality and psychoanalysis: An introduction. *Psychoanalytic Inquiry, 12*, 3–48.

Loftus, E. F. (1993). The reality of repressed memories. *American Psychologist, 48*, 518–537.

Lynn, S. J., & Nash, M. R. (1994). Truth in memory: Ramifications for psychotherapy and hypnotherapy. *American Journal of Clinical Hypnosis, 36*, 198–208.

North, C. S., Ryan, J. E. M., Ricci, D. A., & Wetzel, R. D. (1993). *Multiple personalities, multiple disorders*. New York: Oxford University Press.

Powers, W. T. (1973). *Behavior: The control of perception*. Chicago: Aldine.

Putnam, F. W. (1988). The switch process in multiple personality disorder and other state-change disorders. *Dissociation, 1*, 24–32.

Putnam, F. W. (1989). *Diagnosis and treatment of multiple personality disorder*. New York: Guilford Press.

Putnam, F. W. (1992). Discussion: Are alter personalities fragments or figments? *Psychoanalytic Inquiry, 12*, 95–111.

Putnam, F. W., Guroff, J. J., Silberman, E. K., Barban, L., & Post, R. M. (1986). The clinical phenomenology of multiple personality disorder: A review of 100 recent cases. *Journal of Clinical Psychiatry, 47*, 285–293.

Putnam, F. W., & Loewenstein, R. J. (1993). Treatment of multiple personality disorder: A survey of current practices. *American Journal of Psychiatry, 150*, 1048–1052.

Ross, C. A. (1989). *Multiple personality disorder: Diagnosis, clinical features, and treatment*. New York: John Wiley.

Ross, C. A., & Dua, V. (1993). Psychiatric health care costs of multiple personality disorder. *American Journal of Psychotherapy, 47*, 103–112.

Ross, C. A., Heber, S., Norton, G. R., Anderson, D., Anderson, G., & Barcket, P. (1989). The dissociative disorders interview schedule: A structured interview. *Dissociation, 2*, 169–189.

Ross, C. A., Miller, S. D., Bjornson, L., Reagor, P., Fraser, G. A., & Anderson, G. (1991). Abuse histories in 102 cases of multiple personality disorder. *Canadian Journal of Psychiatry, 36*, 97–101.

Ross, C. A., Miller, S. D., Reagor, P., Bjornson, L., Fraser, G. A., & Anderson, G. (1990). Structured interview data on 102 cases of multiple personality disorder. *American Journal of Psychiatry, 147*, 596–601.

Schultz, R., Braun, B. G., & Kluft, R. P. (1989). Multiple personality disorder: Phenomenology of selected variables in comparison to major depression. *Dissociation, 2*, 45–51.

Skinner, S. T. (1990). Occupational therapy with patients with multiple personality disorder: Personal reflections. *American Journal of Occupational Therapy, 44*, 1024–1027.

Speigel, D. (1984). Multiple personality as a post traumatic stress disorder. *Psychiatric Clinics of North America, 7*, 101–110.

Steele, K. H. (1989). A model for abreation with MPD and other dissociative disorders. *Dissociation, 2*, 151–159.

Steinberg, M. (1993). *Structured Clinical Interview for DSM-IV Dissociative Disorders (SCID-D)*. Washington, DC: American Psychiatric Press.

Steinberg, M., Rounsaville, B., & Cicchetti, D. (1991). Detection of dissociative disorders in psychiatric patients by a screening instrument and a structured diagnostic interview. *American Journal of Psychiatry, 148*, 1050–1054.

Terr, L. (1988). What happens to early memories of trauma? A study of twenty children under the age five at the time of documented traumatic events. *Journal of the American Academy of Child and Adolescent Psychiatry, 27*, 96–104.

Thames, L. (1984, September). *Limit setting and behavioral contracting with the client with multiple personality disorder*. Paper presented at the First International Meeting on Multiple Personality and Dissociative States, Chicago, IL.

Turkus, J. A. (1991). Psychotherapy and case management for multiple personality disorder: Synthesis for continuity of care. *Psychiatric Clinics of North America, 14*, 649–660.

15

Transference and Countertransference Shaping Influences on Dissociative Syndromes

George K. Ganaway

In his 1925 *An Autobiographical Study*, Sigmund Freud recalled an embarrassing incident early in his medical practice that, among other reasons, caused him eventually to abandon formal hypnosis as his primary psychotherapeutic instrument:

> It related to one of my most acquiescent patients, with whom hypnosis had enabled me to bring about the most marvelous results, and whom I was engaged in relieving of her suffering by tracing back her attacks of pain to their origins. As she woke up on one occasion, she threw her arms around my neck. The unexpected entrance of a servant relieved us from a painful discussion, but from that time onwards there was a tacit understanding between us that hypnotic treatment should be discontinued. (1925/1962, p. 27)

By the late 1890s when this incident occurred, Freud already had been troubled by increasing doubt about the efficacy of his and Breuer's technique of hypnotically facilitated catharsis in the treatment of hysteriform conditions. He observed that "even the most brilliant results were liable to be suddenly wiped away if my personal relation with the patient became disturbed," and "such an occurrence proved that the personal emotional relation between doctor and patient was after all stronger than the whole cathartic process, and it was precisely that factor which escaped every effort at control" (1925/1962, p. 27).

In paying close attention to this "mysterious element that was at work behind hypnotism" (p. 27), Freud was laying the groundwork for subsequent theoretical formulations about the phenomenon he called *transference*. Later, students of hypnosis and psychodynamic psychotherapy eventually would echo his concerns about the intense magnification and temporal compression of transference reactions in patients whose treatment focused heavily on hypnotic interventions. Orne and Dinges (1989), for example, recently cautioned that "most of the difficulties encountered when hypnosis is used are associated with transference or countertransference issues that have gone unrecognized because of the speed and intensity with which hypnosis brought about these responses" (p. 1509).

The last two decades have witnessed a revival of Freud and Breuer's century-old technique of actively pursuing, often with the assistance of formal hypnosis, suspected hidden memories of childhood trauma in patients who were once described as suffering from hysteria, but today are diagnosed as having dissociative disorders. In this chapter, I will critically examine the current revival of trauma theory as an explanation for dissociative syndromes and contrast it to conflict theory, which continues to dominate mainstream psychoanalytic thinking with regard to the etiology of neuroses and character pathology. I will attempt to show how transference and countertransference as understood in terms of conflict theory may be influencing clinicians' hypotheses about the suspected traumatic origins of dissociative syndromes, and shaping the actual clinical manifestations of the disorders within the therapeutic dyad.

HYPNOSIS, TRAUMA, AND DISSOCIATIVE DISORDERS

Current theories regarding the etiology of dissociative disorders, in particular Dissociative Identity Disorder (DID) (until recently called Multiple Personality Disorder [MPD]), center around certain predisposing factors thought to be necessary for the development of a dissociative diathesis. These include a high capacity for autohypnotic trance experiences, and exposure to severe, recurrent trauma, usually in the form of physical and/or sexual abuse beginning in early childhood (Braun & Sachs, 1985; Kluft, 1984a, 1984b).

While the evidence for a causative link between exogenous childhood trauma and the later clinical manifestation of multiple "personalities" remains largely anecdotal and equivocal (Frankel, 1993; Ganaway, 1989b, 1992, 1994), experts strongly agree on the high hypnotizability of individuals who meet DID diagnostic criteria (Bliss, 1986; Braun, 1986; Ganaway, 1989b; Kluft, 1984a, 1984b, 1991; Putnam, 1989). Largely as a result of the clinical experiences of a small but prolific group of authors who began publishing in the 1970s and 1980s, the use of formal hypnotic techniques on patients presenting with nonspecific dissociative symptoms (e.g., "losing" time, not remembering behaviors, depersonalization, and derealization) rapidly gained widespread popularity in North America as a method of identifying alternate "personalities," uncovering and facilitating abreactions of perceived childhood trauma memories, and "integrating" the discovered "personalities" or personality states (Allison, 1974; Bliss, 1986; Braun, 1986; Kluft, 1984a, 1984b, 1991; Schreiber, 1973).

Some experts have recommended that hypnosis be used largely as an *adjunct* to a psychodynamically oriented psychotherapy for DID patients (Kluft, 1991; Putnam, 1989). However, many self-appointed specialists in the dissociative disorders field appear to have little knowledge or experience in psychodynamic psychiatry, especially in terms of understanding the importance of intrapsychic conflict, defense, resistance, compromise and transference/countertransference reactions in dissociative-disordered patients. Conversely, clinicians who may use a psychodynamically informed approach often ignore or openly discount experimental hypnosis findings regarding the dissociation-facilitating nature of hypnotic suggestion in trance-prone subjects and the credibility of hypnotically refreshed memories of past experiences (AMA Council on Scientific Affairs, 1985; Orne & Dinges, 1989).

An unfortunate consequence of the above has been the rise of a "cottage industry" in the treatment of alleged victims of childhood abuse who are thought to have completely "repressed" or "dissociated" their trauma memories prior to seeking therapy for puzzling psychological symptoms of various kinds (e.g., depression, anxiety and panic states, phobias, obsessions and compulsions, and chronic relationship problems). These patients discover often through formal hypnosis or quasi-hypnotic "relaxation techniques" involving guided imagery that an impressive accumulation of trauma memories have lain hidden for years among an assortment of alternate "personalities," the existence of which usually was unknown to the patient prior to the DID diagnosis.

It is my intention here to demonstrate how the misinterpretation by well-intentioned but poorly informed therapists of transference and countertransference reactions, particularly in the context of hypnotically enhanced therapy with patients who suffer preexisting disorders of self identity, may foster the creation and perpetuation of an exercise in mutual deception between patient and therapist that reinforces resistance to a genuine understanding of the meaning behind the presenting clinical symptoms. Such a deception may prolong treatment while reducing rather than improving the patient's overall level of adaptive ego functioning (Ganaway, 1992, 1993, 1994).

COMING TO TERMS: TRANSFERENCE, COUNTERTRANSFERENCE, AND THE "REAL RELATIONSHIP"

If controversy exists regarding the significance of transference and countertransference in our theoretical understanding of dissociative disorders, it is but a part of a more generic controversy within the field of psychoanalysis. Abend (1993) notes that "[d]espite universal agreement about the importance of transference, there is no single, comprehensive, generally accepted explanation for the place transference occupies in clinical psychoanalytic theory" (p. 627). To minimize confusion, I will present rather narrow, simplistic definitions of transference and countertransference. The reader should keep in mind that contemporary analysts view these processes as being considerably more complex than described below.

Transference, as defined by Greenson (1967), "is the experience of feeling, drives, attitudes, fantasies, and defenses toward a person in the present which do not befit that person but are a repetition of reactions originating in regard to significant persons of early childhood, unconsciously displaced onto figures in the present" (p. 171). This definition highlights the key mental defense mechanism operative in the transference reaction: *displacement.* Displacement refers to "the shift of feelings, fantasies, etc. from an *object* or *object representation* in the past to an object or object representation in the present" (Greenson, 1967, p. 175). Within psychoanalytic theory, "self" and "object" representations refer to the variety of composite images of self and others that a child has internally constructed based on his or her drives, feelings, and experiences.

Additionally, however, transference may involve the mechanisms of *projection* and *introjection*. In contrast to displacement, the individual who *projects* "is ejecting something from within his *self representation* into or onto another person. *Introjection* is the incorporation of something from an external object into the *self representation*" (Greenson, 1967, p. 175). When these occur during therapy, they typically represent repetitions of similar processes of projection and introjection that previously occurred in relation to historically important persons (Jacobson, 1964).

Characteristic of (but not necessarily limited to) individuals with a more primitive level of ego organization is the tendency to engage in *projective identification*, which is closely related to transference phenomena, and is thought by some to be a hallmark of severe disorders of self identity, such as borderline and primitive narcissistic personality disorders (Kernberg, 1984b). Such personality disorders reflect major disturbances in self and object representations. More will be said later about the relative importance of projection, introjection, and projective identification in our understanding of the influences transference and countertransference may have on the shaping of dissociative syndromes.

The term *countertransference* will be defined here roughly to mean a transference reaction of a therapist to a patient, paralleling the patient's transference to the therapist. Countertransference reactions "can lead to persistent inappropriate behavior toward the patient in the form of constant misunderstanding or some unconscious rewarding, seductive or permissive behavior by the analyst" (Greenson, 1967, p. 348).

Transference and countertransference reactions are to be distinguished from the "real relationship" that also is present between the therapist and patient. Greenson (1971) found it easier to define transference than to provide a clear definition of a "real" relationship, but made an admirable attempt at both. He emphasized that "the two outstanding characteristics of a transference reaction are: (1) it is an indiscriminating, nonselective repetition of the past, and (2) it is inappropriate, it ignores or distorts reality" (p. 89). A "real" relationship, on the other hand, while also consisting of repetitions from the past, "differs from transference in being selective and discriminating in what is repeated. Furthermore, a real relationship is modifiable by internal and external reality" (p. 89). He offered the example of the real relationship between a husband and wife, where the wife may bear a physical resemblance to the husband's mother, but the resemblance "does not bring with it all of the instinctual and emotional components which were originally bound up with the mother" (p. 89).

Greenson (1971) felt that a *working alliance* was essential for successful psychoanalytic treatment. While certain "transference hopes and longings" may contribute to the working alliance, he emphasized that the "reliable, enduring core of the working alliance is the 'real relationship' between the patient and the analyst. . . . The transference feelings, loving or hateful, from the most infantile to the most mature, may be helpful, but transference is an erratic and treacherous ally" (p. 90).

According to classical psychoanalytic theory, transference is of primary importance in analytic treatment. Defensively, it acts as a resistance to insight. At the same time, *analysis of the transference* is the key to achieving insight that leads to lasting changes. In terms of object relations, the transference reaction allows the patient "an opportunity to re-experience all varieties and mixtures of love and hate, oedipal and pre-oedipal" (Greenson, 1967, p. 180) by means of circumscribed regressions.

DISSOCIATION AND TRANSFERENCE REACTIONS

Transference and countertransference are not "created" by the psychotherapist or the patient, respectively; they are *elicited* by the conditions of the therapeutic relationship (Greenson, 1967, p.171). Is it possible, however, for therapists who dogmatically adhere to a fashionable revival of Freud's earliest exogenous trauma theory of neurosis to foster the creation of new symptoms or even complete syndromes in dissociation-prone individuals who are in a particular window of psychological vulnerability through implicit or explicit suggestion within the field of transference?

Based on clinical experience during the past decade in the treatment of more than 350 dissociative-disordered patients, I have arrived at the hypothesis that unrecognized or misunderstood transference and countertransference reactions in many cases may influence the shaping of inchoate dissociative symptom clusters into mutually expected, socioculturally driven stereotypical syndromes or "disorders," including DID, in patients who are "high hypnotizables" and possess a developmentally derived disorder of self identity (most typically borderline or primitive narcissistic character disorders) (Ganaway, 1992, 1993, 1994).

The preconceived "inner cognitive maps" (Michels, 1983) consciously and unconsciously used by all therapists "to look for certain kinds of material, and to search for it when it is not immediately apparent" (pp. 130–131) may result in markedly varied diagnostic formulations and treatment approaches with this patient population, depending on the therapist's knowledge and experience in psychodynamic theories and their application in clinical practice. Furthermore, what is believed by trauma theorists to be an *expressive* form of therapy for alleged childhood trauma survivors may actually be a form of *supportive* therapy, which through the process of symptom substitution acts as a vehicle for prolonged resistance to the resolution of unconscious conflicts ultimately responsible for the presenting clinical symptoms. In order to understand how this can happen, we must examine current theoretical trends in the dissociative disorders and their impact on the meaning of transference for clinicians in the field.

"TRAUMATIC" TRANSFERENCE AND NEW PARADIGMS

To date, Loewenstein (1993) has provided the most comprehensive review of current theoretical trends in the dissociative disorder literature on transference and countertransference reactions in patients with DID and related dissociative syndromes. He credits Cornelia Wilbur, whose pioneering work with Sybil (documented by Schreiber, 1973) became the diagnostic and treatment model for "second generation" therapists such as himself, with inspiring a "scientific revolution" from which "the post-Wilburian paradigm" of DID (MPD) has arisen as a "severe dissociative post-traumatic developmental disorder" (p. 53).

Loewenstein (1993) describes various manifestations of transference encountered in DID patients in keeping with this new paradigm, which necessarily presupposes a history of childhood exposure to repeated actual experiences with abusive and traumatizing figures. In doing so, he follows a trend begun nearly a decade earlier wherein transference reactions in severely dissociative patients were solely defined as forms of "traumatic transference" (Kluft, 1984a; Spiegel, 1988). Such reactions were likened to those manifested in therapy by combat veterans and other survivors of often well-corroborated trauma experiences, who suffer from post-traumatic stress disorders (PTSD). These "often seemingly inexplicable emotional reactions related to dissociative traumatic experiences" (Loewenstein, 1993, p. 57) commonly present as severe mistrust and suspicion based on an unconscious expectation that the ostensibly helpful therapist eventually will "exploit the patient for his or her own narcissistic gratification" (Spiegel, 1986, p. 72). Other traumatic transference reactions may take the form of what Loewenstein (1993) calls the "flashback transference," in which the patient literally experiences the therapist as the personification of a specific abuser via an autohypnotic perceptual illusion.

Countertransference issues in the treatment of DID similarly have been addressed in the literature largely from the perspective of a "dissociative PTSD paradigm." Putnam (1989) has described the problems therapists encounter in relating to the complex internal world of alternate personalities, as well as the difficulties they have in assimilating and working with the often expansive accounts of trauma memories "hidden" among the newly uncovered personalities. Loewenstein summarizes Putnam's list of common countertransference issues to include "fantasies of reparenting the patient; omnipotent grandiosity in the therapist; problems handling erotic feelings toward the patient, as well as from the patient toward the therapist; and difficulties with reactions from [skeptical] colleagues" (1993, p. 57).

Kluft has written extensively about the emotional difficulties therapists encounter in working with DID patients, including initial feelings of excitement, fascination, and overinvestment that eventually yield to "feelings of bewilderment, exasperation, and a sense of being drained by the patient" (Kluft, 1984a, p. 52). Like Putnam, Kluft highlights the difficulty most therapists encounter in empathizing with the DID patient's experience of traumatization, noting that "one is tempted to withdraw, intellectualize, or defensively ruminate about whether or not the events are 'real'" (p. 53). Others have said of those who question the veridicality of DID patients' often extensive abuse histories, which sometimes include bizarre claims such as having been raised in a satanic cult and forced to participate in multiple human sacrifices and cannibalism (Ganaway, 1989b, 1991, 1992), that skeptics are themselves in a complementary state of "dissociation," unable to accept the reality of organized wholesale child abuse.

Counteridentification problems are also cited among the countertransference phenomena not uncommon to therapists working with this patient population. "PTSD by proxy" or "Secondary PTSD" (Olson, Mayton,

& Kowal-Ellis, 1987) are labels given to the syndromes of "nightmares, intrusive images, reenactments, amnesia, estrangement, alienation, irritability, excessive alcohol use, psychophysiological reactions, and survivor guilt" experienced by many therapists who specialize in the treatment of DID and its variants and subscribe to the trauma theory of pathogenesis (Loewenstein, 1993, p. 58).

PROBLEMS WITH THE "POST-WILBURIAN PARADIGM"

So-called "traumatic" transference and countertransference reactions of the types described above likely *do* occur within the field of transference in situations where patients have, in fact, been victims of confirmed exogenous trauma, such as severe childhood physical or sexual abuse. However, therapists who rely on the reductionistic "post-Wilburian paradigm" as a sufficient explanation for these reactions in *all* dissociative disorder patients are blinding themselves to an impressive accumulation of psychoanalytic literature that offers other equally plausible explanations for the same phenomena. The presupposition that patients who react to therapists in the manner previously described must have been exposed to repeated actual abusive experiences with traumatizing figures (Loewenstein, 1993) discounts nearly a century of evolving psychoanalytic theory which emphasizes the combined effects of internal, or psychic, reality and external, or objective, reality when explaining neurotic symptoms and character disorders. Likewise, nature should not be entirely ignored in deference to the seemingly dramatic developmental influences of nurture. Exogenous trauma theory gives short shrift to the important contributing influence of unconscious intrapsychic conflicts over the expression of sexual and aggressive instinctual drives in the creation of compromise symptoms, and the development during psychotherapy of transference reactions that may be phenomenologically indistinguishable from those attributed to exogenous trauma, but serve more complex purposes. From an object relations viewpoint, the new paradigm ignores the likelihood that distortions of historical reality often may be considered an acceptable intrapsychic compromise by the puzzlingly symptomatic, desperately object-seeking dissociative individual with abandonment fears who seeks a promise of perpetual interest, acceptance, approval and caretaking from a therapist who in fantasy has become a wished-for idealized parental surrogate.

Other problems that arise when viewing DID as a "dissociative posttraumatic developmental disorder" involve elevating a more descriptive over a psychodynamic approach to diagnosing and treating these patients' manifest symptom clusters, and failing to consider the impact of high hypnotizability on symptom formation. Despite a wealth of "post-Sybilian" anecdotal accounts of similar abuse histories in the professional and lay literature, a direct causative link between corroborated childhood abuse and the manifestation of a primary dissociative disorder in adult life has not as yet been convincingly demonstrated (Putnam, 1993; Ganaway, 1989b, 1994; Tillman, Nash, & Lerner, Chapter 18, this volume). Nearly all of the recent studies that have attempted to associate child abuse with dissociative disorders have relied upon unverified reconstructed patient memories obtained during therapy sessions, or on reports from patients who have themselves attempted to obtain outside corroboration to validate reconstructed memories (Frankel, 1993; Ganaway, 1992, 1994). Such memories, usually "uncovered" with the patient in a trance state, are subject to distortions and confabulation characteristic of many hypnotically enhanced recollections (AMA Council on Scientific Affairs, 1985). Personal confirmation accounts by patients without independent verification suffer from reporting biases, which are created by the same unconscious defense mechanisms that shape their memory distortions. Patients' reported confirmations, then, may prove to be no more reliable than the memories they originally reconstructed during therapy.

An additional problem involves what Rothstein (1983, p. 24) has labeled "paradigm grandiosity," exemplified here in the mutual expectation by both therapist and patient that the often inchoate, nonspecific dissociative symptom cluster the latter experiences indisputably predicts the eventual "discovery" within the patient of previously undetected alternate identities or "personalities," along with a history of extensive childhood physical and/or sexual abuse that necessarily must exist to account for their presence. In such instances, a preexisting belief in the "post-Wilburian paradigm" may foster an expectation (or even an inferred demand) in psychologically vulnerable dissociative patients that becomes a self-fulfilling prophecy fueled by transference and countertransference wishes and needs (Ganaway, 1993, 1994).

Rothstein (1983) describes how the "narcissistic investment of a theory [by the creator and adherents] contributes an irrational element to paradigm evolution" (p. 12). Consciously or unconsciously, the theory "is felt to be the ultimate provider of answers for the practitioner [and] as such, it assuages his sense of vulnerability and helplessness" (p. 12). Proponents of the "dissociative PTSD" theory, in their enthusiastic zeal for a paradigm revolution, appear to have prematurely closed the debate on the validity of the new paradigm long before sufficient data are available to support or refute it.

Well-trained and experienced psychodynamically informed clinicians realistically maintain a benign skepticism toward *all* theories, especially those that fail to account for the bulk of the clinical findings in each new case, and those for which a more parsimonious explanation of the available data is sufficient (Ganaway, 1989b, 1992, 1993, 1994). My own cumulative clinical experience in attempting to treat dissociative patients initially according to the proposed new paradigm has resulted in growing skepticism on my part regarding the validity of such a simplistic, reductionistic theory. As a result, I have encouraged the consideration of a more integrative etiological theory that incorporates biogenetic factors, drive theory, ego psychology, object relations theory, social psychological theory, sociocultural factors, and experimental hypnosis findings in an attempt to satisfactorily explain the epidemic of newly diagnosed cases of DID that has swept across North America during the last decade (Ganaway, 1994).

TRAUMA THEORY VERSUS CONFLICT THEORY

History teaches us that the "dissociative PTSD" diagnostic and treatment paradigm currently gaining popularity is not new, but represents a simplistic caricature of Freud's earliest psychoanalytic trauma theory, which derived from his hypnotically facilitated treatment of patients with hysteria. Freud originally hypothesized that blocked or "repressed" awareness of trauma memories causes anxiety and other neurotic symptoms. Subsequent data led him to refine and modify his theory; he recognized repression to be the *result* rather than the *cause* of neurotic anxiety. He grew to see repression as a key defense mechanism unconsciously mobilized to keep from conscious awareness anxiety that stemmed from intrapsychic conflicts over the expression of sexual and aggressive instinctual drives (Freud, 1925/1962).

As his *conflict theory* evolved, Freud grew increasingly aware of the importance of transference reactions in therapy both as a resistance to conscious awareness of unresolved intrapsychic conflicts, and as an important vehicle for understanding the infantile origins of those conflicts. He realized as well that a reductionistic trauma theory could not do justice to the complexity of the mind. As Waelder (1967) has noted, perceptions, thoughts, feelings, behaviors, and symptoms all are overdetermined; rarely are they traced to one simple cause. Freud never entirely abandoned his belief that actual childhood trauma (including sexual abuse) could in some cases lead to neurotic symptoms (Freud, 1896/1962, footnote p.168). But he placed far greater emphasis on the importance of the child's conflictual representational world of unconscious and conscious sexual and aggressive fantasies as the main determinant of both normal psychological development and psychopathological syndromes occurring later in life (Gay, 1988).

With respect to the dissociative disorders, while a more complex, integrative theory regarding the origin and clinical manifestations of DID *does not rule out* actual childhood physical and sexual abuse as potential causative antecedents, neither does it *require* such drastic events to explain the phenomenological and transferential aspects of the disorder. *Intrapsychic conflict,* the basic dimension of psychopathology that has been repeatedly documented during a hundred years of psychoanalytic clinical experiences, offers both the necessary and sufficient data to thoroughly understand and explain DID if one is willing to consider as well the added dimension of high hypnotizability. This additional contributing variable may account for enhanced suggestibility to a pathological level in persons already experiencing a chronic disturbance of self identity.

THE REPRESENTATIONAL WORLD

During the evolution of psychoanalytic theory over the past century, Freud and those who followed him observed and documented the now widely recognized finding that children are not just passive recorders of their experiences vis-à-vis the environment. Through fantasy they are *active participants* in the shaping of unconscious internal representations of self and others that later during therapy are inferred through dreams, reconstructed memories about childhood, and transference reactions directed toward the therapist and others.

This implies that adult memories of childhood must be viewed as representing a blend of contributions from an imperfectly perceived external, objective reality, and an unconscious, fantasied psychic reality. Together, they create the subjectively known experiential world that combines sensations derived from external reality with derivatives of unconscious forces (psychic reality), but *is not in itself real* (Michels, 1985). Subjective experience, then, like psychological symptomatology, is multiply determined, and in no way reducible to perceptions of either external reality or psychic reality alone.

The above has important implications for the therapist who is attempting to help a patient comprehend the meaning of his or her subjective experiences of perceived past events and relationships as evoked during therapy through free association and/or hypnotic inquiry, and manifested in transference reactions. The mechanisms of projection and introjection, as described earlier, are necessarily accompanied by distortions in the resulting internal object representations caused by this blend of internal and external reality. For example, a child may transfer much of his or her own aggression to the internal parental representations, "so that they can appear to him to be far more severe and punitive than his parents ever were in reality" (Sandler & Rosenblatt, 1962, p. 138). If the therapist is either psychodynamically uninformed, or chooses to ignore the above in favor of a simplistic assumption that the subjective perceptions of reality in the patient with a severe object relations disturbance represent an accurate, uncontaminated reproduction of the real world as it actually existed, both patient and therapist may be led down a diversionary path of mutual deception in the service of unconscious transference and countertransference needs and wishes. The clinical observation in DID patients of signs of a preexisting diffuse or fragmented sense of identity betrays the presence of a primitive character disorder that *may* or *may not* appear to owe its origin to real as opposed to imagined dangers during infancy and childhood, depending on how the clinical data are interpreted.

THE ROLE OF PROJECTIVE IDENTIFICATION IN DISSOCIATIVE IDENTITY DISORDER

As described earlier, transference reactions are not just displacements; they may also be projections (Greenson, 1967). Representations of the ego, superego, and id, constantly in conflictual tension over sexual and aggressive drive gratification as described in Freud's structural theory, may be played out in fantasies directed toward the therapist. Insofar as the therapist recognizes these projections as such and does not identify with them or act upon them (other than interpreting them to the patient), the process remains *intrapsychic*. However, some feel that the mechanism of *projective identification* allows projection to take on an *interpersonal* dimension as well.

Projective identification is usually classified as a primitive defense mechanism characteristic of individuals with a borderline level of personality organization (Kernberg, 1984a). However, several authors in the dissociative disorders literature have suggested that in particularly complex dissociative syndromes that involve "highly developed forms of [personality] layering and internal secrecy" this defense mechanism is often used both in the field of transference between patient and therapist, and, hypothetically, as form of "internal" projective identification "from one dissociated part-self to another" (Loewenstein, 1993, pp. 55–56).

Closely related to transference and countertransference, the mechanism of projective identification has been observed by Loewenstein (1993), Peebles-Kleiger (1989), Ganaway (1989a) and others to be quite common in DID patients. Like transference, projective identification lacks preciseness in definition, largely a consequence of debate over the intrapsychic versus the interpersonal dimensions of this complex ego mechanism. The more narrow view of projective identification classifies it as "a purely *intrapsychic* defense [mechanism] that may or may not result in a reciprocal response from the clinician" (Gabbard, 1990, p. 34). Kernberg hypothesized that "identification occurs *within the projector,* rather than within the target of the projection. By maintaining this empathic bond or identification with that which has been projected, the projector has the fantasy of control over the projected material" (Gabbard, 1990, pp. 34–35).

A broader conceptualization of projective identification acknowledges an *interpersonal* aspect wherein the therapist becomes a part of the mechanism itself rather than simply a target of projected self- or object representations.

Ogden's (1979) interpersonal definition of projective identification necessarily involves three steps. First, the patient projects an unwanted or unacceptable self- or object-representation onto the therapist (corresponding to transference); secondly, the therapist unconsciously identifies with the projected material and actually begins to feel like or behave as the projected self- or object-representation as a response to coercion from the patient (corresponding to countertransference); and, finally, the projected material gets processed and modified by the therapist, and is then reintrojected by the patient, ultimately resulting in the modification of both the corresponding self- or object-representation and the pattern of interpersonal relatedness with the therapist.

Earlier, I summarized the various manifestations of "traumatic" transference described by proponents of the "dissociative PTSD paradigm." Operating from the perspective of this paradigm, it could be hypothesized that patients who were severely traumatized as children in a home where there was a "conspiracy of silence" might be likely in therapy to generate transference/countertransference patterns that reflect self- and object-representations corresponding to childhood relationships with abusers, abuse enablers (those who suspected or knew of the abuse but appeared either helpless to prevent it or unconcerned about the victim's plight), and rescuing and nurturing protectors (Ganaway, 1989a). Through the mechanism of projective identification, positive and negative self- and object-representations may be projected onto the therapist at times in an unconscious attempt to replicate childhood relationships. On the one hand, the patient may project the unwanted introject of a perceived villainous and abusing figure onto the therapist followed by attempts to provoke him or her into identifying with and acting out a script the patient has unconsciously written, as a form of repetition compulsion of earlier victimization experiences. Succeeding in this, the patient will attempt to control the therapist, who has become the container for the projection, thereby creating the illusion that the unwanted introject itself is being controlled or mastered.

Conversely, the patient may project onto the therapist a fantasied object representation of a loving, caretaking, rescuing, and protecting idealized parental figure who may in fact never have existed, in an effort to provoke the therapist into acting out a wished-for relationship of eternal nurturing, security, and unconditional acceptance. In exchange for this guarantee of specialness, and in the service of perpetuating it, the patient may repeatedly manifest a state of regressive dependency on the therapist that has the appearance of a conditioned helplessness.

Indeed, clinicians working with DID patients encounter such transference and countertransference phenomena so frequently that they view them as ubiquitous in this patient population (Ganaway, 1989a; Loewenstein, 1993), and no doubt there are situations in therapy when historically accurate abuse and fantasied rescue scenarios such as these are acted out in the transference. Problems arise, however, when the simplistic assumption is made that actual severe exogenous trauma with the failure of rescuing, or repair, by nurturing figures represents the *only* logical explanation for these phenomena.

OBJECTIVE VERSUS PSYCHIC REALITY IN PSYCHOANALYSIS

The combination of high hypnotizability (or perhaps more correctly termed "trance-proneness") and a disorder of self identity in the presence of the mutually accepted "dissociative PTSD paradigm" makes both patients *and* therapists particularly vulnerable to the dismissal of alternative psychodynamic explanations to simple exogenous trauma theory. Without independent corroboration, it simply is not possible to know for certain how historically accurate the "good" and "bad" object representations are that DID patients depict in their trauma accounts or in their transference reactions. These internal object representations are understood by the psychodynamically informed clinician *not* to simply represent a passive identification with the outside object (i.e., an exact internal duplication of the significant individual), but rather the introjection of the patient's actively fantasied notions of that significant individual, which can be heavily distorted by compromise formations derived from unconscious conflicts over sexual and aggressive drives and impulses. As noted earlier, then, the recalled image of a villainous abusive parent described by the patient may be more a product of the child's projected aggressive or sexual fantasies than an accurate representation of that parent. Particularly with patients who have primitive character disorders, the therapist is very likely to encounter oversimplified, grossly exaggerated depictions of "good" and "evil" parents (or parent substitutes) of the type described above. This is due to the child's failure to integrate "good" and "bad" self- and object-representations during the early separation and individuation processes (Kernberg, 1984a).

In like manner, childhood experiences that later are reconstructed in therapy as severely traumatic events may contain gross distortions of reality. Abend (1986), for example, cautions that "memories of dramatic events

. . . may be powerfully reorganized and substantially altered later according to the dictates of predominant unconscious fantasies, which in turn reflect the major compromise formations resulting from those patients' unconscious conflicts" (p. 96).

Abend (1986) succinctly summarizes his views on the evolution of psychoanalytic theory in the following statement. In it, he notes that during the course of this evolution abreaction of overwhelming affect associated with traumatic events eventually was set aside as an essential part of the therapeutic action of psychoanalysis:

> Psychoanalysis has come a long way from its earliest days, when the therapeutic task in respect to trauma was conceived as the need to uncover the repressed memories of the trauma in order to permit abreaction. . . . It is the elements of unconscious conflict, and the patterns of compromise formation which these take in the psychic lives of our patients, to which therapeutic attention should always and unfailingly be directed . . . *the actual events themselves, no matter how dramatic and compelling, are of less interest to the analytic therapist than is the task of ascertaining what they have come to mean in the mental lives of patients, and by what pathways they have assumed their significance.* (pp.103–104, emphasis added)

Understanding the *meaning* of a patient's subjective experiences, Rothstein (1986, p. 237) notes, requires the integrative act of "linking present and past, reality and fantasy, idea and affect," an act of a decidedly overdetermined nature.

THE "NEW PARADIGM": EXPRESSIVE OR SUPPORTIVE THERAPY?

It has been suggested by clinicians who stress *meaning* that those who instead emphasize the importance of abreacting and assimilating disturbing affects and perceptions are, in fact, engendering a supportive rather than an expressive psychotherapy (Rothstein, 1986, p. 236). Nowhere does this appear to be more clearly evident, in my opinion, than in the "new paradigm" some authorities in the field have proposed for the treatment of dissociative disorders.

If, as suggested by my clinical experience, we are in fact dealing with a patient population largely composed of individuals with primitive character disorders who are, in addition, exceptionally trance-prone, then a fascination for the hypnotically facilitated retrieval and abreaction of perceived childhood trauma memories encourages avoidance of insight into the rich, multilayered meaning of the patient's perceptions, feelings, and behaviors as played out in the transference.

As Gabbard (1990) has pointed out, "in the psychotherapy of borderline patients, the action is in the transference" (p. 355). Patients who experience split "good" and "bad" internal representations of self and others tend to move from idealizing to devaluing the therapist, or vice versa, sometimes within a single session. Kernberg (1975) has emphasized the importance of focusing on and interpreting this *splitting* defense mechanism as it is manifested in the transference in order to facilitate the integration of split self- and object-representations. This leads to the strengthening of the ego and the establishing of a true therapeutic alliance less encumbered by transference distortions. In some cases, this facilitates in turn a gradual shift to a more traditional analytically oriented expressive psychotherapy, which is usually tolerated only by individuals functioning at a higher, neurotic level of structural organization of the ego.

Fears of loss of object and loss of love seem to be of paramount concern to borderline individuals. These themes also permeate the transference reactions of the dissociative disorder patients I have treated. For these individuals, the dissociative mechanism appears to act not merely as a vehicle for the denial of emotionally painful memories of perceived trauma, but, more importantly, as a primary facilitator in a set of complex defensive behaviors that defend against, while still allowing, the direct expression of consciously unacceptable sexual and aggressive fantasies and impulses. In effect, through dissociation the patient has found a way to verbalize and act out these wishes and impulses with less risk of abandonment or disapproval. He or she does so by attributing responsibility for them to aspects of the mind over which the patient feels no ownership, control, or, sometimes, even awareness.

In accepting the "dissociative PTSD" model for DID as a sufficient explanation both for the splitting-off of parts of the mind and for the unacceptable thoughts, feelings, and behaviors sequestered in them, the therapist and patient become at risk for the development and concretization of a belief in multiple separate identities within the self, as well as a belief in the exogenous traumatic origins of those identities. This in turn allows the patient to focus on passive feelings of victimization rather than exploring the important role of unconscious fantasy in the creation of conflict that eventually leads to compromise through symptoms.

In my opinion, the patient's adoption of the modern stereotypical description of DID based on the "post-Wilburian paradigm" in itself represents a compromise by symptom substitution. In exchange for a promise of the therapist's unfailing interest (often to the point of fascination), nurturing and caretaking, and reassurance that as a child he or she was not responsible for any unacceptable thoughts, impulses, or behaviors, the patient unconsciously meets the therapist's countertransference need to validate the "dissociative PTSD paradigm" by serving up the expected clinical presentation of multiple alternate identities and increasingly expansive stories of severe physical and sexual abuse. The pursuit of what often becomes an endless horizon of newly discovered "personalities" and progressively bizarre and incredible abuse memories serves as a flight from transference, as the patient and therapist place the focus of therapy increasingly on the *content* of abreacted "memories" rather than on the *meaning of the defensive process* that is occurring within the field of transference.

On the surface, such a treatment approach might appear to represent "expressive" dynamic therapy in its most dramatic form, seeming to "render the unconscious conscious" by uncovering apparently long-hidden trauma memories. But insofar as it may instead represent, in some patients, a clever diversion from developing a conscious awareness of unconscious conflicts over sexual and aggressive drives or unresolved severe object relations disturbances, it should more correctly be labeled a supportive approach.

Through countertransference, the therapist unconsciously colludes to create or reinforce in the patient a *new symptom:* the belief in a simplistic, external "traumatic" explanation for the patient's current problems. The new belief system then becomes a substitute for the patient's earlier preoccupation with the distressing original symptoms themselves, diverting him or her away from potentially threatening exploration and understanding of the true, more complex meaning of those symptoms and their underlying defenses. While the patient may experience a temporary decrease in anxiety on having been provided a seemingly logical explanation for puzzling symptoms by an empathic, supportive clinician, and may feel supported emotionally by an identification with the abuse "survivor movement" (whereas previously the patient may have felt he or she had no identity at all), my experience has been that in the long run such a preoccupation prolongs the more important therapeutic task of addressing the underlying severe character disorder, which necessarily involves clarification, gentle confrontation, and interpretation of the complex defensive behaviors representative of unconscious conflict and compromise.

As this process develops, the high hypnotizability (or "trance-proneness"), and hence heightened suggestibility that some authorities believe makes the dissociative disorder patient "the theoretician's best friend" (Ganaway, 1994), greatly enhances the mutual deception between the therapist and patient. Both may find themselves suspending their critical judgment in response to the persuasive delivery in a dissociated state of sometimes purely confabulated yet exquisitely detailed experiences accompanied by intense affect and somatic responses. The magnified nature of the transference and countertransference reactions during such revelations further contributes to a mutual belief in the validity of the memories and of the "new paradigm" for understanding and treating DID and related dissociative syndromes.

On the other hand, when the therapist focuses instead on the *process* as understood through the application of psychoanalytic theory regarding disorders of self-identity, combined with an awareness of the complex interplay of psychodynamics with autohypnotic "trance logic" (Orne, 1959), and takes into consideration as well important interpersonal and sociocultural influences, he or she discovers that what initially may seem to fit the "post-Wilburian paradigm" is not, in fact, nearly so simple to explain after all.

SUMMARY

DID and its variants represent a complex interplay of biogenetic factors (including characteristic high hypnotizability), intrapsychic conflict, defense and compromise formation, object relations disturbances of both intrapsychic and interpersonal origin, and sociocultural factors that may include but are not limited to exposure to actual childhood abuse and/or deprivation. This interplay is reflected in the transference and countertransference reactions within the therapeutic dyad. It is my opinion that transference and countertransference phenomena can and do have shaping influences on theoretical formulations on the childhood origins of DID and on the phenomenology of the disorder. Clinicians in the field should be alert to transference and countertransference pitfalls and should maintain a benign skepticism toward all theories that fail to satisfactorily explain the clinical findings.

A more sophisticated, integrative theory than that provided by the currently popular "dissociative PTSD paradigm" is needed to satisfactorily explain the data emerging as increasing numbers of patients with dissociative disorder diagnoses are being seen and treated by mental health professionals across North America. Further research, both experimental and clinical, clearly is needed if we are ever to fully comprehend these complex disturbances of consciousness, memory, and identity.

REFERENCES

Abend, S. M. (1986). Sibling loss. In A. Rothstein, (Ed.), *The reconstruction of trauma: Its significance in clinical work* (pp. 98–104). New York: International Universities Press.

Abend, S. M. (1993). An inquiry into the fate of transference in psychoanalysis. *Journal of the American Psychoanalytic Association, 41*(3), 627–652.

Allison, R. B. (1974). A new treatment approach for multiple personalities. *American Journal of Clinical Hypnosis, 17,* 15.

AMA Council on Scientific Affairs. (1985). Scientific status of refreshing recollection by the use of hypnosis. *Journal of the American Medical Association, 253,* 1918–1923.

Bliss, E. L. (1986). *Multiple personality, allied disorders and hypnosis.* New York: Oxford University Press.

Braun, B. G. (1986). Issues in the psychotherapy of multiple personality disorder. In B. G. Braun (Ed.), *Treatment of multiple personality disorder* (pp. 1–28). Washington, DC: American Psychiatric Press.

Braun, B. G., & Sachs, R. G. (1985). The development of multiple personality disorder: Predisposing, precipitating, and perpetuating factors. In R. P. Kluft (Ed.), *Childhood antecedents of multiple personality* (pp. 37–64). Washington, DC: American Psychiatric Press.

Frankel, F. H. (1993). Adult reconstruction of childhood events in the multiple personality literature. *American Journal of Psychiatry, 150*(6), 954–958.

Freud, S. (1962). Further remarks on the neuro-psychoses of defence. In J. Strachey (Ed. and Trans.), *The standard edition of the complete psychological works of Sigmund Freud* (Vol. 3, pp. 162–185). London: Hogarth Press. (Original work published 1896)

Freud, S. (1962). An autobiographical study. In J. Strachey (Ed. and Trans.), *The standard edition of the complete psychological works of Sigmund Freud* (Vol. 20, pp. 7–70). London: Hogarth Press. (Original work published 1925)

Gabbard, G. (1990). *Psychodynamic psychiatry in clinical practice.* Washington, DC: American Psychiatric Press.

Ganaway, G. K. (1989a). *The benefits of psychoanalytically informed hospital treatment on a specialized dissociative disorders unit.* Paper presented at the Sixth International Conference on Multiple Personality/Dissociative States, Chicago, IL.

Ganaway, G. K. (1989b). Historical versus narrative truth: Clarifying the role of exogenous trauma in the etiology of MPD and its variants. *Dissociation, 2*(4), 205–220.

Ganaway, G. K. (1991). *Alternative hypotheses regarding satanic ritual abuse memories.* Paper presented at the 99th annual convention of the American Psychological Association, San Francisco, CA.

Ganaway, G. K. (1992). On the nature of memories. *Dissociation, 5*(2), 121–123.

Ganaway, G. K. (1993). *Dissociative disorders and psychodynamic theory: Trauma versus conflict and deficit.* Paper presented in the symposium, Perspectives on Recovered Memories, at the conference, Memory and Reality: Emerging Crisis, Valley Forge, PA.

Ganaway, G. K. (1994). Hypnosis, childhood trauma, and dissociative identity disorder: Toward an integrative theory. *International Journal of Clinical and Experimental Hypnosis.*

Gay, P. (1988). *Freud: A life for our time.* New York: W. W. Norton.

Greenson, R. (1967). *The technique and practice of psychoanalysis.* New York: International Universities Press.

Greenson, R. (1971). The "real" relationship between the patient and the psychoanalyst. In M. Kanzer (Ed.), *The unconscious today* (pp. 213–232). New York: International Universities Press.

Jacobson, E. (1964). *The self and the object world.* New York: International Universities Press.

Kernberg, O. F. (1975). *Borderline conditions and pathological narcissism.* New York: Jason Aronson.

Kernberg, O. F. (1984a). *Internal world and external reality: Object relations theory applied.* New York: Jason Aronson.

Kernberg, O. F. (1984b). *Severe personality disorders: Psychotherapeutic strategies.* New Haven, CT: Yale University Press.

Kluft, R. P. (1984a). Aspects of the treatment of multiple personality disorder. *Psychiatric annals, 14*, 51–55.

Kluft, R. P. (1984b). Treatment of multiple personality. *Psychiatric Clinics of North America, 7*, 9–29.

Kluft, R. P. (1991). Multiple personality disorder. In A. Tasman & S. Goldfinger (Eds.), *American Psychiatric Press review of psychiatry* (Vol. 10, pp. 161–188). Washington, DC: American Psychiatric Press.

Loewenstein, R. L. (1993). Posttraumatic and dissociative aspects of transference and countertransference in the treatment of multiple personality disorder. In R. P. Kluft & C. G. Fine (Eds.), *Clinical perspectives on multiple personality disorder* (pp. 51–85). Washington, DC: American Psychiatric Press.

Michels, R. (1983). The scientific and clinical functions of psychoanalytic theory. In A. Goldberg (Ed.), *The future of psychoanalysis* (pp. 125–135). New York: International Universities Press.

Michels, R. (1985). Introduction to panel: Perspectives on the nature of psychic reality. *Journal of the American Psychoanalytic Association, 33*, 515–519.

Ogden, T. H. (1979). On projective identification. *International Journal of Psycho-Analysis, 60*, 357–373.

Olson, J., Mayton, K., & Kowal-Ellis, N. (1987). Secondary posttraumatic stress disorder: therapist response to the horror. In B. G. Braun (Ed.), *Proceedings of the Fourth International Conference on Multiple Personality Disorder/Dissociative States.* Chicago, IL: Rush University Department of Psychiatry.

Orne, M. T. (1959). The nature of hypnosis: Artifact and essence. *Journal of Abnormal Social Psychology, 58*, 277–299.

Orne, M., & Dinges, D. (1989). Hypnosis. In H. Kaplan & B. Sadock (Eds.), *Comprehensive textbook of psychiatry* (Vol. 5, pp. 1501–1516). Baltimore: Williams and Wilkins.

Peebles-Kleiger, M. J. (1989). Using countertransference in the hypnosis of trauma victims: A model for turning hazard into healing. *American Journal of Psychotherapy, 48*, 518–530.

Putnam, F. W. (1989). *Diagnosis and treatment of multiple personality disorder.* New York: Guilford Press.

Putnam, F. W. (1993). Diagnosis and clinical phenomenology of multiple personality disorder: A North American perspective. *Dissociation, 6*(2/3), 80–86.

Rothstein, A. (1983). *The structural hypothesis: An evolutionary perspective.* New York: International Universities Press.

Rothstein, A. (1986). Conclusion. In A. Rothstein (Ed.), *The reconstruction of trauma: Its significance in clinical work* (pp. 219–230). New York: International Universities Press.

Sandler, J., & Rosenblatt, B. (1962). The concept of the representational world. *Psychoanalytic Study of the Child, 17*, 128–145.

Schreiber, F. R. (1973). *Sybil.* Chicago: Henry Regnery.

Spiegel, D. (1986). Dissociation, double binds, and posttraumatic stress in multiple personality disorder. In B. Braun (Ed.), *Treatment of multiple personality disorder* (pp. 61–78). Washington, DC: American Psychiatric Press.

Spiegel, D. (1988). Dissociation and hypnosis in posttraumatic stress disorders. *Journal of Traumatic Stress, 1,* 17–32.

Waelder, R. (1960). *Basic theory of psychoanalysis.* New York: International Universities Press.

16

Cross-Cultural
Treatment Perspectives
on Dissociative Disorders

Stanley Krippner

Cross-cultural psychologists posit that psychological generalizations cannot be viewed as valid on the basis of research conducted in one sociocultural context, but rather must be demonstrated through cross-cultural research. Further, they feel that psychotherapeutic interventions should not be uniformly applied across different cultural settings. A particular approach might be successful in one society, for example, a Western culture, but inappropriate in another, for example, a non-Western culture. In addition, a comparison of interventions from non-Western cultural settings may yield information that can enhance Western psychotherapy.

Westerners are prone to take terms with which they are familiar and superimpose them on phenomena in other cultures with which they are unfamiliar. Like other psychiatric and psychological terms, "dissociation" is an attempt by members of a social group to describe, explain, or otherwise account for the world in which they live (Gergen, 1985, p. 266). However, "dissociative" phenomena have been constructed differently in other historically situated interchanges among people (Ward, 1980). Some of these alternative concepts will be described in an attempt to preclude the reification of such expressions as "dissociation" and "dissociative disorders," and the noncritical acceptance of the Western construction of these phenomena.

A variety of definitions and descriptions of dissociation exist (see, e.g., Singer, 1990). Janet used the French word *désagrégation* (i.e., "disaggregation," which was modified into "dissociation") to refer to a phenomenon whereby two or more ideas or conscious states become separated and operate with seeming independence (Hilgard, 1992, p. 69), such as occurs with hypnosis, fugue states, and mediumship. Hilgard (1992) and Braun (1988) have pointed out that dissociation may occur at a variety of levels, and is not limited to dysfunctional phenomena. A continuum exists ranging from "highway hypnosis" (in which the attention of a driver becomes focused on the dividing line of a highway, often causing the driver to veer off the road if the line changes suddenly) to multiple personality disorder (MPD), including potential "hidden observers" that are part of the ordinary functioning of the psyche. This range is mirrored in the description of dissociative disorders in the *Diagnostic and Statistical Manual of Mental Disorders*, third edition, revised (DSM III-R; American Psychological Association, 1987). The essential feature is an alteration in the usual integrative functions of identity, memory, or consciousness. This alteration may be sudden or gradual, transient or chronic. A person's customary identity may be temporary forgotten and a new identity may be assumed or imposed (as in Multiple Personality Disorder), or the customary feeling of one's own reality may be lost and replaced by a feeling of unreality (as in Depersonalization Disorder). If the disturbance occurs primarily in memory, a key personal event cannot be recalled (as in Psychogenic Amnesia and Psychogenic Fugue).

The DMS-III-R description is consistent with the definition I have constructed for the purposes of this chapter: *"Dissociation" involves the occurrence of experiences and behaviors that are thought to exist apart from, or to have been disconnected from, the mainstream of one's conscious awareness, behavioral repertoire, and/or self-concept. "Dissociation" is the process by which this disconnection takes place.* This definition is compatible with models of neurological causation (e.g., temporal lobe epilepsy, sleep loss, strokes, severing of the cerebral commissure), the influence of social roles (e.g., Spanos, 1989), and cognitive constructions, such as the one given by Braun (1988), who observed that the psychological doctrine of "association" holds that memories are brought to awareness by means of an association of ideas. Hence, memories that are not available to be associated, are as a consequence dissociated, that is, separated from the mainstream of consciousness and (Tinnin, 1990, p. 157) remaining latent until evoked. My definition also avoids both the overinclusiveness and overrestrictiveness that Braude (1991) detected in previous definitions. He found the following definitions of dissociation to be problematic: "[a] concurrent engagement in two cognitive processes that occur simultaneously," "[a] conflict between two cognitive processes," and "[a] lack of integration between two cognitive processes" (pp. 116–120).

I have selected two examples of dissociation that demonstrate how phenomena that Westerners construct in one fashion may be constructed quite differently in other cultures—"possession" by a discarnate entity and MPD. The former diagnosis is taken quite seriously in many non-Western cultures and is listed in the World Health Organization's (1992) *International Classification of Disease;* the latter is a Western diagnostic construction of which there is little awareness in most non-Western societies. Indeed, Aldridge-Morris (1989) asserts that MPD is a "cultural phenomenon" rather than a "clinical entity," noting that the vast majority of reported cases occur in the United States where they have been presented in such a vast array of books, articles, and films, people start to identify with and, perhaps, begin to play a role that legitimizes negative behaviors.

POSSESSION

The *DSM-IV Options Book* (American Psychiatric Association, 1991) separated "possession" (wherein an individual is taken over by a spirit, power, deity, or other person, an experience accompanied by marked distress and/or social or occupational impairment) from both MPD and "possession" that is viewed as a normal part of a collective cultural or religious practice. The former two are considered to be dissociative disorders while the latter is not. In the *DSM-III-R Casebook* (Spritzer, Gibbon, Skodol, Williams, & First, 1989), Spritzer and colleagues argued that "possessed" persons should be given the diagnosis of "Dissociation Disorder Not Otherwise Specified" because they have a dissociative disorder in that their "experience is similar to a trance state" (p. 378). "Trance" often is defined as an altered state of consciousness with markedly diminished or selectively focused responsiveness to environmental stimuli. In other words, the American Psychiatric Association recognized some types of "possession" as psychopathological but distinguished them from MPD.

Bourguignon (1976) made a further distinction between "trance," "possession," and "possession trance." In her opinion, "possession" does not involve a "trance" or other alterations of consciousness, but an illness purportedly caused by the introjection of malevolent spirits into the mind and body. In "possession trance" there are spirit-induced alterations of consciousness during which the behavior and speech of the possessing entities can be observed. Sometimes the entities are benevolent (as in the case of mediums who "incorporate" their "spirit guides"), and sometimes troublesome (as in the case of malevolent or mischievous entities who talk and act through their victims' bodies). Bourguignon used the term "trance" to refer to induced, altered states of consciousness that are not linked to cultural ideas of possession.

Bourguignon (1989) presented two case studies, one from New York City and one from São Paulo, Brazil, to examine cross-cultural differences in the interpretation of dissociative phenomena. In the former instance, a woman was diagnosed by a psychotherapist as manifesting MPD, and the alter personality was seen as a "split-off" part of the core personality. In the latter instance, the alter personality was conceptualized as a phenomenon in which one of several spirits that possessed the individual at intervals. In both cases, their hosts only dimly or incompletely remembered what transpired when their alters took over, and the alters' behavior tended to violate cultural norms. But in the New York instance, the alter was an embarrassment to the host while, in Brazil, the alter was accepted by the host's social group.

Bourguignon's Brazilian case study is not an anomaly; on the basis of ethnographic reports, she found that spirit embodiment is common in 52% of some 500 societies. I myself have observed these phenomena in Puerto Rico, Haiti, and Brazil, primarily among folk healers and their clients. In all three locations, these spiritists (so named to differentiate them from the spiritualists of the United States) reflect a legacy of African customs and beliefs brought by slaves to the New World. Indeed, incorporating a discarnate entity was considered to be a supreme spiritual experience in West African religion. In addition, many Latin American folk healing practices were influenced by the writings of the French scholar Léon Hippolyte Denizarth Rivail, who wrote seven books about spiritism under the pen name of Allan Kardec (e.g., Kardec, 1868/1983).

Spirit embodiment is often welcome, as when mediums use their spirit guides to "channel" information from their clients' deceased relatives to them. But at times, it is viewed as a disorder in need of treatment, as when "low spirits" attempt to use their host's body to gratify their own impulses or when malevolent spirits possess someone as the result of a sorcerer's hex or an enemy's curse, or when they do so out of their own volition.

Spirit Possession and Incorporation in Puerto Rico

In 1971, Joan Koss-Chioino (1992) was hired as a consultant and a trainer for mental health workers in several Puerto Rican community mental health centers. She developed a therapist–spiritist training project to facilitate meaningful exchanges between allopathic practitioners and folk healers, to offer a curriculum that would provide knowledge and skills to members of both groups, and to develop new psychotherapeutic approaches. In 1979, I visited a community mental health center in Cayey where Koss-Chioino had organized meetings that were held on a bi-weekly basis. The first week was devoted to lectures by representatives from both groups. The second week focused on specific cases wherein both groups gave their input in regard to clients seen at the center. From this point on, the mediums were accepted as members of a team that typically included a physician, a psychologist, a social worker, and, at times, a psychiatrist. Koss-Chioino (Koss, 1987) followed up clients who had received treatment either from Western psychotherapists or from folk healers, and found that the latter group had more success with clients who experienced mood changes and behavioral complaints. Western-oriented psychotherapists were deemed more successful with those who complained of disordered thinking.

Koss-Chioino (1992) questioned the healers about how they enabled their guiding spirits to work through them. Rather than conceptualizing the trance state as a period in which one is dissociated from aspects of oneself and one's world, the practitioners saw the experience as facilitating a "connection to the cosmos" (p. 37). They reported that during the early stages of their development as healers, frequent spontaneous incorporations of spirits occurred, but gradually they were able to exert considerable control over entering the spirit world, and eventually could do so at will, except during periods of emergency or crisis when a guiding spirit might suddenly interrupt the medium's daily activity (p. 38). Koss-Chioino concluded that the medium's experience of incorporating spirit guides "cannot be said to mimic psychotic behavior" (p. 40). Not only was a high degree of control involved, the incorporation led to behavior considered adaptive by the medium's community. Instead of obstructing his or her ability to relate, the medium's alteration in consciousness "function[ed] to enhance interpersonal relating" (p. 39).

Koss-Chioino reported two major types of consciousness alteration among the Puerto Rican spiritists with whom she worked. The principal type paralleled Bourguignon's (1976) concept of the "possession trance." At the beginning of one's mediumship, this experience might be uncomfortable, even painful and disruptive. Eventually, however, the mediums feel only slightly affected during incorporation. For many, the incorporation leads to feelings of well-being, euphoria, and/or tranquility. The second style of altered consciousness identified by Koss-Chioino is more contemplative in nature, and is often preceded by repetitive prayer, which helps the mediums enter the spirit world. There, they report both visual and auditory imagery, leading Koss-Chioino to compare the condition with active daydreaming and self-hypnosis (pp. 38–39).

I have spent time at a number of folk healing centers in Puerto Rico, interacting with several different spiritistic (a word I use to cover both Kardec spiritism and the African-influenced spiritism) groups. The spiritistic movement is widespread; my informants estimated that some 60% of all Puerto Ricans visit a spiritist center at some time. All spiritists share a belief in discarnate entities (e.g., departed relatives and friends, saints, folkloric deities, "earthbound" spirits). Most spiritists believe in reincarnation and in the important role one's past-life activities play in one's current life situation. Communication with the spirit world sometimes occurs in dreams but more often the spirits speak directly through the mediums, who are endowed with special *facultades* (i.e., faculties) such as telepathy, clairvoyance, precognition, and the ability to alter their consciousness and incorporate their spirit guides.

Not infrequently, a spiritist's client will be told that his or her symptoms of distress are actually indications that he or she is developing *facultades*. At that point, counseling will often consist of mediumship training in which the *facultades* are developed under the tutelage of a senior medium. Rather than labeling the spiritist as psychopathological and in need of treatment, he or she is considered an important member of society. Further, the training confirms the social construction of a spiritistic medium and healer. During training, certain internal events are attributed to external sources, and reported sensations and mentations are conceptualized as initiatory ordeals rather than as signs of mental illness. It is likely that "doctrinal compliance" and "demand characteristics" mold and channel the initiate's experiences with regard to imagery, dreams, and other private events. Koss-Chioino (1992, p. 147) reported that rarely are patients selected and groomed to work as mediums who have been diagnosed by Western-oriented therapists as schizophrenic.

I visited a small temple in the western part of the island that typifies Puerto Rico's indigenous folk spiritism. The walls were adorned with pictures of Jesus Christ, American Indian spirit guides, and deceased mediums. A father and son, Samuel and Tomas Vilanovas, were the chief mediums in this temple, which at the time of my visit was filled to its capacity of 30 worshipers. When don Tomas attempted to assist a member of his congregation, he looked into a bowl of water and breathed rapidly, often reporting cold sensations in his neck. This appeared to be an example of the contemplative alteration of consciousness described by Koss-Chioino. The water typically yielded an image that don Tomas used to determine what was affecting the client, and whether it had a physical or spiritual *causa* (i.e., cause). If the former, the client was referred to a physician, or an herbal treatment was prescribed. In the case of a spiritual *causa,* divine punishment, human envy or malevolence, or an "earthbound spirit" who had become the tool of a sorcerer, was held to be responsible. In the latter instance, Tomas attempted to "give light" to the spirit, and assist its ascent to a higher spiritual realm through prayers and offerings. If this did not work, a medium attempted to persuade the spirit to leave its victim in peace (referred to as *trabajando la causa*, or working the cause). Another procedure was to conduct a *despojo* (i.e., exorcism) to forcefully eliminate the offending spirit. I observed a reportedly successful attempt to remove a "low" spirit from its victim; a cigar-smoking medium fumigated the client with tobacco smoke while shaking him and stroking his body with "magnetic passes." I was given a fragrant perfume to rub on my skin as protection against the intruding spirit.

Don Tomas' alteration in consciousness might appear to only be contemplative and not dissociative in nature. However, don Tomas told me that his focus on the container of water often led to an out-of-body experience in which he would enter the spirit world and obtain additional information about his client. Often, don Tomas and his assistants also attempt to enlist the client's spirit guides in the healing; hence, if the spirits have abandoned the client, they will be asked to return. Power objects (e.g., amulets, crucifixes) may be given the client so that self-healing can be facilitated. Don Tomas said that he and his assistants make many suggestions regarding diet and exercise in addition to working with the spirits (Krippner & Welch, 1992, pp. 133–137).

If dissociation involves *experiences and behaviors that exist apart from, or that have been disconnected from the mainstream of one's conscious awareness, behavioral repertoire, and/or self-concept,* do the Puerto Rican spiritists exhibit dissociative states? In cases of involuntary spirit possession, the persons involved usually claim that they lose awareness, feel "violated" by an "intruder," or speak and behave uncontrollably in a way uncharacteristic of them. This is also the case with men and women who are "called" to become mediums through spontaneous possession. One initiate told Koss-Chioino (1992) that during her first experience with spirits, "I seemed to be losing awareness of my surroundings. . . . All of a sudden I felt like something inside me, sort of disassociated with myself, wanted to make me pound my fist on the table and start talking" (p. 60).

Despite the ethereal tone of the vague statements that often characterize their reports (Koss, 1975; Koss-Chioino, 1992, p. 82), experienced mediums contend that they rarely feel out of control during their endeavors. In fact, as a therapeutic device, mediums sometimes attempt to "capture" the pains of a client through experiencing these sensations in their own bodies. Spirit incorporation is often uncomfortable, especially for novices and when *causa* spirits are incorporated; but if a familiar guide is embodied, the experience can be rather pleasant. Some mediums report being "filled up" with "heat" that resides "deep in the body" (p. 82). These mediums reject the suggestion that they are disconnected in any way; on the contrary, they feel they have made a vital connection with a vital part of the universe. Whether an outside observer views the guides as independent entities, "inner self-helpers," subpersonalities (or "ego-states"), imaginative mentations, or archetypal images from the collective unconscious or not, they believe an affiliation is present that reflects integrity rather than separation. However, these experiences are not part of the practitioners' usual behavioral repertoire, nor do the spirit guides neatly fit into their concept of what the self is, and are "dissociative" in nature according to my definition.

Spirit Possession and Incorporation in Haiti

In the 16th and 17th centuries, slave traders brought millions of West African captives to North and South America. These slaves came from many different tribes, but they shared similar religious and magical beliefs, among them the notion that lesser deities did the bidding of the "Supreme Creator." The deities were the gods and goddesses of rivers and mountains, fire and iron, lightning and epidemics, war and peace. Subservient to these deities were the ancestral spirits; their duty was to see that their earthbound descendants carried out the moral precepts handed down to them. West African tribes believed that human behavior was generally predetermined, but occasionally another force, the "divine trickster," would subvert the master plan.

Deities and ancestral spirits visited the living through dreams or through a medium who served as an intermediary. Coincidentally, the hierarchy of the West African religious figures resembled the pantheon of Roman Catholic saints. Indeed, the church's icons, rosary beads, rituals, festivals, and holy communion had their counterparts in the slaves' rituals. Practitioners of religion and magic from West Africa were quick to see the correspondences; for example, they noticed that Legba, the god of entrances, resembled Saint Peter, keeper of the keys. In one of the West African languages, the word for "divinity" was "voudoun." Eventually, the "voudoun" (or "voodoo") religion came into being. It represents an amalgamation of African, European, and Native American beliefs and practices, and can be found today in the American states of Louisiana and South Carolina, and the Republic of Haiti—where voodoo is ubiquitous.

I visited Port-au-Prince, Haiti, in 1980 to meet voodoo mediums and observe their rituals. My guide was Thérèse Roumer, a well-known *mambo* (i.e., female medium). Roumer's fiancé had died suddenly, and I was invited to attend the *dessounin* (i.e., the funeral ritual) in a *peristyle* (i.e., voodoo temple). The *mambos, houngans* (i.e., male mediums), and their apprentices, the *hounsis,* were costumed in white garments. Soon, they announced that they were ready to be "mounted" by the *loa* (i.e., the deities and spirits); in this way, the mediums could pay their respects to the *espirit* (i.e., the soul) of the deceased man. An elaborate *vever* (i.e., a drawing) was traced on the dirt floor with white flour; the frenzied dancing would later erase the *vever,* yet its preparation was an important part of the ceremony, and it served as a ground altar.

I was allowed to tape-record the music, songs, and chants of the *dessounin* up to the time when a special drum beat called upon the *loa* to "mount" the mediums, as riders would "mount" horses—or, in Freudian terms, as the ego would "mount" the unconscious (Bowers, 1961, p. 271). As each *loa* took its turn entering a medium's body, characteristic gestures and movements announced its appearance. The deceased man's *lagu* (i.e., ceremonial food) was placed around the room for his soul to enjoy, which would later be buried toward the end of the ceremony. At about that time, a gourd was broken. After examining the pieces, the *mambos* and *houngans* determined that the soul of the deceased had left its body and had begun its travel to the Lower World.

The Haitians believe that after a year and a day in the Lower World, the soul can become a minor *loa,* returning to the earth to give advice and comfort to the *naga* (i.e., living humans). It is important that people continue to venerate the *loa,* because neglect can cause them to disappear. They also believe that without the *loa,* the world would lose its *espirit* and nature would revert to a mechanistic, amoral state. Voodoo is unusual among religions in that people are dependent on the deities, and the *loa* are also dependent on the *naga.*

Later in the week, I attended a ceremony in the *hounfer* (i.e., the community house) of André Pierre, a well-known Haitian artist. His colorful paintings depict such *loa* as Damballah, the *loa* of the heavens (whose *vever* is a serpent in a field of crosses), and Ghede, the *loa* of sex and of death (whose *vever* is a coffin and a cross). Each *loa* has an African name and an American Indian name; in the American Indian or *preto* tradition, Damballah is Dan Petro while Ghede is Baron Samedi. Pierre is also a *houngan,* and led a group in a libation to each *loa,* spilling a few drops of an alcoholic beverage on the floor in obeisance to their presence (Krippner & Welch, 1992, pp. 131–133).

A major function of the *mambo* and *houngan* is to provide medicine and therapy. Nanan-bouclou is the *loa* of herbs and is called upon when a diagnosis is made (Huxley, 1966, pp. 243–247). The practitioner must determine if an illness is natural or supernatural in origin, which, in turn, determines the nature of the treatment. If the etiology is natural, herbs will be prescribed or the client will be sent to a physician (i.e., if he or she can afford to pay the fees). If the etiology is supernatural, the practitioner may assign the client individual tasks (i.e., sacrifices, prayers), or may bring in the family and/or the community for a healing ritual. For example, if a sorcerer has cast a spell on a client, a *coucher* or purifying sleep may be held at a *hounfer* to counteract the spell. In some cases, a chicken may be sacrificed and the blood used to purify the client. For major exorcisms, a *mambo* might throw bull's bile on the client's face, spit rum on his or her body, set off small explosive devices between his or her legs, and administer an intensive massage (Goodman, 1988). Various *loa* may be asked to assist the client's recovery; no clear dividing line is drawn between the living and the dead as each supports the existence of the other, the living by entering dissociative states where they can be "mounted" by the *loa*.

Spirit Possession and Incorporation in Brazil

In early West African cultures, each person was expected to play his or her part in a web of kinship relations and community networks. Strained or broken social relations were held to be the major cause of sickness; a harmonious relationship with one's community, as well as with one's ancestors, was important for health. At the same time, an ordered relationship with the forces of nature, as personified by the *orixás* or deities, was essential for maintaining the well-being of the individual, the family, and the community. Powerful and terrifying, but so human that they could be talked to, pleaded with, and cajoled through special offerings, the *orixás* were part of the tradition brought by slaves to the New World.

West African healing practitioners felt that they gained access to supernatural power in three ways: by making offerings to the *orixás,* by foretelling the future with the help of an *orixá*, and by incorporating an *orixá* (or even an ancestor), who then diagnosed illnesses, prescribed cures, and provided the community with warnings or blessings. They claimed that such procedures as dancing, singing, or drumming were needed to surrender their mind and body to the discarnate entity (Krippner, 1989, p. 188). The slaves brought these practices to Brazil with them. Despite colonial and ecclesiastical repression, these customs survived over the centuries and eventually formed the basis for a number of robust Afro-Brazilian spiritual movements (Wafer, 1991). Kardec's books were brought to Brazil later, translated into Portuguese, and then became the basis for a related movement, Kardecism. An estimated 60% of Brazilians participate in one of the movements.

Contemporary *mães dos santos* (i.e., mothers of the *orixás*) and *pais dos santos* (i.e., fathers of the *orixás*) teach their apprentices how to sing, drum, and dance in order to incorporate the various deities, ancestors, and spirit guides. They also teach the *iaôs* (i.e., the children of the *orixás*) about the special herbs, teas, and lotions needed to restore health, and about the charms and ceremonies needed to prevent illness. The ceremonies of the various Afro-Brazilian groups (e.g., Candomblé, Umbanda, Batuque, Caboclo, Quimbanda, and Xango) differ, but all share three beliefs: Humans have a spiritual body that generally is reincarnated after physical death; discarnate spirits are in constant contact with the physical world; and humans can learn how to incorporate spirits for the purposes of healing and community service.

In my observations of spirit incorporation among these groups, I have noticed the use of several procedures designed to "call" the spirits. When one medium incorporated an *orixá*, a *preto velho* (i.e., an African slave spirit), a *caboclo* (i.e., an indigenous Indian spirit), or a *criança* (i.e., a girl or boy spirit), I discerned that an entire series of incorporations soon followed, in a domino-like fashion. Just as many participants in hypnotic sessions seem eager to present themselves as "good subjects" (Spanos, 1989), the mediums in Afro-Brazilian or Kardecist healing sessions may be eager to present themselves as "good mediums," and enact behaviors consistent with this interpretation.

I found fairly consistent similarity among the Brazilian mediums I spoke to in their supposed inability to recall the events of the incorporation after the spirits had departed. Spanos (1989) has pointed out that this amnesic quality could be explained as involving a sense of "achievement"; each failure to remember adds legitimacy to a subject's self-presentation as "truly unable to remember," hence as having been deeply in "trance" (p. 101). In other words, interpreting hypnotic phenomena as goal-directed action is helpful when conceiving of mediumship as an activity that meets role demands, since mediums may guide and report their behavior and experience in conformance with these demands. It may not be the case that they lose control over the behavior as they incorporate a spirit, but rather that they engage in an efficacious enactment of a role they are eager to maintain. Bowers (1961) has pointed out that the distinction between "acting" and "actual" possession is a fine one, and that any ability to dramatize the mediums may have further enabled them to intensify the characterization of their role (p. 269).

There are two major categories of dysfunction attributed to hostile spirits; both of them resemble what Western-oriented psychotherapists would label "dissociative disorders." With "obsession," a spirit entity influences an individual's behavior, producing repetitive thoughts, compulsions, phobias, and psychosomatic illnesses. With "possession," the entity is said to actually take control of the individual for short or long periods of time (Lyra, 1984). In the treatment of obsession, the "obsessing spirit" is allowed to express itself through a spiritistic medium in all of its anguish, pain, and ignorance. A different medium dialogues with the obsessing spirit, encouraging it to leave the client. If this "de-obsession" procedure is not successful, the medium uses more force, with bodily gestures, verbal commands, or various rituals, to dismiss the spirit. In some cases, the medium goes into the past lives of the obsessor to determine the most productive therapeutic approach. The medium may find, for instance, that the obsessor may have been mistreated by his or her client in a past life, and, as a result, is attempting to take revenge in the client's current life.

The diagnosis of possession is a more serious matter. In these instances, the possessing spirit has taken over a person's mind and body for longer amounts of time. One commonly used therapeutic procedure is to arrange for a group of mediums to form a circle around the client. One of the mediums temporarily incorporates the offending entity while another one speaks to it. The client is then sent to a different room. The incorporating medium then expunges the spirit from his or her own body, sending it to a higher spiritual dimension. If the spirit entity does not leave easily, other mediums will tempt it to enter their bodies. As the spirit attempts to do so, the mediums visualize a "psychic shield" in front of their bodies, which protects them while the offending spirit is being expelled from the world of human beings.

Once the offending spirit has been expelled, considerable follow-up is required to protect the client against obsession or possession by other spirit entities. Special foods, herbs, and purgatives may be accompanied by rituals, prayers, and/or imagery exercises. Most of the procedures used by Kardecists closely follow the explicit suggestions given by Kardec (e.g., 1857/1968, 1861/1973, 1868/1983) in the 19th century. Likewise, the procedures used by mediums in Afro-Brazilian spiritual groups often have their roots in African tradition (see, e.g., Peek, 1991).

In an attempt to determine how and when the spiritistic mediums originally received their "call," I (Krippner, 1989) interviewed 40 of them (i.e., Kardecist and Afro-Brazilian practitioners) in Brazil. I identified five different but overlapping routes among this group: (1) they come from a family that had a history of mediumship, (2) were "called" by spirits in visions and dreams, (3) succumbed to a malady or "spiritual crisis" from which they recovered in order to serve others, (4) had a revelation while reading spiritistic literature or attending spiritistic worship services, and (5) worked as volunteers in a spiritistic healing center and became inspired by the daily examples of compassion. It is believed that if a "call" is rejected, severe illness or misfortune may result; as one Candomblé medium told me, "Once the *orixá* calls, there is no other path to take" (p. 193).

Once the apprentices begin to receive instruction in mediumship, such experiences as spirit incorporation, automatic writing, out-of-body travel, and the recall of past lives lose their bizarre quality and seem to occur quite naturally. Socialization processes lead to the provision of role models and the support of peers. A number of cues (songs, chants, music, etc.) facilitate spirit incorporation, and a process of social construction teaches control, appropriate role-taking, and a desire to provide the community with support. Richeport (1992) observed several similarities between the mediumistic behaviors and those of many hypnotized subjects, for example, dissociation, the positive use of imagination, and frequent amnesia for the experiences.

But are the dissociative processes Richeport observes indicative of a mental disorder or a socially valuable capacity? The traits most admired in mediums resemble those traits that facilitate ordinary social interactions, such as showing respect for the participants and giving them amicable, friendly advice. I have observed a few instances of bizarre behavior during spiritistic ceremonies; for instance, if a spirit seems to be taking control of the medium too quickly, the other mediums may sing a song that will slow down the process of incorporation (Rouget, 1985). Leacock and Leacock (1972) observed that the Brazilian mediums in their study usually behaved in ways that were "basically rational," communicated effectively with other people, and demonstrated few symptoms that could be considered pathological. They engaged in intensive training and, as mediums, worked so conscientiously that they were often put at risk with seriously ill individuals (p. 212). In other words, their activities are not likely to be the favorite pastimes of fragile-personalities or malingerers.

MULTIPLE PERSONALITY DISORDER

As was mentioned earlier, applying the term "dissociation" is a social group's attempt to describe and explain phenomena its members have observed. However, these phenomena may have been constructed differently in other parts of the world, been given different labels, and been attributed to different etiologies. Martinez-Taboas (1991a) has observed that a wide variety of personal experiences are principally determined by systems of cultural belief, and argued that MPD would be more congruent with a culture in which the self "is expected to be rich in phenomenology and separate in experience," than a culture that promotes the interdependent and the social self (p. 130). Martínez-Taboas further predicted that MPD, because of its association with early physical and sexual abuse, would be rare in societies where children are respected and valued, as well as in societies where dissociation is primarily used to defend the individual self and where "dissociative states are split off into semiotic systems of gods, ghosts, or ancestors" (p. 131).

In surveying the available data, Martínez-Taboas found that MPD cases are similar in such individualistic countries as Canada (Ross, Norton, & Wozney, 1989) and the United States (Coons, Bowman, & Milstein, 1988). He found the rate of MPD in the United States—where there is a high incidence of alleged child abuse—particularly high (Herman, 1992; Kluft, 1985; Martínez-Taboas, 1991b). He found few reports of MPD from Japan (Takahashi, 1990), England (Fahy, 1988), and Russia (Allison, 1991). Topper (personal communication, June 15, 1988) adds that he has never seen a case of MPD in his 12 years among the Navaho Indians. Of the Puerto Rican cases, only 13% of the alters claimed to be supernatural entities, despite the widespread practice of spiritism, but that very statistic confirms Martínez-Taboas's prediction that a "semiotic system of gods, ghosts, or ancestors" will preclude a diagnosis of MPD when so-called spirits are involved.

Both voluntary and involuntary possession are common in Haiti and Brazil but data have not been collected about those activities that would permit a comparison with MPD in such countries as the United States and Canada. The Puerto Rican data suggest that MPD can be detected in a cultural setting quite different from that of Canada, the United States, and Europe, and that "the development and manifestation of MPD is fairly dependent on some environmental and idiosyncratic personal characteristics that, if kept invariable, will probably culminate in a dissociative disorder" (Martínez-Taboas, 1991b, p. 192). I would interpret the findings to suggest that there may be a physiological predisposition to dissociation in general and to MPD specifically which, if activated by trauma in a society where there is an awareness of MPD, spawns alters. If the physiological predisposition is lacking, the trauma may be defended against in another manner.

A Discussion of Cross-Cultural Multiple Personality Disorder Research

What Martínez-Taboas has done is to make predictions regarding the diagnosis of MPD on the basis of several variables. A wide range of Western countries are covered by some of these variables (e.g., individualism), while non-Western countries are covered by others (e.g., "semiotic systems"). What Martínez-Taboas has *not* done is to specifically predict the countries in which MPD would *not* be found. Even if a low incidence of MPD were detected in such countries as Japan, this would not indicate that MPD is completely culture bound. The MPD cases in Japan and other low-incidence countries might indeed be small in number but could still be congruent with the general pattern. In one international survey of 15 detailed case histories, "the symptoms . . . presented were remarkably similar to symptoms of MPD reported previously in the United States and Canada" (Coons, Bowman, Kluft, & Milstein, 1991, p. 125). Child abuse was alleged in each of these cases, and the authors concluded that "MPD is clearly not a culture-bound phenomenon. . . . Since 1840, MPD has been reported in twenty-one different countries plus one territory. . . . This study reports MPD in seven countries where it had not previously been reported" (p. 126). It is interesting that alters in some of the more "atypical cases" reported in this survey resemble the spirits involved in involuntary possession (e.g., a 16th-century priest alter, alters who claim to be Roman Catholic saints, various animal and bird alters).

Aldridge-Morris's (1989) assertion that MPD is more a "cultural phenomenon" than a "clinical entity," also can be evaluated by administering the standardized tests and questionnaires normally used to diagnose MPD. When one of these measures, the Dissociative Experiences Scale (DES; Bernstein & Putnam, 1986) was used to compare MPD cases in the United States and Canada, no significant differences were found (Ross, 1989, p. 136). Another measure, the Dissociative Questionnaire (DIS-Q), has identified "serious dissociative phenomena" among 3% of the population of Belgium and the Netherlands (Vanderlinder, Van Dyck, Vandereycken, & Vertommen, 1991), a percentage similar to that found in the United States and Canada (Ross, Joshi, & Currie, 1990). This procedure shows promise, but cross-cultural work with the DES, the DIS-Q, and similar instruments is only beginning.

Little cross-cultural work has been done with the extraordinary physiological concomitants of some MPD cases, specifically the reported sudden changes that accompany "switching" such as visual refraction, allergic reactions, menstrual irregularities, changes in handedness or handwriting style, cerebral electrical activity, and electrochemical brain conditions (Coons, 1988). Many of these bodily changes are extremely rapid, and go beyond the alterations in gestures, carriage, voice, and facial expressions that could be attributed to conscious or unconscious role playing. I have seen the physiological changes listed above both in cases of voluntary spirit incorporation and involuntary possession. There are also recorded cases of such bodily changes as stigmata and false pregnancies, as well as reports of sudden appearances of rashes, swellings, and tattoo-like patterns among persons who hold the belief that they are divinely favored or malevolently cursed (Murphy, 1992, pp. 233–240). Cross-cultural investigation could yield useful knowledge about the physiological components of dissociative experiences.

In my opinion, the available information suggests that MPD is more than a culture-bound syndrome that is sometimes magnified by iatrogenic catalysts, as it has remarkably similar features wherever it has been reported. Nonetheless, the literature also indicates that MPD is more common in some countries than in others, indicating that cultural factors can increase its occurrence. For instance, in countries with a high incidence of child abuse MPD is more likely to be found since the abuse is a major etiological trigger for the disorder. However, not all instances of actual abuse lead to MPD. It may be that cultural and environmental factors combine with physiological predisposition to determine the sequelae of physical, sexual, verbal, and cultic abuse of children, and that MPD is one of several phenomenon that may result.

Despite the phenomenological similarities noted by Kenny (1981), it seems overly facile to equate MPD with involuntary possession, which most spiritists see as a diagnostic entity in its own right. However, the few folk practitioners who are aware of MPD view the term as closely equivalent to some of the labels they have used for centuries. Western psychotherapy with MPD may take several different forms (Kluft, 1985). Those psychotherapists whose goals are to "fuse" the alters or to achieve some "harmonious" situation (in which the alters move from being separate entities to being cooperative "ego-states" of the individual) would reject the idea of exorcism, but fusion yields the same results as exorcism in that the "alters" cease to have a separate existence (Richeport, 1992, p. 169). Another orientation involves encouraging collaboration among the alters (e.g., Erickson, 1940/ 1980). This procedure is similar to the development of mediumship, wherein the "spirit guides" collaborate with their host and serve as a valuable resource.

While the debate continues over the culture-bound aspects of MPD, there are still patients who need treatment. It is legitimate to ask if there is a practical difference between MPD as role-playing and a special state of consciousness in which MPD occurs? In either instance, clinicians have to deal with the client's dysfunctional behavior, physiologists need to account for the rapid physiological changes that can occur after "switching," and psychologists are required to explain the exotic cognitive activity that differentiates one alter from another. Behavior can be analyzed at three different levels: the social, the biophysical, and the psychological (Kihlstrom, 1991), hence, psychotherapy needs to consider these three levels as well.

Spiritistic Treatment for Multiple Personality Disorder

MPD itself may not be culture bound, but its treatment in North America can be described using that term (Ross, 1989, p. 5). However, the literature contains a few instances where Western-oriented psychotherapists have drawn from folkloric traditions when working with their patients, especially those with a background of spiritism and/or cult ritual abuse. Ronquillo (1991) reports a case of MPD in a Hispanic patient who perceived that her problems arose and were maintained by external forces rather than internal fragmentation. In her case, some of the alters were similar to spiritistic entities. To treat his patient, Ronquillo devised a plan that included both her psychological and cultural profile; for example, the therapist consulted a medium and attended a spiritist meeting with his patient.

Vesper (1991) advocates the use of ceremony with MPD patients and presents a case in which music, poems, symbols, and a fire ceremony were used to successfully treat an MPD patient who claimed that she was being persecuted by malevolent alters, her dominating parents, and memories of a cult ritual in which children were murdered. Goodwin, Hill, and Attias (1990) encourage psychotherapists to familiarize themselves with historical and folk techniques of exorcism, and how they can be adapted when working with MPD patients. They help with confronting the alters, containing destructive impulses, and avoiding psychotherapist burnout. Krippner and Colodzin (1989) describe the use of Native American and Oriental healing methods in the treatment of combat veterans with post-traumatic stress disorders, some of whom demonstrated MPD.

As the concept of MPD becomes better known around the world, various "possession" phenomena may be renamed or given a dual diagnosis. For example, Steinberg (1990) has recommended that the diagnosis of MPD be considered with Hispanics who have a history of the so-called *ataque* syndrome, a transient dissociative disorder. I have had an opportunity to observe this process firsthand in Brazil where some spiritistic healers have heard of MPD, often producing a dual diagnosis in which MPD is associated with involuntary spirit possession and/or past-life evocation. This group differs from both the orthodox psychiatrists and psychologists who employ drugs, hypnosis, psychodrama, and other modalities currently in favor among Western psychotherapists, and the spiritistic practitioners who have never heard of MPD and treat their clients with the same rituals, amulets, and brews that have been used for centuries.

The new practitioners, found primarily among the followers of Allan Kardec, have accepted the Western diagnostic category of MPD as a synonym for certain types of possession. Their clients, however, may or may not be familiar with the MPD label, depending on their level of education and sophistication. They are all familiar with notions about past lives and spirit intrusion. Although no uniformity of practice exists, Kardecist therapy may involve the exorcism of offending "earthbound spirits," the "merging" of interfering "past-life personalities," or a compromise in which some of these personalities remain intact but appear only on circumscribed occasions.

I (Krippner, 1987) have interviewed three Kardecist practitioners in Brazil (Eliezer Mendes, Hernani Andrade, and Carlos Jacob) who claim to have had success in their work with MPD cases. I have also interviewed several of their clients. Eliezer Mendes, a retired surgeon, runs a therapeutic community in the outskirts of Sao Paulo and also sees clients at a São Paulo office on an outpatient basis. Mendes described one case that involved a 12-year-old girl who, at the onset of puberty, began to play boys' games in the street. At the same time, she expressed a dislike of her rapidly developing female physiology. Mendes consulted a group of mediums who diagnosed the client as having been a male in a previous life; this former personality, they maintained, had been evoked by the biological changes accompanying puberty. After about 3 months of psychotherapy, the alleged alter male personality merged with the host female personality. The girl's gender was accepted by what Mendes referred to as the client's "psychological center," a deep-seated aspect of the psyche underlying all personalities, both host and alter.

Mendes prefers the advantages offered by his therapeutic community to seeing clients individually; he refers to the large rooms where the dancing, dramatizations, and exercise sessions take place as the "mad-o-drama" rooms. Both psychotherapists and mediums are present during the group therapy sessions to facilitate the therapeutic process, to "channel" the "crises" that occur, and to pay attention to the alter personalities that become manifest. One person's manifestation of an alter personality might stimulate someone else to uncover his or her unconscious material. Visitors and relatives are urged to join the melee because the inclusion of nondisturbed people is felt to be beneficial to the "energy field" that develops during each therapy session. Folk healers may be invited into group therapy sessions to attempt a "laying on" of hands with receptive clients. Homeopathic practitioners may visit the therapeutic community to prescribe specific remedies for individual clients. If a client's condition deteriorates or does not improve, he or she is sent by Mendes to one of the hospitals run by Brazilian spiritists. In these hospitals, the employees accept the notion that the emergence of past-life personalities and/or possession by a discarnate entity can result in MPD.

Hernani Andrade, an engineer, compares his model of the human psyche to an onion with several layers. Each of the concentric layers represents the same basic "spirit," but that "spirit" can present itself in different forms. Andrade insists that each alter personality has its place in the psyche's "organizing model," and can be evoked during the host personality's lifetime if a need exists. Andrade introduced me to Fiona, a Kardecist medium he had treated. For several years, she had allowed herself to incorporate various discarnate entities. However, in one instance the entity was not a spirit guide but a past-life personality of hers named Carmen, who was a Spanish gypsy. Fiona purportedly exhibited xenoglossy; she spoke a dialect common among gypsies on the Iberian peninsula, of which she had no apparent previous knowledge. Eventually, Fiona learned to cohabit with Carmen rather than attempt a "merging." Carmen was extremely useful during Fiona's mediumistic sessions, and did not manifest unless she was needed.

For Carlos Jacob, an anesthesiologist, MPD has three causes: It can result from traumas in one's current life, "karma" from a past life, or problems originating in the spirit world. In the first instance, his treatment may include allopathic medicine, homeopathic medicine, acupuncture, and/or conventional psychotherapy. In the second instance, past-life therapy is employed in which a purported personality from a former life becomes the client. In the third instance, spiritual exercises (e.g., exorcism, magnetic passes, cleansing the body's "energy centers," mediumship training) are used. Jacob believes that many people who have been institutionalized in mental hospitals are "sensitives," who would derive more benefit from spiritual exercises than from medication.

I have also visited the André Luiz Spiritist Hospital, a psychiatric facility in Belo Horizonte run by Kardec-oriented spiritists. The psychiatrists I interviewed estimated that 12% of their patients are diagnosed with MPD, the major etiological factor being "intruders," but with past-life personalities and sequelae from child abuse playing a role in some cases. At least 50% of them reportedly have achieved some sort of "fusion" or "harmonization" following treatment.

Brazil's spiritistic practitioners would have little difficulty in accepting the DSM-III-R definition of MPD as a dissociative disorder in which the criteria consist of

> the existence within the person of two or more distinct personalities or personality states (each with its own relatively enduring pattern of perceiving, relating to, and thinking about the environment and self) [and in which] at least two of these personalities or personality states recurrently take full control of the person's behavior. (American Psychiatric Association, 1987, p. 272)

Such standard MPD phenomena as "switching," the ignorance the host personality usually has of alter personalities, and the knowledge that alter personalities frequently have of each other have been observed by spiritists as well. They also would agree that practitioners can be at risk when dealing with these cases, as some of the alters tend to engage in dangerous acting-out behaviors including suicide and murder (Watkins & Watkins, 1984, 1988).

PERSPECTIVES ON DISSOCIATIVE DISORDERS

Ellenberger (1970) has traced the historical connection between exorcism and contemporary psychotherapy, finding that psychotherapists' interest in MPD goes in cycles; during some decades, the diagnosis is popular, and at other times, it is rarely used. Kenny (1981) found that 19th-century spiritualism not only favored the development of mediums, some of whom were studied by William James and his colleagues, but also stimulated the appearance of MPD in the same communities. With a declining belief in spirit possession, few cases of MPD were reported. Hacking (1992) claims that child abuse (especially cult ritual abuse) in the United States has taken the place of possession and mediumship as a spur for the diagnosis of MPD. Does this mean that "memories" of cult ritual abuse (Watters, 1992) and MPD itself can be created in the therapeutic office? Many of the pioneering observers of the phenomenon considered the possibility of iatrogenesis in cases of MPD. Janet (1889) noted that once he had named a personality, that personality became more lifelike (p. 318). James (1890) asserted that "It is very easy . . . to suggest during trance the appearance of a secondary personage" (p. 465). Ross (1989, pp. 58–63) convincingly argued that a condition as serious and complex as MPD can not be haphazardly elicited, but the controversy remains. It will no doubt continue, given the current move to reclassify MPD as "dissociative identity disorder."

This issue is a critical one because the diagnosis of MPD, even when accurate, tends to frighten both the patient's caregivers and family members. Herman (1992) documented the harm done to patients by such diagnoses as "somatization disorder," "borderline personality disorder," and "multiple personality disorder," all of which are "charged with pejorative meaning" and evoke suspicion, and even hate, from those around the patients, including psychotherapists who are poorly informed on the topic (p. 123). She stated that the three disorders could be best understood as variants of the complex post-traumatic stress disorder, each deriving its characteristic features from different ways of adapting to a traumatic environment. Gergen (1991) added that the term "dissociation" (and several other terms associated with dissociative disorders) is a negative one, and tends to "discredit the individual [by] drawing attention to problems, shortcomings, or incapacities. To put it more broadly, the vocabulary of human deficit has undergone enormous expansion within the present century" (p. 13). Koss-Chioino (1992) even raised questions concerning "the validity of the concepts behind the definitions of hallucinations and delusions" (p. 140) because "relatively few ideas have been advanced of ways to distinguish hallucinations from visionary experiences" (p. 143).

Dissociation, as I have used the term in this chapter, is not always maladaptively used and the term need not lead to stereotyped reactions. When defined as *experiences and behaviors that exist apart from, or have been disconnected from, the mainstream of one's conscious awareness, behavioral repertoire, and/or self-concept* "dissociative" processes can be viewed as basic skills or capacities similar to imagination and absorption, as well as pathological reactions. Masters (1992) found that marathon runners often use a cognitive style in which they cut themselves off from the sensory feedback they would normally receive from their body. Their deliberate use of this type of dissociation as a running strategy was positively related to scores on a hypnotic susceptibility test. Other positive uses of dissociation include pain control, creative daydreaming, and the "tuning out" of a boring conversation. For Erickson (1940/1980), MPD itself is not necessarily psychopathological, even though a variety of pathologies may characterize some of the alters. In some countries, such as Brazil, "fantasy-proneness" is reinforced by many elements in the society, and the ability to incorporate spirits is highly regarded by any number of people regarded as sagacious (Greenfield, 1991, p. 24).

Dissociation is felt to be dysfunctional in the context of involuntary possession and the so-called "dissociative disorders" such as MPD. But the term can also be applied to voluntary spirit incorporation, which is intentional and—within its cultural context—is, generally speaking, socially adaptive and also serves to empower a number of women who have few other ways of asserting their capabilities. In the Ethiopian Zar cults, many indisposed women are believed to be possessed by spirits. Boddy (1988, p. 19) argued that this interpretation of illness provides an opportunity for the possessed woman to evolve. She described how the "existence of her nonself becomes subjectively real" to the possessed woman, who enters an altered state in order to come to terms with the spirit affecting her health. In describing possession-related illness in Northern Sudanese women, Boddy stated that "it enables a woman to evolve" by providing her with experiences of her "non-self," which "enhanc[e] her sense of personhood" (p. 19). Thus, spirit incorporation can be viewed as therapeutic in some cases as it may release inhibitions and provide a source of esteem for the medium as well as emotional catharsis for the group (Ward, 1980). Finally, Koestler (1964) argued that creativity depends on "bisociation," that is, a mental occurrence wherein two habitually incompatible contexts are simultaneously activited, which is a definition not far removed from some descriptions of "dissociation."

Gergen (1991) reminded us that the "self" is constructed differently by society in various times and places. In traditional Balinese culture, the individual self plays a minimal role in everyday life; rather, the individual is considered representative of a more general social category (Geertz, 1973). It also appears that the human being is extremely malleable: Indeed, MPD research has stimulated a number of writers (e.g., Braude, 1991; Crabtree, 1985; Ornstein, 1986) to propose provocative and innovative theories of the self and the psyche. People can create personalities as required to defend themselves against trauma, to conform to cultural pressures, or to meet the expectations of a psychotherapist, medium, or exorcist. This malleability has both adaptive and maladaptive aspects. One of the beneficial results of renewed interest in MPD and other dissociative reactions is to illustrate the urgent need for more information about them, and to illustrate the important role that cross-cultural research can play in the quest for information about dissociative phenomena.

REFERENCES

Aldridge-Morris, R. (1989). *Multiple personality: An exercise in deception.* Hove, England: Lawrence Erlbaum.

Allison, R. M. (1991). Travel log: In search of multiples in Moscow. *American Journal of Forensic Psychiatry, 12,* 51–66.

American Psychiatric Association. (1987). *Diagnostic and statistical manual of mental disorders* (3rd ed., rev.). Washington, DC: American Psychiatric Association.

American Psychiatric Association. (1991). *DSM-IV options book: Work in progress.* Washington, DC: Author.

Bernstein, E. M., & Putnam, F. W. (1986). Development, reliability, and validity of a dissociation scale. *Journal of Nervous and Mental Disease, 174*, 727–735.

Boddy, J. (1988). Spirits and selves in Northern Sudan: The cultural therapies of possession and trance. *American Ethnologist, 15(1)*, 4–27.

Bourguignon, E. (1976). *Possession.* San Francisco: Chandler & Sharp.

Bourguignon, E. (1989). Multiple personality, possession trance, and the psychic unity of mankind. *Ethos, 17(3)*, 371–384.

Bowers, M. K. (1961). Hypnotic aspects of Haitian voodoo. *International Journal of Clinical and Experimental Hypnosis, 9*, 269–282.

Braude, S. E. (1991). *First person plural: Multiple personality and the philosophy of mind.* New York: Routledge.

Braun, B. G. (1988). The BASK model of dissociation. *Dissociation, 1*, 4–23.

Coons, P. M. (1988). Psychophysiologic aspects of multiple personality disorder: A review. *Dissociation, 1*, 47–53.

Coons, P. M., Bowman, E. S., Kluft, R. P., & Milstein, V. (1991). The cross-cultural occurrence of multiple personality disorder: Additional cases from a recent survey. *Dissociation, 4*, 124–128.

Coons, P. M., Bowman, E. S., & Milstein, V. (1988). Multiple personality disorder: A clinical investigation of 50 cases. *Journal of Nervous and Mental Disease, 176*, 519– 527.

Crabtree, A. (1985). *Multiple man: Explorations in possession and multiple personality.* New York: Praeger.

Ellenberger, H. F. (1970). *The discovery of the unconscious: The history and evolution of dynamic psychiatry.* New York: John Wiley.

Erickson, M. H. (1980). The clinical discovery of a dual personality. In E. Rossi (Ed.), *Hypnotic investigation of psychodynamic processes: The collected papers of Milton H. Erickson on hypnosis* (Vol. 3, pp. 261–270). New York: Irvington. (Original work published circa 1940)

Fahy, T. A. (1988). The diagnosis of multiple personality disorder: A critical review. *British Journal of Psychiatry, 153*, 597–606.

Geertz, C. (1973). *The interpretation of cultures.* New York: Basic Books.

Gergen, K. J. (1985). The social constructionist movement in modern psychology. *American Psychologist, 40*, 266–275.

Gergen, K. J. (1991). *The saturated self: Dilemmas of identity in contemporary life.* New York: Basic Books.

Goodman, F. (1988). *How about demons? Possession and exorcism in the modern world.* Bloomington, IN: University of Indiana Press.

Goodwin, J., Hill, S., & Attias, R. (1990). Historical and folk techniques of exorcism: Applications to the treatment of dissociative disorders. *Dissociation, 3*, 94–101.

Greenfield, S. M. (1991). Hypnosis and trance induction in the surgeries of Brazilian spiritist healer-mediums. *Anthropology of Consciousness, 2(3–4)*, 20–25.

Hacking, I. (1992). Multiple personality disorder and its hosts. *History of the Human Sciences, 5(2)*, 3–31.

Herman, J. L. (1992). *Trauma and recovery*. New York: Basic Books.

Hilgard, E. R. (1992). Dissociation and theories of hypnosis. In E. Fromm & M. R. Nash (Eds.), *Contemporary hypnosis research* (pp. 69–101). New York: Guilford Press.

Huxley, F. (1966). *The invisibles: Voodoo gods in Haiti*. New York: McGraw-Hill.

James, W. (1890). Remarks on M. Prince's "The revelations of hypnotism as a therapeutic agent." *Boston Medical and Surgical Journal, 122,* 475.

Janet, P. (1889). *L'automatisme psychologique*. Paris: Félix Alcan.

Kardec, A. (1968). *The spirits' book*. Sao Paulo: Lake. (Original work published 1857)

Kardec, A. (1973). *The medium's book*. Sao Paulo: Editora Pensamento. (Original work published 1861)

Kardec, A. (1983). *Genesis: The miracles and the predictions*. Boston: Colby and Rich. (Original work published 1868)

Kenny, M. G. (1981). Multiple personality and spirit possession. *Psychiatry, 44,* 337–358.

Kihlstrom, J. F. (1991). The social psychology of hypnosis, warts and all. [Review of *Hypnosis: The cognitive-behavioral perspective*]. *Contemporary Psychology, 36,* 11–13.

Kluft, R. P. (1985). Childhood multiple personality disorder: Predictors, clinical findings, and treatment results. In R. P. Kluft (Ed.), *Childhood antecedents of multiple personality disorder* (pp. 167–196). Washington, DC: American Psychiatric Press.

Koestler, A. (1964). *The act of creation*. New York: Macmillan.

Koss, J. (1975). Therapeutic aspects of Puerto Rican cult practices. *Psychiatry, 38,* 160–171.

Koss, J. (1987). Expectations and outcomes for patients given mental health care or spiritist healing in Puerto Rico. *American Journal of Psychiatry, 144,* 56–61.

Koss-Chioino, J. (1992). *Women as healers, women as patients: Mental health care and traditional healing in Puerto Rico*. Boulder, CO: Westview Press.

Krippner, S. (1987). Cross-cultural approaches to multiple personality disorder: Practices in Brazilian spiritism. *Ethos, 15,* 273–295.

Krippner, S. (1989). A call to heal: Entry patterns in Brazilian mediumship. In C. A. Ward (Ed.), *Altered states of consciousness and mental health: A cross-cultural approach* (pp. 186–206). Newbury Park, CA: Sage.

Krippner, S., & Colodzin, B. (1989). Multi-cultural methods of treating Vietnam veterans with post-traumatic stress disorder. *International Journal of Psychosomatics, 36,* 79–85.

Krippner, S., & Welch, P. (1992). *Spiritual dimensions of healing: From native shamanism to contemporary health care*. New York: Irvington.

Leacock, S., & Leacock, R. (1972). *Spirits of the deep: Drums, mediums and trance in a Brazilian city*. Garden City, NY: Doubleday

Lyra, A. (1984). Psiquiatria, parapsicologia e os fenomenos de obsessao espiritica e possessao demoniaca. *Boletim Medico-Espirita, 1*(2), 35–91.

Martínez-Taboas, M. A. (1991a). Multiple personality disorder as seen from a social constructionist standpoint. *Dissociation, 4,* 129–133.

Martínez-Taboas, M. A. (1991b). Multiple personality disorder in Puerto Rico: Analysis of fifteen cases. *Dissociation, 4,* 189–192.

Masters, K. S. (1992). Hypnotic susceptibility, cognitive dissociation, and runner's high in a sample of marathon runners. *American Journal of Clinical Hypnosis, 34*(3), 193–201.

Murphy, M. (1992). *The future of the body.* Los Angeles: Tarcher.

Ornstein, R. (1986). *Multimind.* Boston: Houghton-Mifflin.

Peek, P. M. (1991). *African divination systems: Ways of knowing.* Bloomington, IN: Indiana University Press.

Richeport, M. M. (1992). The interface between multiple personality, spirit mediumship, and hypnosis. *American Journal of Clinical Hypnosis, 34,* 168–177.

Ronquillo, E. B. Jr. (1991). The influence of "espiritismo" on a case of multiple personality disorder. *Dissociation, 4,* 39–45.

Ross, C. A. (1989). *Multiple personality disorder: Diagnosis, clinical features, and treatment.* New York: John Wiley.

Ross, C. A., Joshi, S., & Currie, R. (1990). Dissociative experiences in the general population. *American Journal of Psychiatry, 147,* 1547–1552.

Ross, C. A., Norton, G. R., & Wozney, K. (1989). Multiple personality disorder: An analysis of 236 cases. *Canadian Journal of Psychiatry, 34,* 413–418.

Rouget, G. (1985). *Music and trance: A theory of the relations between music and possession.* Chicago: University of Chicago Press.

Singer, J. L. (Ed.). (1990). *Repression and dissociation: Implications for personality theory.* Chicago: University of Chicago Press.

Spanos, N. P. (1989). Hypnosis, demonic possession, and multiple personality: Strategic enactments and disavowals of responsibility for actions. In C. Ward (Ed.), *Altered states of consciousness and mental health: A cross-cultural perspective* (pp. 96–124). Newbury Park, CA: Sage.

Spritzer, R., Gibbon, M., Skodol, A., Williams, J., & First, M. (1989). *DSM-III-R casebook.* Washington DC: American Psychiatric Association Press.

Steinberg, M. (1990). Transcultural issues in psychiatry: The *ataque* and multiple personality disorder. *Dissociation, 3,* 31–33.

Takahashi, Y. (1990). Is multiple personality disorder really rare in Japan? *Dissociation, 3,* 57–59.

Tinnin, L. (1990). Mental unity, altered states of consciousness, and dissociation. *Dissociation, 3,* 154–159.

Vanderlinder, J., Van Dyck, R., Vandereycken, W., & Vertommen, H. (1991). Dissociative experiences in the general population in the Netherlands and Belgium: A study with the Dissociative Questionnaire (DIS-Q). *Dissociation, 4,* 180–184.

Vesper, J. H. (1991). The use of healing ceremonies in the treatment of multiple personality disorder. *Dissociation, 4,* 109–114.

Wafer, J. (1991). *The taste of blood: Spirit possession in Brazilian Candomblé.* Philadelphia: University of Pennsylvania Press.

Ward, C. (1980). Spirit possession and mental health: A psycho-anthropological perspective. *Human Relations, 33,* 149–163.

Watkins, J. G., & Watkins, H. H. (1984). Hazards to the therapist in the treatment of multiple personalities. *Psychiatric Clinics of North America, 7,* 111–119.

Watkins, J. G., & Watkins, H. H. (1988). The management of malevolent ego states in multiple personality disorder. *Dissociation, 1,* 67–72.

Watters, E. (1992, January/February). Doors of memory. *Mother Jones,* pp. 24–29, 76–77.

World Health Organization. (1992). *The international classification of mental and behavioural disorders.* Geneva: World Health Organization.

III
ISSUES AND CONTROVERSIES

17

One Hundred Years
of Hysteria

John F. Kihlstrom

A *tough old word like hysteria dies very hard. It tends to out-
live its obituarists.*

—AUBREY LEWIS (1975, p. 12)

Actually, there have been at least 4,000 years of hysteria. Veith (1965, 1977) has traced the history of the syndrome from pharaonic Egypt, where the theory of the migrating uterus was first propounded, through Sydenham (1697), who was first to recognize the emotional cause of the syndrome, to Cullen (1796), who coined the terms *neurology* and *neurosis*, to Charcot (1877/1888), the neurologist who discovered that hysterics were highly suggestible, and, finally, to the beginnings of modern psychiatry in the late 19th century (for other historical treatments, see Merskey 1979, 1983; Micale, 1990). Hysteria has been centrally involved in major conceptual changes in psychiatry and clinical psychology. Ellenberger (1970) has shown how the analysis of hysteria by Freud (Breuer & Freud, 1893–1895/1955; Freud, 1905/1953) and Janet (1889, 1894/1901, 1907)—both of whom studied with Charcot—promoted psychogenic as opposed to somatogenic theories of the origins of mental illness.[1] More recently, analyses of hysteria by Szasz (1961) and of other forms of mental illness by others (Goffman, 1961; Scheff, 1966) laid the foundation for a social-psychological critique of the medical model of psychopathology, and a reinterpretation of mental illness in terms of strategic self-presentation, interpersonal communication, and social control (for a defense of the medical model of psychopathology, which emphasizes that it has nothing to do with somatogenesis, see Siegler & Osmond, 1974; Shagass, 1975).

Although the entire history of hysteria is fascinating, this chapter focuses only on the 100-year period since Charcot's death in 1893, which was also the year Janet's medical thesis on hysteria was accepted, and the year that Breuer and Freud published the "Preliminary Communication" of their *Studies on Hysteria* (1955). (For psychologists interested in hysteria and dissociation, 1993 was a centennial year on three accounts.) It is over this period of time that clinicians and researchers began to develop a nosology for the systematic classification of psychopathology. As Grob (1991) has noted, up until the 19th century physicians were concerned with the diagnosis of individual cases, but not in organizing their diagnoses according to a systematic nosology (there were no psychologists yet, of course). A number of classifica-tory schemes had been proposed by Cullen (1796), Kant (1798/1978), and Pinel (1806/1962), among others. For example, Pinel distinguished between "physical" and "moral" neuroses, anticipating the later division between organic and functional mental illnesses (Spitzer et al., 1992). However, these nosologies did not play a major role in the treatment of individual patients.

Beginning in the mid-19th century, several factors combined to lead psychiatrists (then often known as alienists) to seek agreement on a classification scheme. One of these factors, at least in the United States, was the increasing scope and sophistication of the census and other social databases as instruments of social policy. Another was the need to imitate those branches of medicine that had gained social acceptance by virtue of their actual or perceived scientific rigor. As late as 1917, the Committee on Statistics of the American Medico-Psychological Association (AMPA; the forerunner of the American Psychiatric Association) noted that "The present condition with respect to the classification of mental diseases is chaotic. This condition of affairs discredits the science of psychiatry and reflects unfavorably on our Association" (Salmon, Copp, May, Abbot, & Cotton, 1917, p. 255).

This situation changed quickly. In 1918 the AMPA issued the first edition of the *Statistical Manual for the Use of Institutions for the Insane* (hereafter, referred to as *Statistical Manual*; Committee on Statistics, 1918), which was adopted by the Bureau of the Census in 1920 and went through nine revisions (Committee on Statistics, 1942). This laid the foundation for successive editions of the *Diagnostic and Statistical Manual of Mental Disorders* (DSM; American Psychiatric Association, 1952, 1968, 1980, 1987, 1994). Interestingly, the place of hysteria in these manuals has shifted from one edition to another—it is as if institutional psychiatry does not know quite what to do with it. This is poetic justice, perhaps, for a syndrome that was once attributed to a wandering uterus, but it also reflects deep confusion and misunderstanding within psychiatry. The burden of this chapter is to argue that the mental disorders once grouped under the label "hysteria" are wrongly classified in the latest versions of DSM, and to argue for a new classificatory scheme.

THE HYSTERIA OF CHARCOT AND JANET

For Sydenham (1697), hysteria was characterized by physical symptoms produced by emotional causes (and women were hysterics, while men were hypochondriacs); for Briquet (1859), it was the label for patients with multiple and chronic physical complaints; for Breuer and Freud (1893–1895/1955), it was essentially synonymous with neurosis. However, modern psychopathology owes the classic description of hysteria to Charcot (1877/1888) and Janet (1889, 1894/1901, 1907), and it is to these authorities that we must turn for background on the present-day diagnostic dilemma of hysteria (see also Havens, 1973).

Veith (1965) related the story of how Charcot, a neurologist who was at the time chief of Medical Services at the Salpêtrière hospital in Paris, became interested in hysteria. A reorganization of the hospital led hysterics and nonpsychotic epileptics to be separated from the insane and housed together, after which the hysterical patients quickly began to display epileptiform seizures, which Charcot called *hystero-epilepsy* or *hysteria major*. Closer examination of these patients revealed a number of *stigmata*, or persistent symptoms, of what he called *hysteria minor*, such as disturbances of the tactile sense, including anesthesia and hyperesthesia; disturbances of the special senses, including deafness and tunnel vision; and disturbances of motor function, including paralysis. While the hysterical stigmata mimicked that of organic illnesses, Charcot recognized them as due to emotional disturbances and suggestion. Charcot's theory of hysteria is one of diathesis and stress: a hereditary constitutional weakness combines with a more or less traumatic stress to precipitate "dynamic or functional lesions" (Charcot, 1877/1888, p. 278). These lesions, he maintained, could not be localized with the tools available to him.

Charcot's insistence that hysterical stigmata result from lesions in the central nervous system did not prevent him from understanding the role of psychological factors in their genesis. He noted, for example, that the stressful events precipitating the illness did not always seem traumatic to an objective observer. What was important was that they were *subjectively* traumatic to the patient. This emphasis on what we would now call the mental representation of trauma, as opposed to trauma that is objectively defined, may be viewed as the official beginning of the psychogenic perspective in psychopathology; interestingly, it was put forth by a dedicated neurologist.

Moreover, hysterics were enormously suggestible, as indicated by the hystero-epilepsy observed after the reorganization of the Salpêtrière. The neurologist Babinski, along with Janet and Freud, one of Charcot's most distinguished pupils, even proposed that hysteria be renamed *pithiatism*, after the Greek word *peitho*, meaning "to persuade" (Babinski & Froment, 1918). In addition, it was widely known that the symptoms of hysteria could be artificially produced by means of hypnotic suggestion. In fact, Charcot's demonstrations of hypnosis were the first laboratory models of psychopathology (Kihlstrom, 1979, 1984; Kihlstrom & McGlynn, 1991). Finally, there was the fact that hysterical stigmata conformed to the patients' ideas about the nervous system, rather than to neuroanatomical realities. It can be argued that Charcot's reputation as the most distinguished neurologist of his time lent credibility to the psychogenic theories of mental illness later formulated by Janet, Freud, and others (Havens, 1973; Veith, 1965, 1977).

Janet (1889, 1894/1901, 1907) followed Charcot in emphasizing the importance of a close clinical examination of his patients. His intention was to do for the neuroses what Kraepelin had done for the psychoses, that is, organize them into a coherent nosological scheme. While Kraepelin classified the psychoses into manic–depressive illness and dementia praecox, Janet classified the neuroses into hysteria and psychasthenia. Psychasthenia comprised obsession, anxiety, depression, and hypochondriasis. Janet thought that with each of these, the patient knows precisely what is wrong, and is distressed about it. With hysteria, however, there is a constriction of awareness: the hysterically amnesic does not know what he or she remembers, the hysterically blind and deaf do not know what they see or hear; and, as indicated by *la belle indifférence*, they do not care that they cannot remember, or see, or hear. Thus, Janet (1894/1901) defined anesthesia and amnesia as the primary stigmata of hysteria.

Janet (1889) analyzed mental life into elements known as psychological automatisms, each consisting of a complex act responsive to the details of the stimulus situation, and each including an idea and an emotion. In normal individuals, the entire set of psychological automatisms is bound together and accessible to phenomenal awareness and voluntary control. Under conditions of stress, however, one or more automatisms are split off, or dissociated, from the rest, inaccessible to phenomenal awareness and independent of voluntary control. According to Janet, somnambulistic states, to take one example, represent the involuntary repetition, in fantasy, of some forgotten traumatic experience, followed by amnesia for both the original event and its imagined repetition. In hysterical tunnel blindness, the patients are unaware of objects in the periphery of their visual field, even though their behavior is obviously influenced by these stimuli. Janet's ideas about dissociation were embraced by many of his contemporaries, including William James and Morton Prince in America (Fuller, 1982, 1986), but eventually were superseded by the psychoanalytic theory of Freud and his followers, which emphasized repression and an entirely different, impersonal construal of unconscious mental life.

More recently, Janet's point of view has been revived by Hilgard (1977/ 1986) in the form of the neodissociation theory of divided consciousness. Neodissociation theory conceptualizes the mind as a set of module-like components that monitor, organize, and control mental functioning in various domains. These mental structures are able to seek and avoid certain inputs, and facilitate or inhibit certain outputs, in accordance with global and local demands and intentions. In addition, these structures are subordinate to a central executive structure, which serves as the end point for all stimulus inputs, and as the origin of all motor outputs. This central structure is the cognitive basis for the phenomenal experience of awareness and intentionality. According to neodissociation theory, certain conditions can alter the relations among the various substructures, and between each substructure and the central executive. If, for example, the communication lines that link one substructure with the central executive structure are disrupted, then that substructure will process inputs, and generate outputs, independent of the central executive. This is the sort of thing that happens in hysteria. Indeed, Hilgard's neodissociation theory takes Janet's analysis of hysteria and places it within the conceptual framework of contemporary cognitive psychology.

In his foreword to Janet's *The Mental State of Hystericals* (1894/1901), Charcot the neurologist wrote that "hysteria is largely a mental malady" (p. v). Charcot and Janet differed on the role played by constitutional diathesis and organic lesions in hysteria. But they agreed on one fundamental point: Hysteria, as manifested in the stigmata that are pathognomonic of the disease, is fundamentally a disorder of consciousness. Hysterical patients are unaware of events of which they should, under ordinary circumstances, clearly be cognizant; and they are influenced by ideas, memories, affects, and needs that are excluded from or denied introspective access. This crucial point has been progressively lost over the successive revisions of DSM (for a similar argument, see Nemiah, 1991).

THE OFFICIAL DIAGNOSIS OF HYSTERIA: FROM DSM-I TO DSM-IV

The first edition of the AMPA *Statistical Manual* (Committee on Statistics, 1918) listed 22 categories of mental illness, which mostly consisted of various forms of psychosis (reflecting the somatogenic orientation of psychiatry at the time), but which also included a grouping of "psychoneuroses and neuroses." The 10th edition (Committee on Statistics, 1942) had a more differentiated list of psychoneuroses, including separate subcategories for hysteria, compulsive states, neurasthenia, hypochondriasis, reactive depression, anxiety state, anorexia nervosa, and mixed psychoneuroses. After World War II, a number of social and institutional pressures, including the increasing power of the psychodynamic viewpoint of Freud and the psychosocial perspectives advocated by Adolph Meyer and the brothers Menninger, a concern for reliable (if not necessarily valid) diagnostic procedures, and an expanded interest in less severe forms of mental illness necessitated a revised nosology, which became the American Psychiatric Association's *Diagnostic and Statistical Manual of Mental Disorders* (Grob, 1991).

DSM-I

The first edition of DSM (American Psychiatric Association, 1952), which was heavily influenced by psychoanalysis and other psychodynamic theories of mental illness (Grob, 1991), divided the psychiatric syndromes into three superordinate categories:

1. Disorders caused by impairment of brain tissue function
2. Mental deficiency
3. Disorders of psychogenic origin

The last category was a real catchall; it included any "general difficulty in adaptation of the individual . . . in which any associated brain function disturbance is secondary to the psychiatric disorder" (American Psychiatric Association, 1952, p. 9). It also included psychotic disorders, which were further subdivided into affective reactions, schizophrenic reactions (including the five traditional subtypes of simple, hebephrenic, catatonic, paranoid, and undifferentiated), and paranoid reactions; psychophysiological autonomic and visceral disorders (further classified according to the organ system affected); personality disorders (divided into personality pattern disturbances, personality trait disturbances, and sociopathic personality disturbance); transient situational personality disorders (e.g., adjustment reactions of adulthood, infancy, childhood, adolescence, and late life); and, last, but by no means least, the psychoneurotic disorders.

The psychoneurotic disorders, in turn, consisted of anxiety reaction, dissociative reaction, conversion reaction, phobic reaction, obsessive compulsive reaction, depressive reaction, and a wastebasket category of other forms of psychoneurotic reaction (see Figure 17.1). In line with psychoanalytic theory, the neuroses were characterized by either the conscious experience of anxiety (anxiety reaction, phobic reaction, and obsessive compulsive reaction) or the unconscious control of anxiety by means of certain defense mechanisms. Depressive reaction, in which anxiety is "allayed, and hence partially relieved, by depression and self-depreciation" (p. 33), stood somewhat outside of this dichotomy.

It should be noted that two forms of psychoneurosis were specifically related to the classic concept of hysteria: *dissociative reaction*, which included

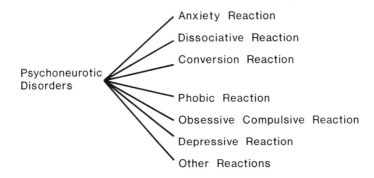

Anxiety Reaction

Dissociative Reaction

Conversion Reaction

Psychoneurotic
Disorders

Phobic Reaction

Obsessive Compulsive Reaction

Depressive Reaction

Other Reactions

FIGURE 17.1. Classification of dissociative and conversion disorders in DSM-I.

"various symptomatic expressions, such as depersonalization, dissociated [multiple] personality, fugue, amnesia, dream state, somnambulism, etc." (p. 32); and *conversion reaction*, which included such "symptomatic manifestations . . . as anesthesia (anosmia, blindness, deafness), paralysis (paresis, aphonia, monoplegia, or hemiplegia), and diskinesis (tics, tremors, posturing, catalepsy)" (p. 33). Again in line with psychoanalytic thought, both dissociative and conversion disorders were attributed to the repression of anxiety-evoking impulses. This schema essentially followed the tradition initiated by Charcot and Janet, which has been abandoned in the latest editions of the DSM.

Moreover, it should be noted that both the dissociative and conversion reactions, being forms of psychoneurosis, were clearly differentiated from the psychophysiological disorders. (DSM-I had no listing for a hysterical personality disorder.) DSM-I explicitly rejected the label of *somatization reaction* for this category, on the grounds that the disorders in question were not simply psychoneurotic in nature. The psychophysiological disorders were further differentiated from the conversion disorders due, in part, to the idea that the symptoms of the latter reflected actual structural changes in the organs involved.

DSM-II

DSM-II (American Psychiatric Association, 1968) represented a rearrangement and expansion of the DSM-I nosology. The ten categories at the highest level of organization were:

1. Mental retardation
2. Organic brain syndromes
3. (Functional) psychoses

4. Neuroses
5. Personality disorders
6. Psychophysiologic disorders
7. Special symptoms (e.g., sleep or eating disorders)
8. Transient situational disturbances
9. Behavior disorders of childhood and adolescence
10. Various nonpsychiatric maladjustments

The changes introduced in DSM-II were subtle but important. For example, the term *reaction* was generally dropped from the nosology. The term *schizophrenia* replaced that of *schizophrenic reaction*, *major affective disorders* that of *affective reaction*, and *anxiety neurosis* that of *anxiety reaction*. The foreword to DSM-II averred that "The change of label has not changed the nature of the disorder" (American Psychiatric Association, 1968, p. ix), but this nosological move must have reflected an emerging construal of the psychoses and neuroses as legitimate medical syndromes, if not full-fledged disease entities.

Nevertheless, the neuroses were still characterized in psychodynamic terms as involving either the direct expression or the unconscious control of anxiety. The subcategories of neurosis were expanded to include neurasthenic neurosis (also known as neurasthenia), depersonalization neurosis (depersonalization syndrome), and hypochondriacal neurosis, as well as the traditional categories of anxiety neurosis, obsessive compulsive neurosis, and depressive neurosis (Figure 17.2). Interestingly, the broad category of neuroses now included a single subcategory of *hysterical neurosis* "characterized by involuntary psychogenic loss or disorder of function" (p. 39). Hysterical neurosis itself was further subdivided into two types: *hysterical neurosis, conversion type*, in which "the special senses or voluntary nervous system are affected, causing such symptoms as blindness, deafness, anosmia, anaesthesias, paraesthesias, paralyses, ataxias, akinesias, and dyskinesias" (pp. 39–40); and *hysterical neurosis, dissociative type*, in which "alterations may occur in the patient's state of consciousness or . . . identity, to produce such symptoms as amnesia, somnambulism, fugue, and multiple personality" (p. 40).

Like DSM-I, DSM-II insisted that *hysterical neurosis, conversion type* be distinguished from the psychophysiological disorders. In part, the distinction was made in terms of the organs involved, that is, those of the central or somatic nervous system versus those of the autonomic nervous system. Another distinction, retained from DSM-I, was that the psychophysiological disorders involved actual changes in organ function.

Similarly, the personality disorders included a subcategory of hysterical personality (also known as histrionic personality disorder), which was "characterized by excitability, emotional instability, over-reactivity, and

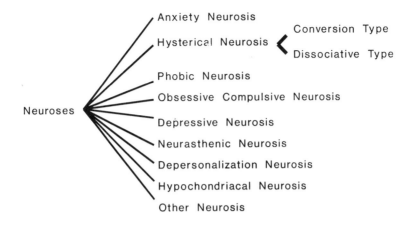

FIGURE 17.2. Classification of dissociative and conversion disorders in DSM-II.

self-dramatization" (p. 43; see also Shapiro, 1965; Horowitz, 1977). DSM-II clearly indicated that hysterical personality should be distinguished from hysterical neurosis, a point repeatedly insisted upon by Chodoff (1954, 1974; Chodoff & Lyons, 1958; see also Ziegler, Imboden, & Meyer, 1960). Nevertheless, the confusion among conversion hysteria, hysterical personality, and other "hysterical" syndromes had begun. For example, a literature review by Temoshock and Atkisson (1977) listed at least 14 different nosological labels related to hysteria (and proposed a psychosocial theory to explain them): dissociated personality, hysterical character disorder, idiosyncratic hysterical psychosis, sociopathy, Briquet's syndrome, anorexia nervosa, conversion symptoms, hysterical personality traits, socially patterned hysterical psychosis, dissociated states, hysterical contagion, millenarian movements, and reactive movements (for a similar list, see Roy, 1982).

DSM-III and DSM-III-R

DSM-III (American Psychiatric Association, 1980) changed everything. As Wilson (1993) has noted, this edition marked a transformation in American (and, for that matter, world) psychiatry, specifically, a return to Kraepelin-style descriptive diagnosis (as opposed to defining syndromes according to speculative theories such as psychoanalysis), and a shift from the psychodynamic, psychosocial, and biopsychosocial models of mental illness to a more strictly biological view. According to the psychosocial model, mental health, neurosis, and psychosis are on a single continuum; mental illness is a "reaction" to environmental events and circumstances. Hence,

Kraepelinian categorical diagnosis are viewed as both arbitrary and irrelevant—useful for statistical reporting and collecting third-party payments, perhaps, but not informative in the treatment of individual cases. Partly in reaction to the antipsychiatry movement, and partly to counter the hegemony of the psychodynamic, psychosocial, and biopsychosocial models of mental illness, DSM-III revived a concern for a theory-neutral descriptive psychopathology, of the sort preferred by Kraepelin, and for the first time canonized a set of diagnostic procedures as well as diagnostic labels.[2] The 17 major classifications of mental illness (18 categories in DSM-III-R) were:

1. Disorders of infancy, childhood, or adolescence
2. Organic mental disorders
3. Substance abuse disorders (in DSM-III-R, "psychoactive")
4. Schizophrenic disorders
5. Paranoid disorders (in DSM-III-R, "delusional" disorders)
6. Psychotic disorders not elsewhere classified
7. Affective disorders (in DSM-III-R, "mood" disorders)
8. Anxiety disorders
9. Somatoform disorders
10. Dissociative disorders
11. Psychosexual disorders (in DSM-III-R, "sexual" disorders)
12. Factitious disorders
13. Disorders of impulse control not elsewhere classified
14. Adjustment disorders
15. Psychological factors affecting physical condition
16. Personality disorders (listed on Axis II)
17. Conditions not attributable to a mental disorder
18. Sleep disorders (added in DSM-III-R).

While acknowledging the superiority of etiological over symptom-based classification, the framers of DSM-III argued that the origins of most mental disorders were unknown, and so merely speculative etiological labels should be abandoned. Accordingly, an attempt was made to eliminate *psychosis* and *neurosis* as superordinate categories (although the terms themselves were marginally preserved, in a political compromise with the psychoanalysts; Grob, 1991). The term *hysteria* was completely eliminated, along with theoretical statements about the unconscious expression of anxiety in dissociative and conversion symptoms. Classification was put on theory-neutral, descriptive grounds. Interestingly, however, DSM-III (and DSM-III-R) retained the far-from-theory-neutral terms *dissociative disorder* and *conversion disorder*, and added another theory-laden term for good measure: *somatization disorder* (for a review, see Kellner, 1990). These terms are the only diagnostic labels remaining in the psychiatric nosology that invoke, or at least imply, a specific etiological mechanism. Obviously, all three are derived from the traditional concept of hysteria. Lewis (1975) was right: Even when the word *hysteria* dies, its underlying concept lives on.

At the same time, however, DSM-III marked a radical departure from the traditional classification of hysteria (Hyler & Spitzer, 1978). Not only was conversion disorder separated from dissociative disorder, conversion disorder was joined to somatization disorder, psychogenic pain disorder, and hypochondriasis under the new rubric of *somatoform* disorder. The somatoform disorders remained clearly separated from the psychophysiological disorders (renamed *psychological disorders affecting physical condition*, a sorry label; hereafter, in this chapter, they will be called *psychosomatic disorders*), hysterical personality disorder (renamed *histrionic personality disorder*), and the new category of *factitious disorders* (including Munchausen's syndrome). The separation between dissociative and conversion disorders was further reinforced by listing them at different levels in the taxonomy: Dissociative disorder was listed in a superordinate category, on the same level as schizophrenia and affective disorder, while conversion disorder was listed as a subset of the somatoform category. This structure was preserved in DSM-III-R (see Figure 17.3).

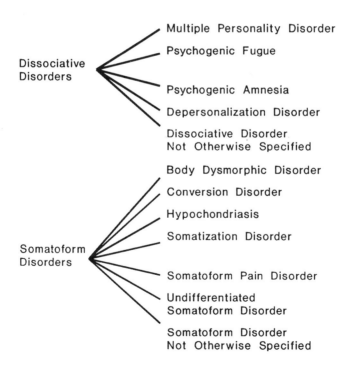

FIGURE 17.3. Classification of dissociative and conversion disorders in DSM-III and DSM-III-R.

So far as the dissociative and somatoform disorders are concerned, the essential structure of the diagnostic system is not changed in DSM-IV (American Psychiatric Association, 1994). In particular, as indicated in Figure 17.4, conversion disorder will remain separated from dissociative disorder, and listed under the rubric of somatoform disorder (Martin, 1992, 1993).

This choice perpetuates what Ryle (1949), in another context, called a category mistake:

> It is not merely an assemblage of particular mistakes. It is one big mistake and a mistake of a special kind . . . It represents the facts of mental life as if they belonged to one logical type or category (or range of types or categories) when they actually belong to another. (p. 17)

ALTERATIONS IN CONSCIOUSNESS IN CONVERSION AND DISSOCIATION

DSM-III created the new superordinate category of somatoform disorder in order to encompass all syndromes characterized by physical symptoms suggesting physical disturbances, but in the absence of organic (anatomical or physiological) findings that would explain the symptoms (for reviews, see Cloninger, 1986; Maxmen, 1986). In somatization disorder, the patient has an extended history of recurrent, multiple bodily complaints. *Somatization disorder* is also known as Briquet's (1859) syndrome, and is frequently identified with classical hysteria (Goodwin & Guze, 1989; Kellner, 1990). Also identified with classical hysteria, of course, is *conversion disorder* (or *hysterical neurosis, conversion type*), which is defined as an alteration or loss of physical function (e.g., paralysis, aphonia, blindness, and anesthesia) expressive of a psychological conflict or need (Ford & Folks, 1985; Lazare, 1981; Martin, 1992, 1993). *Body dysmorphic disorder*, previously known as dysmorphophobia, is diagnosed when the patient is preoccupied with an imagined defect in his or her physical appearance. When the belief is of delusional intensity, the patient may be diagnosed with *delusional* (or paranoid) *disorder, somatic type* (Phillips, 1991; Phillips & Hollander, 1994; Phillips, McElroy, Keck, Pope, & Hudson, 1993). In *somatoform pain disorder*, there is a preoccupation with pain, while in *hypochondriasis* (or hypochondriacal neurosis) there is a preoccupation with serious illness—either the patient believes that he or she has a certain illness, or fears contracting it.

Cloninger (1986) has characterized somatization disorder as *chronic hysteria* (on the basis of its slow onset and poor prognosis) and conversion disorders—along with dissociative disorders—as *acute hysteria* (on the basis

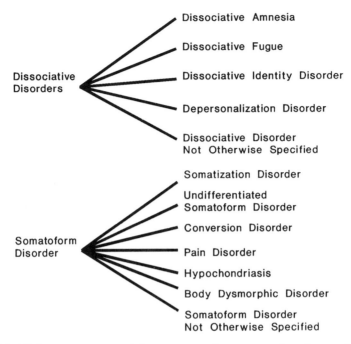

Dissociative Disorders
- Dissociative Amnesia
- Dissociative Fugue
- Dissociative Identity Disorder
- Depersonalization Disorder
- Dissociative Disorder Not Otherwise Specified

Somatoform Disorder
- Somatization Disorder
- Undifferentiated Somatoform Disorder
- Conversion Disorder
- Pain Disorder
- Hypochondriasis
- Body Dysmorphic Disorder
- Somatoform Disorder Not Otherwise Specified

FIGURE 17.4. Classification of dissociative and conversion disorders in DSM-IV.

of rapid onset and remission). However, there is no evidence that individuals who present with conversion symptoms graduate to Briquet's syndrome; hence, the acute–chronic continuum seems inappropriate in this case. As a group, the somatoform disorders are distinguished from other mental disorders involving physical complaints by four criteria (Hyler & Spitzer, 1978): No physical mechanism explains the symptoms; the symptoms are plausibly linked to psychological factors (e.g., traumatic stress or interpersonal conflict) in the patient's life; the initiation of the symptom is not under voluntary control; and the symptom does not necessarily meet an obvious social goal (e.g., financial compensation or insanity defense). Thus, with *factitious disorders* and *malingering* the symptoms are under voluntary control, while with *psychological factors affecting physical condition* and *undiagnosed physical illness* they are not.[3] In factitious disorder and undiagnosed physical illness, there is no environmental goal met by the symptom, while in malingering the goal is obvious. In the case of the psychosomatic disorders, there are obvious physical mechanisms (e.g., chronic autonomic arousal) that explain the symptom (for a discussion of the classification of these disorders, see Looney, Lipp, & Spitzer, 1978).

The rationale for separating dissociative from conversion disorders, and for linking the latter with somatization disorder, hypochondriasis, and the like, was that conversion disorders involve physical symptoms, while the dissociative disorders involve alterations in consciousness affecting memory and identity. This argument misses the essential feature that joins the conversion disorders to the dissociative disorders, and distinguishes them from the somatoform, factitious, and psychosomatic disorders. In the somatoform, factitious, and psychosomatic disorders the symptoms are physical, of the sort usually treated by internal medicine. The somatizer complains of abdominal pain, then pain in the extremities, later shortness of breath and heart palpitations. The patient with dysmorphophobic disorder complains that her nose is bumpy or her lips crooked, that he is losing his hair or his neck is shrinking. Despite all medical assurances, the hypochondriac fears that he has cancer, or AIDS, or has suffered a heart attack, or will soon do so. In the dissociative and conversion disorders, however, the symptoms in question are mental and pseudoneurological. Conversion disorder patients complain of anesthesia or paralysis, deafness or tunnel vision; dissociative disorder patients cannot remember what they have been doing, or even who they are.

Put another way, both the conversion and dissociative disorders are fundamentally disorders involving the monitoring and controlling functions of consciousness. These patients do not consciously perceive, or remember, events that they should be clearly aware of, and they cannot consciously initiate voluntary motor activities. Nothing like these alterations in conscious awareness and control occurs in the case of the somatization, factitious, or psychosomatic disorders.

Dissociative Disorders

The alteration in consciousness is so clearly expressed in what are now called the dissociative disorders that it is incorporated into the very definition of the category: "a disruption in the usually integrated functions of consciousness, memory, identity, or perception of the environment" (American Psychiatric Association, 1994, p. 477; for reviews of the dissociative disorders, see Kihlstrom, 1992a; Kihlstrom, Tataryn, & Hoyt, 1993; Kihlstrom & Schacter, in-press; Schacter & Kihlstrom, 1989; Cardeña, Lewis-Fernandez, Bear, Pakianathan, & Spiegel, 1994). In *dissociative amnesia*, the core symptom is an inability to recollect autobiographical memories, that is, events, including traumatic experiences, from one's personal past. In *dissociative fugue*, knowledge of one's identity is lost, as well as knowledge of one's past. In *dissociative identity disorder* (more familiarly known as *multiple personality disorder*), a single individual alternates between two or more identities, each associated with its own set of autobiographical memories; these identities are separated by a symmetrical or asymmetrical amnesia, so that while the person displays one personality, he or she is unaware of the others, and their associated autobiographical memories. In *depersonalization disorder*, the person perceives him- or herself (depersonalization) or the surrounding environment (derealization) as changed or unreal. As Reed (1974/1988, 1979) has pointed out, this amounts to a failure to recognize objectively familiar objects as such.

That these memory failures are disorders of consciousness is clearly indicated by the fact that they are reversible: When the amnesia or fugue terminates, the person can remember those events that he or she could not remember before. In the case of fugue, the person is now unable to remember events that transpired during the fugue state itself. With multiple personality disorder (MPD), when the multiple personality shifts from one alter ego to another, the memories associated with the new identity are recallable, while those associated with the former identity are not (until the personality shifts again). Reversible memory disorders are disorders of retrieval; they occur because the individual cannot, at the moment, gain access to memories that have been adequately encoded, and remain available in storage. Retrieval, and accessibility, are phenomena of consciousness as they entail bringing available memories into phenomenal awareness.

The role of consciousness in the dissociative disorders is further indicated by the fact that the temporarily inaccessible memories nevertheless exert an impact on the patient's experience, thought, and action outside of awareness. In other words, psychogenic amnesia, fugue, and multiple personality entail a dissociation between two forms of memory, explicit and implicit (Schacter, 1987; Schacter, Chiu, & Ochsner, 1993).[4] Explicit memory refers to the person's conscious, intentional recollection of some event. Implicit memory refers to any change in behavior that is attributable to a past event, independent of conscious recollection of that event. Explicit memory is evident in acts of recall and recognition, which require the person to bring some event into conscious awareness; implicit memory is exemplified by savings in relearning and priming effects, which do not have this constraint. That is to say, subjects can show priming or savings even though they do not remember the events responsible for these effects. Studies of brain-damaged patients with the organic amnesic syndrome, and of intact subjects who studied material under degraded encoding conditions, show that implicit memory can be spared even when explicit memory is grossly impaired.

The same contrast can be observed in patients suffering from the functional amnesia that accompanies dissociative disorders (for comprehensive reviews, see Kihlstrom & Schacter, in press; Kihlstrom et al., 1993; Schacter & Kihlstrom, 1989). For example, Madame D, a patient studied by Janet (1904), lapsed into an amnesic state after being victimized by a practical joke. During her waking hours she had no recollection of the joke, or of anything that had happened during the 6 weeks prior to the event. Nevertheless, she froze in terror whenever she passed the location where the joke had been played, and her nocturnal dreams contained a clear but unrecognized representation of the event itself. Similarly, a rape victim studied by Christianson and Nilsson (1989) became upset whenever she returned to the scene of her assault, a footpath constructed from crumbled bricks; she also reported the frequent intrusion of the words "bricks" and "bricks and the path" into her thoughts. Another patient, Jane Doe, was unable to identify herself or provide any information about her family or place of residence; but when asked on a number of occasions to randomly dial a telephone, she consistently produced a number that proved to belong to her mother (Lyon, 1985).

In a classic experimental case study of multiple personality, Ludwig and his colleagues administered a number of memory tasks to each of several alter egos separated by an interpersonality amnesia (Ludwig, Brandsma, Wilbur, Bendfeldt, & Jameson, 1972). One personality could not recall paired associates taught to the other personalities, of whom he was unaware. Nevertheless, when this personality was asked to memorize, rather than recall, pairs taught to one of the others, it showed a considerable learning advantage. This clearly indicates that the unrecalled items were available in memory, and interacted with ongoing learning processes—albeit outside of awareness. Similarly, a more recent study of MPD showed poor explicit memory when one alter ego was asked to recall paired associates studied by another; however, tests of repetition priming and proactive interference, among others, gave evidence of the transfer of implicit memory across personalities (Nissen, Ross, Willingham, Mackenzie, & Schacter, 1988).

Conversion Disorders

Similar alterations of consciousness, albeit affecting perception in this case, are commonly observed in the conversion disorders, a group of syndromes whose central feature is symptoms or deficits affecting voluntary motor or sensory function" (American Psychiatric Association, 1994, p. 452; for reviews of the conversion disorders, see Kihlstrom, 1992a; Kihlstrom, Barnhardt, & Tataryn, 1992; Martin, 1992, 1993). DSM-IV divides the conversion disorders into three subcategories. *Conversion disorder with sensory symptom or deficit* includes blindness, double and blurred vision, tunnel vision, deafness, tactile anesthesia or analgesia, and hallucinations (including hypersensitivity to both touch and pain). *Conversion disorder with motor symptom or deficit* includes aphonia, impaired balance, paralysis or localized weakness, tremors, urinary retention, difficulty swallowing, and difficulty breathing. *Conversion disorder with seizures or convulsions* includes fainting and other epileptiform behaviors. Although the official definition of conversion disorder does not include the word *consciousness*, it is apparent that all of the disorders listed involve impairments in normal conscious functioning, which affect either the sensory–perceptual system or the voluntary motor system.

Like the dissociative disorders, the conversion disorders are reversible. Patients with functional blindness and deafness eventually recover their sight and hearing; those with functional paralysis eventually regain voluntary movement. Such recuperation is rarely possible in cases of actual lesions in the central nervous system: Rehabilitation of actual nervous system damage involves learning to cope with lost functions rather than the restoration of those functions (Baker & Silver, 1987; Delargy, Peatfield, & Burt, 1986).

The role of consciousness in the conversion disorders is further supported by evidence that unseen, unheard, or unfelt stimuli nevertheless influence the patient's experience, thought, and action. In other words, these patients give evidence of experiencing spared *implicit perception*. Implicit perception is an extension of the concept of implicit memory (Kihlstrom, Barnhardt, & Tataryn, 1992). Explicit perception occurs with everyday acts of seeing and hearing, wherein the person consciously detects the presence of some object in the environment, or consciously perceives its form, motion, or distance from him- or herself. Implicit perception is exemplified by priming effects that are attributable to such stimuli, but which do not require conscious detection, description, or identification. Studies of brain-damaged patients with "blindsight," and of intact subjects who are presented with material under conditions of masking, show that implicit perception can be spared even when explicit perception is grossly impaired.

The distinction between explicit and implicit perception is easy to demonstrate, and in clinical practice constitutes the means by which the differential diagnosis of functional and organic symptoms can be made (Pincus & Tucker, 1985). In functional blindness, optokinetic nystagmus can be induced by slowly rotating a vertically striped drum in the patient's visual field; in cases of unilateral blindness, patients continue to perform visual tasks normally even though a distorting prism has been placed over the ostensibly good eye. And in the case of patients with functional deafness, they will speak more loudly when their speech is masked with white noise. An early series of case studies (which are now recognized as pioneering examples of behavioral assessment and therapy; Yates, 1970) applied the procedures of classical and instrumental conditioning to patients with functional deafness and tactile anesthesias (Cohen, Hilgard, & Wendt, 1933; Hilgard & Marquis, 1940; Malmo, Davis, & Barza, 1952–1953; Sears &

Cohen, 1933). The ability of anesthetic and deaf patients to acquire conditioned responses to tactile and auditory stimuli clearly indicates that the unfelt or unheard stimuli have been processed by the sensory–perceptual system. Hilgard and Marquis (1940) suggested that conditioning techniques permit the measurement of sensory thresholds without reliance on verbal report; apparently, they also permit such measurements without reliance on conscious sensation.

In a classic study, Brady and Lind (1961) employed another learning paradigm, the differential reinforcement of low rates, to investigate and treat a case of functional blindness. The patient was required to press a button every 18–21 seconds; correct responses were signaled by feedback, social approval, or hospital privileges. At the end of the baseline phase, the patient was responding within the target interval on the majority of trials—evidence of temporal conditioning. However, when the experimenters introduced a visual cue, which marked the onset of the target interval, response rate declined precipitously. Although the patient denied that he could see the light, visual perception was implicit in that his behavior was responsive to the stimulus. A follow-up study of this patient by Grosz and Zimmerman (1965), using another visual discrimination task, yielded similar results. In the words of Grosz and Zimmerman (1965, p. 260), the patient "was denying visual functioning while functioning visually" (for further discussion of this case, see Brady, 1966; Zimmerman & Grosz, 1966).

Such paradoxical behavior is evidence of implicit perception, and it has been observed in a number of studies of functional blindness (e.g., Bryant & McConkey, 1989; Grosz & Zimmerman, 1970; Keehn, Keuchler, & Wilkenson, 1973; Miller, 1968, 1986; Theodor & Mandelcorn, 1973) and functional deafness (Barraclough, 1966). Similarly, psychophysiological studies reveal essentially normal somatosensory event-related potentials in cases of functional anesthesia and hemianesthesia (Levy & Behrman, 1970; Levy & Mushin, 1973).

Paradoxes also can be observed in functional paralysis, and again provide the clinical basis for a differential diagnosis (Pincus & Tucker, 1985). Patients may display astasia and abasia while walking, for example, but rarely fall and even more rarely hurt themselves. In the case of functional hemiplegia, patients who are trying to lift their "good" leg while reclining will press down with their "bad" leg, just as intact individuals do. Rehabilitation specialists report that patients with functional paralysis usually show normal muscle tone and dampened reflexes, which clearly indicates that the connections between the effectors and cortical projection areas are intact (Baker & Silver, 1987; Withrington & Wynn-Parry, 1985).

Theorists of a social-psychological persuasion, such as Grosz and Zimmerman (1965; Zimmerman & Grosz, 1966), believe that such patients are malingering—that they see and hear perfectly well while denying vision or audition. Janet (1907) himself rejected such a "crude explanation"

(p. 171). Rather, he argued that the sensory–perceptual deficits observed in hysteria reflected the disconnection of sensations from the person's consciousness: While the sensations were denied representation in phenomenal awareness, they continued to affect reflex behaviors, and voluntary movements, outside of awareness. In other words, the functional anesthesias (defined broadly to include all the sensory modalities) are dissociative in nature.

TOWARD DSM-V: A NEW CLASSIFICATION OF DISSOCIATIVE DISORDERS

The dissociative disorders and conversion disorders share two fundamental features. Both are pseudoneurological in nature, and both involve disruptions in consciousness. Specifically, current and past experiences are temporarily inaccessible to phenomenal awareness, yet they continue to influence the person's experience, thought, and action in the form of implicit percepts and memories; goal-directed actions consciously planned by the individual cannot be executed; and the performance of other actions, planned outside of awareness, is accompanied by the experience of involuntariness. These considerations strongly suggest that the conversion disorders should be separated from the somatoform disorders, and rejoined to the dissociative disorders (their partners in DSM-II) as a major category of psychopathology (for a similar argument, see Nemiah, 1991).

In passing, it must be admitted that the collective label for these disorders, *dissociative*, is somewhat vexatious, because the term has a number of meanings in psychology. Thus, in cognitive psychology, dissociation refers to an experimental outcome in which some condition or manipulation affects one variable and not another. For example, neuropsychological studies of language processing reveal that global dyslexics perform poorly when reading both nonsense and irregular words while surface dyslexics can read nonsense words but not irregular words, and phonological dyslexics can read irregular but not nonsense words. The dissociation between reading irregular and nonsense words indicates that these two functions are served by two somewhat different brain systems. In this sense, dissociation is analogous to the interaction term in the analysis of variance, and does not necessarily implicate consciousness in any way.

Perhaps Janet's own French word *désagrégation* would eliminate confusion, but it is too late for such a move now. Moreover, both *désagrégation* and *dissociation* imply a particular etiology in the syndromes with which the terms are associated. As such, resort to either label would seem to violate the goal, in DSM-III and its successors, of adopting a theory-neutral, purely descriptive nosology. However, it is not necessary to embrace a dissociative explanation for functional amnesia, anesthesia, or paralysis. In what follows, the label *dissociative* will not be construed as referring to some hypothetical underlying mechanism, but rather to the fact that, descriptively, the symptoms in question represent the exclusion of some mental contents or processes from consciousness.

The essential feature of the dissociative disorders, as defined here, is a disruption of the monitoring and controlling functions of consciousness—that is, failures of conscious perception, memory, or motor control—that are not attributable to insult, injury, or disease affecting brain tissue, or to the effects of psychoactive drugs (Kihlstrom & Schacter, in press; Schacter & Kihlstrom, 1989). Further, the disorders are reversible, either temporarily, by means of hypnosis or barbiturates, or permanently, when the crisis resolves and the dissociative process remits. Moreover, careful examination of cases of dissociative disorder usually yields evidence of intact functioning outside of awareness. In this respect, the clinical and experimental meanings of *dissociation* come together: With the dissociative disorders, there is evidence of a dissociation between explicit and implicit expressions of perception, memory, and action. In fact, evidence of such a dissociation might be considered the defining behavioral (as opposed to subjective) feature of the dissociative disorders.

Following this line of reasoning, the dissociative disorders may be further classified according to the specific mental functions affected by the alteration in consciousness: memory and identity, sensation and perception, and voluntary action (see Figure 17.5).

In the *dissociative disorders of memory and identity*, the division of consciousness affects memory, broadly construed to include both episodic knowledge of one's personal history and semantic knowledge of one's identity and self-concept. In *dissociative amnesia*, there is a loss of conscious access to all or part of the individual's autobiographical memory. During the amnestic period, the patient remains cognizant of who he or she is, but cannot bring certain memories into phenomenal awareness. In *dissociative fugue*, there is a temporary loss of identity as well as of autobiographical memory. Again, awareness shifts: During the fugue state, the patient is unaware of his or her premorbid identity and history; after the fugue has resolved, access to premorbid personal knowledge is restored, but awareness of events occurring during the fugue, and any identity adopted in that time, is lost. In *multiple personality disorder*, awareness alternates between two or more identities, each with its own associated fund of autobiographical memories. While the dissociative dysmnesias involve the loss of explicit memory, implicit expressions of memory may often bridge the amnesic barrier.

It should be noted that the memory symptoms of the dissociative disorders fall into two broad classes, negative and positive, paralleling the familiar division between positive and negative symptoms in schizophrenia (Andreason & Olsen, 1982). Thus, dissociative amnesia, and those cases

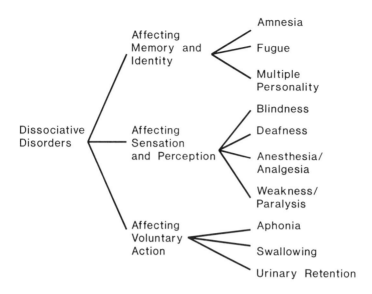

FIGURE 17.5. Classification of dissociative disorders proposed in this chapter: Specific examples listed on the right-hand side of the figure are only meant to serve as illustrations.

of dissociative fugue in which there is a loss but not a shift of identity, involve negative symptoms, that is, the absence of something (memory, identity) that is normally present. Instances of dissociative fugue in which there is an assumption of a new identity, and of MPD (in which there is the assumption of one or more new identities by definition), involve positive symptoms, that is, the presence of something (a second or third identity) that is normally absent. This distinction between positive and negative symptoms is also helpful in classifying the other syndromes of a dissociative nature.

In the *dissociative disorders of sensation and perception*, the division in consciousness affects sensory and perceptual function. The most familiar cases involve negative symptoms: blindness, deafness, tactile anesthesia, analgesia, etc. In each case, the patient is unaware of stimulation in a particular modality, although it should be noted that this unawareness may be partial, as in the case of tunnel vision (which affects the peripheral but not the central visual field), or even content-specific, as in the case of selective deafness to one voice but not another. In any event, it should be understood that the dissociative esthesias affect explicit perception; careful examination will show that implicit perception has been spared, in that the objects and events of which the patient is unaware will continue to influence ongoing experience, thought, and action.

Cases of positive sensory–perceptual symptoms, of which the most familiar type is *psychalgesia*, or functional pain affecting the back, joints, extremities, sexual organs, and bodily orifices should also be placed in the above category. *Psychalgesia* is frequently encountered in the neurological clinic. At first glance, the presence of such positive symptoms would seem to violate the core definition of the dissociative disorders—that they involve a disruption of awareness. If anything, the psychalgic patient has *too much* awareness. From the point of view of neodissociation theory, however, the patient's subjective experience of pain results from the construction of vivid mental images of pain, presumably based on memories of past experience. Hence, dissociation is a relevant term since the patients are unaware that they are generating these experiences for themselves. Because of this failure of reality monitoring, the pains are experienced as sensations rather than as images (for a further discussion, see Kihlstrom, in press).

Finally, the *dissociative disorders of motor function* affect the conscious control of voluntary efferent functions, rather than the conscious monitoring of present or past events. The most familiar instances involve localized weakness, paralysis of the extremities, aphonia, difficulty swallowing (what used to be called *globus hystericus*), and urinary retention. In neodissociative terms, some of these negative symptoms, such as weakness in the extremities, may reflect a failure of communication between the central executive, in which conscious intentions are formed, and the subordinate motor control centers that execute these ideas. Other cases, such as paralysis in the extremities, may reflect the active inhibition of motor activity, although, as in the case of psychalgesia, a dissociative barrier may prevent the person from being aware that this inhibition is the product of his or her own mental activities (Kihlstrom, in press).

The dissociative motor symptoms also include tics, fainting, vomiting, pseudoepileptic convulsions (which, like psychalgia, are rather commonly encountered in the neurological clinic), and the like. Again, it should be clear that despite appearances, these symptoms represent the generation of voluntary motor behaviors on the part of the patient. However, as in the cases of the mental images underlying psychalgia, and the active inhibitions involved in paralysis, the initiation of these behaviors is isolated from the patient's awareness, so that he or she experiences them as involuntary (for a more detailed analysis, see Kihlstrom, in press).

MECHANISM AND PHENOMENOLOGY

The framers of DSM-III and its successors were certainly right to return to Kraepelinian descriptive nosology as the starting place for scientific clinical practice, to emphasize the patient's phenomenology and behavior over clinical inferences and speculations about etiology and underlying mechanisms, and to develop an explicit set of rules that would permit diagnoses to be reliably made. However, in their treatment of the syndromes historically associated with the concept of hysteria, two mistakes have been made and perpetuated.

The first, and less serious, mistake involved retaining the labels *dissociation*, *conversion*, and *somatization*. *Dissociation* can be a purely descriptive term, either referring to a lack of association between or integration of ideas, or to a state in which certain mental contents and processes are excluded from consciousness. Unfortunately, "dissociation" can also refer to the hypothetical process by which this exclusion is achieved—a process that is different from competing alternatives such as repression, suppression, or denial. In contrast *conversion* and *somatization* are exclusively theoretical in nature; they refer to particular processes postulated by psychoanalytic theory, by which unconscious conflicts are symbolically represented as manifest symptoms. *Dissociation* may still have a useful life as a purely descriptive label (Hilgard, 1977/1986), and it may be possible to reconstrue *somatization* in purely descriptive terms as well. But *conversion* appears to be too closely bound to psychoanalysis ever to serve as a theory-neutral descriptive label.

Fortunately, the label *conversion* is unnecessary: The conversion disorders are inherently dissociative in the descriptive sense in that they involve the exclusion of mental contents and processes from conscious awareness and control. At present, the conversion disorders are grouped with the somatoform disorders because they share "physical symptoms suggesting physical disorder" (Martin, 1994). But this is the second mistake. The symptoms of the conversion disorders are not physical, but mental in nature. And they do not suggest physical disorder, but rather a disorder in consciousness. Just as functional amnesia, fugue, and MPD are disorders of consciousness that affect memory and identity, so are functional blindness, deafness, anesthesia, and paralysis disorders of consciousness that affect sensation, perception, and voluntary action. Hence, we can only hope that when DSM-V appears, the term "conversion disorder" will have been abandoned once and for all, and that the syndromes now listed under this label will be returned to the dissociative disorders where they belong.

ACKNOWLEDGMENTS

The point of view represented here is based on research supported by Grant #MH-35856 from the National Institute of Mental Health. I thank John Allen, Melissa Berren, Lawrence Couture, Michael Cyphers, Elizabeth Glisky, Martha Glisky, Heather Law, Chad Marsolek, Shelagh Mulvaney, Victor Shames, Susan Valdiserri, Michael Valdiserri, and Michele Wright for their comments. I am especially grateful to Lucy Canter Kihlstrom for sharing her insights on somatization disorder.

NOTES

1. The earlier role of James Braid in setting the stage for psychogenic theories of psychopathology has been unfairly ignored. See appreciations by Kravis (1988), Kihlstrom (1992b), and Gravitz (1993).

2. Perhaps the most remarkable feature of DSM-III, however, was one that went largely unremarked: A clear change had occurred in the rules by which diagnostic decisions are made. Previous edition of DSM had provided succinct descriptions of the various mental disorders, leaving it up to the individual practitioner to arrive at a diagnosis for the individual case in the absence of specific rules. Before DSM-III, the diagnostic categories were considered, at least implicitly, to be classical proper sets, in which specific symptoms served as singly necessary and jointly sufficient defining features, yielding sharp boundaries between adjacent categories, the perfect nesting of superordinate and subordinate categories, and homogeneity within categories. However, analyses of actual diagnostic judgments showed that practitioners actually treated the syndromes as "fuzzy sets" represented by summary prototypes or sets of exemplars (Cantor & Genero, 1986; Cantor, Smith, French, & Mezzich, 1980; Horowitz, Post, French, Wallis, & Siegelman, 1981; Horowitz, Wright, Lowenstein, & Parad, 1981; Medin, Altom, Edelson, & Freko, 1982), a tendency that is broadly characteristic of natural-object categorization (Medin, 1989; Mervis & Rosch, 1981; Rosch, 1975; Smith & Medin, 1981). By emphasizing correlated rather than defining features, categorization by family resemblance, and within-category heterogeneity, DSM-III implicitly acknowledged that the fuzzy-set view of categorization applied to psychiatric diagnosis as well (Millon, 1991).

3. In DSM-IV, the label for these disorders is *psychological disorders affecting nonpsychiatric medical condition*—a diagnostic term that does not roll easily off the tongue. The Task Force on DSM-IV has solicited proposals for a simpler designation. Dare one propose a simple return to the former *psychophysiological disorders*, or even *psychosomatic disorders*?

4. Other labels for this distinction are direct versus indirect memory (Johnson & Hasher, 1987; Richardson-Klavehn & Bjork, 1988), memory with versus without awareness (Eich, 1984; Jacoby & Dallas, 1981), or declarative versus nondeclarative memory (Squire, Knowlton, & Musen, 1993).

REFERENCES

American Psychiatric Association. (1952). *Diagnostic and statistical manual: Mental disorders*. Washington, DC: Author.

American Psychiatric Association. (1968). *Diagnostic and statistical manual of mental disorders* (2nd ed). Washington, DC: Author.

American Psychiatric Association. (1980). *Diagnostic and statistical manual of mental disorders* (3rd ed). Washington, DC: Author.

American Psychiatric Association. (1987). *Diagnostic and statistical manual of mental disorders* (3rd ed., rev). Washington, DC: Author.

American Psychiatric Association. (1994). *Diagnostic and statistical manual of mental disorders* (4th ed.). Washington, DC: Author.

Andreasen, N. C., & Olsen, S. (1982). Negative versus positive schizophrenia: Definition and validation. *Archives of General Psychiatry, 39*, 789–794.

Babinski, J., & Froment, J. (1918). *Hysteria or pithiatism and reflex nervous disorders in the neurology of war.* London: University of London Press.

Baker, J. H., & Silver, J. R. (1987). Hysterical paraplegia. *Journal of Neurology, Neurosurgery, and Psychiatry, 50*, 375–382.

Barraclough, M. (1966). A method of testing hearing based on operant conditioning. *Behaviour Research and Therapy, 4*, 237–238.

Brady, J. P. (1966). Hysteria versus malingering: A response to Grosz and Zimmerman. *Behaviour Research and Therapy, 4*, 321–322.

Brady, J. P., & Lind, D. L. (1961). Experimental analysis of hysterical blindness. *Archives of General Psychiatry, 4*, 331–339.

Breuer, J., & Freud, S. (1955). *Studies on hysteria.* In J. Strachey (Ed. and Trans.), *The standard edition of the complete psychological works of Sigmund Freud* (Vol. 2). London: Hogarth Press. (Original work published 1893–1895)

Bryant, R. A., & McConkey, K. M. (1989). Visual conversion disorder: A case analysis of the influence of visual information. *Journal of Abnormal Psychology, 98*, 326–329.

Briquet, P. (1859). *Traité clinique et thérapeutique à l'hystérie.* Paris: Ballière et Fils.

Cantor, N., & Genero, N. (1986). Psychiatric diagnosis and natural categorization: A close analogy. In T. Millon & G. L. Klerman (Eds.), *Contemporary directions in psychopathology: Toward the DSM-IV* (pp. 233–256). New York: Guilford Press.

Cantor, N., Smith, E. E., French, R. deS., & Mezzich, J. (1980). Psychiatric diagnosis as prototype categorization. *Journal of Abnormal Psychology, 89*, 181–193.

Cardeña, E., Lewis-Fernandez, R., Bear, D., Pakianathan, I., & Spiegel, D. (1994). Dissociative disorders. In A. Frances & T. Widiger (Eds.), *Source book for DSM-IV.* Washington, DC: American Psychiatric Press.

Charcot, J.-M. (1888). *Clinical lectures on certain diseases of the nervous system.* Detroit: Davis. (Original work published 1877)

Chodoff, P. (1954). A re-examination of some aspects of conversion hysteria. *Psychiatry, 17*, 75–81.

Chodoff, P. (1974). The diagnosis of hysteria: An overview. *American Journal of Psychiatry, 131*, 1073–1078.

Chodoff, P., & Lyons, H. (1958). Hysteria, the hysterical personality, and "hysterical" conversion. *American Journal of Psychiatry, 114*, 734–740.

Christianson, S.-A., & Nilsson, L.-G. (1989). Hysterical amnesia: A case of aversively motivated isolation of memory. In T. Archer & L.-G. Nilsson (Eds.), *Aversion, avoidance, and anxiety* (pp. 289–310). Hillsdale, NJ: Lawrence Erlbaum.

Cloninger, C. R. (1986). Somatoform and dissociative disorders. In G. Winokur & P. Clayton (Eds.), *The medical basis of psychiatry* (pp. 123–151). Philadelphia: W. B. Saunders.

Cohen, L. H., Hilgard, E. R., & Wendt, G. R. (1933). Sensitivity to light in a case of hysterical blindness studied by reinforcement inhibition and conditioning methods. *Yale Journal of Biology & Medicine, 6*, 61–67.

Committee on Statistics. (1918). *Statistical manual for the use of institutions for the insane.* New York: National Committee for Mental Hygiene.

Committee on Statistics. (1942). *Statistical manual for the use of institutions for the insane* (10th ed). New York: National Committee for Mental Hygiene.

Cullen, W. (1796). *First lines of the practice of physic, with practical and explanatory notes by John Rotheram.* Edinburgh: Bell, Bradfute.

Delargy, M. A., Peatfield, R. C., & Burt, A. A. (1986). Successful rehabilitation in conversion paralysis. *British Medical Journal, 292,* 1730–1731.

Eich, E. (1984). Memory for unattended events: Memory with and without awareness. *Memory and Cognition, 12,* 105–111.

Ellenberger, H. F. (1970). *The discovery of the unconscious: The history and evolution of dynamic psychiatry.* New York: Basic Books.

Ford, C. V., & Folks, D. G. (1985). Conversion disorders: An overview. *Psychosomatics, 26,* 371–383.

Freud, S. (1953). *Fragment of an analysis of a case of hysteria.* In J. Strachey (Ed. and Trans.), *The standard edition of the complete psychological works of Sigmund Freud* (Vol. 7, pp. 1–122.). London: Hogarth Press. (Original work published 1905)

Fuller, R. C. (1982). *Mesmerism and the American cure of souls.* Philadelphia: University of Pennsylvania Press.

Fuller, R. C. (1986). *Americans and the unconscious.* New York: Oxford University Press.

Goffman, E. (1961). *Asylums.* New York: Anchor Books.

Goodwin, D. W., & Guze, S. B. (1989). *Psychiatric diagnosis* (4th ed). New York: Oxford University Press.

Gravitz, M. A. (1993). Etienne Felix d'Henin de Cuvillers: A founder of hypnosis. *American Journal of Clinical Hypnosis, 36,* 7–11.

Grob, G. N. (1991). Origins of *DSM-I*: A study in appearance and reality. *American Journal of Psychiatry, 148,* 421–431.

Grosz, H. J., & Zimmerman, J. A. (1965). Experimental analysis of hysterical blindness: A follow-up report and new experimental data. *Archives of General Psychiatry, 13,* 255–260.

Grosz, H. J., & Zimmerman, J. A. (1970). A second detailed case study of functional blindness: Further demonstration of the contribution of objective psychological laboratory data. *Behavior Therapy, 1,* 115–123.

Havens, L. L. (1973). *Approaches to the mind: Movement of the psychiatric schools from sects toward science.* Boston: Little, Brown.

Hilgard, E. R. (1986). *Divided consciousness: Multiple controls in human thought and action* (rev. ed.). New York: Wiley-Interscience. (Original work published 1977)

Hilgard, E. R., & Marquis, D. G. (1940). *Conditioning and learning.* New York: Appleton-Century-Crofts.

Horowitz, L. M., Post, D. L., French, R. d. S., Wallis, K. D., & Siegelman, E. Y. (1981). The prototype as a construct in abnormal psychology: 2. Clarifying disagreement in psychiatric judgments. *Journal of Abnormal Psychology, 90,* 575–585.

Horowitz, L. M., Wright, J. C., Lowenstein, E., & Parad, H. W. (1981). The prototype as a construct in abnormal psychology: I. A method for deriving prototypes. *Journal of Abnormal Psychology, 90,* 568–574.

Horowitz, M. J. (Ed.). (1977). *Hysterical personality.* New York: Jason Aronson.

Hyler, S. E., & Spitzer, R. L. (1978). Hysteria split asunder. *American Journal of Psychiatry, 135*, 1500–1504.

Jacoby, L. L., & Dallas, M. (1981). On the relationship between autobiographical memory and perceptual learning. *Journal of Experimental Psychology: General, 110*, 306–340.

Janet, P. (1889). *L'automatisme psychologique.* Paris: Felix Alcan.

Janet, P. (1901). *The mental state of hystericals.* New York: Putnam's Sons. (Original work published 1894)

Janet, P. (1904). Amnesia and the dissociation of memories by emotion. *Journal de Psychologie, 1*, 417–453.

Janet, P. (1907). *The major symptoms of hysteria.* New York: Macmillan.

Johnson, M. K., & Hasher, L. (1987). Human learning and memory. *Annual Review of Psychology, 38*, 631–668.

Kant, I. (1978). *Anthropology from a pragmatic point of view.* Carbondale, IL: Southern Illinois University Press. (Original work published 1798)

Keehn, J. D., Keuchler, H. A., & Wilkenson, D. A. (1973). Behavior therapy in a transactional context: The case of a blind drunk. *Behavior Therapy, 4*, 147–149.

Kellner, R. (1990). Somatization: Theories and research. *Journal of Nervous and Mental Disease, 178*, 150–160.

Kihlstrom, J. F. (1979). Hypnosis and psychopathology: Retrospect and prospect. *Journal of Abnormal Psychology, 88*, 459–473.

Kihlstrom, J. F. (1984). Conscious, subconscious, unconscious: A cognitive perspective. In K. S. Bowers & D. Meichenbaum (Eds.), *The unconscious reconsidered* (pp. 149–211). New York: John Wiley.

Kihlstrom, J. F. (1992a). Dissociative and conversion disorders. In D. J. Stein & J. Young (Eds.), *Cognitive science and clinical disorders* (pp. 247–270). San Diego: Academic Press.

Kihlstrom, J. F. (1992b). Hypnosis: A sesquicentennial essay. *International Journal of Clinical and Experimental Hypnosis, 40*, 301–314.

Kihlstrom, J. F. (in press). Conscious awareness and the awareness of control. In H. J. Crawford (Ed.), *Consciousness and dissociation: Esssays in honor of Ernest R. Hilgard* Washington, DC: American Psychological Association.

Kihlstrom, J. F., Barnhardt, T. M., & Tataryn, D. J. (1992). Implicit perception. In R. F. Bornstein & T. S. Pittman (Eds.), *Perception without awareness* (pp. 17–54). New York: Guilford Press.

Kihlstrom, J. F., & McGlynn, S. M. (1991). Experimental research in clinical psychology. In M. Hersen, A. E. Kazdin, & A. S. Bellack (Eds.), *Clinical psychology handbook* (2nd ed., pp. 239–257). New York: Pergamon.

Kihlstrom, J. F., & Schacter, D. L. (in press). Functional disorders of autobiographical memory. In A. Baddeley, F. Watts, & B. Wilson (Eds.), *Handbook of memory disorders.* London: John Wiley.

Kihlstrom, J. F., Tataryn, D. J., & Hoyt, I. P. (1993). Dissociative disorders. In P. J. Sutker & H. E. Adams (Eds.), *Comprehensive handbook of psychopathology* (2nd ed., pp. 203–234). New York: Plenum Press.

Kirmayer, L. J. (1986). Somatization and the social construction of illness experience.

In S. McHugh & T. M. Vallis (Eds.), *Illness behavior: A multidisciplinary model* (pp. 111–133). New York: Plenum Press.

Kluft, R. P., Steinberg, M., & Spitzer, R. L. (1988). DSM-II-R revisions in the dissociative disorders: An exploration of their derivation and rationale. *Dissociation, 1*, 39–46.

Kravis, N. M. (1988). James Braid's psychophysiology: A turning point in the history of dynamic psychiatry. *American Journal of Psychiatry, 145*, 1191–1206.

Lazare, A. (1981). Conversion symptoms. *New England Journal of Medicine, 305*, 745–748.

Levy, R., & Behrman, J. (1970). Cortical evoked responses in hysterical hemianaesthesia. *Electroencephalography and Clinical Neurophysiology, 29*, 400–402.

Levy, R., & Mushin, J. (1973). The somatosensory evoked response in patients with hysterical anaesthesia. *Journal of Psychosomatic Research, 17*, 81–84.

Lewis, A. (1975). The survival of hysteria. *Psychological Medicine, 5*, 9–12.

Looney, J. G., Lipp, M. R., & Spitzer, R. L. (1978). A new method of classification for psychophysiologic disorders. *American Journal of Psychiatry, 135*, 304–308.

Ludwig, A. M., Brandsma, J. M., Wilbur, C. B., Bendfeldt, F., & Jameson, D. H. (1972). The objective study of a multiple personality: Or, Are four heads better than one? *Archives of General Psychiatry, 26*, 298–310.

Lyon, L. S. (1985). Facilitating telephone number recall in a case of psychogenic amnesia. *Journal of Behavior Therapy and Experimental Psychiatry, 16*, 147–149.

Malmo, R. B., Davis, J. F., & Barza, S. (1952–1953). Total hysterical deafness: An experimental study. *Journal of Personality, 21*, 188–204.

Martin, R. L. (1992). Diagnostic issues for conversion disorder. *Hospital and Community Psychiatry, 43*, 771–773.

Martin, R.L. (1994). DSM-IV diagnostic options for conversion disorder, proposed autonomic arousal disorder and pseudocyesis. In A. Frances & T. Widiger (Eds.), *Source book for DSM-IV*. Washington, DC: American Psychiatric Press.

Maxmen, J. S. (1986). *Essential psychopathology*. New York: W. W. Norton.

Medin, D. L. (1989). Concepts and conceptual structure. *American Psychologist, 44*, 1469–1481.

Medin, D. L., Altom, M. W., Edelson, S. M., & Freko, D. (1982). Correlated symptoms and simulated medical classification. *Journal of Experimental Psychology: Learning, Memory, and Cognition, 8*, 37–50.

Merskey, H. (1979). *The analysis of hysteria*. London: Bailliere Tindall.

Merskey, H. (1983). Hysteria: The history of an idea. *Canadian Journal of Psychiatry, 28*, 428–433.

Mervis, C. B., & Rosch, E. (1981). Categorization of natural objects. *Annual Review of Psychology, 32*, 89–115.

Micale, M. S. (1990). Hysteria and its historiography: The future perspective. *History of Psychiatry, 1*, 33–124.

Miller, E. (1968). A note on the visual performance of a subject with unilateral functional blindness. *Behaviour Research and Therapy, 6*, 115–116.

Miller, E. (1986). Detecting hysterical sensory symptoms: An elaboration of the forced choice technique. *British Journal of Clinical Psychology, 25*, 231–232.

Millon, T. (1991). Classification in psychopathology: Rationale, alternatives, and standards. *Journal of Abnormal Psychology, 100*, 245–261.

Nemiah, J. C. (1991). Dissociation, conversion, and somatization. *Annual Review of Psychiatry, 10*, 248–260.

Nissen, M. J., Ross, J. L., Willingham, D. B., Mackenzie, T. B., & Schacter, D. L. (1988). Memory and awareness in a patient with multiple personality disorder. *Brain and Cognition, 8*, 117–134.

Phillips, K. A. (1991). Body dysmorphic disorder: The distress of imagined ugliness. *American Journal of Psychiatry, 148*, 1138–1149.

Phillips, K. A., & Hollander, E. (1994). Body dysmorphic disorder: DSM-IV source book review. In A. Frances & T. Widiger (Eds.), *Source book for DSM-IV*. Washington, DC: American Psychiatric Press.

Phillips, K. A., McElroy, S. L., Keck, P. E., Pope, H. G., & Hudson, J. I. (1993). Body dysmorphic disorder: 30 cases of imagined ugliness. *American Journal of Psychiatry, 150*, 302–308.

Pincus, J. H., & Tucker, G. J. (1985). *Behavioral neurology* (3rd ed.). New York: Oxford University Press.

Pinel, P. (1962). *A treatise on insanity* (2nd. ed.). New York: Hafner. (Original work published 1806)

Reed, G. (1979). Anomalies of recall and recognition. In J. F. Kihlstrom & F. J. Evans (Eds.), *Functional disorders of memory* (pp. 1–28). Hillsdale, NJ: Lawrence Erlbaum.

Reed, G. (1988). *The psychology of anomalous experience* (rev. ed.). Buffalo, NY: Prometheus. (Original work published 1974)

Richardson-Klavehn, A., & Bjork, R. A. (1988). Measures of memory. *Annual Review of Psychiatry, 39*, 475–543.

Rosch, E. (1975). Cognitive representations of semantic categories. *Journal of Experimental Psychology: General, 104*, 192–223.

Roy, A. (Ed.). (1982). *Hysteria*. Chichester: John Wiley.

Ryle, G. (1949). *The concept of mind*. London: Hutchinson.

Salmon, T. W., Copp, O., May, J. V., Abbott, E. S., & Cotton, H. A. (1917). Report of the Committee on Statistics of the American Medico-Psychological Association. *American Journal of Insanity, 74*, 255–260.

Schacter, D. L. (1987). Implicit memory: History and current status. *Journal of Experimental Psychology: Learning, Memory, and Cognition, 13*, 501–518.

Schacter, D. L., Chiu, C.-Y. P., & Ochsner, K. N. (1993). Implicit memory: A selective review. *Annual Review of Neuroscience, 16*, 159–182.

Schacter, D. L., & Kihlstrom, J. F. (1989). Functional amnesia. In F. Boller & J. Graffman (Eds.), *Handbook of neuropsychology* (Vol. 3, pp. 209–231). Amsterdam: Elsevier.

Scheff, T. J. (1966). *Being mentally ill: A sociological theory*. Chicago: Aldine.

Sears, R. R., & Cohen, L. H. (1933). Hysterical anesthesia, analgesia, and astereognosis. *Archives of Neurology and Psychiatry, 29*, 260–271.

Shapiro, D. (1965). *Neurotic styles*. New York: Basic Books.

Siegler, M., & Osmond, H. (1974). *Models of madness, models of medicine*. New York: Harper & Row.

Shagass, C. (1975). The medical model in psychiatry. *Comprehensive Psychiatry, 16*, 405–413.

Smith, E. E., & Medin, D. L. (1981). *Categories and concepts*. Cambridge: Harvard University Press.

Spitzer, R. L., First, M. B., Williams, J. B. W., Kendler, K., Pincus, H. A., & Tucker, G. (1992). Now is the time to retire the term "organic mental disorders." *American Journal of Psychiatry, 149,* 240–244.

Squire, L. R., Knowlton, B., & Musen, G. (1993). The structure and organization of memory. *Annual Review of Psychology, 44,* 453–495.

Sydenham, T. (1697). *Dr. Sydenham's method of curing almost all diseases, and description of their symptoms, to which are now added five discourses of the same author concerning the pleurisy, gout, hysterical passion, dropsy, and rheumatism* (3rd. ed.). London: Newman & Parker.

Szasz, T. S. (1961). *The myth of mental illness.* New York: Harper & Row.

Temoshock, L., & Atkisson, C. C. (1977). Epidemiology of hysterical phenomena Evidence for a psychosocial theory. In M. J. Horowitz (Ed.), *Hysterical personality* (pp. 143–222). New York: Jason Aronson.

Theodor, L. H., & Mandelcorn, M. S. (1973). Hysterical blindness: A case report and study using a modern psychophysical technique. *Journal of Abnormal Psychology, 82,* 552–553.

Veith, I. (1965). *Hysteria: The history of a disease.* Chicago: University of Chicago Press.

Veith, I. (1977). Four thousand years of hysteria. In M. J. Horowitz (Ed.), *Hysterical personality* (pp. 7–93). New York: Jason Aronson.

Wilson, M. (1993). DSM-III and the transformation of American psychiatry: A history. *American Journal of Psychiatry, 150,* 399–410.

Withrington, R. H., & Wynn-Parry, C. B. (1985). Rehabilitation of conversion paralysis. *Journal of Bone and Joint Surgery, 67,* 635–637.

Yates, A. J. (1970). *Behavior therapy.* New York: John Wiley.

Ziegler, F. F., Imboden, J. B., & Meyer, E. (1960). Contemporary conversion reactions: A clinical study. *American Journal of Psychiatry, 116,* 901–910.

Zimmerman, J., & Grosz, H. J. (1966). "Visual" performance of a functionally blind person. *Behaviour Research and Therapy, 4,* 119–134.

18

Does Trauma Cause Dissociative Pathology?

Jane G. Tillman
Michael R. Nash
Paul M. Lerner

Most contemporary clinical theorists studying the psychological effects of trauma have adopted models similar to those of Breuer and Freud (Breuer & Freud, 1895/1955). They contend that early childhood trauma leads to the repeated overuse of dissociation until it becomes the individual's primary psychological defense, manifesting itself in dramatic alterations in the experience of self and world (Frischholz, 1985; Kluft, 1987; Putnam, 1985; Spiegel, Hunt, & Dondershine, 1988). Based on a wealth of clinical observations, these models define a causal continuity between trauma in childhood and subsequent adult symptoms of dissociation. What is so appealing about these traumagenic models of psychopathology is that they also chart a sure course for treatment, involving a therapeutic regression to the developmental stage in question, a reemergence of long repressed (or dissociated) memories, and a gradual resumption of development from that point. Thus, the assumption of a causal link between trauma and later dissociative pathology is fundamental to how these clinical theorists explain dissociation *and* how they treat it. Yet the idea that trauma causes dissociative pathology is almost never seriously questioned.

This chapter critically evaluates the conceptual, methodological, and empirical evidence for, and against, trauma as cause of dissociation. First, we explore the nature of causality; second, we define the nature of trauma and dissociation from a psychoanalytic perspective; third, we review the relevant empirical literature on trauma and dissociation; and, finally, we offer some tentative conclusions about how trauma may, or may not, be causally linked to dissociation.

THE NATURE OF CAUSALITY

Causes are the building blocks of theory, hence the more we understand causes and their nature, the richer our theories will be. Aristotle outlined four types of causes that contribute to our understanding of the world. Briefly, he put forth the following four causes: (1) the material cause, (2) the efficient cause, (3) the formal cause, and (4) the final cause. The material cause is the underlying and static essence of a thing, such as cellular or molecular structure, genes, matter, or material. For human behavior, the material cause would consist of neurotransmitters, and other biochemical bases of behavior. The efficient cause refers to the succession of events across time, which Aristotle thought originates or sustains motion. Examples of the efficient cause are activating, making happen, or impelling events. In terms of human behavior, the efficient cause may be understood as the agency or action of human beings (Wallace, 1974). The formal cause is the underlying structure or framework of an object or an experienced event. Examples of formal causes are blueprints, personality types, outlines, or other form-based descriptive features. Lastly, the final cause is the reason for, or the end to which, an event occurs, or the purpose for which an object exists. The final cause would also include the idea of why certain behaviors take place, and an understanding of their adaptive value (Rychlak, 1981).

Due to the reductionism of the Scientific Revolution, the final and formal causes were subsumed under the categories of material and efficient cause. Philosophers such as Hobbes, Locke, Berkeley, and Hume emphasized that the interpretation of cause should be limited to material and efficient causation, which they understood to be externally observable phenomena in the world of objects in motion. In attempting to understand the mission of social scientists, Wallace (1974) states:

> If the physical and biological sciences have made the greatest progress in recent times through the study of matter's substructure, and in this sense have shed new light on material and formal causality, it is perhaps to be expected that the sciences of man, examining anew the concepts of action and purpose, may shed equal light on efficient and final causality. (p. 320)

Thus, in his opinion, an examination of the internal world of agency, action, volition, and narrative should be an important aspect of the research enterprise.

In the study of human behavior and its aberrations, understanding the efficient cause in terms of an external event is short-sighted. However, using the efficient cause to examine dissociative phenomena from the view of human agency, action, and purpose seems especially well-suited to scholars of human behavior. When most dissociation researchers delineate causes of dissociation, they typically rely on somewhat constricted versions of material, efficient, and formal causation: They view the material cause in terms of a genetically determined capacity to dissociate (Braun, 1989); the efficient cause in terms of a direct linkage between external trauma and dissociative pathology (Briere & Runtz, 1988, 1989; Kluft, 1987; Sanders & Giolas, 1991; Spiegel, 1986); and the formal cause in terms of a descriptive counting of dissociative symptoms, rather than trying to cogently explain the process of traumatization and its effects (a point made by Kendall-Tackett, Williams, & Finkelhor, 1993).

Missing from the above are two potentially rich conceptualizations of cause, wherein efficient cause is framed in terms of human agency or action, not just external events; and final cause as the purpose of the dissociative defense. In elaborating the contribution of individuals to the dissociative process, and their agency in creating their own narrative structure, psychologists are able to work with a richer model of efficient cause. This has great significance for psychologists who understand not just external events but the internal contributions of agency as well. In terms of dissociation, emphasizing the role of the individual in addition to understanding the external traumatic event, allows for a more complete theory. In a similar manner, the final cause or the reason for dissociative symptoms has been theorized as related to their survival value (Spiegel, 1986). This certainly appears to be true when the event is happening. However, the continued use of dissociation must also have a purpose. Why is the dissociative defense operating years after the traumatic event(s) has occurred? In the study of defense mechanisms, psychodynamic theorists are able to contribute to an understanding of cause.

UNDERSTANDING TRAUMA AND DISSOCIATION

Defining Trauma

By primarily operating from a notion of external efficient causation, dissociation theorists have attempted to construe trauma as limited to the event. These theorists sometimes articulate forms of maladaptive response to trauma (e.g., anxiety, depression, hypnoidal state), but rarely is the patient's construction of the event considered (an aspect of internal efficient cause). While we object to this narrow definition, our review of the empirical literature will examine the evidence bearing on traumatic events as external efficient causes of dissociation. In addition to this, we will also discuss the methodological and conceptual consequences of defining trauma in terms of external efficient causes alone. Surely internal efficient causes such as how the individual constructs and perceives an event, and how it is integrated into existing psychic structures of meaning must be considered as a part of any satisfying definition of trauma.

Defining Dissociation

In reviewing the literature on dissociation, Lerner (1992) suggests that the concept of dissociation remains poorly understood and tends to be descriptive rather than explanatory. He discusses dissociation from the vantage point of psychoanalytic ego psychology and seeks to outline a comprehensive theory of dissociation that includes four perspectives: defense, memory, consciousness, and self. Integrating these four domains, Lerner defines dissociation as a defensive process in which experiences are split off and kept unintegrated through alterations in memory and consciousness, with a resulting impairment of the self. It is Lerner's definition that will serve as our working definition of dissociation.

As a defense, dissociation has commonalties with, as well as distinctions from, other defenses such as repression, splitting, and denial. Splitting and dissociation both involve an active maintaining of distance between mental contents, both are used to defensively ward off anxiety, and both contribute to a disturbance in identity or self. The separation of conscious from unconscious is not operative in the case of either splitting or dissociation. Kernberg's (1975) theory of splitting involves polarizing object and self-representations into "good" and "bad," and then attempting to keep these apart from one another. In contrast, dissociation tends to be a broader process and involves a variety of divisions that are not typically polarized into good or bad.

With dissociation, disturbances of memory are often reported. Specifically, forgetting is the memory disturbance that attends dissociation. In classic psychoanalytic thinking, forgetting is also operative in repression. However, not all instances of forgetting are the result of repression or dissociation. Here, it is useful to avoid construing memory as a unitary mechanism, and to instead utilize George Klein's (1970) theory of memory as comprised of four components: (1) registration, (2) storage or retention, (3) coding or categorization within schemata, and (4) retrieval or reconstruction. In recognizing the various subfunctions of memory, it follows that the effects of dissociation on memory will vary according to the particular function(s) involved.

Different theorists have speculated about how dissociation affects the processes of memory storage and retrieval. Examining the effects of psychic trauma on the mind, Horowitz (1992) suggested that memories of the trauma are registered and retained but are difficult to integrate with existing meaning structures and the self schema. In terms of Klein's model, Horowitz postulated that with psychic trauma, the memory structure as a whole is not impaired, but the subfunction of categorization within existing schemata is impeded.

Rapaport (1952) drew a distinction between states of consciousness and ways of experiencing consciousness. States of consciousness, he argued, exist along the continuum of waking through sleep. The ways of experiencing consciousness refers to the mode by which the contents of consciousness are experienced. For example, the contents of consciousness may be experienced as memories, as illusions, as facts, or as wishes. The dimension of attributed qualities of realness underlies these ways of experiencing consciousness.

Klein applied Rapaport's distinction between states of consciousness and ways of experiencing consciousness to his understanding of the processes of memory. In his paradigm, the state of consciousness provides the context for the memory, and the experiential mode of consciousness determines how the memory is registered, stored, organized, and retrieved, including its subjective sense of realness. When examined from the perspective of this paradigm, what is normally viewed as a loss of memory, forgetting, or a failure in retrieval, is not that, but instead represents a distortion in the mode of experiencing. One may respond to a stored representation of an actual event as something not real, but as imagined. Or, conversely, a vividly imagined event may be falsely experienced as an actual happening, rather than as a fantasy. Klein's theory provides a useful framework through which to better understand the internal processes that contribute to a dissociative event, and helps explain some of the difficulty in distinguishing what is an imagined event from an actual happening. Persons experiencing dissociative episodes often report being confused as to what is real, not through a loss of memory content, but by a clouding of the experiential mode through which content is remembered.

Memory is also a substantial contributor to one's sense of identity. Hilgard (1977) noted that memory is an essential prerequisite for maintaining a sense of identity over time, which provides a sense of continuity and stability. Conversely, Rapaport and Gill (1942/1967) asserted that personal identity is an important component of memory. They suggested that without a sense of identity, memories become either logically deductible knowledge or else unavailable for recall. They argued that personal identity provides the necessary context for the entrance of a memory into consciousness. Thus, when a memory is in conflict with personal identity it is excluded from consciousness. Implicit in the phenomena of memory loss is a loss of personal identity. Such a loss of identity can be experienced as fragmentation or as moments of discontinuity in the experience of time, self, and place.

Rapaport (1951/1967) distinguished consciousness from states of consciousness. Consciousness, he maintained, is a complex process that can be broken down into components such as awareness, reflectiveness, content, experiential mode, and state of consciousness. Descriptions of dissociative patients often include references to the patient's state of consciousness. The patient's experience may be described as dreamlike, or hypnoticlike in quality. These descriptions typically do not include or expand on Rapaport's other dimensions of consciousness. Rapaport (1951/1967) noted that both awareness and reflectiveness (reflexive awareness) are related to the effectiveness of one's control over one's impulses. From this ego psychological perspective, maximal awareness correlates with an optimal control of impulses, whereas limited awareness correlates with a lack of or excessive and rigid impulse control. Disturbances in the experience of the thematic contents of consciousness effects the degree and adequacy of reality testing. Further, compromised reality testing may be related to an inappropriate experiencing of an event. As with memory, the experiential modes of consciousness may be understood to lie along a continuum of realness. Via an alteration in the experiential mode, the sense of realness of an experience may be compromised, (i.e., the real may be mistaken for unreal; the unreal mistaken for real).

Almost all contemporary descriptions of dissociation include a disturbance in self-cohesion. Spiegel (1988) suggested that dissociation results in the loss of self or in self-fragmentation. Nemiah (1981) identified two hallmarks of pathological dissociation. The first marker is a disturbance of personal identity or self. Putnam (1989) identified two overriding features characteristic of all dissociative disorders, one of which is a disturbance in the individual's sense of self.

Concerns with the self are also prominent in contemporary psychoanalytic literature. However, dissociation theorists tend not to approach disturbances of self from a psychoanalytic perspective, meaning that although they associate a disruption in self or identity with the dissociative disorders, they often fail to elaborate upon what they mean when speaking of the self. By examining current dissociation theorists writings in light of various psychoanalytic conceptions of self, we can look at various disturbances of self from several structural vantage points.

Following Lerner's model, we suggest approaching the self from three perspectives: structure, contents, and functions. According to this formulation, the issue of coherence relates to structure, while that of self-concept and self-image relates to content. The impact of dissociation on both the structure and content of the self has been addressed (Beahrs, 1982; Putnam, 1989). What has received less attention is the effect of dissociation on the self's functions. Spiegel (1988) represents an exception to this omission as he examined the relationship between dissociation and the self-functions of regulating and mediating experiences. Spiegel noted that with dissociation the self loses its awareness of its mediating functions.

Two functions of the self are impaired by dissociation: The function of immediately experiencing something and the function of self-observation. When an individual experiences a painful event as happening to a different self, the participating self seems especially separate and estranged from the observing self. When an individual is absorbed in a special state such as a hypnotic like trance, the observing self seems to all but diminish with the experiencing self's increasing absorption, which serves to protect the self from memories of a traumatic experience. While the functions of the self usually operate in a harmonious and integrated manner, in dissociation the experiencing and observing functions are split and operate separately. Most commonly, what happens is the experiencing self becomes distant and estranged while the observing self becomes acutely aware.

Dissociation is a complex defensive process, distinct from other defenses such as repression, splitting, and denial. The subfunctions of memory, consciousness, and the self all play an integral part in the experience of dissociation, with disturbances occurring in different functions and subfunctions. The contribution of psychodynamic theory to dissociation is that it adds internal efficient causation to the existing material and formal causes associated with dissociative phenomena. Likewise, through conceiving of defenses as adaptive measures, a psychoanalytic approach to defensive operations contributes to an understanding of final causes.

EMPIRICAL RESEARCH
ON TRAUMA AND DISSOCIATION

We will first review the research often cited as supporting the idea that trauma causes dissociation, and we will follow that with a consideration of methodological and evidential matters that mitigate against accepting the conventional thinking about this linkage.

Evidence Supporting Trauma
as an External Efficient Cause

Much, though not all, of the research we review examines the effects of early sexual trauma. It is important to note that researchers and clinical theorists investigating early sexual abuse have claimed that this type of trauma is associated with a variety of psychiatric disorders (Herman, Perry, & van der Kolk, 1989; Ogata et al., 1990; Pribor & Dinwiddie, 1992; Walker et al., 1988). Thus, dissociative pathology is only one of a host of syndromes cited as resulting from early sexual trauma: Broad spectrum symptoms and pathology across both Axis I and Axis II of the *Diagnostic and Statistical*

Manual of Mental Disorders, third edition, revised (DSM-III-R; American Psychiatric Association, 1987) are also included, such as anxiety, depression, self-destructiveness, object relations pathology, substance abuse, antisocial personality, borderline personality, and somatization (Briere & Runtz, 1988; Bryer, Nelson, Miller, & Krol, 1987; Walker et al., 1988; Fromuth, 1986; Alexander & Lupfer, 1987).

There are two relatively noninteracting clinical research traditions that have examined the relationship between trauma and dissociation:

The MPD, PTSD, and hypnosis research. Many clinical theorists who have concerned themselves with multiple personality disorder (MPD) and posttraumatic stress disorder (PTSD) claim that high hypnotizability is a sensitive indicator of dissociation, and may be a reliable marker of a pathological process that presumably begins with trauma (Bliss, 1984; Frischholz, 1985; Spiegel, 1986). MPD anchors the extreme end of the scale of dissociative pathology. In patients with MPD the prevalence of early trauma is reported to be from 85–97% (Coons & Milstein, 1986; Kluft, 1987; Putnam, Guroff, Silberman, Barban, & Post, 1986). Bliss (1980) speculated that MPD is created by the unknowing use of autohypnosis, which is linked to dissociative phenomena. Indeed, other investigators report that high hypnotizability is a characteristic of most, and perhaps all, MPD patients (Bliss, 1984; Frischholz, 1985; Frischholz, Lipman, Braun, & Sachs, 1992).

Combat veterans with PTSD have been found to have significantly higher levels of hypnotizability when compared to non-PTSD Vietnam veterans (Spiegel et al., 1988). Spiegel (1986) reported that the experience of involuntariness may be the common link between hypnotizability, dissociation, and trauma. Hence, he suggested a hypnotizability measure may be quite helpful as a diagnostic tool when suspected cases of dissociative disorder or MPD are part of the clinical picture.

Research on the association between trauma and the exaggerated use of dissociation. Chu and Dill (1990) studied 98 female psychiatric inpatients in an attempt to understand the relationship between childhood physical/sexual abuse and dissociative experiences. As measured by the Dissociative Experiences Scale (DES), they found that childhood abuse was associated with higher levels of adult dissociative experiences. They did not control for family environment or the age at which the abuse first occurred. The main effects were examined for survivors of physical abuse alone and sexual abuse alone, with patients who reported both physical and sexual abuse having the highest mean score on the DES (Bernstein & Putnam, 1986). The researchers also found that 63% of a group of general female psychiatric inpatients reported histories of childhood physical and/or sexual abuse. In a study of adolescents undergoing psychiatric hospitalization, Sanders and

Giolas (1991) found that scores on the DES correlated significantly with self-reported physical abuse or punishment, sexual abuse, psychological abuse, neglect, and a negative home atmosphere. Again, covariates were not considered.

In the area of adult trauma, investigators in a recent study (Bremner et al., 1992) examined 85 Vietnam veterans, 53 of whom had a diagnosis of PTSD and were receiving treatment for PTSD symptoms, and 32 of whom were receiving treatment for medical disorders. The researchers administered the DES, the Combat Exposure Scale, and a modified DES that was used in an attempt to measure dissociative experiences during the time of a combat-related event. This group found that PTSD-diagnosed veterans reported a significantly higher number of dissociative experiences than the medical group. This difference persisted even when analysis controlled for combat exposure. Their finding that PTSD patients report a higher number of dissociative experiences is consistent with the clinical experience with this population and its widespread report of "flashbacks."

Carlson and Rosser-Hogan (1991) examined dissociative symptoms, PTSD, and depression in Cambodian refugees. Fifty Cambodian refugees who had settled in the United States were randomly selected from a list of 500 potential subjects. Of the 50 subjects in the study, 49 had never received professional mental health care. The instruments used included the DES, the Post-Traumatic Inventory (Meinhardt, Tom, Tse, & Yu, 1986), and a measure of depression and anxiety. In this study, 96% of the refugees had high dissociation scores, 80% could be classified as suffering from clinical depression, and 86% met the DSM-III-R criteria for PTSD. Dissociation was widely prevalent, again across diagnostic categories. In addition, the scores on the DES were positively correlated with the amount of trauma experienced, as measured by the Post-Traumatic Inventory.

From a nonclinical sample of 278 adult university women, Briere and Runtz (1988) found that 15% reported having had sexual contact with a significantly older person before the age of 18. This group of women (defined as sexually traumatized) also reported higher levels of dissociation, somatization, anxiety, and depression than did the nonabused women. In a large survey study of relatively affluent professional women, Elliott and Briere (1992) found that nonabused subjects reported less family disturbance in their families of origin than did abused subjects. Abused subjects scored higher than nonabused subjects on the Trauma Symptom Checklist even when the effects of family pathology were controlled for. The authors concluded that family pathology moderates the causal relationship between trauma and symptomatology but does not explain it. However, serious design problems involving method variance and subtest selection render these conclusions suspect.

Evidential and Methodological Considerations That Mitigate against Construing Trauma as an External Efficient Cause

With regard to methodological considerations, first comes the problem of defining trauma in the literature. For instance, many theorists have assumed that childhood sexual abuse is by definition traumatic. Yet a more recent review questions whether all cases of sexual abuse necessarily involve overwhelming affect, fear for safety, and helplessness (Kendall-Tackett et al., 1993).

Second, there are also some problems in defining and operationalizing dissociation. The DES (Bernstein & Putnam, 1986) is widely employed in assessing dissociative symptoms, and it does demonstrate satisfactory split-half and test–retest reliability. In addition, there is reason to believe that patients with and without dissociative disorders score differentially on the scale (Frischholz, Braun, Sachs, & Hopkins, 1990). However, there is some evidence that a large component of an individual's DES score can be attributed not to dissociative pathology specifically, but to gross psychopathology in general. Norton, Ross, and Novotny (1990); Sandberg and Lynn (1992); and Nash, Hulsey, Sexton, Harralson, and Lambert (1993) all detected a confound between general psychological impairment and DES scores, wherein high DES scores were associated with greater psychopathology. In the Nash et al. study the DES correlated .70 with the F scale of the MMPI. Similar findings were obtained for two other scales: The Dissociation Content Scale (Boswell, Sanders, & Hernandez, 1985, cited in Sanders, 1986), and The Indiana Dissociative Symptom Scale (Levitt, 1989). Thus, when the DES scores of traumatized patients exceed those of nontraumatized patients, it is possible that the difference has less to do with dissociation per se, and more to do with gross pathology.

Third, all too often current research in the area of sexual trauma fails to consider the baseline reports of abuse among *all* female patients in a clinical setting. The incidence of childhood abuse in the MPD population is reported to be from 85–90% (Coons & Milstein, 1986; Kluft, 1987; Putnam et al., 1986), but among women in a general clinical setting the base rate for sexual abuse is between 44–77% (Briere & Zaidi, 1989; Bryer et al., 1987). The overlap of the upper end of estimates of sexual abuse in the clinical population with those of MPD patients with a reported history of sexual and/or physical abuse is considerable and further calls into question the direct link between sexual and/or physical abuse and dissociative disorders.

Fourth, the research design in existing studies on the link between sexual trauma and patterns of resulting psychopathology is sometimes weak. (Browne & Finkelhor, 1986; Kendall-Tackett et al., 1993; Nash et al., 1993). Specifically, it is flawed in the following respects: (1) It consists of weak control groups wherein nonclinical abused subjects are typically compared with nonclinical nonabused subjects, and (2) it consists of weak dependent measures.

Fifth, most researchers claiming trauma as a cause of dissociative pathology have neglected to consider other pathogenic factors in the child's environment that might explain subsequent pathology. Families in which abuse occurs are more pathological than nonabusing families, with higher levels of role or boundary confusion, more rigid behavioral control, and less cohesiveness and adaptability (Alexander & Lupfer, 1987; Harter, Alexander, & Neimeyer, 1988; Hoagwood & Stewart, 1988). Thus, differences between abused and nonabused samples on measures of psychopathology in general (and dissociation in particular) may be due, not to the effects of trauma per se, but to the nonspecific effects of living in a pathogenic home environment. Indeed, recent empirical work suggests that some adult pathology associated with childhood sexual trauma may reflect the effects of a broadly pathogenic family environment rather than the effects of sexual abuse per se (Harter et al., 1988; Fromuth, 1986; Wyatt & Newcomb, 1990). Nash and his colleagues (Nash et al., 1993) found that subjects who were sexually traumatized in childhood were significantly more dissociative than nonabused subjects. However, when family environment was used as a covariate, the effect for early trauma receded to the point of nonsignificance. These findings bring into question the conclusions of previous researchers who failed to control for important pathogenic contextual features of the victim's environment.

Sixth, there is a growing realization that the validity of at least some reports of abuse is marginal. Clinicians have long recognized the problem of false negatives (i.e., not remembering trauma when it actually *did* occur). Now we are faced with the problem of false positives (remembering trauma when it *did not* in fact occur). Noting the dramatic increase in reports of bizarre satanic ritual abuse, especially among dissociative patients, Loftus (1993) has drawn attention to the problem of false memory. Ganaway (1991) found that up to 50% of dissociative-disordered patients report satanic ritualistic abuse involving heinous, even cannibalistic crimes, carried out by an organized network of secret covens. These fantastic accounts, although compellingly rendered, have never been confirmed by law enforcement authorities. If the reports of dissociative-disordered patients can be so profoundly compromised, the conclusions of Bliss (1984) and others (Coons & Milstein, 1986; Kluft, 1987; Putnam et al., 1986) on the prevalence of early sexual trauma among MPD patients must also be reevaluated. This all has had a chilling effect on the internal validity of retrospective studies and raises the specter that dissociation confounds the accuracy of reports of early trauma, that is, dissociative symptomatology may predispose some patients to confound fantasy, dream, and mnemonic experience.

Nonsupportive Empirical Findings

In addition to the methodological and conceptual issues listed above, some empirical work is quite at odds with the conventional view that trauma causes dissociation. First, a relationship among dissociation, hypnotizability, and trauma is not found in many studies. For instance, three studies report no significant correlation between measures of hypnotizability and measures of dissociation (Nash et al. 1993; Putnam, Helmers, & Trickett, 1992). Second, in recent, well-designed research studies, one with children (Putnam et al., 1992) and one with adults (Nash et al., 1993), individuals who reported sexual abuse in childhood were no more hypnotizable than controls. Further, while in both studies traumatized subjects scored marginally higher than controls on measures of dissociation, in the one study that controlled for the chaotic family environment of abused subjects, no effect was obtained.

Epidemiological studies of MPD in nonclinical populations cast some doubt on the generalizability of earlier studies that examined psychiatric patients. Ross (1991) studied dissociative phenomena, MPD, and self-report histories of childhood trauma in clinical as well as nonclinical populations using the DES. He estimated that between 5–10% of the general population is affected by a dissociative disorder. Ross also found incidents of MPD in the general population at a rate of 3.1% based on a 450-person sample to which he administered the Dissociative Disorder Interview Schedule (DDIS; Ross, Heber, Norton, & Anderson, 1989). Ross stated that the data of individuals with MPD in the general population were radically different from the data of the clinical MPD patients. In the clinical MPD population, 85–97% of patients report a history of severe sexual and physical abuse (Coons & Milstein, 1986; Kluft, 1987; Putnam et al., 1986). In Ross's (1991) study, MPD subjects in the general population rarely reported histories of abuse, and reported experiencing little psychopathology. This is an interesting report of a supposedly extremely pathological condition resulting from severe childhood abuse; it reveals that MPD in the general population is relatively disconnected from a history of abuse and profound distress. Earlier studies claiming to find evidence of a trauma/hypnotizability/dissociative link (Bliss, 1980,1984; Coons & Milstein, 1986; Kluft, 1987; Putnam et al., 1986) may need to be reexamined in light of Ross's findings.

In a recent comprehensive review of childhood sexual abuse and subsequent psychopathology, Kendall-Tackett et al. (1993) maintained that abused children who are asymptomatic may be truly less affected by abuse. Fully one-third of the victims across studies were found to have little or no measurable impairment. Kendall-Tackett et al. concluded that although some children suffer from dissociative-like symptoms (specifically PTSD symptoms), empirical research does not support the notion that PTSD symptomatology is an inevitable consequence of sexual trauma, or is even the most prevalent pattern of symptomatology. Although sexualization and PTSD are frequent postsex abuse findings, they are not universal. In the studies examined, Kendall-Tackett et al. conclude among children who were found to be symptomatic, there are a host of diagnostic categories associated with sexual trauma.

According to many studies, other events known to be traumatic have rarely involved dissociation. In his research on the survivors of Nazi concentration camps, Krystal (1991) generally found that although the trauma endured was severe, and the subsequent psychological disturbance sometimes quite substantial, dissociation was not a prominent post-traumatic symptom. In Holocaust survivors the post-traumatic symptoms researchers have observed include greatly restricted cognitive and affective capacities or alexithymia, depression, survivor guilt, sleep disturbances, repetitive dreams, chronic pain syndromes, and chronic anxiety as well as characterological difficulties (Eitinger, 1980). In short, although the trauma experienced by Holocaust survivors is agreed to be severe, it has not been associated with dissociation in the clinical or empirical literature.

In studying the aftereffects of the Chowchilla kidnapping, Terr (1985) outlined the signs and symptoms of childhood trauma, which she termed the "four Cs." These hallmarks are: (1) cognitive–perceptual errors, (2) collapse of early developmental achievements, (3) compulsive repetition, and (4) contagion. This last symptom, contagion, refers to the contagious nature of the post-traumatic symptoms that were observed among the Chowchilla children. Although the event was traumatic for the children who were kidnapped, Terr notes that via the mechanism of contagion, post-traumatic symptoms were transmitted to the victims' family members and friends, who had not endured the direct trauma of the kidnapping. This finding regarding contagion is supported by second-generation Holocaust survivors, who report post-traumatic symptoms from bearing witness to the suffering and trauma endured by their parents. In this case, the pathology resulted despite no direct experiencing of the traumatic event. The mechanism operating in cases of contagion may be identification with the victim or the aggressor, a defensive strategy that can be construed as an internal efficient cause.

In summation, while theories of a linear relationship between trauma and dissociative disorders are intuitively attractive, empirical research has not produced a clear demonstration of this link. There does appear to be some kind of a relationship between childhood trauma and later dissociative disorders, but many studies have failed to control for other contributing pathogenic factors that could explain this association. Hence, researchers have yet to pinpoint the relationship. The connection between hypnotizability and dissociation has also been called into question by recent studies (Nash et al., 1993; Putnam et al., 1992). Likewise, current research in the area of memory (Loftus, 1993) poses challenging questions for future research design.

Recent methodological reviews and empirical findings have revealed that the dissociation literature is burdened with conceptual and design problems. Indeed, the very definitions of trauma and dissociation are quite unsatisfactory. In the case of trauma, events that the public eye views as unusually appalling, tragic, victimizing, or brutal are generally accepted as traumatic in nature (American Psychiatric Association, 1987), but events that do not seem so out of the ordinary are *not* viewed as traumatic. Without recourse to the patient's construction of the event (internal efficient cause) and the social/environmental context in which the event is embedded (external efficient cause), one can imagine clinical researchers making errors in both directions: They might define an event as traumatic when it is not, as well as not define an event as traumatic when it is. We would suggest that researchers might consider reframing the questions they ask. For instance, instead of asking, "What are the effects of trauma?", they might ask: "What is it about an event, and an individual's construction of that event that renders it pathogenic?"

The problem of defining dissociation is no less complex. In an eloquent presentation and subsequent article, Frankel (1990) cautioned the MPD/dissociation disorder professional community that the fate of dissociation in the late 20th century may resemble that of hysteria in the late 19th century. Specifically, its boundaries may become so permeable that it will eventually mean everything and therefore nothing. Indeed, the considerable statistical overlap between the "gold standard" of dissociation measures (the DES), and measures of general psychopathology is sobering. Again, through only relying on the descriptive features of dissociation (i.e., the formal cause), without a broad theoretical framework, we may be prevented from developing the precise and discriminating measures we need.

Methodological problems like failing to consider baseline rates of trauma across all psychiatric diagnostic groups; confounding trauma with other environmental pathogenic factors; the presence of weak, or absence of, control groups; and the questionable reliability of some reports of trauma all compromise what can be inferred from trauma research. When these problems are corrected, findings are often quite at odds with predictions based on traumagenic theories. But of these methodological problems, the most important, and widely overlooked, is the failure to control for other contextual features of the victim's family and social environment that may also cause impairment. For some victims, the traumatic event(s) may be a signal variable that the home environment is profoundly and broadly pathogenic. Subsequent adult impairment may result from not the trauma alone, but the context in which it was embedded. To this we add another caution: As Conte (1986) pointed out, attributional distortions made by trauma victims about their family environment could complicate the interpretation of retrospective studies; that is, traumatized individuals may overestimate the degree of disruption in their family precisely *because* they were abused. In fact, no amount of technical manipulation of cross-sectional correlational data can yield definitive causal information. Only prospective, longitudinal studies can begin to unravel the problem of how trauma relates to psychopathology in general.

Finally, we note the fervor with which some dissociation theorists and the lay press adhere to the trauma–dissociation link. One might anticipate that the, at best, equivocal research basis for this view would inspire skepticism, or at least serve to mute the grand conclusions about univariate cause and effect between trauma and dissociation that abound in the professional and lay literatures—but it does not. Convictions concerning this issue may be stubbornly resistant to change due to the operation of a common type of error in human inference: The "representativeness heuristic" (Nisbett & Ross, 1980). In other words, dramatic and salient events so completely capture the attention of observers that lay persons and clinicians alike fail to take into account more mundane disconfirming information, like baseline data. For example, as a result of dramatic airline crashes, many people infer that great danger attends airplane flight, despite all the baseline evidence to the contrary. In the present case, trauma (especially sexual abuse) and dissociative pathology (especially MPD) are both immensely dramatic and salient events that may lead even the most discerning thinker to: (1) overlook disconfirmatory data (e.g., dissociative-disordered individuals who were not traumatized; non-dissociative-disordered individuals who were traumatized, or (2) overemphasize the confirmatory data (e.g., cases where there is a victim of violent or abhorrent acts who eventually manifests MPD).

SUMMARY

In this chapter, the relevant literature on the link between trauma and dissociation has been reviewed and the puzzling and occasionally contradictory findings outlined. What is clear is that the relationship between trauma and dissociation does not appear to be linear. In reviewing the existing literature, we outlined methodological weaknesses that often stem from the current conceptualization of the relationship between trauma and dissociation. We proposed a psychoanalytic formulation, which we believe incorporates both the efficient and final cause into an understanding of how dissociative pathology might emerge as a potential response to traumatic events.

There are currently two streams of thought in psychiatry that contribute to our understanding of various psychopathological entities, one being descriptive and the other theory-based. The two differ as far as conceptualization, points of emphasis, values, and methodology are concerned. In general, descriptive psychiatry emphasizes discrete and observable behaviors, exclusive nosological categories, and empirical studies with minimal underlying theoretical structure. In contrast, the theory-based perspective that we espouse (psychoanalytic) considers disturbances in terms of structural, dynamic, and developmental roots, and spurns research that is highly conceptually based.

As a logical consequence of the above, descriptive efforts tend to lead to linear thinking and linear studies in which the findings tend to be interpreted in linear ways. By contrast, psychoanalysis emphasizes both multideterminism and various points of view instead of linear thinking. By multideterminism, we mean that any underlying single motive can be expressed in various pieces of behavior and that any one piece of behavior can reflect various motives. By various points of view, we mean that any one piece of behavior may be viewed from several perspectives, including the dynamic, the economic, the structural, the genetic, and the adaptive. In this paper, we have offered a psychoanalytic conceptualization of both trauma and dissociation.

While the existing research is quite valuable, it fails to capture the complexity of the relationship between trauma and dissociation implied in a psychoanalytic conceptualization. To complement this existing research then, empirical studies are needed that are based firmly in theory and that also attend to internal efficient cause and final cause. Studies examining internal efficient cause should examine individual perceptual differences, or organizing schematas for processing traumatic events. Psychodynamic theory can be used to inform the design of empirical studies examining the internal efficient cause in terms of economic and dynamic functions. Likewise, the final cause can be studied in terms of the long-term adaptive function of dissociation in the processing of traumatic events.

REFERENCES

Alexander, P., & Lupfer, S. (1987). Family characteristics and long-term consequences associated with sexual abuse. *Archives of Sexual Behavior, 16*, 235–245.

American Psychiatric Association (1987). *Diagnostic and statistical manual of mental disorders* (3rd ed., rev.). Washington DC: Author.

Beahrs, J. O. (1982). *Unity and multiplicity: Multilevel consciousness of self in hypnosis, psychiatric disorder, and mental health.* New York: Brunner/Mazel.

Bernstein, E. M., & Putnam, F. W. (1986). Development, reliability, and validity of a dissociation scale. *Journal of Nervous and Mental Disease, 174* (12), 727–735.

Bliss, E. L. (1980). Multiple personalities: A report of 14 cases with implications for schizophrenia and hysteria. *American Journal of Psychiatry, 39*, 1388–1397.

Bliss, E. L. (1984). A symptom profile of patients with multiple personalities, including MMPI results. *Journal of Nervous and Mental Disease, 172*, 197–201.

Braun, B. G. (1989). Psychotherapy of the survivor of incest with a dissociative disorder. *Psychiatric Clinics of North America, 12* (2), 307–324.

Bremner, J. D., Southwick, S., Brett, E., Fontana, A., Rosenheck, R., & Charney, D. S. (1992). Dissociation and posttraumatic stress disorder in Vietnam combat veterans. *American Journal of Psychiatry, 149* (3), 328–332.

Breuer, J., & Freud, S. (1955). *Studies in hysteria*. In J. Strachey (Ed. and Trans.), *The standard edition of the complete psychological works of Sigmund Freud* (Vol. 2, pp. 1–181). London: Hogarth Press. (Original work published 1895)

Briere, J., & Runtz, M. (1988). Post sexual abuse trauma. *Journal of International Violence, 2*, 367–379.

Briere, J., & Runtz, M. (1989). The trauma symptom checklist (TSC-33): Early data on a new scale. *Journal of Interpersonal Violence, 4* (2), 151–163.

Briere, J., & Zaidi, L. Y. (1989). Sexual abuse histories and sequelae in female psychiatric emergency room patients. *American Journal of Psychiatry, 146*, 1602–1606.

Browne, A., & Finkelhor, D. (1986). Impact of child sexual abuse: A review of the research. *Psychological Bulletin, 99*, 66–77.

Bryer, J., Nelson, B., Miller, J., & Krol, P. (1987). Childhood sexual abuse as factors in adult psychiatric illness. *American Journal of Psychiatry, 144*, 1426–1430.

Carlson, E. B., & Rosser-Hogan, R. (1991). Trauma experiences, posttraumatic stress, dissociation, and depression in Cambodian refugees. *American Journal of Psychiatry, 148*(11), 1548–1551.

Chu, J. A., & Dill, D. L. (1990). Dissociative symptoms in relation to childhood physical and sexual abuse. *American Journal of Psychiatry, 147* (7), 887–892.

Conte, J. R. (1986). Sexual abuse and the family: A critical analysis. In T. Trepper & M. J. Barrett (Eds.), *Treating incest: A multiple systems perspective* (pp. 113–126). New York: Haworth Press.

Coons, P. M., & Milstein, V. (1986). Psychosexual disturbances in multiple personality: Characteristics, etiology, and treatment. *Journal of Clinical Psychiatry, 47*, 106–110.

Eitinger, L. (1980). The concentration camp syndrome and its late sequelae. In J. Dimsdale (Ed.), *Survivors, victims and perpetrators* (pp. 127–162). Washington, DC: Hemisphere.

Elliott, D. M., & Briere, J. (1992, August). *Child sexual abuse and family environment: Combined impacts and the effects of statistical control*. Paper presented at the 100th annual meeting of the American Psychological Association, Washington, DC.

Frankel, F. H. (1990). Hypnotizability and dissociation. *American Journal of Psychiatry, 147*, 823–829.

Frischholz, E. J. (1985). The relationship among dissociation, hypnosis, and child abuse in the development of multiple personality. In R. P. Kluft (Ed.), *Childhood antecedents of multiple personality* (pp. 99–120), Washington, DC: American Psychiatric Press.

Frischholz, E. J., Lipman, L. S., Braun, B. G., & Sachs, R. G. (1992). Psychopathology, hypnotizability and dissociation. *American Journal of Psychiatry, 149*, 1521–1525.

Frischholz, E. J., Braun, B. G., Sachs, R. G., & Hopkins, L. (1990). The dissociative experiences scale: Further replication and validation. *Dissociation Progress in the Dissociative Disorders, 3*, 151–153.

Fromuth, M. E. (1986). The relationship of childhood sexual abuse with later psychological and sexual adjustment in a sample of college women. *Child Abuse and Neglect, 10,* 5–15.

Ganaway, T. (1991, August). *Alternative hypotheses regarding satanic ritual abuse memories.* Paper presented at the 99th annual meeting of the American Psychological Association, San Francisco.

Harter, S., Alexander, P., & Neimeyer, R. A. (1988). Long-term effects of incestuous child abuse in college women: Social adjustment, social cognition, and family characteristics. *Journal of Consulting and Clinical Psychology, 56,* 5–8.

Herman, J., Perry, C., & van der Kolk, B. (1989). Childhood trauma in borderline personality disorder. *American Journal of Psychiatry, 146,* 490–495.

Hilgard, E. R. (1977). *Divided consciousness: Multiple controls in human thought and action.* New York: John Wiley.

Hoagwood, K., & Stewart, J. M. (1988, August). *Family structural factors in cases of child sexual abuse.* Paper presented at the annual meeting of the American Psychological Association, Atlanta, GA.

Horowitz, M. (1992). The effects of psychic trauma on the mind: Structure and process of meaning. In J. Barron, M. Eagle, & D. Wolitzky (Eds.), *Interface of psychoanalysis and psychology* (pp. 489–500). Washington, DC: American Psychological Association.

Kendall-Tackett, K. A., Williams, L. M., & Finkelhor, D. (1993). Impact of sexual abuse on children: A review and synthesis of recent empirical studies. *Psychological Bulletin, 113,* 164–180.

Kernberg, O. F. (1975). *Borderline conditions and pathological narcissism.* New York: Jason Aronson.

Klein, G. S. (1970). *Perception, motives, and personality.* New York: Jason Aronson.

Kluft, R. P. (1987). An update on multiple personality disorder. *Hospital and Community Psychiatry, 38,* 363–373.

Krystal, H. (1991). Integration and self-healing in post-traumatic states: A ten-year retrospective. *American Imago, 48* (1), 93–118.

Lerner, P. M. (1992). *Some preliminary thoughts on dissociation.* Unpublished manuscript.

Levitt, E. E. (1989). *The clinical application of MMPI special scales.* Hillsdale, NJ: Lawrence Erlbaum.

Loftus, E. F. (1993). The reality of repressed memories. *American Psychologist, 48* (5), 518–537.

Meinhardt, K., Tom, S., Tse P., & Yu, C. Y. (1986). Southeast Asian refugees in the "Silicon Valley": The Asian health assessment project. *Amerasia; 12,* 43–65.

Nash, M. R., Hulsey, T. L., Sexton, M. C., Harralson, T. L., & Lambert, W. (1993). Long-term sequelae of childhood sexual abuse: Perceived family environment, psychopathology, and dissociation. *Journal of Clinical and Consulting Psychology, 61* (2), 276–283.

Nemiah, J. C. (1981). Dissociative disorders. In A. M. Freedman & H. I. Kaplan (Eds.), *Comprehensive textbook of psychiatry* (3rd ed.). Baltimore: Williams & Williams.

Nisbett, R., & Ross, L. (1980). *Human inference: Strategies and short-comings of social judgment.* Englewood Cliffs, NJ: Prentice Hall.

Norton, G. R., Ross, C. A., & Novotny, M. F. (1990). Factors that predict scores on the Dissociative Experiences Scale. *Journal of Clinical Scale, 46,* 273–277.

Ogata, S., Silk, K., Goodrich, S., Lohr, N., Westen, D., & Hill, E. (1990). Childhood sexual and physical abuse in adult patients with borderline personality disorder. *American Journal of Psychiatry, 147,* 1008–1013.

Pribor, E. F., & Dinwiddie, S. H. (1992). Psychiatric correlates of incest in childhood. *American Journal of Psychiatry, 149,* 52–56.

Putnam, F. W. (1985). Dissociation as a response to extreme trauma. In R. P. Kluft (Ed.), *Childhood antecedents of multiple personality* (65–98). Washington, DC: American Psychiatric Press.

Putnam, F. W. (1989). *Diagnosis and treatment of multiple personality disorder.* New York: Guilford Press.

Putnam, F. W., Guroff, J. J., Silberman, E. K., Barban, L., & Post, R. M. (1986). The clinical phenomenology of multiple personality disorder: A review of 100 recent cases. *Journal of Clinical Psychiatry, 47,* 285–293.

Putnam, F. W., Helmers, K., & Trickett, P. K. (1992). *Hypnotizability and dissociativity in sexually abused girls.* Unpublished manuscript, Laboratory of Developmental Psychology, National Institute of Mental Health, Bethesda, MD.

Rapaport, D. (1967). States of consciousness: A psychopathological and psychodynamic view. In M. Gill (Ed.), *The collected papers of David Rapaport* (pp. 385–404). New York: Basic Books. (Original work published 1951)

Rapaport, D. (1952). Projective techniques and the theory of thinking. *Journal of Projective Techniques, 16,* 269–275.

Rapaport, D., & Gill, M. (1967). A case of amnesia and its bearing on the theory of memory. In M. Gill (Ed.), *The collected papers of David Rapaport* (pp. 113-119). New York: Basic Books. (Original work published 1942)

Ross, C. A. (1991). Epidemiology of multiple personality disorder and dissociation. *Psychiatric Clinics of North America, 14* (3), 503–517.

Ross, C. A., Heber, S., Norton, G. R., & Anderson, G. (1989). Differences between multiple personality disorder and other diagnostic groups on the structured interview. *Journal of Nervous and Mental Disease, 177*(8), 487–491.

Rychlak, J. F. (1981). *Introduction to personality and psychotherapy.* Boston: Houghton Mifflin.

Sandberg, D. A., & Lynn, S. J. (1992). Dissociative experiences, psychopathology and adjustment, and adolescent maltreatment in female college students. *Journal of Abnormal Psychology, 101,* 717–723.

Sanders, S. (1986). The perceptual alteration scale: A scale measuring dissociation. *American Journal of Clinical Hypnosis, 29,* 95–102.

Sanders, B., & Giolas, M. H. (1991). Dissociation and childhood trauma in psychologically disturbed adolescents. *American Journal of Psychiatry, 148* (1), 50–54.

Spiegel, D. (1986). Dissociating damage. *American Journal of Clinical Hypnosis, 29* (2), 123–131.

Spiegel, D. (1988). Dissociation and hypnosis in post-traumatic stress disorder. *Journal of Traumatic Stress, 1,* 17–33.

Spiegel, D. T., Hunt, T., & Dondershine, H. F. (1988). Dissociation and hypnotizability in posttraumatic stress disorder. *American Journal of Psychiatry, 145,* 301–305.

Terr, L. (1985). Psychic trauma in children and adolescents. *Psychiatric Clinics of North America, 8* (4), 815–835.

Walker, E., Katon, W., Harrop-Griffiths, J., Holm, L., Russo, J., & Hickok, L. (1988). Relationship of chronic pain to psychiatric diagnoses and childhood sexual abuse. *American Journal of Psychiatry, 145* (1), 75–80.

Wallace, W. A. (1974). *Causality and scientific explanation.* Ann Arbor: University of Michigan Press.

Wyatt, G. E., & Newcomb, M. D. (1990). Internal and external mediators of women's sexual abuse in childhood. *Journal of Consulting and Clinical Psychology, 58,* 758–767.

19
Recovered Memories of Childhood Abuse: A Source Monitoring Perspective

Robert F. Belli
Elizabeth F. Loftus

The flight had been uneventful. Two passengers were engaged in casual conversation. One passenger began discussing his work as an experimental psychologist researching memory. Suddenly, the other passenger switched the conversation to a discussion of his adult children, in particular, a daughter who was having weight problems. She had been seeing a therapist. She was accusing him and his wife of having sexually abused her as a child. "Nothing like that ever happened," he said, "Why would she remember such a terrible thing about us?"

This chance incident was for one of us (Belli) the first exposure to a rapidly growing phenomenon of adults claiming, often during therapy, that they had recovered once-repressed memories of their parents having abused them as children. Some of these claims are rather bizarre, such as those that include themes of satanic rituals and murder (Braun & Sachs, 1988; Ganaway, 1989, 1991). There usually is no corroborating physical evidence. Yet, these claims have led to dire consequences such as legal action, in which both the accused and the accusers suffer.

Along with these claims, a growing debate has arisen among those lay persons involved and professionals alike about whether these claims are veridical memories of actual events or honest fabrications, due to suggestions introduced by therapists, or such sources such as self-help books, of events that never occurred. Either scenario bespeaks tragedy.

There seems to be no doubt that sexual (and other forms of) childhood abuse occur with alarming frequency and lead to severe psychological trauma among their victims (Daro, 1988; Finkelhor, 1986; LaFontaine, 1990). If the repressed memories are veridical, the frequency of childhood abuse may be even greater than previously believed. If the memories are honest fabrications, both the accused and the accuser have been victimized: Family relationships have been damaged or destroyed, reputations have been ruined, and extensive financial loss often follows. Moreover, the accuser's memories of childhood have been invaded and harmed.

The self-help book *The Courage to Heal* (Bass & Davis, 1988) discusses the suffering that a discoverer of repressed memories must endure: "If you maintained the fantasy that your childhood was 'happy,' then you have to grieve for the childhood you thought you had. . . . You must give up the idea that your parents had your best interest at heart. . . . You may have to grieve over the fact that you don't have an extended family for your children . . . that you don't have family roots" (pp. 118–119). Although such suffering is sadly warranted if the memories are veridical, it is a total tragedy if the memories are fabrications induced through suggestion. Given the severity of the consequences that these claims engender, there needs to be a close examination of the different possibilities.

Many professionals believe the authenticity of these reports, arguing that repression is a common defense mechanism used to shelter victims from traumatic experiences (see Loftus, 1993). Dissociative disorders have been particularly linked with individuals who repress memories of traumatization (Chu, 1988). In fact, some therapists are inclined to infer the existence of a repressed traumatic history in clients who have the symptoms of a dissociative disorder and who appear to be unable to remember many childhood events (see Lynn & Nash, 1994).

Others are skeptical that each and every one of these reports is veridical; they believe that some people may have been influenced by suggestion. In searching for a traumatic past in their clients, some therapists may be inadvertently encouraging the "recovery" of memories of traumatic events that in actuality never happened (Loftus, 1993; Lynn & Nash, 1994). The psychological literature, including experimental research that we have conducted, has shown that people can be persuaded to remember events that never took place. Moreover, the kinds of techniques used by some therapists to uncover repressed memories resemble the techniques that have led to false memories in controlled laboratory work. One goal of this chapter is to discuss some of the factors that lead to false memories in the laboratory, and to explore the extent to which these findings might shed light on how some claims of repressed childhood abuse could represent honest mistakes.

THE EXPERIMENTAL EVIDENCE

The Misinformation Effect

A great deal of research on suggestibility has focused on the role of misinformation in altering reports about past events. When subjects witness an event, and are later misinformed about some aspects of what occurred, their final reports about the event contain more errors than reports from control subjects who were not misinformed, a finding known as the *misinformation effect*. A typical experiment exploring the misinformation effect involves three phases. In the first phase, subjects are shown a series of slides depicting some event, such as a robbery. In this phase critical *event items* (such as a stolen diamond ring) may be shown. In the second phase, some subjects are verbally misinformed, often by reading a narrative, that *postevent items* (such as a pearl necklace) were stolen during the event. Control subjects are not misinformed during the second phase. Finally, in the third phase, subjects are tested on what they remember seeing during the event. The test might involve, for example, a cued-recall test or a forced-choice test involving event and postevent items. Researchers have become particularly interested in two types of errors associated with the misinformation effect. One error involves an inability to remember what was originally experienced, a process called *memory impairment* (e.g., Belli, 1989; Belli, Lindsay, Gales, & McCarthy, 1994; Lindsay, 1990; Loftus, Hoffman, & Wagenaar, 1992; Loftus, Miller, & Burns, 1978). A second error involves the subjects' remembering the misinformation as something seen in the event itself, a process called *source misattribution* (e.g., Belli, 1989; Belli et al., 1994; Johnson, Hashtroudi, & Lindsay, 1993; Lindsay, 1990; Lindsay & Johnson, 1989; Loftus & Hoffman, 1989; Zaragoza & Lane, 1991, 1992).

Memory impairment and source misattribution may occur together, or they may be independent of one another (Lindsay, 1994; Zaragoza & Lane, 1992). In the former case, remembering that the misinformation was part of the event may impair the ability to remember the original information (Belli et al., 1994). For example, the suggestion that a pearl necklace was stolen may impair the ability to remember that it actually was a diamond ring that was stolen. Additionally, misinformation may induce memory impairment without source misattribution. Subjects may correctly remember that the misinformation (pearl necklace) was presented only after the event, yet be unable to remember the original information (diamond ring) because memory for it is blocked by having remembered the misinformation (Belli, Windschitl, McCarthy, & Winfrey, 1992; Chandler, 1991). Finally, source misattribution may occur without memory impairment, when, for example, the original event information (diamond ring) was never encoded in the first place (and thus there is no original memory to impair), yet subjects incorrectly remember that the misinformation (pearl necklace) occurred during the event (Loftus & Hoffman, 1989).[1] Of these processes, source misattribution is more important to the present discussion since it involves people remembering having seen things that were only suggested to them.

In comparison to control subjects, misled subjects more often report having seen postevent items, which by design were never shown at all.[2] Subjects have falsely reported seeing yield signs instead of the stop signs that were actually shown (Loftus et al., 1978), screwdrivers instead of hammers (McCloskey & Zaragoza, 1985), *Vogue* magazine instead of *Mademoiselle* (Tversky & Tuchin, 1989), eggs instead of breakfast cereal (Ceci, Ross, & Toglia, 1987), blue plastic pitchers instead of green ones (Belli, 1988), a man sporting a mustache instead of being clean-shaven (Gibling & Davies, 1988), and the word "Nixon" on a T-shirt instead of the word "Yukon" (Sheehan & Tilden, 1986), among numerous other examples. The research leaves little doubt that false reports are easy to induce.

Yet, these false reports of postevent items may not involve actual source misattribution. As one possibility, misled subjects may remember that postevent items were presented only verbally, yet report having seen postevent items, reasoning that the experimenter who prepared the narrative must have known what was in the slides, and that the postevent items serve as probable candidates of what was shown (Belli, 1989; Lindsay, 1990; McCloskey & Zaragoza, 1985). However, evidence exists that indicates at least some postevent reports involve genuine misattributions of source. Loftus, Donders, Hoffman, and Schooler (1989) found that misled subjects respond as quickly and confidently to postevent items as they do to event items regarding whether the objects were seen, and subjects have been shown to be willing to bet substantial sums of money on having seen the postevent items (Weingardt, Toland, & Loftus, 1994). In addition, subjects may continue to make the source misattribution that they remember having seen postevent items despite strong warnings that the items came only from the verbal postevent information and not from the original visual event (Belli et al., 1994; Zaragoza & Lane, 1992). Postevent items must share characteristics in common with event items for people to have such a high degree of confidence in them.

Other evidence reveals that the characteristics of memories about the sources of event and postevent items may be similar but not identical (see Schooler, Gerhard, & Loftus, 1986). Reports of postevent items are reduced among misled subjects when they are specifically queried and encouraged to evaluate the sources of remembered items (the "source monitoring test," see Lindsay & Johnson, 1989; Zaragoza & Koshmider, 1989). Nevertheless, source misattributions have been shown to occur even with source monitoring tests (Ackil & Zaragoza, 1992; Carris, Zaragoza, & Lane, 1992;

Zaragoza & Lane, 1992; Zaragoza & Moore, 1990). Thus, misled subjects at times do remember having seen items that were only suggested to them.

Using "logic of opposition" instructions, Lindsay (1990) provided especially convincing evidence that subjects truly do remember having seen postevent items. Lindsay used a cued-recall test (e.g., what type of tool did the man place in his tool box?) that specifically requested that subjects report only those items seen in the slides, and in which any response that involved reporting a postevent item was incorrect. Most importantly, with the "logic of opposition" instructions, subjects were correctly informed that there was no question on the test for which a correct answer was an item from the postevent narrative. Thus, if subjects remembered that the source of an item was the narrative, they were instructed not to report that item since it would be incorrect. Despite the "logic of opposition" instructions, subjects in the misled condition significantly reported having seen postevent items more often (27% of all responses) in comparison to the control condition (9% of all responses, reflecting a guessing rate). Lindsay's study highlights the extent to which suggested details may become incorporated into people's memories of eyewitnessed events.

Source Misattribution of Events with Greater Complexity

Research on the misinformation effect has shown that people will remember having seen details of events that had only been suggested to them. However, the situation is obviously much more complex when adults suddenly remember having been sexually abused as children. Such memories involve whole events or a whole series of events, not, as some have emphasized, the relatively minor details in the events included with the misinformation effect studies (Darton, 1991; Franklin & Wright, 1991). In addition, memories of sexual abuse involve one's own participation (even if it is unwilling) in the event, as opposed to being an uninvolved witness, as is the case with most of the studies on the misinformation effect. Thus, one potential difficulty in generalizing from the misinformation effect to memories of abuse is the pallid nature of the suggested items used in the typical laboratory research.

On the other hand, there is research that has shown source misattribution with events of considerably great complexity. In one experiment, Intraub and Hoffman (1992) showed subjects color photographs of rich and complex scenes, such as a father holding a son at a zoo to look at an elephant. Subjects also read paragraphs describing scenes that were and were not shown visually. In a follow-up test conducted 1 week later, in which subjects were presented with the same paragraphs that they had read earlier with some additional new paragraphs, and were asked to determine if they had seen a corresponding photograph for each paragraph, subjects often claimed (38%

of the time) they had seen color photographs corresponding to paragraphs that had actually not been associated with any photograph. In addition, when asked to freely recall only those photographs they had seen, and to be careful to exclude any scenes presented only in paragraph form, 29% of all the free recalls were of scenes that the subject only read about. Finally, a few subjects were asked to draw remembered photographs, and again, some of the drawings were of scenes presented only in paragraph form. Clearly, subjects were remembering having seen complex scenes that were presented solely in verbal form.

Other research has shown that subjects will misremember actions that they imagined themselves as performing as actions they actually did perform. Foley and Johnson (1985), and Lindsay, Johnson, and Kwon (1991), had subjects either perform simple actions (such as touching one's toes or crossing one's arms) or imagine themselves as performing these actions. Although children were more likely than adults to confuse imagined actions with real ones, adults also showed source misattributions. In related work, Anderson (1984) presented adult subjects with line drawings of common objects, and had the subjects actually trace the outline of half of the drawings and imagine themselves tracing the outline of the remaining half. In a follow-up test, among the drawings that were correctly remembered as having been presented earlier, the adult subjects remembered having actually traced 39% of the drawings that they had only imagined tracing. In short, these experiments show that people have difficulty determining that their imagined actions are not real.

The above evidence shows that people sometimes will remember simple imagined actions as real events. Yet, a report of sexual abuse involves a considerably more extensive degree of self-involvement in the activity. Recent evidence (Loftus & Coan, in press) from five individuals, two 8-year-old children, one 14-year-old, and two adults, has shown that an extensive childhood memory of an incident that never really happened can be implanted in a person. In this study, the five subjects were each told by a trusted relative of an incident occurring when they were around 5 years of age in which they had been briefly lost. The trusted relative initially provided some details, such as where the event happened, how the person was found, and that the event had been scary for all involved. All subjects were asked if they remembered the incident at some point later. The older subjects were instructed to attempt to remember the incident every day for several days; some of the subjects were also asked about the incident several weeks later. Four of the subjects produced additional details about the event, such as the color of a flannel shirt that a stranger wore, or the existence of an elevator bell. One subject was so convinced of the genuineness of the memory that during debriefing he strongly resisted accepting the fact that the memory was implanted.

Taken together, the experimental evidence shows that subjects sometimes remember events that never happened, ranging from the trivial to the profound, from the simple to the complex, from their witnessing another's actions to their remembering their own actions. Given the extent to which subjects will misattribute suggested or imagined events as real in the laboratory, raises questions about the veridicality of some reports of repressed sexual abuse memories "recovered" through the assistance of a therapist or self-help guide.

THE SOURCE MONITORING FRAMEWORK

The experimental literature highlights the ease with which subjects can be encouraged to misattribute the source of their remembered experiences, so that events that were either suggested or imagined are remembered as having actually occurred. Yet, the literature simultaneously shows that subjects can also be accurate in identifying the sources of their memories (e.g., see Ackil & Zaragoza, 1992; Foley & Johnson, 1985; Lindsay & Johnson, 1989; Lindsay et al., 1991; Zaragoza & Koshmider, 1989). Any attempt to evaluate whether particular memories are accurate or inaccurate with respect to their source (especially when the particular memories involve adults providing recently evoked reports of childhood sexual abuse), requires an understanding of the conditions necessary for source misattribution to occur.

One theoretical approach that has been very helpful for predicting the accuracies and errors in remembering the source of past experiences has been the *source monitoring* framework, developed by Johnson et al. (1993), and other colleagues (e.g., Johnson, Foley, Suengas, & Raye, 1988; Johnson & Raye, 1981). According to this framework, the source of one's memories is not directly specified in the memories themselves, but rather, source information is inferred from various aspects of the content contained in the memories. In other words, determining the source of one's memories involves an attribution process. The process can be more or less deliberative, and appears to be based on the characteristics of the remembered information.

One particular attribution that people must make involves determining whether a particular item of remembered information was originally generated externally, such as in the case of perceptual experience, or whether it was originally generated internally, such as through the acceptance of suggestion or through imagination. This process has been called *reality monitoring* (Johnson, 1985, 1988a, 1988b; Johnson, Foley, Suengas, & Raye, 1988; Johnson & Raye, 1981). In other words, "reality monitoring" deals with choosing whether to attribute the source of remembered information to external reality or to internal generation.

As in the case of all source monitoring, reality monitoring attributions are based on the characteristics of the remembered information. During encoding (when an event is originally acquired), information that originates from an external source is likely to be encoded with rich perceptual information (e.g., visual and acoustic detail) that is associated with perceptually experiencing a real world event. On the other hand, information that originates internally, such as through fantasy, is likely to be heavily encoded with information resulting from cognitive, thinking, and reflective processes, which the individual uses to generate the images. Consider, for example, the different experiences of an individual who actually travels in space and one who simply imagines such an event. The real space traveler *perceptually* experiences weightlessness, whereas the person who fantasizes must *think* about what weightlessness would be like (e.g., "If I were in space; I'd float around the space ship"). Although the real space traveler may also think about the experience, and the imaginary space traveler may be able to conjure up a perceptual sense that approximates what actual weightlessness might be like, the space travel events as encoded by these individuals would nevertheless consist of information that differs with respect to perceptual and cognitive characteristics.

In addition, not only are the characteristics that are encoded different depending on source, but to some degree, these characteristics are preserved in memory over time. Thus, during later remembering, events that originated externally are likely to have richer perceptual information than events internally generated, whereas internally originated events are likely to have richer information about cognitive operations than events externally experienced (Johnson, Foley, Suengas, & Raye, 1988; Schooler et al., 1986). Using relatively nondeliberative processes, people are often correct in their attributions of source; they are likely to attribute a memory with rich perceptual information to an external source, whereas they are likely to attribute a memory richer in information on cognitive operations to an internal source (Johnson et al., 1993).

Source Misattributions

Despite the above information, source misattributions often occur when the characteristics of the remembered information are not reliable indicants of source. Misattributing an internally generated event to an external experience is likely to arise either when a memory of the event has few characteristics that mark the presence of cognitive operations typically associated with the imagination, or there is an abundance of perceptual aspects typically associated with an external experience.

With regard to cognitive operations, dreams are internally generated events but they lack information about cognitive operations because they are generated unconsciously, and thus are not thought about or reflected upon consciously. Consistent with the source monitoring framework, Johnson, Kahan, and Raye (1984) found that memories of one's own dreams are not particularly easy to differentiate from memories of another person's dreams. Relatedly, in degrading the conditions of either the encoding or the testing process, by dividing subjects' attention at encoding or by forcing subjects to make rapid source decisions at testing, a greater likelihood exists that subjects will misattribute internally generated stimuli as being externally generated (Jacoby, Woloshyn, & Kelley, 1989; Zaragoza & Lane, 1991). In other words, people will think they perceived something they only imagined. Subjects apparently make these source misattributions because when faced with degraded conditions they are less able to encode, or to process at testing, information about the cognitive activity associated with the memories. As a consequence, subjects base their attributions on less reliable source information such as familiarity.

With regard to perceptual information, substantive evidence reveals the crucial role played by the quality or quantity of the imagery or visualization employed in the internal generation of an event. For instance, increasing the similarity of perceptual information about an imagined event to that of an external event enhances the likelihood the source will be misattributed as a real external event. Subjects are relatively good at differentiating the source of their memories for words they actually said from words they imagine another saying, and also good at discriminating words actually said by another person from words they imagine themselves as saying. However, they do significantly poorer with source judgments that require their discriminating words they actually said from words they only imagined themselves as saying (Foley, Santini, & Sopasakis, 1989), or those that require discriminating words another person actually said from words they imagined being said in that other person's voice (Johnson, Foley, & Leach, 1988). The perceptual information associated with another's voice is quite different from that associated with one's own voice, and people less often confuse reality with imagination when it comes to different voices. However, the perceptual information involved in a genuine perception is quite similar to the perceptual information generated in imagination when a voice from the same person is experienced in reality and used in imagination.

Relatedly, subjects are relatively good at differentiating the sources of memories of objects they actually drew from those they merely looked at, but much poorer at differentiating the sources of memories of actual tracings from imagined ones (Anderson, 1984). Apparently, in imagining that one is tracing an object, similar perceptual information is created to that which results from actually tracing an object, in both quantity and quality.

The misinformation effect is likely to be, at least partly, the result of subjects' visualizing the misleading postevent information. Encouraging the additional visualization of postevent misinformation, either by having subjects answer questions that may implicitly encourage them to visualize misinformation (Zaragoza & Lane, 1992), or by explicitly instructing them to visualize postevent information read in a narrative (Carris et al., 1992), has also been shown to exacerbate the misattribution of the source of the misinformation to the original event.

Asymmetries in source monitoring errors also reveal the important role that visualization plays in encouraging source misattributions. Subjects are more likely to misattribute the source of an imagined or suggested memory to a memory for an actual event, than to misattribute the source of a memory of an actual event to an imagined or suggested event (Anderson, 1984; Belli et al., 1994; Foley, Durso, Wilder, & Friedman, 1991). In other words, people are more likely to think that they have perceived an event they have only imagined than to think they have only imagined an event that they have actually perceived. Through their imagination, people can often visualize the perceptual details that would occur if they were doing or witnessing something. Apparently, it is much more difficult when one is actually doing or witnessing something to visualize the cognitive processes that would occur if one were only imagining the act.

In summary, although source attributions are often accurate when based on the qualitative characteristics of memories, misattributions may arise when these characteristics are not reliable indices of source. Moreover, conditions that degrade the characteristic reliability of the source of information will enhance source misattributions, as illustrated by the experimental evidence. In the next section, we show that, in general, memories of childhood experiences can often be inaccurate when those qualitative characteristics that lead to accurate source attributions are deficient. More specifically, we hypothesize that therapy and self-help sources may introduce conditions that enhance the likelihood of source confusion.

Childhood Memories

An abundance of experimental research on source misattributions has tested our ability to discriminate internally from externally generated *recent* events. Most of the research on source misattribution has examined memory for *recent* events. As we have noted, the qualitative characteristics of memories for recent events will tend to be different for internally generated experiences in comparison to those externally perceived. Nevertheless, source misattributions with the memories of recently experienced events can be readily produced in the laboratory by using techniques that encourage the characteristics of memories for internally and externally generated experiences to be more alike.

Interestingly, the extent of differentiation in the qualitative characteristics of real and imagined events is much less pronounced for memories of childhood than for recent events. For instance, Johnson, Foley, Suengas, and Raye (1988) had subjects remember perceived (e.g., a visit to a library) and imaginary (e.g., a fantasy) events that occurred both recently and in childhood. Subjects then rated each memory on a wide range of characteristics, including those of a perceptual, affective, and cognitive nature. Importantly, and consistent with the source monitoring framework, perceived significantly differed from imagined recent events on most (20 of 37) of the characteristics, with perceived events having higher ratings on perceptual characteristics (e.g., visual detail, sound, smell, taste, spatial arrangement of objects and people), while imagined events had higher ratings on cognitive characteristics (e.g., implications, complexity). For childhood events, however, perceived significantly differed from imagined events on only 3 of the 37 characteristics. Moreover, for perceived events, recent experiences received higher ratings than childhood experiences on 13 of the 37 characteristics, which mostly dealt with perceptual information (e.g., visual detail, vividness, and spatial arrangement of objects and people). Thus, largely because of the lack of perceptual information about childhood memories, memories of perceived and imagined childhood events are more similar to each other with respect to qualitative characteristics than are memories of perceived and imagined recent events. Given that people often determine the source of remembered information on the basis of qualitative characteristics, the study by Johnson, Foley, Suengas, and Raye (1988) highly suggests that misattributing the source of an imagined event to an actual event ought to occur more readily for childhood memories than for memories of recent events. "One might require a substantial amount of perceptual detail before accepting an experience as a memory of an actual recent event and require less to accept it as a memory of an actual long-ago event" (Johnson et al., 1993, p. 5).

Given that memories of childhood perceptual events tend to be lacking in perceptual information, any addition of imagery and visualization to an imaginary event, which will increase the amount of perceptual information associated with an imaginary event, ought to be quite effective in leading one to misattribute the source of an imaginary event to reality. As noted above, Loftus and Coan (in press) were able to induce false childhood memories by encouraging subjects to visualize perceptual details that were part of an imagined experience. In therapy as well, therapists may encourage clients to visualize events that never happened through suggestion (Loftus, 1993). Some therapists have been documented asking leading questions that encourage adult clients to visualize having been abused as children. They may ask questions such as, "You know, in my experience, a lot of people who are struggling with many of the same problems you are have often had some kind of really painful things happen to them as kids—maybe they were beaten and molested. And I wonder if anything like that ever happened to you?" (Forward & Buck, 1988, p. 161). Or they may say, "Your symptoms sound like you've been abused when you were a child. What can you tell me about that?" (Trott, 1991, p. 18), or even more suggestively, "You sound to me like the sort of person who must have been sexually abused. Tell me what that bastard did to you" (Davis, 1991, p. 82).

If no particular memories are revealed, therapists may encourage their clients to guess about possible abuse or to tell a story regarding abuse (Olio, 1989). Other techniques include interpreting client dreams in such a way the clients are encouraged to visualize abuse memories (Poston & Lison, 1990; Watters, 1991). As noted above, dream memories lack a cognitive dimension, which is unusual for memories that lack an internal source during the waking state. Due to this lack, the source of dreams may be fairly easily misattributed to external reality. Indeed, it is a common experience to be confused about whether what has happened in a dream is real. Despite the uncertainty in the reality of dreams, therapists may encourage clients to interpret the content of dreams as including themes of abuse, which are, in turn, reflections of real events (Williams, 1987). Although it is true that dreams often do contain content that elaborates upon what is happening in daily life (Hall & Van deCastle, 1966), such a fact raises a most troubling possibility. Dreams containing abuse themes may emerge in therapy as the *result* of an initial suggestion to the client that he or she is the victim of abuse (Loftus, 1993).

Perhaps the use of hypnosis and hypnotic age regression is the most potent solicitor of abuse allegations. In general, the reliability of hypnotically enhanced memory has been extensively questioned in the literature (Smith, 1983). In particular, hypnotic age regression is suspected to be disturbingly unreliable in producing authentic memory (Nash, 1987). It even has occasionally led to such bizarre memories as being abducted by extraterrestrial aliens (Gordon, 1991). Relatedly, hypnotically induced false memories have been readily produced in controlled conditions (Laurence & Perry, 1983).

Visualizing abuse is not the only manner by which a source attribution of reality can be induced. Some therapists also encourage clients to focus on how they feel given the supposed abuse. Interestingly, remembering feelings tends to make imagined and perceived events more alike, thus enhancing the danger of source misattribution (Johnson, 1988; Suengas & Johnson, 1988). Clients routinely report recovering abuse memories associated with an extensive degree of strong feeling. Although people may become convinced of the authenticity of these reports because of the overwhelming affect associated with them (Loftus, 1993), strong emotion has not been clearly demonstrated to be a reliable signal for authenticity.

Strategic Processes

The "source monitoring" framework (Johnson, 1988; Johnson et al., 1993; Johnson & Raye, 1981) emphasizes that attributions of source are not based on the characteristics of remembered experiences alone. People may engage in deliberate strategic processes when making determinations of source, such as retrieving other memories or evidence that supports the source attribution, or evaluating the semantic content of their memories and the likelihood that such memories may have come from particular sources. For example, consider that you remember having read that life was discovered on Mars. If you are fairly well-versed in astronomy, you would be aware that no reputable astronomy source would make such a claim when deliberating on the potential source of this memory. You might then attribute the source to an irresponsible publication, perhaps a popular tabloid.

When subjects are encouraged (as opposed to not encouraged) to specify the source of a remembered item or event, they are more likely than not to employ strategic processes so as to promote better source discriminations between event and misleading postevent information (Lindsay, 1994; Lindsay & Johnson, 1989; Zaragoza & Koshmider, 1989; Zaragoza & Lane, 1992). When asked to do so, subjects apparently do employ stricter criteria in attributing the source of postevent misinformation to an event. In addition, strategic processes have been shown to help subjects correctly identify the source of information as imagined memory when that is the case. One subject, for example, knew that a childhood memory was a fantasy because the subject remembered being a doctor at the time, yet realized that the event originally happened when the person was too young to have been a doctor (Johnson, Foley, Suengas, & Raye, 1988).

Strategic processes may also be used in therapy by clients who begin to develop memories of being sexually abused as children, as they attempt to determine whether these memories originated in imagination or reality. If, for example, a client remembers having had an overall happy childhood with loving parents, a memory of abuse may be so dissonant with these other memories that the client may attribute the source of the memory to imagination or suggestion. Certainly, some clients reject the suggestion of abuse.

On the other hand, despite the experimental evidence (Anderson, 1984; Belli et al., 1994) that reporting a real event as imaginary occurs more frequently than reporting an imaginary event as real, therapists often attempt to convince their clients of the authenticity of abuse when clients sense that a visualization is not authentic (Petersen, 1991). For instance, they may inform their clients that not accepting the visualizations as real is part of the resistance associated with keeping an authentic memory of a traumatic event out of full awareness (Bass & Davis, 1988). They may seek to support any visualizations as authentic memories with other evidence, such as explaining the abuse in terms of the client's precipitating problem. Clients usually view therapists as experts who know the cause of their discomfort, and thus may be motivated to accept suggestions from them.

In other instances, clients may come into therapy with no memories of abuse, but may have had, or currently have, strained relations with their parents. In this situation, any discovered memories of abuse could be supported by other memories associated with the strained relationship. Finding memories consistent in tone with abuse may contribute to encouraging clients to conclude that the abuse actually occurred (cf. Johnson et al., 1993).

In many instances, despite encouragement from therapists, clients will not conjure up any memories of abuse (Loftus, 1993), which may be understood by therapists as a sign of continued repression (Blume, 1990). Yet, through faulty reasoning, many other clients may come to believe that they were abused as children when, in fact, they were not. Therapists may encourage clients to consider supporting evidence. They may emphasize that the symptoms are characteristic of abuse victims, and that any uncomfortable feeling, whether physical or psychological, is a sign of abuse. Thus, despite having no clear memory of any abuse incident, clients will come to believe that they had an abusive past. Consider the following comments from *The Courage to Heal* (Bass & Davis, 1988): "If you are unable to remember any specific instances . . . but still have a feeling that something abusive happened to you, it probably did. . . . If you think you were abused and your life shows the symptoms, then you were" (pp. 21–22).[3]

In summary, although strategic processes may initially lead clients to question the authenticity of abuse, therapists may encourage them to focus on aspects of their experiences that support the belief abusive events really took place. Unfortunately, there are no firm criteria by which the authenticity of abuse claims can be judged, since determining whether the source of memories is the imagination or reality is an error-prone attributional process.

CONCLUSION

The literature on experimental psychology has shown that false memories are relatively easy to produce in the laboratory through suggestion and encouraging the use of the imagination. We have begun to understand the factors associated with the promotion of false memories. Visualizing perceptual detail while imagining something facilitates the later misattribution that the source of a memory is reality. In addition, providing evidence that is believed to be consistent with an abuse theme may lead one to develop a false memory through strategic processes. Finally, discriminating the sources of real and imagined events is more difficult when the events occurred during childhood than if they occurred more recently.

We have also suggested that those factors that are implicated in promoting false memories in the laboratory may resemble those used by therapists, who may be inadvertently intent on uncovering repressed memories of abuse. Particularly with the symptoms associated with dissociative disorders, therapists may be inclined to posit the existence of a traumatic past and infer the presence of repressed memories. In order to uncover these inferred memories, clients may then be encouraged to visualize being abused and may be presented with arguments that support an interpretation that abuse has occurred. Moreover, childhood memories appear particularly vulnerable to false claims regarding their reality. These considerations make us skeptical about the authenticity of some reports of repressed childhood abuse memories.

Although we are concerned that false reports of abuse often may be honest fabrications, we do not deny the possibility of authentic repressed memories. However, given the attributional nature of determining the source of memories, there simply is no reliable means to correctly judge when a memory is based in reality and when it is not. In our view, the practice by some therapists of encouraging adult clients to recover memories of childhood abuse is creating the very real danger that child abuse incidents are being misreported. In addition to the tragic consequences for the accusers and accused involved with false reports, such misreporting also drains needed resources away from the genuine victims. Further, society may come to doubt the experiences of actual victims given a climate wherein the abuse reports of clients are uncritically accepted and encouraged during the course of therapy, no matter how dubious. If anyone is a victim, then no one is.

ACKNOWLEDGMENT

We thank Steve Lindsay for his very helpful comments on an earlier version of this chapter.

NOTES

1. Researchers (e.g., Lindsay & Johnson, 1989; Zaragoza & Lane, 1992) have also pointed out that subjects also commit source misattributions when they remember that misinformation occurred both during and after the event.

2. Of course, any reports of postevent items among control subjects represent guesses, since they were not exposed to any misinformation.
3. The symptoms mentioned include low self-esteem, suicidal or self-destructive thoughts, depression, and sexual dysfunction, among others. Although sexual abuse may lead to such symptoms, there are a number of other causes of them. An additional passage in *The Courage to Heal* expresses the suggestive theme that one must believe having been abused despite contradictory evidence: "Even if your memories are incomplete, even if your family insists nothing ever happened, you still must believe yourself. Even if what you experienced feels too extreme to be possible or too mild to be abuse, even if you think 'I must have made it up' . . . you have to come to terms with the fact that someone did those things to you. This is something you will have to acknowledge again and again" (p. 87).

REFERENCES

Ackil, J., & Zaragoza, M. S. (1992, November). *Developmental differences in source monitoring and eyewitness suggestibility.* Poster presented at the meeting of the Psychonomic Society, St. Louis, MO.

Anderson, R. E. (1984). Did I do it or did I only imagine doing it? *Journal of Experimental Psychology: General, 113,* 594–613.

Bass, E., & Davis, L. (1988). *The courage to heal.* New York: Harper & Row.

Belli, R. F. (1988). Color blend retrievals: Compromise memories or deliberate compromise responses? *Memory and Cognition, 16,* 314–326.

Belli, R. F. (1989). Influences of misleading postevent information: Misinformation interference and acceptance. *Journal of Experimental Psychology: General, 118,* 72–85.

Belli, R. F., Lindsay, D. S., Gales, M. S., & McCarthy, T. T. (1994). Memory impairment and source misattribution in postevent misinformation experiments with short retention intervals. *Memory and Cognition, 22,* 40–54.

Belli, R. F., Windschitl, P. D., McCarthy, T. T., & Winfrey, S. E. (1992). Detecting memory impairment with a modified test procedure: Manipulating retention interval with centrally presented event items. *Journal of Experimental Psychology: Learning, Memory, and Cognition, 18,* 356–367.

Blume, E. S. (1990). *Secret survivors: Uncovering incest and its aftereffects in women.* New York: Ballantine.

Braun, B. G., & Sachs, R. G. (1988, October). *Recognition of possible cult involvement in MPD patients.* Paper presented at the Fifth International conference on Multiple Personality/Dissociative States, Chicago, IL.

Carris, M., Zaragoza, M. S., & Lane, S. (1992, May). *The role of visual imagery in source misattribution errors.* Paper presented at the meeting of the Midwestern Psychological Association, Chicago, IL.

Ceci, S. J., Ross, D. F., & Toglia, M. P. (1987). Suggestibility in children's memory: Psycholegal implications. *Journal of Experimental Psychology: General, 116,* 38–49.

Chandler, C. C. (1991). How memory for an event is influenced by related events: Interference in modified recognition tests. *Journal of Experimental Psychology: Learning, Memory, and Cognition, 17,* 115–125.

Chu, J. A. (1988). Ten traps for therapists in the treatment of trauma survivors. *Dissociation, 1,* 24–32.

Daro, D. (1988). *Confronting child abuse.* New York: Free Press.

Darton, N. (1991, Oct. 7). The pain of the last taboo. *Newsweek,* pp. 70–72.

Davis, L. (1991). Murdered memory. *In Health, 5,* 79–84.

Finkelhor, D. (1986). *A sourcebook on child sexual abuse.* Newbury Park, CA: Sage.

Foley, M. A., Durso, F. T., Wilder, A., & Friedman, R. (1991). Developmental comparisons of explicit versus implicit imagery and reality monitoring. *Journal of Experimental Child Psychology, 51,* 1–13.

Foley, M. A., & Johnson, M. K. (1985). Confusions between memories for performed and imagined actions. *Child Development, 56,* 1145–1155.

Foley, M. A., Santini, C., & Sopasakis, M. (1989). Discriminating between memories: Evidence for children's spontaneous elaborations. *Journal of Experimental Child Psychology, 48,* 146–169.

Forward, S., & Buck, C. (1988). *Betrayal of innocence: Incest and its devastation.* New York: Penguin.

Franklin, E., & Wright, W. (1991). *Sins of the father.* New York: Crown.

Ganaway, G. K. (1989). Historical versus narrative truth: Clarifying the role of exogenous trauma in the etiology of MPD and its variants. *Dissociation, 2,* 205–220.

Gibling, F., & Davies, G. (1988). Reinstatement of context following exposure to post-event information. *British Journal of Psychology, 79,* 129–141.

Gordon, J. S. (1991). The UFO experience. *The Atlantic Monthly, 268,* 82–92.

Hall, C. S., & Van deCastle, R. L. (1966). *The content analysis of dreams.* New York: Appleton-Century-Crofts.

Intraub, H., & Hoffman, J. E. (1992). Reading and visual memory: Remembering scenes that were never seen. *American Journal of Psychology, 105,* 101–114.

Jacoby, L. L., Woloshyn, V., & Kelley, C. (1989). Becoming famous without being recognized: Unconscious influences of memory produced by dividing attention. *Journal of Experimental Psychology: General, 118,* 115–125.

Johnson, M. K. (1985). The origin of memories. In P. C. Kendall (Ed.), *Advances in cognitive-behavioral research and therapy* (Vol. 4, pp. 1–26). New York: Academic Press.

Johnson, M. K. (1988a). Discriminating the origin of information. In T. F. Oltmanns & B. A. Maher (Eds.), *Delusional beliefs: Interdisciplinary perspectives* (pp. 34–65). New York: John Wiley.

Johnson, M. K. (1988b). Reality monitoring: An experimental phenomenological approach. *Journal of Experimental Psychology: General, 117,* 390–394.

Johnson, M. K., Foley, M. A., & Leach, K. (1988). The consequences for memory of imagining in another person's voice. *Memory and Cognition, 16,* 337–342.

Johnson, M. K., Foley, M. A., Suengas, A. G., & Raye, C. L. (1988). Phenomenal characteristics of memories for perceived and imagined autobiographical events. *Journal of Experimental Psychology: General, 117,* 371–376.

Johnson, M. K., Hashtroudi, S., & Lindsay, D. S. (1993). Source monitoring. *Psychological Bulletin, 114,* 3–28.

Johnson, M. K., Kahan, T. L., & Raye, C. L. (1984). Dreams and reality monitoring. *Journal of Experimental Psychology: General, 113,* 329–343.

Johnson, M. K., & Raye, C. L. (1981). Reality monitoring. *Psychological Review, 88*, 67–85.

LaFontaine, J. (1990). *Child sexual abuse.* Cambridge, England: Polity Press.

Laurence, J. R., & Perry, C. (1983). Hypnotically created memory among highly hypnotizable subjects. *Science, 222*, 523–524.

Lindsay, D. S. (1990). Misleading suggestions can impair eyewitnesses' ability to remember event details. *Journal of Experimental Psychology: Learning, Memory, and Cognition, 16*, 1077–1083.

Lindsay, D. S. (1994). Memory source monitoring and eyewitness testimony. In D. F. Ross, J. D. Read, & M. P. Toglia (Eds.), *Adult eyewitness testimony: Current trends and developments* (pp. 27–55). New York: Cambridge University Press.

Lindsay, D. S., & Johnson, M. K. (1989). The eyewitness suggestibility effect and memory for source. *Memory and Cognition, 17*, 349–358.

Lindsay, D. S., Johnson, M. K., & Kwon, P. (1991). Developmental changes in memory source monitoring. *Journal of Experimental Child Psychology, 52*, 297–318.

Loftus, E. F. (1993). The reality of repressed memories. *American Psychologist, 48*, 518–537.

Loftus, E. F., & Coan, J. (in press). The construction of childhood memories. In D. Peters (Ed.), *The child witness in context: Cognitive, social, and legal perspectives.* New York: Kluwer.

Loftus, E. F., Donders, K., Hoffman, H. G., & Schooler, J. W. (1989). Creating new memories that are quickly accessed and confidently held. *Memory and Cognition, 17*, 607–616.

Loftus, E. F., & Hoffman, H. G. (1989). Misinformation and memory: The creation of new memories. *Journal of Experimental Psychology: General, 118*, 100–104.

Loftus, E. F., Hoffman, H. G., & Wagenaar, W. A. (1992). The misinformation effect: Transformations in memory induced by postevent information. In M. L. Howe, C. J. Brainerd, & V. F. Reyna (Eds.), *Development of long-term retention* (pp. 159–183). New York: Springer-Verlag.

Loftus, E. F., Miller, D. G., & Burns, H. J. (1978). Semantic integration of verbal information into a visual memory. *Journal of Experimental Psychology: Human Learning and Memory, 4*, 19–31.

Lynn, S. J., & Nash, M. (1994). Truth in memory: Ramifications for psychotherapy and hypnotherapy. *American Journal of Clinical Hypnosis, 36*, 194–208.

McCloskey, M., & Zaragoza, M. (1985). Misleading postevent information and memory for events: Arguments and evidence against memory impairment hypotheses. *Journal of Experimental Psychology: General, 114*, 1–16.

Nash, M. (1987). What, if anything, is regressed about hypnotic age regression? A review of the empirical literature. *Psychological Bulletin, 102*, 42–52.

Olio, K. A. (1989). Memory retrieval in the treatment of adult survivors of sexual abuse. *Transactional Analysis Journal, 19*, 93–94.

Petersen, B. (1991). *Dancing with Daddy: A childhood lost and a life regained.* New York: Bantam.

Poston, C., & Lison, K. (1990). *Reclaiming our lives: Hope for adult survivors of incest.* New York: Bantam.

Schooler, J. W., Gerhard, D., & Loftus, E. F. (1986). Qualities of the unreal. *Journal of Experimental Psychology: Learning, Memory, and Cognition, 12*, 171–181.

Sheehan, P. W., & Tilden, J. (1986). The consistency of occurrences of memory distortion following hypnotic induction. *International Journal of Clinical and Experimental Hypnosis, 34*, 122–137.

Smith, M. (1983). Hypnotic memory enhancement of witnesses: Does it work? *Psychological Bulletin, 94*, 387–407.

Suengas, A. G., & Johnson, M. K. (1988). Qualitative effects of rehearsal on memories for perceived and imagined complex events. *Journal of Experimental Psychology: General, 117*, 377–389.

Trott, J. (1991). The grade five syndrome. *Cornerstone, 20*, 16–18.

Tversky, B., & Tuchin, M. (1989). A reconciliation of the evidence on eyewitness testimony: Comments on McCloskey and Zaragoza. *Journal of Experimental Psychology: General, 118*, 86–91.

Watters, E. (1991). The devil in Mr. Ingram. *Mother Jones, 16*, 30–33, 65–68.

Weingardt, K. R., Toland, H. K., & Loftus, E. F. (1994). Reports of suggested memories: Do people truly believe them? In D. F. Ross, J. D. Read, & M. P. Toglia (Eds.), *Adult eyewitness testimony: Current trends and developments* (pp. 3–26). New York: Cambridge University Press.

Williams, M. (1987). Reconstruction of an early seduction and its aftereffects. *Journal of the American Psychoanalytic Association, 15*, 145–163.

Zaragoza, M. S., & Koshmider, J. W. III. (1989). Misled subjects may know more than their performance implies. *Journal of Experimental Psychology: Learning, Memory, and Cognition, 15*, 246–255.

Zaragoza, M. S., & Lane, S. (1991, November). *The role of attentional resources in suggestibility.* Paper presented at the meeting of the Psychonomic Society, San Francisco, CA.

Zaragoza, M. S., & Lane, S. M. (1992). *Source misattributions and the suggestibility of eyewitness memory.* Unpublished manuscript.

Zaragoza, M. S., & Moore, K. (1990, November). *Source misattributions in eyewitness memory.* Poster presented at the meeting of the Psychonomic Society, New Orleans, LA.

20

Dissociation and Multiple Personality: Conflicts and Controversies

Richard Horevitz

The topic of clinical dissociative disorders, especially Multiple Personality Disorder (MPD) and its more attenuated forms, has become the focus of a lively, though often acrimonious, debate. Today, as occurred a hundred years ago, professional viability and scientific esteem are at stake (cf. Ellenberger, 1970; van der Hart & van der Kolk, 1991; Frankel, 1993; Bowers & Davidson, 1991; McHugh, 1992; Orne & Dinges, 1989; Orne & Bates, 1992; Mersky, 1992). The question of the "reality" of MPD is most often the focus of the debate, which occurs in a polemical climate (Dell, 1988; Hilgard, 1988) and impedes scientific study (Putnam, 1991).

MPD once thought to be rare, is being diagnosed with ever increasing frequency.[1] Its mention in the clinical and scientific literature has grown exponentially: averaging from just under one citation per year between 1791 and 1970; to nine citations per year between 1971 and 1980; to 60 citations per year between 1981 and 1990 (Gotteman, Greaves, & Coons, 1992). Multiple personality is now commonly featured in popular media publications, television and documentary specials, feature articles, and talk shows.

A century ago, the diagnosis and scientific exploration of MPD also was very much in vogue. Scientific work in this area appeared to provide a unique window to the nature of human consciousness (Ellenberger, 1970). Moral and legal concerns also were raised due to the idea that MPD patients may or may not be personally responsible for their actions (cf. Sutcliffe & Jones, 1962, pp. 236–243). MPD patients were all viewed as highly hypnotizable and were often, though not always, discovered to have MPD in the course of hypnosis or hypnotic treatment. Thus, investigators interested in either hypnosis or MPD became involved in the other (Ellenberger, 1970;

Sutcliffe, 1961). Set in the larger intellectual ferment of the times, interest in MPD and hypnosis engendered both "credulity" and "skepticism" (Sutcliffe, 1960; Ellenberger, 1970); credulity because the phenomena of both hypnosis and MPD are astonishing and quite compelling, and skepticism because so much of what astonishes and compels, on closer examination, appears other than it first seemed.

THE CONTROVERSY

The dramatic increase in the diagnosis of MPD has led to a controversy that centers on the *meaning* of this increase. Are we in the midst of a form of social hysteria akin to the periodic eruptions of witchcraft and possession passions that have characterized European (and American) culture over the years (Spanos, 1989; Aldridge-Morris, 1989)? Have some clinicians become so fascinated with the *possibility* of multiplicity in patients that they covertly elicit it during therapy (Orne, Dinges, & Orne, 1984; Halleck, 1990; Bowers, 1991; Kampman, 1992; Frankel, 1990)? Or, have some clinicians, attuned to the complex social pathology that results from the pervasive and perverse abuse of children, become better diagnosticians of the secret inner worlds of childhood trauma survivors, which are characterized by fragmented, autonomous self-structures heretofore hidden under an adaptive veneer of reasonably solid adult functioning (Goodwin, 1985; Kluft, 1985a; Putnam, 1989; Ross, Anderson, Fleisher, & Norton, 1991)?

A controversy that "generat[es] heated polemics at professional meetings and protracted running battles in the correspondence sections of the leading journals" (Putnam, 1991, p. 490) inevitably hampers genuine scientific discovery and understanding. Nonetheless, it is possible to step back and assess the controversy in terms of a potential common ground, genuine conflicts, as well as the philosophical and scientific problems that underlie the conflict.

In this chapter, I will particularly address the issues that have their origins in the controversies of a century ago. I do so from the perspective of a clinician working on a daily basis with MPD patients who seeks to achieve a deeper scientific understanding of trauma and dissociation.

COMMONALITIES AMONG COMPETING MODELS

There are competing models and metaphors among investigators of MPD, since, in part, not all subscribe to similar theoretical perspectives. Likewise, among critics and skeptics, there is little unanimity in how the disorder is conceptualized, since they possess different theoretical stances.

Nonetheless, I believe three key areas exist in which there is potential for a common ground, which are:

1. A modern flexible process account of personality and personality identity.
2. A recognition that differences exist between clinical dissociation and hypnotic dissociation, as well as the acceptance of the importance of suggestibility, fantasy-proneness, social influence, and acculturation (among other factors) in the development of MPD symptomatology.
3. An awareness of the constructive nature of memory, its proneness to error, and the particular vulnerability of the highly hypnotizable to pseudomemory creation and confabulation.

WHAT IS "PERSONALITY" IN MULTIPLE PERSONALITY DISORDER?

The irreducible core of MPD is the simultaneous existence within an individual of more than one *distinct organization of personal identity*, where *distinct* denotes *"a sense of {one's} own personal existence"* (Kluft, 1991, p. 609). In other words, each identity has a sense of its own personal experience that differs from that of some other identity that "coincidentally" may "inhabit" the same body or somehow share in the same life (Mulhern, 1991). Since such an assertion violates the common sense understanding of terms such as self, individual, and personality (cf. Strawson, 1959), it is difficult to precisely describe what this "distinct organization" might be.[2] Historically, it has been variously labeled "alter personality," "personality," "alter," "entity," "disaggregated self-state," "ego-state," or some other *nonprocess* nominative that attempts to denote fully separate, coexisting individual selves or permanent personality states. While the above labels may capture the 19th-century vision of dissociation, they fail to express a more current understanding.

Kluft and his colleagues (Kluft, Steinberg, & Spitzer, 1988, p. 51) and Putnam (1989, p. 103) made serious attempts to wrangle with providing process rather than state/trait descriptions of personality processes in MPD. Kluft (1991) approached the topic again more recently:

> Putnam and I described reconfigurations rather than reified divisions, emphasizing the personalities should be understood as ways the mind may be organized rather than as "pieces of a pie." From this flows an appreciation that the number of personalities can be quite large because they constitute configurations rather than portions of a unity. (pp. 610–611)

Such formulations are within the scope of many contemporary redefinitions of consciousness (Hilgard, 1977, 1991; Kihlstrom, 1984, 1987), personality processes (e.g., Bandura, 1978; Mischel, 1973, 1979, 1983; Mahoney, 1991; Buss, 1991; Magnusson & Törestad, 1993), cognitive processes (especially the distributed process—Kihlstrom, 1987; McClelland & Rumelhart, 1985; Ratcliff, 1990; Yates & Nasby, 1993), and the complexities of personal identity (Maddi, 1984; Dixon, Brunet, & Laurence, 1990).

However reasonable such formulations may be, they are not without problems. Orne and his colleagues (Orne & Bauer-Manley, 1991; Orne & Bates, 1992) looked at the way in which *metaphors* of the mind and of cognitive organization become reified by the MPD clinicians. "The road between theory and practice," Orne wrote, "is as treacherous as it is important . . . particularly when theory is stated metaphorically" (Orne & Bauer-Manley, 1991, p. 94). He also argued that "Multiple personality disorder (MPD) is a uniquely powerful example of what can happen when theoretical or clinical metaphors are reified and treated as if they were *literally* true" (p. 95). Orne criticized MPD clinicians who ask their patients to provide the names, functions, ages, sex, handedness, or idiosyncratic traits of the "discrete states of consciousness" or "reconfigurations," or ask to speak to a particular part (cf. Braun, 1986). He assumed based on such behavior that MPD clinicians hold the view that there are several competing real individuals (Orne & Dinges, 1989) in the patient. Orne argued that it is the therapist's behavior toward the patient that leads to the imperceptible slide from metaphor to literalism, and that complex theoretical formulations offer no protection against this confusion. Orne is certainly on strong ground here—how one behaves surely has much greater impact than what one says about the behavior. He cautions MPD investigators not to repeat the chimeric agenda of earlier hypnosis researchers who sought to prove that hypnosis was some very special, unique, and real state.

These concerns must be addressed by MPD researchers if conceptual clarity and intellectual rapprochement are to be achieved. Contemporary MPD clinicians hold that direct work with alter identities is essential to treatment. They believe that in order to establish the normal integrative functions of learning, memory, identity, and consciousness, they must pay attention to the separate, distinctly organized self-identities. Should this therapuetic approach and the speculation that underlies it prove valid and enduring, then the study of MPD holds the promise of shedding light on the cognitive processes by which imaginative experience is transduced into compelling reality.

We need to know much more about how, when, under what conditions, and with whom these processes are genuinely therapeutic and when they are countertherapeutic. MPD clinical investigators need to integrate into their treatment the many subtle ways in which identity is continually reformulated to respond to situational demands (e.g. Schlenker, 1985; Schlenker & Weigold, 1992; Mead, 1934; Baumeister, Stillwell, & Wotman, 1990; Goffman, 1959) and therefore, to *design appropriate clinical studies to assess these effects*. This is not as daunting a process as it seems. Theoretical work on the metaphoric and symbolic processes occurring in psychotherapy has a long history (e.g., Bateson, 1972; Langer, 1967; Haley, 1963; Watzlawick, 1978; Whitaker & Malone, 1953). Further, cognitive-behavioral treatments of anxiety and depression have been carefully viewed from the perspective of cognitive change in response to situational demands (for a review, see Brewin, 1989). Hence, a high priority should be placed on investigating the impact of the demand characteristics and expectancies placed on the expression of MPD in treatment.

DISSOCIATION

The distinguishing clinical features of multiple personality disorder are the *dissociative* processes, such as *identity alteration, identity confusion, depersonalization, fugue* and *trancelike states*, and *amnesia*. Since the 19th century, MPD patients have been recognized as highly hypnotizable. A large body of experimental literature confirms this association (e.g., Frischholz, Lipman, Braun, & Sachs, 1992; Frischholz, 1985; Lipman, Braun, & Frischholz, 1984; Lynn, Rhue, & Green, 1988; Nash, Lynn, & Givens, 1984; Bliss, 1984; to name a few). The high hypnotizability found with MPD and other dissociative-disordered patients was thought to be explained by common, underlying dissociative processes (cf. Braun, 1986).

There is an emerging consensus, however, that a link between hypnotizability and MPD was too readily assumed and may be illusory. For example, Frankel (1990), Hilgard (1987, 1991), Carlson and Putnam (1989), van der Hart and Friedman, (1989), and Lynn and colleagues (e.g., Mare, Lynn, Kvall, Sivec, & Sanderberg, 1991), from differing perspectives, all suggest that clinical dissociation should be clearly distinguished from the "dissociative" processes involved in hypnosis.

Little evidence exists of a causal relation between hypnotizability and dissociative disorders, even though childhood abuse has been linked with increased hypnotizability. Early findings (e.g., J.R. Hilgard, 1962) that suggest this connection have not stood up under further investigation (Nash & Lynn, 1986; Nash, Sexton, Hulsey, Harralson & Lambert, 1993; Council, 1987; Johnson, Kirsch, & Irving, 1991). Many investigators (Frischholz & Braun, 1991; Frischholz, Braun, Sachs, & Hopkins, 1991; Nadon, Hoyt, Register, & Kihlstrom, 1991; Putnam, personal communication, March 23, 1992) found only low to modest correlations between scores on the Dissociative Experiences Scale (DES) and hypnotizability. Further, Putnam's data (Putnam, 1992; personal communication, March 23, 1992) failed to uphold the abuse–hypnotizability–dissociation connection. Since measured hypnotizability increases during childhood development, a history of abuse, in light of this connection, should predict greater increases in both hypnotizability and dissociation in abused over nonabused children. Putnam did not find any difference between a group of sexually abused children and nonabused matched controls as to increases in measured hypnotizability over a 3-year period. Between the two samples, however, marked differences have appeared over time in the development of dissociative processes, as measured by the Child Dissociative Checklist (Putnam, 1992; personal communication, March 23, 1992).

Recently, hypnosis investigators have become intrigued with the possibility of a connection between Wilson and Barber's (1983) construct of "fantasy-proneness," childhood abuse, and possible substrates for MPD. Lynn and colleagues (Lynn, Rhue, & Green, 1988; Rhue & Lynn, 1988; Lynn, Milano, & Weekes, 1992) have found "fantasy-proneness" to be more highly correlated with abuse histories and DES scores than hypnotizability per se. They point to many of the characteristics shared by both the highly fantasy prone and MPD patients, as well as their similar early and adult experiences, and suggest that the active cognitive processes underlying fantasy-proneness may be the essence of dissociation. They argue that MPD might well represent the "crossing of a fine line" between the creation of an inner character and the development of a persona that comes to be viewed as a separate self. They suggest that from one perspective, pathological dissociation can be thought of as an "imagination-based cognitive strategy."

MPD investigators, first Kluft with his "Four Factor" theory (Kluft, 1984; Kluft, Steinberg, & Spitzer, 1988), and, later, Young (1988) and Ganaway (1989), have suggested that imaginative processes, including active fantasy, play a central role in the lives of MPD patients and in the elaboration of both symptoms and internal experience. Janet argued much the same point 100 years ago in his essay on suggestibility in hysterics, (Ellenberger, 1970; Perry & Laurence, 1984; van der Hart, personal communication, June 6, 1992).

Most MPD investigators appear to view *clinical dissociation* as involving much more than suggestion or an "imaginative-based cognitive strategy." Putnam (1989), Kluft (1985a, 1991), Spiegel and associates (Spiegel, Hunt, & Dondershine, 1988; Spiegel, 1991), and Braun (Braun, 1986) suggest an individual might inherit a dissociative capacity. Whatever such a capacity might be, it would differ from those that underlie the ability to enter trance; rather it would involve the ability to segregate and idiosyncratically encode experience into separated psychological or psychobiological processes with great fluidity in identity. This capacity may, perhaps, affect the processes of early autobiographical memory (cf. Nelson, 1993; Howe & Courage, 1993). However compelling, the idea of a dissociative capacity remains purely speculative.

Dissociation is also thought to be a mechanism by which overwhelming experience is processed in an unintegrated manner. It is believed that the unintegrated or parallel-processed experience is not lost, but rather encoded not only in terms of emotion (state dependency) but also in terms of personal identity (identity alteration). Functionally, dissociation is thought to protect the child from experiencing the full impact of experience or behavior on his or her emerging personal identity (Putnam, 1989; Donovan & McIntyre, 1990). Despite this seemingly highly conservative system, it is clear that children who are severely traumatized are affected regardless of the levels of memory or dissociation operating (e.g., Terr, 1991; Herman, 1992; Pynoos, 1990; Trickett & Putnam, 1993; Briere & Runtz, 1988a; Briere & Runtz, 1988b; Browne & Finkelhor, 1986; Bryer, Nelson, Miller, & Krol, 1987; Wolfe, 1985, 1987). These models of clinical dissociation, whether or not they stand up to scientific scrutiny, better explain the overall pattern of dissociative handicaps, daily experiences, and disabilities of MPD patients than the single-factor theory of how fantasy leads to "personality" elaboration or suggestion to the self-perception that one is a "multiple." Investigators not working directly with MPD patients tend to focus on the problems of explaining multiplicity or dissociation in isolation from the pervasive patterns of deficits, and interpersonal and cognitive styles common to these patients. Dissociation remains the critical problem to understand, but needs to be examined not only from the perspective of child development, but from the broader context of the effects of trauma on cognitive processing and identity (Spiegel, 1990).

MEMORY

MPD patients have problems with memory (Braun & Frischholz, 1992). Amnesia, a frequently reported feature of the disorder, can consist of several different types: (1) dense, but intermittent, childhood amnesia; (2) amnesia for present-life behaviors; (3) "intra-personality" agnosia; (4) episodes of very brief, but disturbing, "micro" amnesias; and (5) dramatic hypermnesia, characterized by "flashbulb" memories, dramatic recall of "long-forgotten" events, flashbacks, so-called "somatic memories," memory intrusions of various sorts, and sensitivity to unpredicted stimuli (cf. van der Kolk & van der Hart, 1991).

Despite the persistent belief among some clinicians that memory is a vast video storehouse and hypnosis the ideal software retrieval system, experimental studies have demonstrated beyond any doubt, under a wide variety conditions with a wide range of stimuli, that hypnotically enhanced recall is fraught with difficulty. Virtually all experimental studies demonstrate that increased recall comes at the expense of accuracy, which is further complicated by the fact the subjects report greater confidence in the veracity of hypnotically and retrieved information for *both* accurate and inaccurate information (e.g. Sheehan, 1988; Dywan & Bowers, 1983; Nogrady, McConkey, & Perry, 1985; Laurence & Perry, 1983). The problem is not related solely to the use of hypnosis. Similar effects are found during non-hypnotic-memory-for-events testing (Loftus, 1982, 1992; Loftus & Hoffman, 1989; Geiselman, Bjork, & Fishman, 1983; Kihlstrom, 1983; Roediger & Payne, 1982, 1985; also see Anderson, 1984, on imagination and reality monitoring).

We now also know that high hypnotizability is a predictor of increased vulnerability to suggested pseudomemories (Barnier & McConkey, 1992; Lynn, Weekes, & Milano, 1989; McCann & Sheehan, 1988; Labelle, Laurence, Nadon, & Perry, 1990). Hypnotizability, however, is not the only factor affecting the production of pseudomemories. Expectancies, instructional sets, the type of memory task (e.g., objectively verifiable versus subjective and unverifiable) all influence the rates of pseudomemory production, which range from 0% to 80% (Lynn, Milano, & Weekes, 1992, p. 356).

While it is possible that those patients who are more apt to be diagnosed with MPD likely have the cognitive capacities to readily absorb environmental information and interpersonal suggestion and transform it into personal memory, significant false memory problems in MPD patients have yet to be demonstrated. On the other hand, Frankel (1993) observed quite trenchantly that, significant verification of childhood abuse memories also have not been demonstrated. Verification of abuse memories is a simpler task for children alleging sexual abuse and, in general, while some false allegations surely exist, the preponderance of evidence supports that this occurs at low levels. Likewise, although false memory is likely a problem in human life and a demonstrable laboratory finding, Christianson (1992) concludes that the "loss of clarity and detail over time seems to be far less in memories of real life events than can be expected from the forgetting curve typically found in basic memory research" (p. 31).

Thus, while a serious investigator of MPD must acknowledge that memories, especially early memories, are subject to distortions, confabulations, displacement and other vagaries of the rewriting of personal history, there is actually little support for the level of doubt expressed by some critics (e.g., Orne & Bauer-Manley, 1991; Bowers, 1991). The problem is only significant when the conceptual and clinical error is made in thinking that past trauma is the treatment issue rather than the pathological dissociative processes. This error leads to a focus on trauma and retribution and, occasionally, "healing by litigation." The standard of proof for abuse allegations must be much higher here (Horevitz, 1992).

Nonetheless, clinicians working with MPD patients and others alleging childhood abuse should make systematic efforts to confirm allegations independent of the therapeutic situation. Unfortunately, many record sources are unavailable. Schools rarely will release their confidential records; hospitals and pediatricians do not hold onto chart data from 20 or 30 years before; and few if any incidents of abuse are ever reported from before the most recent past. Further, no one has addressed the complex ethical dilemma of approaching family members systematically, *as a matter of routine treatment*, rather than on an occasional or random basis.

The formation of autobiographical memory in childhood is still poorly understood. The study of trauma memory (Trickett & Putnam, 1993), as well as normal autobiographical memory and forgetting, is in its infancy (Fivush, 1988; Wetzler & Sweeney, 1986; Fivush & Hudson, 1990; Horowitz & Reidbord, 1992; Ross & Conway, 1986; Ross, 1989). Clinical studies, (e.g., Terr, 1988, 1991) appear to show that very early and forgotten trauma is preserved and enacted in play. While infants learn and retain memory in nonverbal modes along the way to acquiring language (e.g., Mandler, 1990, 1992; Meltzoff, 1988; Hall & Oppenheim, 1987; Rovee-Collier, 1990), and demonstrate enduring and highly specific sensory and motor learning (see Rovee-Collier, 1990), this evidence does not provide convincing proof that clients' very early infancy reports of abuse are accurate. Clinicians' facile acceptance of these reports can only heighten the doubts regarding their judgment, inadvertent reinforcement of abuse reports, and the provision of contextual expectancies that raise the rates of false memory, and thus cast doubt on all clinically derived data.

A SUMMARY OF COMMONALITIES

The question of the reality of MPD has stirred controversy in many areas of psychology and psychiatry. I have argued that unrecognized common ground exists across the various conceptualizations of MPD. This common ground has been obscured by clinicians and experimentalists' general lack of familiarity with each other's domains of inquiry and lingering doubts about what constitutes the relevant reference point for MPD (e.g., the work of the few leading clinical investigators, the "clinical lore" of private-practice clinicians, or the sensationalized presentations in the media). I identified three areas in which the basis for a common ground can be found:

In the area of personality and personal identity, MPD theorists have proposed that MPD be thought of in terms of alternating identity configurations. These configurations are thought to be relatively plastic, permeable, and malleable in childhood (Kluft, 1985a; Putnam, 1989), and increasingly rigid and fixed in adulthood, leading to the unique patterns of MPD symptomatology.

In the area of consciousness and dissociation, it is now commonly assumed that there is a distinction between clinical or pathological dissociation and the dissociative processes found in hypnosis. The implication of this emergent consensus is that hypnosis research, which for so long provided the basis for exploring pathological dissociation, can no longer be expected to provide insights across various domains. Entirely new research strategies involving clinical dissociation with patient populations will have to be developed to ascertain the validity of those conceptual models that have come to dominate the field of dissociation.

In the area of memory, MPD investigators and cognitive psychologists are likely to agree that clinical work with MPD patients often overlooks the complexity of memory as revealed in research, and that memory distortions, pseudomemories, suggestibility factors, and context-dependent effects all affect these patients in treatment. Unfortunately, many clinicians working with MPD patients exhibit an almost "blind faith" in the veridicality of patient reports and have little knowledge of the complex nature of memory, which research continues to reveal. The question remains of the significance of the memory problems that cognitive science has pointed out. While little doubt exists that memory is reconstructive and extremely context sensitive in its retelling (Loftus, 1992, 1993; Ceci & Bruck, 1993), the evidence to date suggests that psychopathology itself does not contribute to the distortion of early childhood memories and that the memories of patients in treatment are reasonably adequate (Brewin, Andrews, & Gotlib, 1993; Christianson & Loftus, 1991).

Given the commonalities detailed above, it is possible to envision a time when sufficient evidence will have accumulated to satisfy both the critical skepticism of the experimental scientist and the necessary acceptance of the clinician. In short, we will come to live with the middle ground. The difficulty, as mentioned earlier, will be in devising ethical and practical means for verifying early childhood memories that involve parental abuse, given that even at their best parents are poor historians of their children's lives (cf. Brewin, Andrews, & Gotlib, 1993, for a review).

INCOMMENSURABILITIES

In the first part of this chapter, I explored areas where conceptual clarification and good empirical research could provide a common ground for discourse and the reasonable investigation of the phenomena known as MPD. In this section, I briefly cover some of the difficulties I see in attaining the clarity requisite for the resolution of the *conflict* surrounding MPD or its transformation into reasoned *controversy*.

Some of the difficulties to attaining a consensus are neither empirical, conceptual, nor scientific. MPD patients present stories that are painful to hear and elicit feelings in the therapist or investigator that are difficult to tolerate. The intensity of this experience can lead to many responses, ranging from an overwhelming desire to right the wrongs the patient describes to an outright denial that the patient's stories or experiences are true. This range of response has little to do with either the veracity of the patient report or the validity of the diagnosis of MPD. There are clinician (or investigator) variables that predispose a person to specific beliefs or responses to reports of extreme human experience. These variables have been discussed elsewhere (Goodwin, 1985).

The class of problems I address here as "incommensurable" have to do with the beliefs and basic assumptions clinicians (or investigators) possess, with their difficulties in reasoning and logic, with their rhetorical and moral concerns, as well as with core issues about the practice of science. These issues have less to do with empirical investigation than they do with habits of the mind in understanding the data currently available. Thus, these problems are, in Ryle's words, philosophical because they require us to "rectify the logical geography of the knowledge we already possess" (1949, p. 7).

1. *Paradigms.* Loewenstein and Ross (1992) suggested that Kuhn's sense of a "paradigm shift" in science can be applied to the current conflict over the reality of MPD. In Kuhn's (1970) opinion, when a science is not yet fully established, anomalies to paradigms lead to new theories that threaten the established paradigms, and a major conflict of values occurs. In his view, science changes not merely by the gradual accretion of empirical data and well-reasoned arguments but by shifts of allegiances that parallel shifts in political or religious allegiance. In other words, rhetoric, more than logic, leads to "conversion" experiences on an all-or-none basis.[3]

Loewenstein and Ross (1992) suggest there is a new *traumaterigic* paradigm, which is competing with the older *psychodynamic* and *psychosocial* paradigms. This model addresses the poorly understood impact of profound trauma on the developing child's neurobiological and psychobiological processes, cognitive and motoric development, and the vagaries of personality development. According to this model, the prototypical MPD patient is not the "classic" multiple with florid symptoms and "alters" of polar moral/personal styles, but the treatment refractory, polysymptomatic, post-traumatic stress disorder patient, who is enshrouded in a pathology of secrecy. Dissociative processes are seen as largely hidden and rarely revealed without direct inquiry. Even when they exhibit overt dissociative behaviors, MPD patients, much like obsessive compulsive disordered patients, will almost never voluntarily report their main fears, experiences, and feelings of distress.

The traumatergic paradigm dramatically differs from the psychodynamic paradigm wherein MPD is construed as the result of unconscious defenses serving a weak ego in the face of intolerable affects, which leads to the hysterical presentation of "split-off" aspects of the self (MPD). According to the old paradigm, "split-off" aspects of the self represent *failures* of experiential integration, the disavowal of responsibility, and false presentations of self (Spanos, Weekes, & Bertrand, 1985; Halleck, 1990). From this perspective, MPD is best treated by the suppression of dissociative symptoms and a refusal to "reify" part-personalities by addressing them directly or allowing them to be the focus of treatment. Overall treatment is determined by other self-psychological practices common to the treatment of borderline personality (Orne & Bates, 1992; Kernberg, 1975; personal communication, May 20, 1992).

According to the new paradigm, the impact of trauma on development has less to do with the "shattering" of a unitary mind, self, or ego structure than with a complex phenomenon involving the development of alternative versions of the self to adapt to unrelenting and unremediated trauma wherein little is predictable. As childhood plasticity gives way to adult rigidity, flexible (if sequestered) identities become increasingly fixed and less fluid. However, they all represent manifestations of the total person; there is no "true person" with false selves. This perspective leads to a treatment in which the clinician attempts to deepen the qualities of personhood across the separate, distinct cores of identity in order to promote the true integration of self-parts in severely compromised and damaged patients.

2. *"Overgeneralization."* Science requires that we do not overgeneralize from the limited conclusions empirical experimentation generates. Bowers and Hilgard (1988) state the formal problem:

> It is the nature of experiments to select from a larger domain of knowledge certain limited aspects that can be subjected to measurement and used to establish lawful relationships among selected variables. . . . However, caution is needed in generalizing from any one series of experiments because of their selective nature—a selectivity often determined by the theoretical orientation of the investigator. Unless such dangers are kept in perspective, we can become victimized by the so-called "cult of empiricism." (Toulman & Leary, quoted in Bowers & Hilgard, 1988, pp. 9–10)

In his early work on the "hidden observer" phenomenon in hypnotic pain control, Hilgard (1977) saw parallels between his empirical findings and the clinical findings on MPD that had implications for his neodissociation theory. Since then, Hilgard (personal communication, April, 1992) has clearly rethought the matter, perhaps because so much theorizing about MPD has leaned on his "hidden observer" work. Today, he says that his investigations with such phenomena as the "hidden observer" are much too limited in scope to use when drawing conclusions about MPD. Bower (personal communication, May 12, 1992) advocated a similar restraint based on the present status of knowledge in the cognitive sciences. Still, other distinguished cognitive and neural scientists, for example, Edelman (1989) and Pribram (personal communication, October 29, 1992), have found critical use for MPD research in their larger theories of brain functioning and cognitive processes.

Skeptical scientists are particularly likely to focus on the experimental findings from hypnosis, attribution, and the rich memory research, as well as that from the social psychology of influence research, when drawing conclusions about MPD. Proponents of MPD are likely to look at the sociological realities of the extent of child abuse, including the profoundly disturbing incidence of the bizarre exploitation of children. Further, they tend to accept the patient's self-presentation and take his or her tortured secrecy as evidence against the existence of "false positives." In this way, both critics and proponents of MPD strain the limits to which empirical studies can be generalized.

3. *Language and its uses.* Much of the confusion that so distorts the manner in which MPD is viewed has to do with the power of words to ignite and capture the imagination. Word-pictures, more than anything else, are at the root of the problem. Just when we think reason is being invoked, we cannot see beyond the pictures language elicits (Wittgenstein, 1953). For instance, the mental picture evoked by the words "multiple personalities" is hard to get beyond and hard to accept. Even the very large improvement that comes with renaming MPD Dissociative Identity Disorder in the fourth edition of the *Diagnostic and Statistical Manual of Mental Disorders* (DSM-IV; American Psychiatric Association, 1994) cannot traverse the problem. Though it is easier to *imagine* multiple identities than multiple personalities, we are still left with the linguistic difficulty of talking sensibly about these "multiple identities."

Critics find their ideas about and pictures of MPD so intellectually and aesthetically unacceptable that they appear to take a hostile rather than an intellectually curious attitude toward what seems to be such a terrible disorder. In trying to make this unwanted picture disappear, important psychological constructs or understandings are often given *special* status in relation to MPD. For instance, suggestibility, social and interpersonal influence, expectancy effects, and demand characteristics, which surely are a part of all human interactions, are used to explain MPD even though they are not used to explain other forms of psychopathology, even in the absence of sufficient evidence. Likewise, the use of language and metaphor in the framing of problems and their solutions, which is a core element of change in all forms of psychotherapy (Watzlawick, Beavin, & Jackson, 1967; Watzlawick, 1978), is thought to be *inherently* problematic with these patients. In short, a form of folie à deux (Mersky, 1992) emerges in ways one would never think to routinely apply to the treatments of other patient categories.

On the other hand, MPD clinicians, in my experience, often display the most astonishing lack of awareness of the complex processes accompanying social and interpersonal influences. They appear uninformed about the problems of clinical judgement and decision-making biases, described by cognitive scientists and decision theorists, which affect them every day (Dumont, 1993; Einhorn, 1988; Fischhoff, 1982; Kelley, 1967; Kelley, 1992; Tversky & Kahnemann, 1981). Clinicians routinely give meaning and veracity to the most minimal client cues, as if they were detectives examining evidence rather than persons interacting with others. The large literature on the problem of base rate fallacy (Meehl & Rosen, 1955; Kahneman & Tversky, 1973; Dawes, 1988) and its impact on diagnostic decision making is virtually unknown among clinicians and contributes to our ill-repute.

4. *Misunderstandings about diagnoses and their validity.* Psychiatric and psychological diagnoses are established by consensus (Spitzer & Williams, 1985). Reliability and validity are central considerations in establishing diagnoses beyond the mere coherence of a syndrome of signs and symptoms. Evidence of symptom cohesiveness, differential responsiveness to treatment, a particular family history, a predictable course or life history, and for a unique etiology and contributing factors is essential to establishing categories that can be judged for reliability and validity (Goodwin & Guze, 1984; Cloninger, 1989). By all standards, MPD has matched and even exceeded the requirements demanded of all psychiatric or psychological conditions (Horevitz, 1987; Putnam, 1991).

Critics who claim MPD is nonexistent, rare, iatrogenic, or overdiagnosed may be right or they may be wrong. However, no data at present exists to directly support these contentions. Data supporting the reliability and validity of the diagnosis of MPD and other dissociative disorders have been forthcoming thanks largely to the development of three valid and reliable screening instruments for the dissociative disorders: the DES, the Dissociative Disorders Interview Schedule (DDIS), and the Structured Clinical Interview for DSM-IV Dissociative Disorders (SCID-D; Steinberg, Rounsaville, & Cicchetti, 1990; Steinberg, 1993).

With the development of reliable and valid instruments, epidemiological studies have become feasible. Studies of the incidence of MPD and the dissociative disorders are underway that resemble the community stratified population samplings, wherein the "gold standard" is used. More readily obtained differential studies are also being done wherein MPD patients are compared with other psychiatric populations and normal groups. Using such a study, Ross arrived at a prevalence figure of 1.3% for MPD. Thus the prevalence rate of MPD appears, from this first study, to be slightly greater than that of schizophrenia in the general population (Ross, Joshi, & Currie, 1990; Ross, Anderson, Fleisher, & Norton, 1991; Ross, 1991). Interestingly, in the general population sample, Ross found an incidence rate of 2% for individuals who met DSM-III-R MPD criteria but who demonstrated little overt psychopathology characteristic of clinical post-traumatic MPD, and who also denied any history of abuse.

The validity of diagnoses should be scrutinized in a very tough-minded manner. Goodwin and Guze (1984) state this idea well: "Knowing that it is more difficult to eliminate or reduce observer bias in studies of psychological processes, we should demand more rather than less in the way of repeatedly demonstrated, systematic, controlled evidence" (p. 277).

In conclusion, more work needs to be done to further establish convergent and discriminant validity. Further, the real test for establishing the validity of a psychopathological diagnosis will involve demonstrating the existence of psychological processes critical to the disorder in nonpathological populations. In addition, a well-grounded theoretical model of psychological processes needs to be established that will generate testable hypotheses.

5. *Moral, professional, and emotional concerns.* The single most common criticism of the diagnosis of MPD in patients is that it encourages patients who are already prone to disavow responsibility for their actions to further retreat from taking responsibility for them (cf. Spanos, Weekes, & Bertrand, 1985; Spanos, 1989; Orne & Bates, 1992; Hallek, 1990; Bowers, 1991). This criticism is ethical and moral in nature. From this perspective, in tolerating a continued disavowal of responsibility clinicians promote psychological and moral ill-health and contribute to a further perversion of personal values in the culture at large.

The question here is not whether these are worthy sentiments, but whether (a) diagnosing MPD in practice actually does lead to a diminished sense of responsibility, and if so when? and whether (b) this problem of responsibility involves *how* people treat MPD patients or whether an exogenous explanation (e.g., the trauma itself)?

6. *Honesty in science problems.* Few critics have bothered to read the MPD literature deeply and impartially; and few of the critiques are untainted by emotionalism or present good experimental *hypotheses* for MPD researchers to test. It is simply not good enough to argue against MPD based on the

false characterization of what MPD clinicians do or believe. If there are logical, empirical, or methodological failures in the way MPD investigation is being conducted, then critics would help advance science by illustrating these errors in well-researched responses rather than those that are well-argued.

Likewise, few MPD investigators take the criticism seriously and look judiciously for errors in their reasoning or clinical methods. Indeed, few have mastered the relevant experimental literature and considered the extent to which it is relevant to clinical practice. As I suggested earlier, it appears that many of those who are most concerned with elucidating a well-formulated and well-grounded theory of dissociation and MPD have pursued a "pick-and-choose" method of dealing with the scientific and experimental literature so that previously held beliefs and favored hypotheses are validated (Kluft, 1993).

7. *Housekeeping failures.* As abuse stories of patients become increasingly bizarre, clinicians in the field of MPD treatment need to keep the house in order, which they have failed to do. Our colleagues "outside the home" are telling us that we have a "siege mentality": We will defend almost any pro-survivor, pro-patient claim; tolerate almost any hair-brained conceptualization; publish without scrutiny any "clinically relevant" paper; and tolerate the proliferation of a range of therapeutic behaviors of absolutely unknown quality and minimal training. Quite independent of the reality or validity of the diagnosis of MPD, the manner of its handling by professionals has alarmed many. Perhaps it should not be surprising that in the treatment of this most difficult and frightening disorder many significant treatment errors occur (cf. Chu, 1988, 1991; Greaves, 1988) that are compounded by the astonishingly unscientific and naive attitudes often found in clinicians.

CONCLUSION

To resolve the 100-year-old debate about the authenticity of MPD, underlying normative biases will have to surface so their roles in the debate can be clarified. For instance, Saks (1992) discussed the social-psychological literature on obedience to authority in light of the normative biases of researchers. He pointed to Asch's (1952, 1956) implicit assumption in all his work that conformity to norms is bad because it leads to error. Likewise, Milgram's (1974) experiments were regarded as "horrific" because they showed how easily "good people" can do "bad things." Saks suggested that "we should learn how people actually respond when investigators are unsure of what the correct or proper response is" (1992,

p. 222). Conflicting rule systems are inevitable in difficult social situations, therefore he suggested, the best question is: "How do people respond to these different layers of rules and differing calls for loyalty from different authorities" (1992, p. 223). What is it, and how is it, that clinicians working with MPD patients "see" and respond to particular aspects of patient presentations that others might not?

When we look at the whole mosaic of problems involved in the hypnosis/MPD connection, we see that many are due to the conflicting rule systems of clinical practice, of experimental and clinical science, and to the subsystems of conflicting rules within each. How do we recognize the influence of these competing claims and find our way through them? Surely not by reason alone.

Simon (1990), reflecting on a lifetime of studying rationality and expert decision making, recently argued that rationality is bounded by the slow speed with which we process phenomena and the limits of short-term memory. It is augmented by our capacity to store vast amounts of memory, rules, and algorithms. But as familiarity with a subject decreases, rationality breaks down and conventional heuristics take over. It is not possible to cross this chasm that divides us through discourse unless we become *true* experts in each other's domain.

In an essay on William James, Kihlstrom and McConkey (1990) demonstrated that James's genius was great enough to encompass the theoretical split between so-called special state and social-psychological positions. Today, when resolution again seems possible, perhaps we will have yet again a psychologist capable of integrating the two paradigms. Perhaps we shall someday be fortunate in the same way when addressing the problems and controversies surrounding MPD so that we can get down to both a serious investigation of the disorder and an unhampered state-of-the-art care of MPD patients.

ACKNOWLEDGMENTS

An earlier version of this chapter was presented as the Presidential Address for Division 30 of the 100th Annual American Psychological Association Meeting, August 18, 1992. In the course of the preparation of this chapter, I wrote to many of the significant contributors in the field regarding their views on many of the subjects covered in the address. I would like to thank each of them for their help: Gordon Bower, Kenneth Bowers, Bennett Braun, James Chu, Helen Crawford, Fred Frankel, George Frazer, Erika Fromm, Edward Frischholz, Jean Goodwin, Ernest Hilgard, Otto Kernberg, John Kihlstrom, Irving Kirsch, Richard Loewenstein, Elizabeth Loftus, Steven Lynn, John Nemiah, Martin Orne, Gary Peterson, Frank Putnam, David Spiegel, Marlene Steinberg, Moshe Torem, and Onno van der Hart. Steven Lynn, Benjamin Kleinmuntz, and Mary Ann Redeker provided invaluable editorial assistance.

NOTES

1. In DSM-IV, MPD was renamed Dissociative Identity Disorder. It is hoped that this change will serve to refocus discussion on the validity and frequency of the occurrence of the syndrome. The new designation may still leave something to be desired but no longer sounds like an oxymoron, as MPD did to some critics.
2. Recent contributions to attribution theory (e.g., Au, 1986; Semin & Fiedler, 1988) have emphasized the centrality of language for the process of attribution. "Words that people use to describe simple, everyday actions and states carry with them powerful implications for the causal explanations of those events" (Edwards & Potter, 1993, p. 23). It seems likely that some of the heat in the controversy of MPD can be understood as relating to causal attributions surrounding the words central to the argument (e.g., "alter identities," "personality fragments," "multiple personalities," "repressed memory," "trauma," "dissociation"), all of which readily lend themselves to mind pictures and causal attributions thought to be accurate descriptions of reality rather than metaphors of language (Wittgenstein, 1953).
3. An argument can be made that Kuhn's model does not explain as well as others do (e.g., those of Laudan and Lakatos) the history of physics or psychology (Gholson & Barker, 1985). However, Kuhn's emphasis on metaphysics and rhetoric can aptly be applied to the history of clinical psychology as well as its problematic relationship to scientific psychology.

REFERENCES

Aldridge-Morris, R. (1989). *Multiple personality: An exercise in deception.* Hillside, NJ: Lawrence Erlbaum.

American Psychiatric Association (1994). *Diagnostic and statistical manual of mental disorders* (4th ed.). Washington, DC: Author.

Anderson, R. E. (1984). Did I do it or did I only imagine doing it? *Journal of Experimental Psychology, 113*(4), 594–615.

Asch, S. E. (1952). Effects of group pressure upon the modification and distortions of judgement. In G. E. Swanson, T. M. Newcomb, & E. Hartley (Eds.), *Readings in social psychology* (rev. ed, pp. 2–11). New York: Holt, Rinehart & Winston.

Asch, S. E. (1956). Studies of independence and conformity: A minority of one against a unanimous majority. *Psychological Monographs, 70*(9, Serial No. 416).

Au, T. K. (1986). A verb is worth a thousand words: The causes and consequences of interpersonal events implicit in language. *Journal of Memory and Language, 25*, 104–122.

Bandura, A. (1978). The self system in reciprocal determinism. *American Psychologist, 33*, 344–358.

Barnier, A., & McConkey, K. (1992). Reports of real and false memories: The relevance of hypnosis, hypnotizability, and test context. *Journal of Abnormal Psychology, 101*, 521–527.

Bateson, G. (1972). *Steps to an ecology of mind: Collected essays in anthropology, psychiatry, evolution, and epistemology.* San Francisco: Chandler.

Baumeister, A., Stillwell, A., & Wotman, S. (1990). Victim and perpetrator accounts of interpersonal conflict: Autobiographical narratives about anger. *Journal of Personality and Social Psychology, 59*, 994–1005.

Bliss, E. L. (1984). A symptom profile of patients with multiple personalities, including MMPI results. *Journal of Nervous and Mental Disease, 172*, 197–202.

Bowers, K. (1991). Dissociation in hypnosis and multiple personality disorder. *International Journal of Clinical and Experimental Hypnosis, 39*(3), 155–176.

Bowers, K. S., & Davidson, T. M. (1991). A neodissociative critique of Spanos's social-psychological model of hypnosis. In S. J. Lynn & J. W. Rhue (Eds.), *Theories of hypnosis: Current models and perspectives* (pp. 105–143). New York: Guilford Press.

Bowers, K. S., & Hilgard, E. R. (1988). Some complexities in understanding memory. In H. M. Pettinati (Ed.), *Hypnosis and memory* (pp. 3–20). New York: Guilford Press.

Braun, B. G. (1986). *Treatment of multiple personality disorder.* Washington, DC: American Psychiatric Press.

Braun, B. G., & Frischholz, E. J. (1992). Remembering and forgetting in patients suffering from multiple personality disorder. In S. Christianson (Eds.), *The handbook of emotion and memory: Research and theory* (pp. 411–427). Hillsdale, NJ: Lawrence Erlbaum.

Brewin, C. R. (1989). Cognitive change processes in psychotherapy. *Psychological Review, 96*(3), 379–394.

Brewin, C. R., Andrews, B., & Gotlib, I. H. (1993). Psychopathology and early experience: A reappraisal of retrospective reports. *Psychological Bulletin, 113*, pp. 82–98.

Briere, J. D., & Runtz, M. (1988a). Multivariate correlates of childhood psychological and physical maltreatment among university women. *Child Abuse and Neglect, 12*, 331–341.

Briere, J., & Runtz, M. (1988b). Post sexual abuse trauma. In G. Wyatt & G. Powell (Eds.), *The lasting effects of child sexual abuse* (pp. 85–99). Beverly Hills, CA: Sage.

Browne, A., & Finkelhor, D. (1986). Impact of child sexual abuse: A review of the research. *Psychological Bulletin, 99*, 66–77.

Bryer, J. B., Nelson, B. A., Miller, J. B., & Krol, P. A. (1987, November). Childhood sexual and physical abuse as factors in adult psychiatric illness. *American Journal of Psychiatry, 144*(11), 1426–1430.

Buss, D. M. (1991). Evolutionary personality psychology. In M. R. Rosenzweig & L. W. Porter (Eds.), *Annual review of psychology* (Vol. 42, pp. 459–491). Palo Alto, CA: Annual Review Press.

Carlson, E. B., & Putnam, F. W. (1989). Integrating research on dissociation and hypnotizability: Are there two pathways to hypnotizability? *Dissociation, 2*, 32–38.

Ceci, S. J., & Bruck, M. (1993). Suggestibility of the child witness: A historical review and synthesis. *Psychological Bulletin, 113*(3), 403–439.

Christianson, S. A. (1992). Remembering emotional events. In S. Christianson (Eds.), *The handbook of emotion and memory: Research and theory* (pp. 307–342). Hillsdale, NJ: Lawrence Erlbaum.

Christianson, S. A., & Loftus, E. F. (1991). Remembering emotional events: The fate of detailed information. *Cognition and Emotion, 5*, 81–108.

Chu, J. A. (1988). Ten traps for therapists in the treatment of trauma survivors. *Dissociation, 1*(1), pp. 24–32.

Chu, J. A. (1991). On the misdiagnosis of multiple personality disorder. *Dissociation, 4*, 200–204.

Cloninger, C. R. (1989). Establishment of diagnostic validity in psychiatric illness: Robins and Guze's method revisited. In L. Robins & J. Barrett (Eds.), *The validity of psychiatric diagnoses* (pp. 9–16). New York: Raven Press.

Coons, P. M., Bowman, E. S., & Milstein, V. (1988). Multiple personality disorder: A clinical investigation of 50 cases. *Journal of Nervous and Mental Disease, 176*, 519–527.

Council, J. R. (1987). *Patterns of fantasy arising from childhood sexual abuse.* Paper presented at the 97th Annual Convention of the American Psychological Association, New York, New York.

Dawes, R. M. (1988). *Rational choice in an uncertain world.* San Diego: Harcourt, Brace & Jovanovich.

Dell, P. F. (1988). Professional skepticism about multiple personality. *Journal of Nervous and Mental Diseases, 176*, 528–531.

Dixon, M., Brunet, A., & Laurence, J. (1990). Hypnotizability and automaticity: Toward a parallel distributed processing model of hypnotic responding. *Journal of Abnormal Psychology, 99*, 336–343.

Donovan, D. M., & McIntyre, D. (1990). *Healing the hurt child: A developmental–contextual approach.* New York: W.W. Norton.

Dumont, F. (1993). Inferential heuristics in clinical problem formulation: Selective review of their strengths and weaknesses. *Professional Psychology: Research and Practice, 24*(2), 196–205.

Dywan, J., & Bowers, K. S. (1983). The use of hypnosis to enhance recall. *Science, 222*, 184–185.

Edelman, G. M. (1989). *The remembered present: A biological theory of consciousness.* New York: Basic Books.

Edwards, D., & Potter, J. (1993). Language and causation: A discursive action model of description and attribution. *Psychological Review, 100*(1), 23–41.

Einhorn, H. J. (1988). Diagnosis and causality in clinical and statistical prediction. In D. C. Turk & P. Salovey (Eds.), *Reasoning, inference and judgement in clinical psychology* (pp. 51–70). New York: Free Press.

Ellenberger, H. F. (1970). *The discovery of the unconscious: The history and evolution of dynamic psychiatry.* New York: Basic Books.

Fischhoff, B. (1982). For those condemned to study the past: Heuristics and biases in hindsight. In D. Kahenman, P. Slovic, & A. Tversky (Eds.), *Judgement under uncertainty: Heuristics and biases* (pp. 335–351). New York: Cambridge University Press.

Fivush, R. (1988). The functions of event memory: Some comments on Nelson and Barsalou. In U. Neisser & E. Winograd (Eds.), *Remembering reconsidered: Ecological and traditional approaches to the study of memory* (pp. 277–282). New York: Cambridge University Press.

Fivush, R., & Hudson, J. (1990). *Knowing and remembering in young children.* New York: Cambridge University Press.

Frankel, F. H. (1990). Hypnotizability and dissociation. *American Journal of Psychiatry, 147*, 823–829.

Frankel, F. H. (1993). Adult reconstruction of childhood events in the multiple personality literature. *American Journal of Psychiatry, 150*, 954–958.

Frischholz, E. J. (1985). The relationship among dissociation, hypnosis, and child abuse in the development of multiple personality disorder. In R. P. Kluft (Ed.), *Childhood antecedents of multiple personality disorder* (pp. 99–126). Washington, DC: American Psychiatric Press.

Frischholz, E. J., & Braun, B. G. (1991, August 8). *Diagnosing dissociative disorders: New methods.* Paper presented at the 99th Annual Convention of the American Psychological Association, San Francisco, CA.

Frischholz, E. J., Braun, B. G., Sachs, R. G., & Hopkins, L. (1991). The Dissociative Experiences Scale: Further replication and validation. *Dissociation, 4*(4), 151–153.

Frischholz, E. J., Lipman, L. S., Braun, B. G., & Sachs, R. G., (1992). Psychopathology, hypnotizability, and dissociation. *American Journal of Psychiatry, 149*(11), 1521–1525.

Ganaway, G. K. (1989). Historical truth versus narrative truth: Clarifying the role of exogenous trauma in the etiology of multiple personality disorder and its variants. *Dissociation, 2*, 205–220.

Geiselman, R. E., Bjork, R. A., & Fishman, D. L. (1983). Disrupted retrieval in directed forgetting: A link with post hypnotic amnesia. *Journal of Experimental Psychology, 112*(1), 58–72.

Gholson, B., & Barker, P. (1985). Kuhn, Lakatos, and Laudan: Applications in the history of physics and psychology. *American Psychologist, 40*(7), 755–769.

Goffman, E. (1959). *The presentation of self in everyday life.* Garden City, NY: Doubleday.

Goodwin, J. (1985). Credibility problems in multiple personality and abused children. In R. Kluft (Ed.), *Childhood antecedents of multiple personality* (pp. 1–19). Washington, DC: American Psychiatric Press.

Goodwin, D. W., & Guze, S. B. (1984). *Psychiatric diagnosis* (3rd ed.). New York: Oxford University Press.

Gotteman, C., Greaves, G., B., & Coons, P. M. (1992). *Multiple personality and dissociation, 1791–1990: A complete bibliography.* Atlanta, GA: George Greaves.

Greaves, G. B. (1988). Common errors in the treatment of multiple personality disorder. *Dissociation, 1*, 61–66.

Haley, J. (1963). *Strategies of psychotherapy.* New York: Grune & Stratton.

Hall, W., & Oppenheim, R. (1987). Developmental psychobiology: Prenatal, perinatal, and early postnatal aspects of behavioral development. In M. R. Rosenzweig & L. W. Porter (Eds.), *Annual review of psychology* (Vol. 38, pp. 91–128). Palo Alto, CA: Annual Review Press.

Halleck, S. L. (1990). Dissociative phenomena and the question of responsibility. *International Journal of Clinical and Experimental Hypnosis, 38*, 298–314.

Herman, J. L. (1992). *Trauma and recovery.* New York: Basic Books.

Herman, J. L., & Schatzow, E. (1987). Recovery and verification of memories of childhood sexual trauma. *Psychoanalytic Psychology, 4*, 1–14.

Hilgard, E. R. (1977). *Divided consciousness: Multiple controls in human thought and action.* New York: John Wiley.

Hilgard, E. R. (1987). Multiple personality and dissociation. In *Psychology in America: A historical survey* (pp. 303–315). San Diego, CA: Harcourt Brace Jovanovich.

Hilgard, E. R. (1988). Commentary: Professional skepticism about multiple personality. *Journal of Nervous and Mental Disease, 176*, 532.

Hilgard, E. R. (1991). A neodissociation interpretation of hypnosis. In S. J. Lynn & J. W. Rhue (Eds.), *Theories of hypnosis: Current models and perspectives* (pp. 83–104). New York: Guilford Press.

Horevitz, R. P. (1987). *Multiple personality and borderline personality disorders: Differential diagnosis and differential treatment.* Paper presented at the 95th Annual Convention of the American Psychological Association, Washington, DC.

Horevitz, R. P. (1994). *Psychological indices and corroborative facts of a history of abuse in multiple personality disorder patients.* Unpublished manuscript.

Horowitz, M. J., & Reidbord, S. P. (1992). Memory, emotion, and response to trauma. In S. Christianson (Eds.), *The handbook of emotion and memory: Research and theory* (pp. 342–357). Hillsdale, NJ: Lawrence Erlbaum.

Howe, M. L., & Courage, M. L. (1993). On resolving the enigma of infantile amnesia. *Psychological Bulletin, 113*, 305–326.

Johnson, G., & Kirsch, I. (1991). *Dissociation, hypnotizability, and fantasy proneness in a clinical sample of survivors of abuse.* Paper presented at the 99th Annual Convention of the American Psychological Association, Washington, DC.

Kahneman, D., & Tversky, A. (1973). On the psychology of prediction. *Psychological Review, 80*, 237–251.

Kampman, R. (1992). [Review of *Multiple personality disorder: An exercise in self deception*]. *International Journal of Clinical and Experimental Hypnosis, 60*(1), 44–46.

Kelley, H. H. (1967). Attribution theory in social psychology. In D. Levine (Eds.), *Nebraska symposium on motivation* (pp. 192–238). Lincoln, NE: University of Nebraska Press.

Kelley, H. H. (1992). Common-sense psychology and scientific psychology. In M. Rosenzweig & L. Porter (Eds.), *Annual review of psychology* (Vol. 43, pp. 1–23). Palo Alto, CA: Annual Review Press.

Kernberg, O. F. (1975). *Borderline conditions and pathological narcissism.* New York: Jason Aronson.

Kihlstrom, J. F. (1983). Instructed forgetting: Hypnotic and nonhypnotic. *Journal of Experimental Psychology: General, 112*(1), 73–79.

Kihlstrom, J. F. (1984). Conscious, subconscious, unconscious: A cognitive perspective. In K. S. Bowers & D. Meichenbaum (Eds.), *The unconscious reconsidered* (pp. 149–210). New York: John Wiley.

Kihlstrom, J. F. (1987). Introduction to the special issue: Integrating personality and social psychology. *Journal of Personality and Social Psychology, 53*, 989–992.

Kihlstrom, J. F., & McConkey, K. M. (1990). William James and hypnosis: A centennial reflection. *Psychological Science, 1*(2), 174–178.

Kluft, R. P. (1984). Aspects of the treatment of multiple personality disorder. *Psychiatric Annals, 14*, 51–55.

Kluft, R. P. (1985a). The natural history of multiple personality disorder. In R. P. Kluft (Ed.), *Childhood antecedents of multiple personality* (pp. 197–238). Washington, DC: American Psychiatric Press.

Kluft, R. P. (Ed.). (1985b). *Childhood antecedents of multiple personality disorder.* Washington, DC: American Psychiatric Press.

Kluft, R. P. (1991). Multiple personality disorder. In A. Tasman & S. Goldfinger (Eds.), *American Psychiatric Press review of psychiatry* (Vol. 10, pp. 161–188). Washington, DC: American Psychiatric Press.

Kluft, R. P. (1993). Basic principles in conducting the treatment of multiple personality disorder. In R. P. Kluft & C. Fine (Eds.), *Clinical perspectives on multiple personality disorder* (pp. 53–73). Washington, DC: American Psychiatric Press.

Kluft, R. P., Steinberg, M., & Spitzer, R. L. (1988). DSM-III-R revisions in the dissociative disorders: An exploration of their derivation and rationale. *Dissociation, 1*, 39–46.

Kuhn, T. S. (1970). *The structure of scientific revolutions*. Chicago: University of Chicago Press.

Labelle, L., Laurence, J., Nadon, R., & Perry, C. (1990). Hypnotizability, preference for an imagic cognitive style, and memory creation in hypnosis. *Journal of Abnormal Psychology, 99*, 222–228.

Langer, S. K. (1967). *Mind: An essay on human feeling* (Vol. 1). Baltimore: John Hopkins University Press.

Laurence, J., & Perry, C. (1983). Hypnotically created pseudomemories among highly hypnotizable subjects. *Science, 222*, 523–524.

Lipman, L. S., Braun, B. G., & Frischholz, E. J. (1984). Hypnotizability and multiple personality disorder: I. Overall hypnotic responsivity. In B.G. Braun (Ed.), *Dissociative disorders 1984: Proceedings of the First International Conference on Multiple Personality/Dissociative States* (p. 100). Chicago: Rush–Presbyterian–St.Luke's Medical Center.

Loewenstein, R. L., & Ross, D., R. (1992). Multiple personality and psychoanalysis: An introduction. *Psychoanalytic Inquiry, 12*(1), 3–48.

Loftus, E. F. (1982). Remembering recent experiences. In L. S. Cermak (Ed.), *Human memory and amnesia* (pp. 239–255). Hillside, NJ: Lawrence Erlbaum.

Loftus, E. F. (1992). When a lie becomes memory's truth: Memory distortion after exposure to misinformation. *Current directions in psychological science, 1*(4), 121–123.

Loftus, E. F. (1993). The reality of repressed memories. *American Psychologist, 48*(5), 518–537.

Loftus, E. F., & Hoffman, H. G. (1989). Misinformation and memory: The creation of new memories. *Journal of Experimental Psychology: General, 118*(1), 100–104.

Lynn, S. J., Milano, M., & Weekes, J. (1992). Hypnosis and pseudomemories: The effects of prehypnotic expectancies. *Journal of Personality and Social Psychology, 60*, 318–326.

Lynn, S. J., Rhue, J. W., & Green, J., P. (1988). Multiple personality and fantasy proneness: Is there an association or dissociation. *British Journal of Experimental and Clinical Hypnosis, 5*(3), 138–142.

Lynn, S. J., Weekes, J. R., & Milano, M. J. (1989). Reality versus suggestion: Pseudomemory in hypnotizable and simulating subjects. *Journal of Abnormal Psychology, 98*, 137–144.

Maddi, S. R. (1984). Personology for the 1980's. In R. Zucker, J. Aronoff, & A. Rabin (Eds.), *Personality and the prediction of behavior* (pp. 7–41). New York: Academic Press.

Magnusson, D., & Törestad, B. (1993). A holistic view of personality: A model revisited. In M. R. Rosenzweig & L. W. Porter (Eds.), *Annual review of psychology* (Vol. 44, pp. 427–452). Palo Alto, CA: Annual Review Press.

Mahoney, M. J. (1991). *Human change processes: The scientific foundations of psychotherapy.* New York: Basic Books.

Mandler, J.M. (1990). Recall of events by preverbal children. In, A. Diamond (Ed.), *The development and neural bases of higher cognitive functions: Annals of the New York Academy of Sciences* (Vol. 608, pp. 485–516). New York: New York Academy of Sciences.

Mare, C., Lynn, S. J., Kvall, S., Sivec, H., & Sanderberg, D. (1991, August 17). *Dissociation and hypnotizability: A rigorous test.* Paper presented at the 99th annual convention of the American Psychological Association, San Francisco.

McCann, T., & Sheehan, P. (1988). Hypnotically induced pseudomemories: Sampling their occurrence among hypnotizable subjects. *Journal of Personality and Social Psychology, 58.*

McClelland, J. L., & Rumelhart, D. (1985). Distributed memory and the representation of general and specific information. *Journal of Experimental Psychology: General, 114,* 159–188.

McHugh, P. R. (1992). Psychiatric misadventures. *The American Scholar,* 497–510.

Mead, G. H. (1934). *Mind, self, and society.* Chicago: University of Chicago Press.

Meehl, P. E., & Rosen, A. (1955). Antecedent probability and the efficiency of psychometric signs, patterns, or cutting scores. *Psychological Bulletin, 52,* 194–216.

Meltzoff, A. (1988). Infant imitation after a 1-week delay: Long-term memory for novel acts and multiple stimuli. *Developmental Psychology, 24*(4), 470–476.

Mersky, H. (1992). The manufacture of personalities: The production of multiple personality disorder. *British Journal of Psychiatry, 160,* 327–340.

Milgram, S. (1974). *Obedience to authority.* New York: Harper & Row.

Mischel, W. (1973). Toward a cognitive social learning reconceptualization of personality. *Psychological Review, 80,* 252–283.

Mischel, W. (1979). On the interface of cognition and personality: Beyond the person–situation debate. *American Psychologist, 34*(9), 740–754.

Mischel, W. (1983). Convergences and challenges in the search for consistency. *American Psychologist, 39*(4), 351–364.

Mulhern, S. (1991). Embodied alternative identities: Bearing witness to a world that might have been. *Psychiatric Clinics of North America, 14,* 769–786.

Nadon, R., Hoyt, I., Register, P. A., & Kihlstrom, J. F. (1991). Absorption and hypnotizability: Context effects reexamined. *Journal of Personality and Social Psychology, 60,* 144–153.

Nash, M. R., Lynn, S. J., & Givens, D. L. (1984). Adult hypnotic susceptibility, childhood punishment, and childhood abuse: A brief communication. *International Journal of Clinical and Experimental Hypnosis, 32,* 6–11.

Nash, M. R., & Lynn, S. J. (1986). Child abuse and hypnotic ability. *Imagination, Cognition, and Personality, 5,* 211–218.

Nash, M. R., Sexton, M., Hulsey, T., Harralson, T., & Lambert, W. (1993). Long-term sequelae of childhood sexual abuse: Perceived family environment psychopathology, and dissociation. *Journal of Consulting and Clinical Psychology, 61*(2), 276–283.

Nelson, K. (1993). The psychological and social origins of autobiographical memory. *Psychological Science, 4*(1), 7–11.

Nogrady, H., McConkey, K. M., & Perry, C. W. (1985). Enhancing visual memory: Trying hypnosis, trying imagination, and trying again. *Journal of Abnormal Psychology, 94,* 195–204.

Orne, M. T., & Bates, B. L. (1992). Reflections on multiple personality disorder: A view from the looking-glass of hypnosis past. In C. Pierce, M. Greenblatt, & A. Kales (Eds.), *The mosaic of contemporary psychiatry in perspective.* New York: Springer Verlag.

Orne, M. T., & Bauer-Manley, N. (1991). Disorders of self: Myths, metaphors, and the demand characteristics of treatment. In J. Strauss & G. Goethals (Eds.), *The self: Interdisciplinary approaches* (pp. 93–106). New York: Springer-Verlag.

Orne, M. T., & Dinges, D. F. (1989). Hypnosis. In H. Kaplan & B. Sadock (Eds.), *Comprehensive textbook of psychiatry* (Vol. 5, pp. 1501–1516). Baltimore: Williams & Wilkins.

Orne, M. T., Dinges, D. F. & Orne, G. C. (1984). On the differential diagnosis of multiple personality in the forensic context. *International Journal of Clinical and Experimental Hypnosis, 32,* 118–169.

Perry, C., & Laurence, J. (1984). Mental processing outside of awareness: The contributions of Freud and Janet. In K. S. Bowers & D. Meichenbaum (Eds.), *The unconscious reconsidered* (pp. 9–48). New York: John Wiley.

Putnam, F. W. (1989). *Diagnosis and treatment of multiple personality disorder.* New York: Guilford Press.

Putnam, F. W. (1991): Recent research on multiple personality disorder. *Psychiatric Clinics of North America, 14*(3), 489–502.

Putnam, F. W. (1992). Discussion: Are alter personalities fragments or figments? *Psychoanalytic Inquiry, 12*(1), 95–111.

Pynoos, R. S. (1990). Post-traumatic stress disorder in children and adolescents. In B. Garfinkel, G. Carlson, & E. Weller (Eds.), *Psychiatric disorders in children and adolescents* (pp. 48–63). Philadelphia: Saunders.

Ratcliff, R. (1990). Connectionist models of recognition memory: Constraints imposed by learning and forgetting functions. *Psychological Review, 97,* 285–308.

Rhue, J. W., & Lynn, S. J. (1988). Fantasy proneness: The ability to hallucinate "as real as real." *British Journal of Experimental and Clinical Hypnosis, 6,* 173–180.

Roediger, H. L. I., & Payne, D. (1982). Hypermnesia: The role of repeated testing. *Journal of Experimental Psychology: Learning, Memory, and Cognition, 8,* 66–72.

Roediger, H. L. I., & Payne, D. (1985). Recall criterion alone does not affect recall level or hypermnesia: A puzzle for generate/recognize theories. *Memory and Cognition, 13,* 1–7.

Ross, C. A. (1989). *Multiple personality disorder: Diagnosis, clinical features, and treatment.* New York: John Wiley.

Ross, C. A. (1991). Epidemiology of multiple personality disorder and dissociation. *Psychiatric Clinics of North America, 14*(3), 503–517.

Ross, C. A., Anderson, G. R., Fleisher, W. P., & Norton, G. R. (1991). The frequency of multiple personality disorder among psychiatric inpatients. *American Journal of Psychiatry, 148*, 1717–1720.

Ross, M., & Conway, M. (1986). Remembering one's own past: The construction of personal histories. In R. M. Sorrentino & E. T. Higgins (Eds.), *Handbook of motivation and cognition: Foundations of social behavior* (Vol. 1, pp. 122–144). New York: Guilford Press.

Ross, C. A., Joshi, S., & Currie, R. (1990). Dissociative experiences in the general population. *American Journal of Psychiatry, 147*, 1547–1552.

Rovee-Collier, C. (1990). The "memory system" of prelinguistic infants. In A. Diamond (Ed.), *The development and neural bases of higher cognitive functions.* New York: New York Academy of Sciences.

Ryler, G. (1949). *The concept of mind.* New York: Barnes and Noble.

Saks, M. J. (1992). Commentary: Obedience versus disobedience to legitimate versus illegitimate authorities issuing good versus evil directives. *Psychological Science, 3*(4), 221–223.

Schlenker, B. R. (1985). Identity and self-identification. In B. R. Schlenker (Ed.), *The self and social life* (pp. 65–99). New York: McGraw-Hill.

Schlenker, B. R., & Weigold, M. F. (1992). Interpersonal processes involving impression regulation and management. In M. S. Rosenzweig & L. W. Porter (Eds.), *Annual review of psychology* (Vol. 43, pp. 133–168). Palo Alto, CA: Annual Review Press.

Semin, G., & Fiedler, K. (1988). The cognitive functions of linguistic categories in describing persons: Social cognition and language. *Journal of Personality and Social Psychology, 58*, 558–568.

Sheehan, P. W. (1988). Confidence, memory, and hypnosis. In H. M. Pettinati (Ed.), *Hypnosis and memory* (pp. 96–127). New York: Guilford Press.

Simon, H. A. (1990). Invariants of human behavior. In M. R. Rosenzweig & L. Porter (Eds.), *Annual review of psychology* (Vol. 41, pp. 1–19). Palo Alto, CA: Annual Reviews Press.

Spanos, N. P., Weekes, J. R., & Bertrand, L. D. (1985). Multiple personality: A social psychological perspective. *Journal of Abnormal Psychology, 94*(3), 362–376.

Spanos, N. P. (1989). Hypnosis, demon possession and multiple personality: Strategic enactments and disavowals of responsibility for actions. In C. Ward (Ed.), *Altered states of consciousness and mental health: A cross cultural perspective* (pp. 96–124). Newbury Park, CA: Sage.

Spiegel, D. (1990). Hypnosis, dissociation, and trauma. In J. L. Singer (Ed.), *Repression and dissociation: Implications for personality theory, psychopathology, and health* (pp. 121–142). Chicago: University of Chicago Press.

Spiegel, D. (1991). Dissociation and trauma. In A. Tasman & S. Goldfinger (Eds.), *American Psychiatric Press review of psychiatry* (Vol. 10, 261–266). Washington, DC: American Psychiatric Press.

Spiegel, D., Hunt, T., & Dondershine, H. E. (1988). Dissociation and hypnotizability in posttraumatic stress disorder. *American Journal of Psychiatry, 145*(3), 301–305.

Spitzer, R. L., & Williams, J. B. (1985). Classification in psychiatry. In H. Kaplan & B. Sadock (Eds.), *Comprehensive textbook of psychiatry* (Vol. 4, pp. 591–598). Baltimore: Williams & Wilkins.

Steinberg, M. (1993). *Structured Clinical Interview for DSM-IV Dissociative Disorders (SCID-D)*. Washington, DC: American Psychiatric Press.

Steinberg, M., Rounsaville, B., & Cicchetti, D. V. (1990). The structured clinical interview for DSM-III-R dissociative disorders: Preliminary report on a new diagnostic instrument. *American Journal of Psychiatry, 147*, 76–82.

Strawson, P. (1959). *Individuals: An essay in descriptive metaphysics*. Garden City, NY: Anchor Doubleday.

Sutcliffe, J. (1960). "Credulous" and "skeptical" views of hypnotic phenomena: A review of certain evidence and methodology. *International Journal of Clinical and Experimental Hypnosis, 8*, 73–101.

Sutcliffe, J. (1961). "Credulous" and "skeptical" views of hypnotic phenomena: Experiments on esthesia, hallucination and delusion. *Journal of Abnormal and Social Psychology, 62*, 189–200.

Sutcliffe, J. P., & Jones, J. (1962). Personal identity, multiple personality, and hypnosis. *The International Journal of Clinical and Experimental Hypnosis, 10*(4), 231–269.

Terr, L. C. (1988). What happens to early memories of trauma? A study of 20 children under age five at the time of documented trauma events. *Journal of the American Academy of Child and Adolescent Psychiatry, 27*, 96–104.

Terr, L. A. (1991). Childhood traumas: An outline and overview. *American Journal of Psychiatry, 148*(1), 1–20.

Trickett, P. K., & Putnam, F. W. (1993). Impact of child sexual abuse on females: Toward a developmental, psychobiological integration. *Psychological Science, 4*(2), 81–87.

Tversky, A., & Kahnemann, D. (1981). The framing of decisions and the psychology of choice. *Science, 221*, 453–458.

van der Hart, O., & Friedman, B. (1989). A reader's guide to Pierre Janet on dissociation: A neglected intellectual heritage. *Dissociation, 2*, 3–16.

van der Hart, O., & van der Kolk, B. (1991). Hypnotizability and dissociation [letter to the editor]. *American Journal of Psychiatry, 148*(8), 1105.

Watzlawick, P. (1978). *The language of change*. New York: Basic Books.

Watzlawick, P., Beavin, J. H., & Jackson, D. D. (1967). *Pragmatics of human communication: A study of interactional patterns, pathologies, and paradoxes*. New York: W. W. Norton.

Wetzler, S., & Sweeney, J. (1986). Childhood amnesia: An empirical demonstration. In D. Rubin (Eds.), *Autobiographical memory* (pp. 191–201). New York: Cambridge University Press.

Whitaker, C. A., & Malone, T. P. (1953). *The roots of psychotherapy*. New York: The Blakiston Company.

Wilson, S. C., & Barber, T. (1983). The fantasy-prone personality: Implications for understanding imagery, hypnosis, and parapsychological phenomena. In A. Sheikh (Ed.), *Imagery: Current theory, research, and application* (pp. 340–387). New York: John Wiley.

Wittgenstein, L. (1953). *Philosophic investigations*. New York: Macmillan.

Wolfe, D. A. (1985). Child-abusive parents: An empirical review and analysis. *Psychological Bulletin, 97*(3), 462–482.

Wolf, D. A. (1987). *Child abuse: Implications for child development and psychopathology.* Newbury Park, CA: Sage.

Yates, J. L., & Nasby, W. (1993). Dissociation, affect, and network models of memory: An integrative proposal. *Journal of Traumatic Stress, 6*(3), 305–326.

Young, W. C. (1988). Observations on fantasy in the formation of multiple personality disorder. *Dissociation, 1,* 13–20.

Index